Nurse as Educator

PRINCIPLES OF TEACHING AND LEARNING FOR NURSING PRACTICE

Third Edition

Susan B. Bastable, EdD, RN
Professor and Chair
Department of Nursing
Le Moyne College
Syracuse, NY

JONES AND BARTLETT PUBLISHERS

Sudbury, Massachusetts

BOSTON   TORONTO   LONDON   SINGAPORE

World Headquarters

Jones and Bartlett Publishers
40 Tall Pine Drive
Sudbury, MA 01776
978-443-5000
info@jbpub.com
www.jbpub.com

Jones and Bartlett Publishers Canada
6339 Ormindale Way
Mississauga, Ontario L5V 1J2
Canada

Jones and Bartlett Publishers International
Barb House, Barb Mews
London W6 7PA
United Kingdom

Jones and Bartlett's books and products are available through most bookstores and online booksellers. To contact Jones and Bartlett Publishers directly, call 800-832-0034, fax 978-443-8000, or visit our website, www.jbpub.com.

Substantial discounts on bulk quantities of Jones and Bartlett's publications are available to corporations, professional associations, and other qualified organizations. For details and specific discount information, contact the special sales department at Jones and Bartlett via the above contact information or send an email to specialsales@jbpub.com.

The authors, editor, and publisher have made every effort to provide accurate information. However, they are not responsible for errors, omissions, or for any outcomes related to the use of the contents of this book and take no responsibility for the use of the products and procedures described. Treatments and side effects described in this book may not be applicable to all people; likewise, some people may require a dose or experience a side effect that is not described herein. Drugs and medical devices are discussed that may have limited availability controlled by the Food and Drug Administration (FDA) for use only in a research study or clinical trial. Research, clinical practice, and government regulations often change the accepted standard in this field. When consideration is being given to use of any drug in the clinical setting, the health care provider or reader is responsible for determining FDA status of the drug, reading the package insert, and reviewing prescribing information for the most up-to-date recommendations on dose, precautions, and contraindications, and determining the appropriate usage for the product. This is especially important in the case of drugs that are new or seldom used.

Production Credits
Executive Editor: Kevin Sullivan
Acquisitions Editor: Emily Ekle
Associate Editor: Amy Sibley
Editorial Assistant: Patricia Donnelly
Production Director: Amy Rose
Production Editor: Carolyn F. Rogers
Associate Marketing Manager: Rebecca Wasley
Associate Marketing Manager: Ilana Gordon
Manufacturing & Inventory Control Supervisor: Amy Bacus
Composition: Auburn Associates, Inc.
Cover Design: Kristin E. Ohlin
Cover Image: © Brand X Pictures/age fotostock
Printing and Binding: Malloy, Inc.
Cover Printing: Malloy, Inc.

Library of Congress Cataloging-in-Publication Data
Nurse as educator : principles of teaching and learning for nursing practice / [edited by] Susan B. Bastable. — 3rd ed.
    p. ; cm.
  Includes bibliographical references and index.
  ISBN-13: 978-0-7637-4643-8 (pbk. : alk. paper)
  ISBN-10: 0-7637-4643-6 (pbk. : alk. paper)
1. Health education. 2. Teaching. 3. Learning. I. Bastable, Susan Bacorn.
  [DNLM: 1. Education, Nursing—methods. 2. Learning—Nurses' Instruction. 3. Patient Education—methods. 4. Teaching—Nurses' Instruction. WY 18 N9715 2008]
RT90.N86 2008
613—dc22
                                                                    2007042254

6048

Printed in the United States of America
12 11 10 09   10 9 8 7 6 5 4

To the past, present, and future students in my undergraduate and graduate nursing education courses

and

To my mentors, M. Louise Fitzpatrick, M. Janice Nelson, Margaret M. Braungart, and Mary S. Collins, for their professional advice and guidance and their constant friendship.

Contents

Part Two: *Characteristics of the Learner* *91*

Foreword

Throughout the development of American nursing, a distinguishing characteristic has been its consistent emphasis on the education of its students, its clinicians, and the consumers of nursing care. Since the early 20th century, education has been viewed as a fundamental part of nursing practice and the primary means to prevent disease and to improve the health of the country's diverse communities.

Advances in the profession over many decades reflect the importance placed on education in the promotion and maintenance of health and its essential role in addressing the challenges of global health. Although substantively more complex and mired in the web of politics and economics, the nature of our contemporary health concerns are reminiscent of those faced at the turn of the 20th century. They include the plight of new immigrants, the increased threat of communicable diseases of epidemic proportion, and the issues that affect environmental health and affordability of health care. The Public Health Movement of the early 1900s was a response to these problems and a defining moment for nursing. Education was identified as the primary strategy for dealing with the multiplicity of health concerns and the nurse in the community was the instrument of that strategy. That response was rooted in the belief that education was the critical vehicle for delivering health information based on scientific advances, and if effectively applied by providers and recipients of care, would make a discernable difference in the quality of life. Today, we continue to believe that education is an important and potentially transformational instrument in the provision of nursing care.

Since the first publication of *Nurse as Educator: Principles of Teaching and Learning* in 1997, we have experienced an explosion of technology that affects every aspect of everyday life. Its impact on health care and the education of nurses is enormous. The use of technology in diagnosis and treatment has changed and advanced nursing science. Its use significantly supports the art of nursing and delivery of care. Nursing is currently taught and practiced with great reliance on technology. It permits students to study selectively, at their own pace, to deal with the ambiguities of clinical situations in simulated environments, and to access courses through a variety of distance learning possibilities. Surfing the Web provides immeasureable amounts of information to both healthcare providers and consumers. Simultaneous with the expansion of technology has been a shift of emphasis in the educational paradigm from teaching to learning and a greater focus on measurable outcomes of education, not only attention to its process.

The value of Susan Bastable's work continues to be demonstrated in this third edition because it is an outstanding resource and foundation for grounding nurses in the timeless principles that influence effective learning and the achievement of desirable outcomes, regardless of their settings or positions. At a time in our history when the shortage of nurses is exceeded by an even more critical dearth of well-prepared nursing faculty, this scholarly yet practical book is especially needed. It is an exemplary contribution to nursing and to the preparation of those who are the architects of the educational process, as well as those who are its implementers. *Nurse as Educator* shares the expertise of its contributors to the benefit of faculty and graduate students, in particular. It also has the potential to influence the ability of undergraduates and practicing nurses to effectively assist the public in learning how to maintain their health. It supports the nursing profession's ultimate claim that one of its primary purposes is the health education of the people it serves.

M. Louise Fitzpatrick, EdD, RN, FAAN
Connelly Endowed Dean and Professor
College of Nursing, Villanova University

Preface

Given the critical nursing faculty shortage nationwide, the growing demand for more nurses to deliver the highest quality of care possible, the significant problem of consumer health literacy in this country, and the increasing recognition of the importance of client education to improve health outcomes, this third edition of *Nurse as Educator* is a timely resource to address these pressing issues. This text is intended for use by nurses teaching in academic programs, by staff nurses practicing in any setting as caregivers or as staff educators, and by upper-level undergraduate and graduate nursing students who are to become the future professionals of tomorrow. No matter what their role or status, it is a legal, ethical, and moral responsibility of nurses in practice to teach others, whether their audience consists of clients, fellow colleagues, or prospective members of the profession.

Educating others has been an essential component of nursing practice for many years, yet the majority of nurses acknowledge that they have not had the formal preparation to successfully and securely assume the educator role. In today's healthcare arena, the unique holistic perspective of nursing practice mandates that nurses possess the knowledge and skills necessary to educate various audiences in a variety of settings with efficiency and effectiveness as well as with competency and confidence. This text was written to assist nurses to become proficient in their roles as educators by understanding the principles of teaching and learning. It is comprehensive in scope and depth, taking into consideration the basic foundations of the education process, the needs and characteristics of learners, the appropriate techniques and strategies for instruction, and the methods to evaluate the achievement of educational outcomes. In essence, this text addresses answers to questions that pertain to the education process—who, what, where, when, how, and why.

This third edition represents a major revision of the preceding edition by incorporating new models and theories, new ideas, and new perspectives on the principles and practices of teaching and learning. All chapters include updated references, but the classic references relevant to the field of education have been retained. Many chapters have been reformatted to enhance the organization of content; current statistics reflect changes in population trends; and new tables have been added to summarize information. In addition, Web sites are provided as sources for further information on particular topics, such as literacy, special populations, and learning styles. Of particular importance is the inclusion of a new section at the end of each chapter, entitled "State of the Evidence," which reviews the evidence from research and expert opinion as the basis for making decisions about possible changes in various approaches to teaching and learning.

Accompanying this third edition is a companion Web site at **http://nursing.jbpub.com/ nursingeducation** which offers various resources for instructors and students. Faculty will find tools to assist them with the delivery of content as well as with the assessment and evaluation of students who are learning the educator role. These online materials include test items, learning activities, and PowerPoint slides that correspond to the respective chapters in the textbook. The availability and easy accessibility of such materials allow faculty to deliver information in a flexible manner and at their convenience. Students will find learning objectives, Web links, an interactive glossary, critical thinking questions, small group discussion questions, and case studies. Faculty can also assign these student elements as homework or as content for an online course.

Acknowledgments

It is so true that accomplishments are difficult, if not impossible, to achieve without the constant love and support of family. The ability to complete this text could never have been realized without the patience, understanding, and encouragement of my husband, Jeffrey, who endured (once again) the many long months I spent on writing and editing these third edition chapters. To him I am especially indebted. Also, it is with a deep sense of pride that I extend recognition to my son, Garrett, and my daughter, Leigh, who are serving our country as officers in the United States Navy. My preoccupation with preparing this revision actually helped me get through their long absences while both were on military deployment in the Middle East. And, it is with special appreciation that I acknowledge my parents, Robert and Dorrie Bacorn, and my "other" mother, Gerry Bastable, who have always been and will always be my sources of inspiration.

In addition, a most sincere thank you is expressed to each of my contributors for their knowledge and expertise in the principles of teaching and learning. They have been loyal and steadfast throughout the process of revising and editing their respective chapters. Special gratitude, too, is extended to Jackie Utton, Department of Nursing Assistant at Le Moyne College, who spent countless hours typing, copying, and mailing chapter materials and managing the office affairs in my absence. Also instrumental in the revision of this text was the assistance provided to me by Kari Zhe-Heimerman, the Science Librarian at Le Moyne College, who devoted much effort in locating articles and books to update the references used for each chapter.

Finally, praise is given to the editorial staff of Jones and Bartlett Publishers, in particular Kevin Sullivan (Executive Editor), Carolyn Rogers (Production Editor), Tricia Donnelly (Editorial Assistant), and Amy Sibley (Associate Editor), for providing consistent guidance and expert advice, and for always being available whenever I needed them. They truly are a wonderful, talented team!

Contributors

Susan B. Bastable, EdD, RN
Professor and Chair
Department of Nursing
Le Moyne College
Syracuse, New York

Margaret M. Braungart, PhD
Professor of Psychology
Center for Bioethics and Humanities
State University of New York
Upstate Medical University
Syracuse, New York

Richard. G. Braungart, PhD
Professor Emeritus of Sociology and International
    Relations
Maxwell School of Citizenship and Public Affairs
Syracuse University
Syracuse, New York

Michelle A. Dart, MS, PNP, CDE
Nurse Consultant
Intellicare
Portland, Maine

**Kirsty Digger, MS, RN, CEN, Doctoral
    Candidate**
Lecturer
Department of Nursing
State University of New York at New Paltz
New Paltz, New York

Julie A. Doody, BS, RN
Community Health Nurse
Division of Maternal and Child Health
Onondaga County Health Department
Syracuse, New York

Kathleen Fitzgerald, MS, RN, CDE
Patient Educator
St. Joseph's Hospital Health Center
Syracuse, New York

Diane S. Hainsworth, MS, RN-C, ANP
Clinical Case Manager—Oncology
University Hospital
State University of New York
Upstate Medical University
Syracuse, New York

Sharon Kitchie, PhD, APRN, BC
Patient Education Coordinator and Nurse
    Educator at the Health Information Center
University Hospital
State University of New York
Upstate Medical University
Syracuse, New York

M. Janice Nelson, EdD, RN
Professor and Dean Emeritus
College of Nursing
State University of New York
Upstate Medical University
Syracuse, New York

Eleanor Richards, PhD, RN
Associate Professor and Chair
Department of Nursing
State University of New York at New Paltz
New Paltz, New York

Deborah L. Sopczyk, PhD, RN
Dean of Health Sciences
Excelsior College
Albany, New York

Kay Viggiani, MS, RN, CNS
Associate Professor (Retired) and Adjunct
Nursing Division
Keuka College
Keuka Park, New York

Priscilla Sandford Worral, PhD, RN
Coordinator of Nursing Research
University Hospital
State University of New York
Upstate Medical University
Syracuse, New York

About the Author

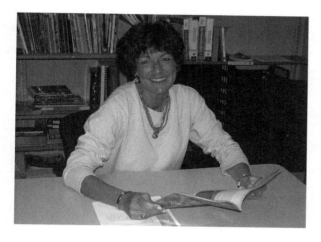

Susan Bacorn Bastable earned her MEd in community health nursing and her EdD in curriculum and instruction in nursing at Teachers College, Columbia University, in 1976 and 1979 respectively. She received her diploma from Hahnemann Hospital School of Nursing (now known as Drexel University of the Health Sciences) in Philadelphia in 1969 and her bachelor's degree in nursing from Syracuse University in 1972.

Dr. Bastable is currently Professor and founding Chair of the Department of Nursing at Le Moyne College in Syracuse, New York. She began her academic career in 1979 as Assistant Professor at Hunter College, Bellevue School of Nursing, in New York City where she remained on the faculty for two years. From 1987 to 1989, she was Assistant Professor in the College of Nursing at the University of Rhode Island. In 1990, she joined the faculty of the College of Nursing at Upstate Medical University of the State University of New York (SUNY) in Syracuse, where she was Associate Professor and Chair of the Undergraduate Program for 14 years. In 2004, she assumed her present leadership position at Le Moyne and has successfully established an RN-BS completion program, created an innovative 4-year undergraduate Dual Degree Partnership in Nursing with the associate's degree program at St. Joseph's College of Nursing in Syracuse, and instituted an MS program and two Post-MS Certificate programs with tracks in nursing education and nursing administration.

Dr. Bastable has taught undergraduate courses in nursing research, community health, and the role of the nurse as educator, and courses at the master's and post-master's level in the academic faculty role, curriculum and program development, and educational assessment and evaluation. For the past 26 years, she has been a consultant and external faculty member for Excelsior College (formerly known as Regents College of the University of the State of New York). Her clinical practice includes experience in community health, oncology, rehabilitation and neurology, occupational health, and medical/surgical nursing.

Dr. Bastable has been recognized with the 1996 President's Award for Excellence in Teaching at Upstate Medical University, the SUNY 1999 Chancellor's Award for Excellence in Teaching, and the 2001 Nursing Education Alumni Association Award. Also in 2001, she was inducted into the Nursing Education Alumni Association's Hall of Fame at Teacher's College, Columbia University.

Part One

Perspectives on Teaching and Learning

Chapter 1

Overview of Education in Health Care

Susan B. Bastable

CHAPTER HIGHLIGHTS

Historical Foundations for the Teaching Role of Nurses

Social, Economic, and Political Trends Affecting Health Care

Purposes, Goals, and Benefits of Client and Staff Education

The Education Process Defined

Role of the Nurse as Educator

Barriers to Teaching and Obstacles to Learning

Factors Impacting the Ability to Teach

Factors Impacting the Ability to Learn

Questions to Be Asked About Teaching and Learning

State of the Evidence

KEY TERMS

❑ education process
❑ teaching/instruction
❑ learning
❑ patient education

❑ staff education
❑ barriers to teaching
❑ obstacles to learning

OBJECTIVES

After completing this chapter, the reader will be able to

1. Discuss the evolution of the teaching role of nurses.
2. Recognize trends affecting the healthcare system in general and nursing practice in particular.
3. Identify the purposes, goals, and benefits of client and staff/student education.
4. Compare the education process to the nursing process.

5. Define the terms *education process*, *teaching*, and *learning*.
6. Identify reasons why client and staff/student education is an important duty for professional nurses.
7. Discuss the barriers to teaching and the obstacles to learning.
8. Formulate questions that nurses in the role of educator should ask about the teaching–learning process.

Education in health care today—both patient education and nursing staff/student education—is a topic of utmost interest to nurses in every setting in which they practice. Teaching is a major aspect of the nurse's professional role (Carpenter & Bell, 2002). The current trends in health care are making it essential that clients be prepared to assume responsibility for self-care management. Also, these trends make it imperative that nurses in the workplace be accountable for the delivery of high-quality care. The focus is on outcomes that demonstrate the extent to which patients and their significant others have learned essential knowledge and skills for independent care, or that staff nurses and nursing students have acquired the up-to-date knowledge and skills needed to competently and confidently render care to the consumer in a variety of settings.

The need for nurses to teach others and to help others learn will continue to increase in the healthcare environment (Carpenter & Bell, 2002). With changes rapidly occurring in the system of health care, nurses are finding themselves in increasingly demanding, constantly fluctuating, and highly complex positions (Gillespie & McFetridge, 2006). Nurses in the role of educators must understand the forces, both historical and present day, that have influenced and continue to influence their responsibilities in practice.

One purpose of this chapter is to shed light on the historical evolution of teaching as part of the professional nurse's role. Another purpose is to offer a perspective on the current trends in health care that make the teaching of clients a highly visible and required function of nursing care delivery. Also addressed are the continuing education efforts required to ensure ongoing practice competencies of nursing personnel.

In addition, this chapter clarifies the broad purposes, goals, and benefits of the teaching–learning process; focuses on the philosophy of the nurse–client partnership in teaching and learning; compares the education process to the nursing process; identifies barriers to teaching and obstacles to learning; and highlights the status of research in the field of patient education as well as staff and student education. The focus is on the overall role of the nurse in teaching and learning, no matter who the audience of learners may be. Nurses must have a basic prerequisite understanding of the principles and processes of teaching and learning to carry out their professional practice responsibilities with efficiency and effectiveness.

Historical Foundations for the Teaching Role of Nurses

Patient education has long been considered a major component of standard care given by nurses. The role of the nurse as educator is deeply entrenched in the growth and development of the profession. Since the mid-1800s, when nursing was first acknowledged as a unique discipline, the responsibility for teaching has been recognized as an important role of nurses as caregivers. The focus of teaching efforts by nurses has not only been on the care of the sick and on promoting the health of the well public, but also on educating other nurses for professional practice.

Florence Nightingale, the founder of modern nursing, was the ultimate educator. Not only did she develop the first school of nursing, but she also devoted a large portion of her career to teaching nurses, physicians, and health officials about the importance of proper conditions in hospitals and homes to improve the health of people. She also emphasized the importance of teaching patients of the need for adequate nutrition, fresh air, exercise, and personal hygiene to improve their well-being. By the early 1900s, public health nurses in this country clearly understood the significance of the role of the nurse as teacher in preventing disease and in maintaining the health of society (Chachkes & Christ, 1996).

For decades, then, patient teaching has been recognized as an independent nursing function. Nurses have always educated others—patients, families, and colleagues. It is from these roots that nurses have expanded their practice to include the broader concepts of health and illness (Glanville, 2000).

As early as 1918, the National League of Nursing Education (NLNE) in the United States (now the National League for Nursing [NLN]) observed the importance of health teaching as a function within the scope of nursing practice. Two decades later, this organization recognized nurses as agents for the promotion of health and the prevention of illness in all settings in which they practiced (National League of Nursing Education, 1937). By 1950, the NLNE had identified course content in nursing school curricula to prepare nurses to assume the role as teachers of others. Most recently, the NLN developed the first certified nurse educator (CNE) exam (National League for Nursing, 2006) to raise "the visibility and status of the academic nurse educator role as an advanced professional practice discipline with a defined practice setting" (Klestzick, 2005, p. 1).

So, too, the American Nurses Association (ANA) has for years put forth statements on the functions, standards, and qualifications for nursing practice, of which patient teaching is a key element. In addition, the International Council of Nurses (ICN) has long endorsed the nurse's role as educator to be an essential component of nursing care delivery.

Today, all state nurse practice acts (NPAs) include teaching within the scope of nursing practice responsibilities. Nurses, by legal mandate of the NPAs, are expected to provide instruction to consumers to assist them to maintain optimal levels of wellness and manage illness. Nursing career ladders often incorporate teaching effectiveness as a measure of excellence in practice (Rifas, Morris, & Grady, 1994). By teaching patients and families as well as healthcare personnel, nurses can achieve the professional goal of providing cost-effective, safe, and high-quality care.

In recognition of the importance of patient education by nurses, the Joint Commission (JC), formerly the Joint Commission on Accreditation of Healthcare Organizations (JCAHO), established nursing standards for patient education as early as 1993. These standards, known as mandates, describe the type and level of care, treatment, and services that must be provided by an agency or organization to receive accreditation. Required accreditation standards have provided the impetus for nursing service managers to put greater emphasis on unit-based clinical staff education activities for the improvement of nursing care interventions to achieve expected client outcomes (Joint Commission on Accreditation of Healthcare Organizations, 2001). Positive outcomes of patient care are to be achieved by nurses through teaching activities that must be patient centered and family oriented.

More recently, the JC has expanded its expectations to include an interdisciplinary team approach in the provision of patient education as well as evidence that patients and their significant others participate in care and decision making and understand what they have been taught. This requirement means that providers must consider the literacy level, educational background, language skills, and culture of every client during the education process (Cipriano, 2007; Davidhizar & Brownson, 1999; JCAHO, 2001).

In addition, the Patient's Bill of Rights, first developed in the 1970s by the American Hospital Association, has been adopted by hospitals nationwide. It establishes the guidelines to ensure that patients receive complete and current information concerning their diagnosis, treatment, and prognosis in terms they can reasonably be expected to understand.

The Pew Health Professions Commission (1995), influenced by the dramatic changes surrounding health care, published a broad set of competencies it believed would mark the success of the health professions in the 21st century. Shortly thereafter, the commission (1998) released a fourth report as a follow-up on health professional practice in the new millennium. Numerous recommendations specific to the nursing profession have been proposed by the commission. More than one half of them pertain to the importance of patient and staff education

and to the role of the nurse as educator. These recommendations for the practice of nursing include the need to:

- Provide clinically competent and coordinated care to the public
- Involve patients and their families in the decision-making process regarding health interventions
- Provide clients with education and counseling on ethical issues
- Expand public access to effective care
- Ensure cost-effective and appropriate care for the consumer
- Provide for prevention of illness and promotion of healthy lifestyles for all Americans

In 2006, the Institute for Healthcare Improvement announced the 5 Million Lives campaign. The campaign's objective is to reduce the 15 million incidents of medical harm that occur in U.S. hospitals each year. Such an ambitious campaign has major implications for teaching patients and their families as well as nursing staff and students the ways they can improve care to reduce injuries, save lives, and decrease costs of health care (Berwick, 2006).

Another recent initiative was the formation of the Sullivan Alliance to recruit and educate staff nurses to deliver culturally competent care to the public they serve. Effective health care and health education of our patients and their families depends on a sound scientific base and cultural awareness in an increasingly diverse society. This organization's goal is to increase the racial and cultural mix of nursing faculty, students, and staff, who will be sensitive to the needs of clients of diverse backgrounds (Sullivan & Bristow, 2007).

Accomplishing the goals and meeting the expectations of these various organizations calls for a redirection of education efforts. Since the 1980s, the role of the nurse as educator has undergone a paradigm shift, evolving from what once was a disease-oriented approach to a more prevention-oriented approach. In other words, the focus is on teaching for the promotion and maintenance of health. Education, once done as part of discharge plans at the end of hospitalization, has expanded to become part of a comprehensive plan of care that occurs across the continuum of the healthcare delivery process (Davidhizar & Brownson, 1999).

As described by Grueninger (1995), this transition toward wellness has entailed a progression "from disease-oriented patient education (DOPE) to prevention-oriented patient education (POPE) to ultimately become health-oriented patient education (HOPE)" (p. 53). This new approach has changed the role of the nurse from one of wise healer to expert advisor/teacher to facilitator of change. Instead of the traditional aim of simply imparting information, the emphasis is now on empowering patients to use their potentials, abilities, and resources to the fullest (Glanville, 2000).

Also, the role of today's educator is one of training the trainer—that is, preparing nursing staff through continuing education, in-service programs, and staff development to maintain and improve their clinical skills and teaching abilities. It is essential that professional nurses be prepared to effectively perform teaching services that meet the needs of many individuals and groups in different circumstances across a variety of practice settings. The key to the success of our profession is for nurses to teach other nurses. We are the primary educators of our fellow colleagues and other healthcare staff personnel (Donner, Levonian, & Slutsky, 2005). In addition, the demand for educators of nursing students is at an all-time high.

Another very important role of the nurse as educator is serving as a clinical instructor for students in the practice setting. Many staff nurses function as clinical preceptors and mentors to ensure that nursing students meet their expected learning outcomes. However, evidence indicates that nurses in the clinical and academic settings feel inadequate as mentors and preceptors due to poor preparation for their role as teachers. This challenge of relating theory learned in the classroom setting to the practice environment requires nurses not only to be up to date with clinical skills and innovations in practice, but to possess the knowledge and skills of the principles of teaching and learning. However, knowing the practice field is not the same thing as knowing how to teach the field. The role of the clinical educator is a dynamic one that requires the teacher to actively engage students to become competent and caring professionals (Gillespie & McFetridge, 2006).

Social, Economic, and Political Trends Affecting Health Care

In addition to the professional and legal standards put forth by various organizations and agencies, many social, economic, and political trends nationwide affecting the public's health have led to increased attention to the role of the nurse as teacher and to the importance of client and staff education. The following are some of the significant forces influencing nursing practice in particular and the healthcare system in general (Birchenall, 2000; Bodenheimer, Lorig, Holman, & Grumbach, 2002; Cipriano, 2007; DeSilets, 1995; Glanville, 2000; U.S. Department of Health and Human Services, 2000; Zikmund-Fisher, Sarr, Fagerlin, & Ubel, 2006):

- The federal government has published *Healthy People 2010: Understanding and Improving Health*, a document that put forth national health goals and objectives for the future. These goals and objectives include the development of effective health education programs to assist individuals to recognize and change risk behaviors, to adopt or maintain healthy practices, and to make appropriate use of available services for health care. Achieving these national priorities would dramatically cut the costs of health care, prevent the premature onset of disease and disability, and help all Americans lead healthier and more productive lives. Nurses, as the largest group of health professionals, play an important role in making a real difference by teaching clients to attain and maintain healthy lifestyles.

- The growth of managed care has resulted in shifts in reimbursement for healthcare services. Greater emphasis has been placed on outcome measures, many of which can be achieved primarily through the health education of clients.

- Health providers are recognizing the economic and social values of reaching out to communities, schools, and workplaces to provide education for disease prevention and health promotion.

- Politicians and healthcare administrators alike recognize the importance of health education to accomplish the economic goal of reducing the high costs of health services. Political emphasis is on productivity, competitiveness in the marketplace, and cost-containment measures to restrain health service expenses.

- Healthcare professionals are increasingly concerned about malpractice claims and disciplinary action for incompetence. Continuing education, either by legislative mandate or as a requirement of the employing institution, has come to the forefront in response to the challenge of ensuring the competency of practitioners. It is a means to transmit new knowledge and skills as well as to reinforce or refresh previously acquired knowledge and abilities for the continuing growth of staff.

- Nurses continue to define their professional role, body of knowledge, scope of practice, and expertise, with client education as central to the practice of nursing.

- Consumers are demanding increased knowledge and skills about how to care for themselves and how to prevent disease. As people are becoming more aware of their needs and desire a greater understanding of treatments and goals, the demand for health information is expected to intensify. The quest for consumer rights and responsibilities, which began in the 1990s, continues into the 21st century.

- Demographic trends, particularly the aging of the population, are requiring an emphasis to be placed on self-reliance and maintenance of a healthy status over an extended lifespan. As the percentage of the U.S. population over 65 years climbs dramatically in the next 20 to 30 years, the healthcare needs of the baby boom generation of the post–World War II era will become greater as members deal with degenerative illnesses and other effects of the aging process.

- Among the major causes of morbidity and mortality are those diseases now recognized as being lifestyle related and preventable through educational intervention. In addition, millions of incidents of medical harm occur every year in U.S. hospitals, making it imperative that clients, nursing staff, and nursing students be educated about preventive measures that will reduce these incidents (Berwick, 2006).

- The increase in chronic and incurable conditions requires that individuals and families become informed participants to manage their own illnesses. Patient teaching can facilitate an individual's adaptive responses to illness.

- Advanced technology is increasing the complexity of care and treatment in home and community-based settings. More rapid hospital discharge and more procedures done on an outpatient basis are forcing patients to be more self-reliant in managing their own health. Patient education is necessary to assist them to independently follow through with self-management activities.

- Healthcare providers are becoming increasingly aware that client health literacy is an essential skill if health outcomes are to be improved nationwide. Nurses must attend to the education needs of their clients to be sure that they adequately understand the information required for independence in self-care activities to promote, maintain, and restore their health.

- There is a belief on the part of nurses and other healthcare providers, which is supported by research, that client education improves compliance and, hence, health and well-being. Better understanding by clients and their families of the recommended treatment plans can lead to increased cooperation, decision making, satisfaction, and independence with therapeutic regimens. Health education will enable patients to independently solve problems encountered outside the protected care environments of hospitals, thereby increasing their independence.

- An increasing number of self-help groups exist to support clients in meeting their physical and psychosocial needs. The success of these support groups and behavioral change programs depends on the nurse's role as teacher and advocate.

Nurses recognize the need to develop their expertise in teaching to keep pace with the demands of patient and staff education. As they continue to define their role, body of knowledge, scope of practice, and professional expertise, nurses realize more than ever before that their role as educator is central to the practice of nursing and should be captured to even a greater extent as part of their professional domain. Nurses are in a key position to carry out health education. They are the healthcare providers who have the most continuous contact with clients, are usually the most accessible source of information for the consumer, and are the most highly trusted of all health professionals. In Gallup polls taken since 1999, nurses continue to be ranked No. 1 in honesty and ethics among 45 occupations (Mason, 2001; McCafferty, 2002; Saad, 2006).

Purposes, Goals, and Benefits of Client and Staff Education

The purpose of patient education is to increase the competence and confidence of clients for self-management. The goal is to increase the responsibility and independence of clients for self-care. This can be achieved by supporting patients through the transition from being invalids to being self-sustaining in managing their own care; from being dependent recipients to being involved participants in the care process; and from being passive listeners to active learners. An interactive, partnership education approach provides clients the opportunity to explore and expand their self-care abilities (Cipriano, 2007).

The single most important action of nurses as caregivers is to prepare clients for self-care. If they cannot independently maintain or improve their health status when on their own, we have failed to help them reach their potential (Glanville, 2000). The benefits of client education are many. Effective teaching by the nurse has demonstrated the potential to:

- Increase consumer satisfaction
- Improve quality of life
- Ensure continuity of care
- Decrease client anxiety
- Effectively reduce the complications of illness and the incidence of disease
- Promote adherence to treatment plans
- Maximize independence in the performance of activities of daily living
- Energize and empower consumers to become actively involved in the planning of their care

Because many health needs and problems are handled at home, there truly does exist a need to educate people on how to care for themselves—both to get well and to stay well. Illness is a natural life process, but so is mankind's ability to learn. Along with the ability to learn comes a natural curiosity that allows people to view new and difficult situations as challenges rather than as defeats. As Orr (1990) observed, "Illness can become an educational opportunity . . . a 'teachable moment' when ill health suddenly encourages [patients] to take a more active role in their care" (p. 47). This observation remains relevant today.

Numerous studies have documented the fact that informed clients are more likely to comply with medical treatment plans, find innovative ways to cope with illness, and are less likely to experience complications. Overall, clients are more satisfied with care when they receive adequate information about how to manage for themselves. One of the most frequently cited complaints by patients in litigation cases is that they were not adequately informed (Reising, 2007).

Just as the need exists for teaching clients to help them become participants and informed consumers to achieve independence in self-care, the need also exists for staff nurses to be exposed to up-to-date information with the ultimate goal of enhancing their practice. The purpose of staff and student education is to increase the competence and confidence of nurses to function independently in providing care to the consumer. The goal of our education efforts is to improve the quality of care delivered by nurses. Nurses play a key role in improving the nation's health, and they recognize the importance of lifelong learning to keep their knowledge and skills current (DeSilets, 1995).

In turn, the benefits to nurses in their role as educators include increased job satisfaction when they recognize that their teaching actions have the potential to forge therapeutic relationships with clients, enhanced patient–nurse autonomy, increased accountability in practice, and the opportunity to create change that really makes a difference in the lives of others.

Our primary aims, then, as educators should be to nourish clients, mentor staff, and serve as teachers and clinical preceptors for nursing students. We must value our role in educating others and make it a priority for our clients, our fellow colleagues, and the future members of our profession.

The Education Process Defined

The *education process* is a systematic, sequential, logical, scientifically based, planned course of action consisting of two major interdependent operations, teaching and learning. This process forms a continuous cycle that also involves two interdependent players, the teacher and the learner. Together, they jointly perform teaching and learning activities, the outcome of which leads to mutually desired behavior changes. These changes foster growth in the learner and, it should be acknowledged, growth in the teacher as well. Thus, the education process is a framework for a participatory, shared approach to teaching and learning (Carpenter & Bell, 2002).

The education process has always been compared to the nursing process—rightly so, because the steps of each process run parallel to one another, although they have different goals and objectives. Both processes provide a rational basis for nursing practice rather than an intuitive one. The education process, like the nursing process, consists of the basic elements of assessment, planning, implementation, and evaluation. The two are different in that the nursing process focuses on the planning and implementation of care based on the assessment and diagnosis of the physical and psychosocial needs of the patient. The education process, on the other hand, focuses on the planning and implementation of teaching based on an assessment and prioritization of the client's learning needs, readiness to learn, and learning styles (Carpenter & Bell, 2002). The outcomes of the nursing process are achieved when the physical and psychosocial needs of the client are met. The outcomes of the education process are achieved when changes in knowledge, attitudes, and skills occur. Both processes are ongoing, with assessment and evaluation perpetually redirecting the planning and implementation phases of the processes. If mutually agreed-on outcomes in either process are not achieved, as determined by evaluation, then the nursing process or the education process can and should begin again through reassessment, replanning, and reimplementation (**Figure 1–1**).

It should be noted that the actual act of *teaching* or *instruction* is merely one component of the education process. Teaching and instruction, terms often used interchangeably with one another, are deliberate interventions that involve sharing information and experiences to meet intended learner outcomes in the cognitive, affective, and psychomotor domains according to an education plan. Teaching and instruction, both one and the same, are often formal, structured, organized activities prepared days in advance, but they can be performed informally on the spur of the moment during conversations

Figure 1–1 Education process parallels nursing process.

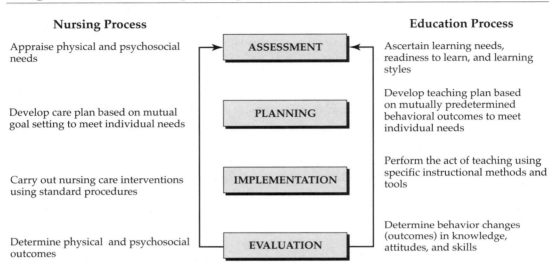

Nursing Process		**Education Process**
Appraise physical and psychosocial needs	ASSESSMENT	Ascertain learning needs, readiness to learn, and learning styles
Develop care plan based on mutual goal setting to meet individual needs	PLANNING	Develop teaching plan based on mutually predetermined behavioral outcomes to meet individual needs
Carry out nursing care interventions using standard procedures	IMPLEMENTATION	Perform the act of teaching using specific instructional methods and tools
Determine physical and psychosocial outcomes	EVALUATION	Determine behavior changes (outcomes) in knowledge, attitudes, and skills

or incidental encounters with the learner. Whether formal or informal, planned well in advance or spontaneous, teaching and instruction are nevertheless deliberate and conscious acts with the objective of producing learning (Carpenter & Bell, 2002).

The fact that teaching and instruction are intentional does not necessarily mean that they have to be lengthy and complex tasks, but it does mean that they comprise conscious actions on the part of the teacher in responding to an individual's need to learn. The cues that someone has a need to learn can be communicated in the form of a verbal request, a question, a puzzled or confused look, a blank stare, or a gesture of defeat or frustration. In the broadest sense, then, teaching is a highly versatile strategy that can be applied in preventing, promoting, maintaining, or modifying a wide variety of behav-

iors in a learner who is receptive, motivated, and adequately informed (Duffy, 1998).

Learning is defined as a change in behavior (knowledge, attitudes, and/or skills) that can be observed or measured and that occur at any time or in any place as a result of exposure to environmental stimuli. Learning is an action by which knowledge, skills, and attitudes are consciously or unconsciously acquired such that behavior is altered in some way (see Chapter 3). The success of the nurse educator's endeavors at teaching is measured not by how much content has been imparted, but rather by how much the person has learned (Musinski, 1999).

Specifically, *patient education* is a process of assisting people to learn health-related behaviors that can be incorporated into everyday life with the goal of optimal health and independence in self-care. *Staff education*, by contrast, is the process of influencing the behavior of nurses by producing changes in their knowledge, attitudes, and skills to help nurses maintain and improve their competencies for the delivery of quality care to the consumer. Both patient and staff education involve forging a relationship between the learner and the educator so that the learner's information needs (cognitive, affective, and psychomotor) can be met through the process of education (see Chapter 10).

A useful paradigm to assist nurses to organize and carry out the education process is the ASSURE model (Rega, 1993). The acronym stands for:

- **A**nalyze the learner
- **S**tate the objectives
- **S**elect the instructional methods and materials
- **U**se the instructional methods and materials
- **R**equire learner performance
- **E**valuate the teaching plan and revise as necessary

Role of the Nurse as Educator

For many years, organizations governing and influencing nurses in practice have identified teaching as an essential responsibility of all registered nurses in caring for both well and ill clients. For nurses to fulfill the role of educator, no matter whether their audience consists of patients, family members, nursing students, nursing staff, or other agency personnel, they must have a solid foundation in the principles of teaching and learning.

Legal and accreditation mandates as well as professional nursing standards of practice have made the educator role of the nurse an integral part of high-quality care to be delivered by all registered nurses licensed in the United States, regardless of their level of nursing school preparation. Given this fact, it is imperative to examine the present teaching role expectations of nurses, irrespective of their preparatory background. The role of educator is not primarily to teach, but to promote learning and provide for an environment conducive to learning—to create the teachable moment rather than just waiting for it to happen (Wagner & Ash, 1998). Also, the role of the nurse as teacher of patients and families, nursing staff, and students certainly should stem from a partnership philosophy. A learner cannot be made to learn, but an effective approach in educating others is to actively involve learners in the education process (Bodenheimer et al., 2002).

Although by license all nurses are expected to teach, few have ever had formal preparation in the principles of teaching and learning (Donner et al., 2005). As you will see in this textbook, there is much knowledge and there are skills to be acquired to carry out the role as educator with efficiency and effectiveness. Although all nurses are able to function as givers of information, they need to acquire the skills of being a facilitator of the learning process (Musinski, 1999). Consider the following questions posed:

- Is every nurse adequately prepared to assess for learning needs, readiness to learn, and learning styles?
- Can every nurse determine whether information given is received and understood?

- Are all nurses capable of taking appropriate action to revise the approach to educating the client if the information provided is not comprehended?
- Do nurses realize the need to transition their role of educator from being a content transmitter to being a process manager, from controlling the learner to releasing the learner, and from being a teacher to becoming a facilitator (Musinski, 1999)?

A growing body of evidence suggests that effective education and learner participation go hand in hand. The nurse should act as a facilitator, creating an environment conducive to learning that motivates individuals to want to learn and makes it possible for them to learn (Musinski, 1999). The assessment of learning needs, the designing of a teaching plan, the implementation of instructional methods and materials, and the evaluation of teaching and learning should include participation by both the educator and the learner. Thus, the emphasis should be on the facilitation of learning from a nondirective rather than a didactic teaching approach (Knowles, Holton, & Swanson, 1998; Musinski, 1999; Mangena & Chabeli, 2005; Donner et al., 2005).

No longer should teachers see themselves as simply transmitters of content. Indeed, the role of the educator has shifted from the traditional position of being the giver of information to that of a process designer and coordinator. This role alteration from the traditional teacher-centered to the learner-centered approach is a paradigm shift that requires skill in needs assessment as well as the ability to involve learners in planning, link learners to learning resources, and encourage learner initiative (Knowles et al., 1998; Mangena & Chabeli, 2005).

Instead of the teacher teaching, the new educational paradigm focuses on the learner learning. That is, the teacher becomes the guide on the side, assisting the learner in his or her effort to determine objectives and goals for learning, with both parties being active partners in decision making throughout the learning process. To increase comprehension, recall, and application of information, clients must be actively involved in the learning experience (Kessels, 2003; London, 1995). Glanville (2000) describes this move toward assisting learners to use their own abilities and resources as "a pivotal transfer of power" (p. 58).

Certainly patient education requires a collaborative effort among healthcare team members, all of whom play more or less important roles in teaching. However, physicians are first and foremost prepared "to treat, not to teach" (Gilroth, 1990, p. 30). Nurses, on the other hand, are prepared to provide a holistic approach to care delivery. The teaching role is a unique part of our professional domain. Because consumers have always respected and trusted nurses to be their advocates, nurses are in an ideal position to clarify confusing information and make sense out of nonsense. Amidst a fragmented healthcare delivery system involving many providers, the nurse serves as coordinator of care. By ensuring consistency of information, nurses can support clients in their efforts to achieve the goal of optimal health (Donovan & Ward, 2001). They also can assist their colleagues in gaining knowledge and skills necessary for the delivery of professional nursing care.

Barriers to Teaching and Obstacles to Learning

It has been said by many educators that adult learning takes place not by the teacher's initiating and motivating the learning process, but rather by the teacher's removing or reducing obstacles to learning and enhancing the process after it has begun. The educator should not limit learning to the information that is intended but should clearly make possible the potential for informal, unintended learning that can occur each and every day with each and every teacher–learner encounter (Carpenter & Bell, 2002).

Unfortunately, nurses must confront many barriers in carrying out their responsibilities for educating others. Also, learners face a variety of potential obstacles that can interfere with their learning. For the purposes of this textbook, *barriers to teaching* are defined as those factors that impede the nurse's ability to deliver educational services. *Obstacles to learning* are defined as those factors that negatively affect the ability of the learner to pay attention to and process information.

Factors Impacting the Ability to Teach

The following include the major barriers interfering with the ability of nurses to carry out their roles as educators (Carpenter & Bell, 2002; Casey, 1995; Chachkes & Christ, 1996; Duffy, 1998; Glanville, 2000; Honan, Krsnak, Petersen, & Torkelson, 1988):

1. Lack of time to teach is cited by nurses as the greatest barrier to being able to carry out their educator role effectively. Early discharge from inpatient and outpatient settings often results in nurses and clients having fleeting contact with one another. In addition, the schedules and responsibilities of nurses are very demanding. Finding time to allocate to teaching is very challenging in light of other work demands and expectations. In one survey by the Joint Commission, 28% of the nurses claimed that they were not able to provide patients and their families with the necessary instruction because of lack of time during their shifts at work (Stolberg, 2002). Nurses must know how to adopt an abbreviated, efficient, and effective approach to client and staff education by first adequately assessing the learner and then by using appropriate instructional methods and instructional tools at their disposal. Discharge planning plays an ever more important role in ensuring continuity of care across settings.

2. Many nurses and other healthcare personnel admit that they do not feel competent or confident with their teaching skills. As stated previously, although nurses are expected to teach, few have ever taken a specific course on the principles of teaching and learning. The concepts of patient education are usually integrated throughout nursing curricula rather than being offered as a specific course of study. As early as 1965, Pohl found that one third of 1,500 nurses, when questioned, reported that they had no preparation for the teaching they were doing, while only one fifth felt

they had adequate preparation. Almost 30 years later, Kruger (1991) surveyed 1,230 nurses in staff, administrative, and education positions regarding their perceptions of the extent of nurses' responsibility for and level of achievement of patient education. Although all three groups strongly believed that client and staff education is a primary responsibility of nurses, the vast majority of them rated their ability to perform educator role activities as unsatisfactory. Few additional studies have been forthcoming on the nurses' perceptions of their educator role (Trocino, Byers, & Peach, 1997). Today, the role of the nurse as educator still needs to be strengthened in undergraduate nursing education, but fortunately an upswing in interest and attention to the educator role has been gaining significant momentum in graduate nursing programs across the country.

3. Personal characteristics of the nurse educator play an important role in determining the outcome of a teaching–learning interaction. Motivation to teach and skill in teaching are prime factors in determining the success of any educational endeavor (see Chapter 11).

4. Until recently, low priority was often assigned to patient and staff education by administration and supervisory personnel. With the strong emphasis on Joint Commission mandates, the level of attention paid to the educational needs of consumers as well as healthcare personnel has changed significantly. However, budget allocations for educational programs remain tight and can

interfere with the adoption of innovative and time-saving teaching strategies and techniques.

5. The environment in the various settings where nurses are expected to teach is not always conducive to carrying out the teaching–learning process. Lack of space, lack of privacy, noise, and frequent interferences due to client treatment schedules and staff work demands are just some of the factors that negatively affect the nurse's ability to concentrate and to effectively interact with learners.

6. An absence of third-party reimbursement to support patient education relegates teaching and learning to less than high-priority status. Nursing services within healthcare facilities are subsumed under hospital room costs and, therefore, are not specifically reimbursed by insurance payers. In fact, patient education in some settings, such as home care, often cannot be incorporated as a legitimate aspect of routine nursing care delivery unless specifically ordered by a physician.

7. Some nurses and physicians question whether patient education is effective as a means to improve health outcomes. They view patients as impediments to teaching when patients do not display an interest in changing behavior, when they demonstrate an unwillingness to learn, or when their ability to learn is in question. Concerns about coercion and violation of free choice, based on the belief that patients have a right to choose and that they cannot be forced to comply, explain why some professionals feel frustrated in their efforts to teach. Unless all healthcare members buy into the utility

of patient education (that is, they believe it can lead to significant behavioral changes and increased compliance to therapeutic regimens), then some professionals may continue to feel absolved from their responsibility to provide adequate and appropriate patient education.

8. The type of documentation system used by healthcare agencies has an effect on the quality and quantity of patient teaching. Both formal and informal teaching are often done (Carpenter & Bell, 2002) but not written down because of insufficient time, inattention to detail, and inadequate forms on which to record the extent of teaching activities. Many of the forms used for documentation of teaching are designed to simply check off the areas addressed rather than allow for elaboration of what was actually accomplished. In addition, most nurses do not recognize the scope and depth of teaching that they perform on a daily basis. Communication among healthcare providers regarding what has been taught needs to be coordinated and appropriately delegated so that teaching can proceed in a timely, smooth, organized, and thorough fashion.

Factors Impacting the Ability to Learn

The following are some of the major obstacles interfering with a learner's ability to attend to and process information (Glanville, 2000; Weiss, 2003):

1. Lack of time to learn due to rapid patient discharge from care and the amount of information a client is expected to learn can discourage and frustrate the learner, impeding the ability and willingness to learn.

2. The stress of acute and chronic illness, anxiety, and sensory deficits in patients are just a few problems that can diminish learner motivation and interfere with the process of learning. However, it must be pointed out that illness alone seldom acts as an impediment to learning. Rather, illness is often the impetus for patients to attend to learning, make contact with the healthcare professional, and take positive action to improve their health status.

3. Low literacy and functional health illiteracy has been found to be a significant factor in the ability of clients to make use of the written and verbal instructions given to them by providers. Almost half of the American people read and comprehend at or below the eighth-grade level and an even higher percentage suffer from health illiteracy (see Chapter 7).

4. The negative influence of the hospital environment itself, resulting in loss of control, lack of privacy, and social isolation, can interfere with a patient's active role in health decision making and involvement in the teaching–learning process.

5. Personal characteristics of the learner have major effects on the degree to which behavioral outcomes are achieved. Readiness to learn, motivation and compliance, developmental-stage characteristics, and learning styles are some of the prime factors influencing the success of educational endeavors.

6. The extent of behavioral changes needed, both in number and in complexity, can overwhelm learners and dissuade them from attending to and accomplishing learning objectives and goals.
7. Lack of support and lack of ongoing positive reinforcement from the nurse and significant others serve to block the potential for learning.
8. Denial of learning needs, resentment of authority, and lack of willingness to take responsibility (locus of control) are some psychological obstacles to accomplishing behavioral change.
9. The inconvenience, complexity, inaccessibility, fragmentation, and dehumanization of the healthcare system often result in frustration and abandonment of efforts by the learner to participate in and comply with the goals and objectives for learning.

Questions to be Asked About Teaching and Learning

To maximize the effectiveness of client and staff/student education by the nurse, it is necessary to examine the elements of the education process and the role of the nurse as educator. Many questions arise related to the principles of teaching and learning. The following are some of the important questions that the chapters in this textbook address:

- How can members of the healthcare team work together more effectively to coordinate educational efforts?

- What are the ethical, legal, and economic issues involved in patient and staff education?
- Which theories and principles support the education process, and how can they be applied to change the behaviors of learners?
- What assessment methods and tools can be used to determine learning needs, readiness to learn, and learning styles?
- Which learner attributes negatively and positively affect an individual's ability and willingness to learn?
- What can be done about the inequities (in quantity and quality) in the delivery of education services?
- Which elements need to be taken into account when developing and implementing teaching plans?
- Which instructional methods and materials are available to support teaching efforts?
- Under which conditions should certain teaching methods and materials be used?
- How can teaching be tailored to meet the needs of specific populations of learners?
- What common mistakes are made when teaching others?
- How can teaching and learning be best evaluated?

State of the Evidence

The literature on patient and staff education is extensive from both a research- and nonresearch-based perspective. The nonresearch literature on patient education is prescriptive in nature and tends to give anecdotal tips on how to take individualized approaches to teaching and learning.

A computer literature search, for example, reveals literally thousands of nursing and allied health articles and books on teaching and learning that are available from the general to the specific.

However, many research-based studies are being conducted on teaching specific population groups about a variety of topics, but only recently has attention been focused on how to most effectively teach those with long-term chronic illnesses. Much more research must be conducted on the benefits of patient education as it relates to the potential for increasing the quality of life, leading a disability-free life, decreasing the costs of health care, and managing independently at home through anticipatory teaching approaches. Studies from acute-care settings tend to focus on preparing a patient for a procedure, with emphasis on the benefits of information to alleviate anxiety and promote psychological coping. Evidence does suggest that patients cope much more effectively when taught exactly what to expect (Donovan & Ward, 2001; Duffy, 1998; Mason, 2001).

More research is definitely needed on the benefits of teaching methods and instructional tools using the new technologies of computer-assisted instruction, online and other distance learning modalities, cable television, and Internet access to health information for both patient and staff education. These new approaches to information require a role change of the educator from one of teacher to resource facilitator as well as a shift in the role of the learner from being passive to an active recipient. The rapid advances in technology for teaching and learning also will require a better understanding of generational orientations and experiences of the learner (Billings & Kowalski, 2004). Also, the effectiveness of videotapes and audiotapes with

different learners and in different situations must be further explored (Kessels, 2003). Given the significant incidence of low-literacy rates among patients and their family members, much more investigation needs to be done on the impact of printed versus audiovisual materials as well as written versus verbal instruction on learner comprehension (Weiss, 2003).

Gender issues, the influence of socioeconomics on learning, and the strategies of teaching cultural groups and special populations need further exploration as well. Unfortunately, primary sources of information from nursing literature on the issues of gender and socioeconomic attributes of the learner are scanty, to say the least, and the findings from interdisciplinary research on the influence of gender on learning remain inconclusive.

Nevertheless, nurses are expected to teach diverse populations with complex needs and a range of abilities in both traditional settings and nontraditional, unstructured settings. For more than 30 years, nurse researchers have been studying how best to teach patients, but much more research is required (Mason, 2001). Also, few studies have examined nurses' perceptions about their role as educators in the practice setting (Trocino et al., 1997). We need to establish a stronger theoretical basis for intervening with clients throughout "all phases of the learning continuum, from information acquisition to behavioral change" (Donovan & Ward, 2001, p. 211). Also, emphasis needs to be given to research in nursing education to ensure that the nursing workforce is prepared for "a challenging and uncertain future" in health care (Stevens & Valiga, 1999, p. 278).

In addition, further investigation should be undertaken to document the cost effectiveness of educational efforts in reducing hospital stays, decreasing readmissions, improving the personal quality of life, and minimizing complications of illness and therapies. Furthermore, given the number of variables that can potentially interfere with the teaching–learning process, additional studies must be conducted to examine the effects of environmental stimuli, the factors involved in readiness to learn, and the influences of learning styles on learner motivation, compliance, comprehension, and the ability to apply knowledge and skills once they are acquired. One particular void is the lack of information in the research database on how to assess motivation. The author of Chapter 6 proposes parameters to assess motivation but notes the paucity of information specifically addressing this issue.

Although it was almost 20 years ago that Oberst (1989) delineated the major issues in patient education studies related to the evaluation of the existing research base and the design of future studies, the following four broad problem categories she identified remain pertinent today:

1. Selection and measurement of appropriate dependent variables (educational outcomes)
2. Design and control of independent variables (educational interventions)
3. Control of mediating and intervening variables
4. Development and refinement of the theoretical basis for education

Summary

Nurses are considered information brokers— educators who can make a significant difference in how patients and families cope with their illnesses, how the public benefits from education directed at prevention of disease and promotion of health, and how staff and student nurses gain competency and confidence in practice through education activities that are directed at continuous, lifelong learning. Many challenges and opportunities are ahead for nurse educators in the delivery of health care as this nation moves forward in the 21st century.

The teaching role is becoming even more important and more visible as nurses respond to the social, economic, and political trends impacting on health care today. The foremost challenge for nurses is to be able to demonstrate, through research and action, that definite links exist between education and positive behavioral outcomes of the learner. In this era of cost containment, government regulations, and healthcare reform, the benefits of client, staff, and student education must be made clear to the public, to healthcare employers, to healthcare providers, and to payers of healthcare benefits. To be effective and efficient, nurses must be willing and able to work collaboratively with other members of the healthcare team to provide consistently high-quality education to the audiences they serve.

The responsibility and accountability of nurses for the delivery of care to the consumer can be accomplished, in part, through education based on solid principles of teaching and learning. The key to effective education of our audiences of learners is the nurse's understanding of and ongoing commitment to the role of educator.

REVIEW QUESTIONS

1. How far back in history has teaching been a part of the professional nurse's role?
2. Which nursing organization was the first to recognize health teaching as an important function within the scope of nursing practice?
3. What legal mandate universally includes teaching as a responsibility of nurses?
4. How have the ANA, NLN, ICN, AHA, JC, and PEW Commission influenced the role and responsibilities of the nurse as educator?
5. What current social, economic, and political trends make it imperative that clients and nursing staff be adequately educated?
6. What are the similarities and differences between the education process and the nursing process?
7. What are three major barriers to teaching and three major obstacles to learning?
8. What common factor serves as both a barrier to education and as an obstacle to learning?
9. What is the current status of research- and non-research-based evidence pertaining to education?

References

Berwick, D. (2006, December 12). *IHI launches national campaign to reduce medical harm in U.S. hospitals: Building on its landmark 100,000 lives campaign.* Retrieved December 21, 2006, from http://www.ihi.org

Billings, D., & Kowalski, K. (2004). Teaching learners from varied generations. *The Journal of Continuing Education in Nursing, 35*(3), 104–105.

Birchenall, P. (2000). Nurse education in the year 2000: Reflection, speculation and challenge. *Nurse Education Today, 20*, 1–2.

Bodenheimer, T., Lorig, K., Holman, H., & Grumbach, K. (2002). Patient self-management of chronic disease in primary care. *JAMA, 288*(19), 2469–2475.

Carpenter, J. A., & Bell, S. K. (2002). What do nurses know about teaching patients? *Journal for Nurses in Staff Development, 18*(3), 157–161.

Casey, F. S. (1995). Documenting patient education: A literature review. *Journal of Continuing Education in Nursing, 26*(6), 257–260.

Chachkes, E., & Christ, G. (1996). Cross cultural issues in patient education. *Patient Education & Counseling, 27*, 13–21.

Cipriano, P. F. (2007). Stop, look, and listen to your patients and their families. *American Nurse Today, 2*(6), 10.

Davidhizar, R. E., & Brownson, K. (1999). Literacy, cultural diversity, and client education. *Health Care Manager, 18*(1), 39–47.

DeSilets, L. D. (1995). Assessing registered nurses' reasons for participating in continuing education. *Journal of Continuing Education in Nursing, 26*(5), 202–208.

Donner, C. L., Levonian, C., & Slutsky, P. (2005). Move to the head of the class: Developing staff nurses as teachers. *Journal of Nurses in Staff Development, 21*(6), 277–283.

Donovan, H. S., & Ward, S. (2001, third quarter). A representational approach to patient education. *Journal of Nursing Scholarship*, 211–216.

Duffy, B. (1998). Get ready—Get set—Go teach. *Home Healthcare Nurse, 16*(9), 596–602.

Gillespie, M., & McFetridge, B. (2006). Nursing education—The role of the nurse teacher. *Journal of Clinical Nursing, 15,* 639–644.

Gilroth, B. E. (1990). Promoting patient involvement: Educational, organizational, and environmental strategies. *Patient Education and Counseling, 15,* 29–38.

Glanville, I. K. (2000). Moving towards health oriented patient education (HOPE). *Holistic Nursing Practice, 14*(2), 57–66.

Grueninger, U. J. (1995). Arterial hypertension: Lessons from patient education. *Patient Education and Counseling, 26,* 37–55.

Honan, S., Krsnak, G., Petersen, D., & Torkelson, R. (1988). The nurse as patient educator: Perceived responsibilities and factors enhancing role development. *Journal of Continuing Education in Nursing, 19*(1), 33–37.

Joint Commission on Accreditation of Healthcare Organizations. (2001). *Patient and family education: The compliance guide to the JCAHO standards* (2nd ed.). Retrieved January 25, 2001, from http://www.accreditinfo.com/news/index.cfm?artid=2011

Kessels, R. P. C. (2003). Patients' memory for medical information. *Journal of the Royal Society of Medicine, 96,* 219–222.

Klestzick, K. R. (2005). *Results from landmark nurse educator certification examination.* Retrieved December 20, 2005, from http://www.nln.org/news

Knowles, M. S., Holton, E. F., & Swanson, R. A. (1998). *The adult learner: The definitive classic in adult education and human resource development* (5th ed., pp. 198–201). Houston, TX: Gulf Publishing.

Kruger, S. (1991). The patient educator role in nursing. *Applied Nursing Research, 4*(1), 19–24.

London, F. (1995). Teach your patients faster and better. *Nursing, 95,* 68, 70.

Mangena, A., & Chabeli, M. M. (2005). Strategies to overcome obstacles in the facilitation of critical thinking in nursing education. *Nurse Education Today, 25,* 291–298.

Mason, D. (2001). Promoting health literacy: Patient teaching is a vital nursing function. *American Journal of Nursing, 101*(2), 7.

McCafferty, L. A. E. (2002, January 7). Year of the nurse: More than four out of five Americans trust nurses. *Advance for Nurses,* 5.

Musinski, B. (1999). The educator as facilitator: A new kind of leadership. *Nursing Forum, 34*(1), 23–29.

National League of Nursing Education. (1937). *A curriculum guide for schools of nursing.* New York: The League.

National League for Nursing. (2006). Certified nurse educator (CNE) 2006 candidate handbook. Retrieved July 21, 2007, from http://www.nln.org/facultycertification/index.htm

Oberst, M. T. (1989). Perspectives on research in patient teaching. *Nursing Clinics of North America, 24*(2), 621–627.

Orr, R. (1990). Illness as an educational opportunity. *Patient Education and Counseling, 15,* 47–48.

Pew Health Professions Commission. (1995). *Critical challenges: Revitalizing the health professions for the twenty-first century: The Third Report of the Pew Health Professions Commission.* San Francisco: University of California.

Pew Health Professions Commission. (1998). *Recreating health professional practice for a new century: The Fourth Report of the Pew Health Professions Commission, Center for the Health Professions.* San Francisco: University of California.

Pohl, M. L. (1965). Teaching activities of the nursing practitioner. *Nursing Research, 14*(1), 4–11.

Rega, M. D. (1993). A model approach for patient education. *MEDSURG Nursing, 2*(6), 477–479, 495.

Reising, D. L. (2007, February). Protecting yourself from malpractice claims. *American Nurse Today,* 39–44.

Rifas, E., Morris, R., & Grady, R. (1994). Innovative approach to patient education. *Nursing Outlook, 42*(5), 214–216.

Saad, L. (2006, December 14). Nurses top list of most honest and ethical professions. *The Gallup Poll.* Retrieved September 15, 2007, from http://www.galluppoll.com/content/?ci=25888&pg-i

Stevens, K. R., & Valiga, T. M. (1999). The national agenda for nursing education research. *Nursing and Health Care Perspectives, 20*(5), 278.

Stolberg, S. G. (2002, August 8). Patient deaths tied to lack of nurses. *New York Times.* Retrieved August 8, 2002, from, http://www.nytimes.com/2002/08/08/health/08NURS.html

Sullivan, L. W., & Bristow, L. R. (2007, March 13). *Summary proceedings of the national leadership symposium on increasing diversity in the health professions.* Washington, DC: The Sullivan Alliance, 1–12.

Trocino, L., Byers, J. F., & Peach, A. G. (1997). Nurses' attitudes toward patient and family education: Implications for clinical nurse specialists. *Clinical Nurse Specialist: A Journal for Advanced Nursing Practice, 11*(2), 77–84.

U.S. Department of Health and Human Services. (2000). *Healthy people 2010: Objectives for improving health.* (Vol. II). Washington, DC: U.S. Government Printing Office.

Wagner, S. P., & Ash, K. L. (1998). Creating the teachable moment. *Journal of Nursing Education, 37*(6), 278–280.

Weiss, B. D. (2003). *Health literacy: A manual for clinicians.* Chicago: American Medical Association and American Medical Association Foundation, 1–12.

Zikmund-Fisher, B. J., Sarr, B., Fagerlin, S., & Ubel, P. A. (2006). A matter of perspective: Choosing for others differs from choosing for yourself in making treatment decisions. *Journal of General Internal Medicine, 21*, 618–622.

Chapter 2

Ethical, Legal, and Economic Foundations of the Educational Process

M. Janice Nelson

CHAPTER HIGHLIGHTS

A Differentiated View of Ethics, Morality, and the Law

Evolution of Ethical and Legal Principles in Health Care

Application of Ethical and Legal Principles to Patient Education
- *Autonomy*
- *Veracity*
- *Confidentiality*
- *Nonmalfeasance*
- *Beneficence*
- *Justice*

Legality of Patient Education and Information Documentation

Economic Factors of Patient Education: Justice and Duty Revisited

Financial Terminology
- *Direct Costs*
- *Indirect Costs*

Cost Savings, Cost Benefit, and Cost Recovery

Program Planning and Implementation

Cost-Benefit Analysis and Cost-Effectiveness Analysis

State of the Evidence

KEY TERMS

- ❑ ethical
- ❑ moral
- ❑ legal
- ❑ autonomy
- ❑ veracity
- ❑ confidentiality
- ❑ nonmalfeasance
- ❑ negligence
- ❑ malpractice

- ❑ beneficence
- ❑ justice
- ❑ *respondeat superior*
- ❑ direct costs
- ❑ fixed costs
- ❑ variable costs
- ❑ indirect costs
- ❑ cost savings
- ❑ cost benefit

❑ cost recovery
❑ revenue generation
❑ cost-benefit analysis

❑ cost-benefit ratio
❑ cost-effectiveness analysis

OBJECTIVES

After completing this chapter, the reader will be able to

1. Identify the six major ethical principles.
2. Distinguish between ethical and legal dimensions of the healthcare delivery system, including patient and staff education.
3. Describe the importance of nurse practice acts.
4. Describe the legal and financial implications of documentation.
5. Delineate the ethical, legal, and economic importance of federal, state, and accrediting body regulations and standards in the delivery of healthcare services.
6. Differentiate among financial terms associated with the development, implementation, and evaluation of patient education programs.

Today as never before in the evolution of the healthcare field, there is a critical consciousness of individual rights stemming from both natural and constitutional law. Healthcare organizations are laden with laws and regulations ensuring clients' rights to a quality standard of care, to informed consent, and subsequently to self-determination. Consequently, it is crucial that the providers of care be equally proficient in both educating the public and in educating nursing students and staff who are or will be the practitioner educators of tomorrow.

Although the physician is primarily held legally accountable for the medical regimen, it is a known fact that patient education generally falls to the nurse. Indeed, given the close relationship of the nurse to the client, the role of the nurse in this educational process is absolutely essential and mandated as such through a variety of state nurse practice acts.

We are indeed living in an age of an enlightened public that is not only aware, but also demands recognition of individual constitutional rights regarding freedom of choice and rights to self-determination. In fact, it may seem curious to some that federal and state governments, accrediting bodies, and professional organizations find it necessary to legislate, regulate, or provide standards and guidelines to ensure the protection of human rights when it comes to matters of health care. The answer, of course, is that the federal government has abandoned its historical hands off policy toward physicians and other health professionals in the wake of serious breaches of public confidence and shocking revelations of abuses of human rights in the name of biomedical research.

These issues of human rights are fundamental to the delivery of quality healthcare services. They are equally fundamental to the education process, in that the intent of the educator should be to empower the client to make informed choices and to be in control of the consequences of those choices regardless of the outcome. Thus, in explicating the role of the nurse in the teaching–learning process, it would be remiss to omit the ethical and legal foundations of that process. Also, in the interest of justice, which refers to the equal distribution of benefits and burdens, it is important to acknowledge the relationship of costs to the healthcare facility in the provision of such services. Teaching and learning principles, with their inherent legal and ethical dimensions, apply to any situation in which the educational process is occurring.

The purpose of this chapter is to provide the ethical, legal, and economic foundations that underpin the patient education initiative on the one hand and the rights and responsibilities of the provider on the other. This chapter explores the differences between and among ethical, moral, and legal concepts. It explores the ethical and legal foundations of human rights, and it reviews the ethical and legal dimensions of health care. Furthermore, this chapter examines the importance of documentation of patient teaching while highlighting the economic factors that must be considered in the delivery of patient education in healthcare settings. An additional section provides a brief discussion of evidence-based practice and its relationship to quality and evaluation of patient education programs.

A Differentiated View of Ethics, Morality, and the Law

Although ethics as a branch of classical philosophy has been studied throughout the centuries, by and large these studies were left to the domains of philosophical and religious thinkers. More recently, due to the complexities of modern-day living and the heightened awareness of an educated public, ethical issues related to health care have surfaced as a major concern of both healthcare providers and recipients of these services. Thus, it is a widely held belief that the client has the right to know his or her medical diagnosis, the treatments available, and the expected outcomes. This information is necessary so that informed choices by clients relative to their respective diagnoses can be made in concert with advice offered by health professionals.

Ethical principles of human rights are rooted in natural laws, which, in the absence of any other guidelines, are binding on human society. Inherent in these natural laws are, for example, the principles of respect for others, truth telling, honesty, and respect for life. Ethics as a discipline interprets these basic principles of behavior in broad terms that guide moral decision making in all realms of human activity (Tong, 2007).

Although multiple perspectives on the rightness or wrongness of human acts exist, among the most commonly referenced are the writings of the 16th-century German philosopher, Immanuel Kant, and those of the 19th-century English scholar and philosopher, John Stuart Mill (Edward, 1967). Kant proposed that individual rights prevail and openly proclaimed the deontological notion of the "Golden Rule." Deontology (from the Greek word *deon*, which means duty) is the ethical belief system that stresses the importance of doing one's duty and following the rules. Thus, respect for individual rights is key and one person should never be treated merely as a means to another person's benefit or a group's well-being (Tong, 2007). Mill, on the other hand, proposed the teleological notion or utilitarian approach to ethical decision making that allows for the sacrifice of one or more individuals so that a group of people can benefit in some important way. He believed that given the alternatives, choices should be made that result in the greatest good for the greatest number of people.

Likewise, the legal system and its laws are based on ethical and moral principles that, through experience and over time, society has accepted as behavioral norms (Hall, 1996; Lesnick & Anderson, 1962). This relationship accounts in part for the fact that the terms *ethical, moral,* and *legal* are so often used in synchrony. It should be made clear, however, that while these terms are certainly interrelated, they are not necessarily synonymous.

Ethics refers to the guiding principles of behavior, and *ethical* refers to norms or standards of behavior. Although the terms moral or morality are generally used interchangeably with the terms ethics or ethical, one can differentiate the notion of moral rights and duties from the notion of ethical rights and duties. *Moral* refers to an internal value system (the moral fabric of one's being) and this value system, defined as *morality*, is expressed externally through ethical behavior. Ethical principles deal with intangible moral values, so they are not enforceable by law, nor are these principles laws in and of themselves. *Legal* rights and duties, on the other hand, refer to rules governing behavior or conduct that are enforceable under threat of punishment or penalty, such as a fine, imprisonment, or both.

The intricate relationship between ethics and the law explains why ethics terminology, such as informed consent, confidentiality, nonmalfeasance, and justice, can be found within the language of the legal system. In keeping with this practice, nurses may cite professional commitment or moral obligation to justify the education of clients as one dimension of their role. In reality, the legitimacy of this role stems from the nurse practice act that exists in the particular state where the nurse resides, is licensed, and is employed. In essence, the nurse practice act is not only legally binding, but it is also protected by the police authority of the state in the interest of protecting the public (Brent, 2001; Mikos, 2004).

Evolution of Ethical and Legal Principles in Health Care

In the past, ethics was relegated almost exclusively to the philosophical and religious domains. Likewise, from a historical vantage point, medical and nursing care was considered a humanitarian, if not charitable, endeavor. Often it was provided by members of religious communities and others considered to be generous of spirit, caring in nature, courageous, dedicated, and self-sacrificing in their service to others. Public sentiment was so strong in this regard that for many years healthcare organizations, which were considered to be charitable institutions, were largely immune from legal action "because it would compel the charity to divert its funds for a purpose never intended" (Lesnik & Anderson, 1962, p. 211). In the same manner, healthcare practitioners in the past—who were primarily physicians and nurses—were usually regarded as Good Samaritans who acted in good faith.

Although there are numerous court records of lawsuits involving hospitals, physicians, and nurses dating back to the early 1900s, those numbers pale in comparison with the volumes being generated on a daily basis in today's world

(Reising & Allen, 2007). Further, despite the horror stories that have been handed down through the years regarding inhumane and often torturous treatment of prisoners, the mentally infirm, the disabled, and the poor, there was limited focus in the past on ethical aspects of that care. In turn, there was little thought of legal protection for the rights of such mentally, physically, or socioeconomically challenged people.

Clearly, this situation has changed dramatically. Informed consent, for example, which is a basic tenet of ethical thought, was established in the courts as early as 1914 by Justice Benjamin Cardozo. Cardozo determined that every adult of sound mind has a right to protect his or her own body and to determine how it shall be treated (Hall, 1992; *Schloendorff v. Society of New York Hospitals,* 1914). Although the Cardozo decision was of considerable magnitude, governmental interest in the bioethical underpinnings of human rights in the delivery of healthcare services did not really surface until after World War II.

Over the years, legal authorities such as federal and state governments maintained a hands-off posture when it came to issues of biomedical research or physician–patient relationships. However, human atrocities committed by the Nazis in the name of biomedical research during World War II shocked the world into critical awareness of gross violations of human rights. Unfortunately, such abuses were not confined to wartime Europe alone. On United States soil, for example, the nontreatment of syphilitic African Americans in Tuskegee, Alabama; the injection of live cancer cells into uninformed, nonconsenting older adults at the Brooklyn Chronic Disease Hospital; and the use of institutionalized mentally retarded children to test hepatitis vaccines at Willowbrook Developmental Center on Staten Island, New York, shocked the nation and raised a critical consciousness of disturbing breaches in the physician–patient relationship (Brent, 2001; Centers for Disease Control and Prevention, 2005; Rivera, 1972; Thomas & Quinn, 1991; Weisbard & Arras, 1984).

Stirred to action by these disturbing phenomena, in 1974 Congress moved with all due deliberation to create the *National Commission for the Protection of Human Subjects of Biomedical and Behavioral Research* (Department of Health and Human Services [DHHS], 1983). As an outcome of this unprecedented act, an institutional review board for the protection of human subjects (IRBPHS) was rapidly established at the local level by hospitals, academic medical centers, and any agency or organization where research on human subjects was being conducted. To this day, the primary emphasis of these review boards is on confidentiality, truth telling, and informed consent, with specific concern for vulnerable populations such as infants, children, prisoners, and the mentally ill. Every proposal for biomedical research that involves human subjects must be submitted to a local IRBPHS for intensive review and approval before proceeding with a proposed study (DHHS, 1983). Further, in response to its concern about the range of ethical issues associated with medical practice and a perceived need to regulate biomedical research, in 1978 Congress established the President's Commission for the Study of Ethical Problems in Medicine and Biomedical and Behavioral Research (Brent, 2001; DHHS, 1983; Thomas & Quinn, 1991).

Interestingly, as early as 1950, the American Nurses Association (ANA) developed and adopted an ethical code for professional practice that has since been revised and updated several times (ANA, 1976, 1985, 2001). The latest revision of the ANA's code, now entitled the *Code of*

Ethics for Nurses With Interpretive Statements, was released in 2001 for implementation in the new millennium. This code represents an articulation of professional values and moral obligations in relation to the nurse–patient relationship and in support of the profession and its mission.

In 1975, the American Hospital Association (AHA) followed suit by disseminating a document entitled *Patient's Bill of Rights,* which was revised in 1992 (Association of American Physicians and Surgeons, 1995). A copy of these patient rights is framed and posted in a public place in every healthcare facility across the United States. In addition, federal standards developed by the Center for Medicare and Medicaid Services (CMS)—an arm of the Health Care Financing Administration (HCFA)—require that the patient be provided with a personal copy of these rights either at the time of admission to the hospital or long-term care facility or prior to the initiation of care or treatment when admitted to a surgicenter, an HMO, home care, or a hospice. As a matter of fact, many states have adopted the statement of patient rights as part of their state health code. Thus these rights fall under the jurisdiction of the law, rendering them legally enforceable by threat of penalty.

Application of Ethical and Legal Principles to Patient Education

In considering the ethical and legal responsibilities inherent in the process of patient education, six major ethical principles are intricately woven throughout the ANA's *Code of Ethics* (2001), the AHA's *Patient's Bill of Rights* (1992), and similar documents promulgated by other healthcare organizations as well as the federal government. These principles, which encompass the very issues that precipitated federal intervention into healthcare affairs, are autonomy, veracity, confidentiality, nonmalfeasance, beneficence, and justice.

Autonomy

The first of these principles, *autonomy*, is derived from the Greek words *auto* (self) and *nomos* (law) and refers to the right of self-determination (Tong, 2007). Laws have been enacted to protect the patient's right to make choices independently. Federal mandates, such as informed consent, must be evident in every application for federal funding to support biomedical research. The local IRBPHS assumes the role of judge and jury to ascertain adherence to this enforceable regulation (Dickey, 2006).

The Patient Self-Determination Act (PSDA), which was passed by Congress in 1991 (Ulrich, 1999), is a clear example of the principle of *autonomy* enacted into law. Any healthcare facility, such as acute- and long-term care institutions, surgicenters, HMOs, hospices, or home care, that receives Medicare and/or Medicaid funds, must comply with the PSDA. The law requires, either at the time of hospital admission or prior to the initiation of care or treatment in a community health setting, "that every individual receiving health care be informed in writing of the right under state law to make decisions about his or her health care, including the right to refuse medical and surgical care and the right to initiate advance directives" (Mezey, Evans, Golob, Murphy, & White, 1994, p. 30). These authors readily acknowledge the nurse's responsibility to ensure informed decision making by patients, which includes but is certainly not limited to advance directives (e.g., living wills, durable power of attorney, and designation of a healthcare proxy). Documentation of such instruction must appear in the patient's record, which is the legal document validating that informed consent took place.

One principle worth noting in the ANA's *Code of Ethics* is that which addresses collaboration "with members of the health professions and other citizens in promoting community and national efforts to meet the health needs of the public" (New York State Nurses Association, 2001, p. 6). Although not specified in such detail in the ANA document, this principle certainly provides a justification for patient education both within and outside the healthcare organization. It provides an ethical rationale for health education classes open to the community, such as childbirth education courses, smoking cessation classes, weight reduction sessions, discussions of women's health issues, and positive interventions for preventing child abuse. While health education, per se, is not an interpretive part of the principle of autonomy, it certainly lends credence to the ethical notion of assisting the public to attain greater autonomy when it comes to matters of health promotion and high-level wellness. In fact, consistent with the *Model Nurse Practice Act* (ANA, 1978), all contemporary nurse practice acts contain some type of statements identifying health education as a legal duty and responsibility of the registered nurse.

Veracity

Veracity, or truth telling, is closely linked to informed decision making and informed consent. The early 20th-century landmark decision by Justice Benjamin Cardozo (*Schloendorff v. Society of New York Hospitals,* 1914) specified an individual's fundamental right to make decisions about his or her own body. This ruling provided a basis in law for patient education or instruction regarding invasive medical procedures. Nurses are often confronted with issues of truth telling,

as was exemplified in the Tuma case (Rankin & Stallings, 1990). In the interest of full disclosure of information, the nurse (Tuma) had advised a cancer patient of alternative treatments without consultation with the client's physician. Tuma was sued by the physician for interfering with the medical regimen that he had prescribed for care of this particular patient. Although Tuma was eventually exonerated from professional misconduct charges, the case emphasized a significant point of law to be found in the New York State Nurse Practice Act (1972), which states, "A nursing regimen shall be consistent with and shall not vary from any existing medical regimen." In some instances, this creates a double bind for the nurse. Creighton (1986) emphatically explained that failure or omission to properly instruct the patient relative to invasive procedures is tantamount to battery.

Cisar and Bell (1995) addressed this concept of battery related to medical treatment exceedingly well. In addition to explaining Curtin's (1978) *Ethical Decision-Making Model*, which serves as a guide for healthcare providers facing an ethical dilemma, the authors offered the following explanation of the four elements making up the notion of informed consent that are such vital aspects of patient education:

1. *Competence*, which refers to the capacity of the patient to make a reasonable decision.
2. *Disclosure of information*, which requires that sufficient information regarding risks and alternative treatments be provided to the patient to enable him or her to make a rational decision.
3. *Comprehension*, which speaks to the individual's ability to understand or to grasp intellectually the information being provided. A child, for example, may not yet be of an age to understand

any ramifications of medical treatment and must, therefore, depend on his or her parents to make a decision that will be in the child's best interest.

4. *Voluntariness*, which indicates that the patient has made a decision without coercion or force from others.

While all four of these elements might be satisfied, the client might still choose to reject the regimen of care suggested by healthcare providers. This decision could be due to the exorbitant cost of a treatment or to certain personal or religious beliefs. Whatever the case, it must be recognized by all concerned that a competent, informed client cannot be forced to accept treatment as long as he or she is aware of the alternatives as well as the consequences of any decision (Cisar & Bell, 1995).

A final dimension of the legality of truth telling relates to the role of the nurse as expert witness. Professional nurses who are recognized for their skill or expertise in a particular area of nursing practice may be called on to testify in court on behalf of either the plaintiff (the one who initiates the litigation) or the defendant (the one being sued). In any case, the concept of expert testimony speaks for itself. Regardless of the situation, the nurse must always tell the truth and the client (or his or her health proxy) is always entitled to the truth (Hall, 1996).

Confidentiality

Confidentiality refers to personal information that is entrusted and protected as privileged information via a social contract, healthcare standard or code, or legal covenant. Such information may not be disclosed by healthcare providers when acquired in a professional capacity from a patient without consent of that patient. If sensitive information were not to be protected, patients would lose trust in their providers and would be reluctant to openly share problems with them.

A distinction must be made between the terms anonymous and confidential. Information is *anonymous*, for example, when researchers are unable to link any subject's identity in their records. Information is *confidential* when identifying materials appear on subjects' records, but can only be accessed by the researchers (Tong, 2007).

Only under special circumstances may secrecy be ethically broken, such as when a patient has been the victim or subject of a crime to which the nurse or doctor is a witness (Lesnick & Anderson, 1962). Other exceptions to confidentiality occur when professionals suspect or are aware of child or elder abuse, narcotic use, communicable diseases, gunshot or knife wounds, or the threat of violence toward someone. To protect the welfare of others, professionals are permitted to breach confidentiality. Another example occurs when a patient tests positive for HIV/AIDS and has no intention of telling his or her spouse about this diagnosis. In this instance, the physician is obligated to warn the spouse directly or indirectly of the risk of potential harm (Tong, 2007). According to Brent (2001), "this area of legislation concerned with health care privacy and disclosure reveals the tension between what is good for the individual vis-à-vis what is good for society" (p. 141).

The 2003 updated Health Information Portability and Accountability Act (HIPAA) ensures nearly absolute confidentiality related to dissemination of patient information, unless the patient himself or herself authorizes release of such information (Kohlenberg, 2006). One goal of the HIPAA policy, first enacted by Congress in 1996, is to limit disclosure of patient health-care information to third parties, such as insurance companies or employers. This law, which requires patients' prior written consent for release of their health information, was never meant to interfere with consultation between professionals, but is intended to prevent elevator conversations about private matters of individuals entrusted to our care. In an open, liberal, and technologically advanced society such as ours, this law is a must to ensure confidentiality (Tong, 2007). Today, in some states and under certain conditions, such as death or impending death, a spouse or members of the immediate family can be apprised of the patient's condition if this information was previously unknown to them. Despite federal and state legislation protecting the confidentiality rights of individuals, the issue of the ethical/moral obligation of the person with HIV/AIDS or genetic disease, for example, to *voluntarily* divulge his or her condition to others who may be at risk remains largely unresolved (Legal Action Center, 2001).

Nonmalfeasance

Nonmalfeasance means "do no harm" and constitutes the ethical fabric of legal determinations encompassing negligence and/or malpractice. According to Brent (2001), *negligence* is defined as "conduct which falls below the standard established by law for the protection of others against unreasonable risk of harm" (p. 54). She further asserts that the concept of professional *negligence* "involves the conduct of professionals (e.g., nurses, physicians, dentists, and lawyers) that fall [sic] below a professional standard of due care" (p. 55). As clarified by Tong (2007), due care is "the kind of care healthcare professionals give patients when they treat them attentively and vigilantly so as to avoid mis-

takes" (p. 25). For negligence to exist, there must be a duty between the injured party and the person whose actions (or nonactions) caused the injury. A breach of that duty must have occurred, it must have been the immediate cause of the injury, and the injured party must have experienced damages from the injury (Brent, 2001).

The term *malpractice*, by comparison, still holds as defined by Lesnick and Anderson in 1962. *Malpractice*, these authors asserted, "refers to a limited class of negligent activities committed within the scope of performance by those pursuing a particular profession involving highly skilled and technical services" (p. 234). More recently, *malpractice* has been specifically defined as "negligence, misconduct, or breach of duty by a professional person that results in injury or damage to a patient" (Reising & Allen, 2007). Thus, *malpractice*, per se, is limited in scope to those whose life work requires special education and training as dictated by specific educational standards. In contrast, negligence embraces all improper and wrongful conduct by anyone arising out of any activity. Reising and Allen (2007) describe the most common causes for malpractice claims against nurses:

1. Failure to follow standards of care
2. Failure to use equipment in a responsible manner
3. Failure to communicate
4. Failure to document
5. Failure to assess and monitor
6. Failure to act as patient advocate
7. Failure to delegate tasks properly

The concept of duty is closely tied to the concepts of negligence and malpractice. Nurses' duties are spelled out in job descriptions at their places of employment. Policy and procedure manuals of a particular facility exist certainly to protect the patient, but they also exist to protect the employee, in this instance, the nurse, and the employer against litigation. Policies are more than guidelines. Policies and procedures determine standards of behavior (duties) expected of employees of a particular institution and can be used in a court of law in the determination of negligence.

Expectations of professional nursing performance are also measured against the nurse's level of education and concomitant skills, standing orders of the physician, institution-specific protocols, standards of care upheld by the profession (ANA), and standards of care adhered to by the various clinical specialty organizations of which the nurse may be a member. If the nurse is certified in a clinical specialty or is identified as a "specialist" although not certified, he or she will be held to the standards of that specialty (Yoder Wise, 1995).

In the instance of litigation, the key operational principle is that the nurse is not measured against the optimal or maximum of professional standards of performance; rather, the yardstick is laid against the prevailing practice of what a prudent and reasonable nurse would do under the same circumstances in a given community. Thus, the nurse's duty of patient education (or lack thereof) is measured against not only prevailing policy of the employing institution, but also against prevailing practice in the community. In the case of clinical nurse specialists (CNSs), nurse practitioners (NPs), or clinical education specialists (CESs), for example, the practice is measured against institutional policies for this level of worker as well as against prevailing practice of nurses performing at the same level in the community or in the same geographic region.

Beneficence

Beneficence is defined as "doing good" for the benefit of others. It is a concept that is legalized through adherence to critical tasks and duties contained in job descriptions; in policies, procedures, and protocols set forth by the healthcare facility; and in standards and codes of ethical behaviors established by professional nursing organizations. Adherence to these various professional performance criteria and principles, including adequate and current patient education, speaks to the nurse's commitment to acting in the best interest of the patient. Such behavior emphasizes patient welfare, but not necessarily to the detriment of the well-being of the healthcare provider. That is, the effort to save lives and relieve human suffering is a duty to do good only within reasonable limits. For example, when AIDS first appeared, the cause and control of this fatal disease was unknown. Some healthcare professionals protested that the duty of beneficence did not include caring for patients who put them at risk for this deadly, infectious, and untreatable disease. Once it became clear that transmission through occupational exposure was quite small, the majority of healthcare practitioners concurred with the opinion of the American Medical Association that they "... may not ethically refuse to treat a patient whose condition is within [their] current realm of competence solely because the patient is seropositive" (Tong, 2007).

Justice

The sixth and final ethical principle, *justice*, speaks to the fairness and equal distribution of goods and services. The law is the justice system. The focus of the law is the protection of society; the focus of health law is the protection of the consumer. It is unjust to treat a person better or worse than another person in a similar condition or circumstance, unless a difference in treatment can be justified with good reason. In today's healthcare climate, professionals must be as objective as possible in allocating scarce medical resources in a just manner. Decision making for the fair distribution of resources includes the following criteria as defined by Tong (2007):

1. To each, an equal share
2. To each, according to need
3. To each, according to effort
4. To each, according to contribution
5. To each, according to merit
6. To each, according to the ability to pay (p. 30)

According to Tong, healthcare professionals may have second thoughts about the application of these criteria in particular circumstances because one or more of the criteria could be at odds with the concept of justice. "To allocate scarce resources to patients on the basis of their social worth, moral goodness, or economic condition rather than on the basis of their medical condition is more often than not wrong" (p. 30).

As noted earlier, adherence to the *Patient's Bill of Rights* is legally enforced in most states. This means that the nurse or any other health professional can be subjected to penalty or to litigation for discrimination in provision of care. Regardless of his or her age, gender, physical disability, sexual orientation, or race, for example, the client has a right to proper instruction regarding risks and benefits of invasive medical procedures. S/he also has a right to proper instruction regarding self-care activities, such as home dialysis, for example, that are beyond normal activities of daily living for most people.

Furthermore, when a nurse is employed by a particular healthcare facility, she or he enters into a contract, written or tacit, to provide nurs-

ing services in accordance with the policies of the facility. Failure to provide nursing care (including educational services) based on patient diagnosis or persistence in providing substandard care based on client age, diagnosis, culture, national origin, sexual preference, and the like, can result in liability for breach of contract with the employing institution.

Most recently, the U.S. Congress has wrestled with another version of patients' rights within which every American carrying health insurance is guaranteed access to emergency room care, to treatment by medical specialists, and to government-run clinical trials (Abood, 2001; President's Advisory Commission on Consumer Protection and Quality in the Healthcare Industry, 1998). Also, considerable argument has ensued among members of Congress over the extent to which health maintenance organizations (HMOs) can be sued for delay or denial of care, and what limits, if any, should be placed on the damages (Zuckerman, 2001). This federal legislation adds an interesting dimension to the notion of justice as it applies to health care. The proposed patients' rights legislation is intended only for those covered by health insurance. This restriction raises serious questions for the uninsured regarding the right of access to health care and subsequently the right of access to health education. Emanuel (2000) raises a critical point in asserting that "the diffuseness of decision making in the American health care system precludes a coherent process for allocating health care resources" (p. 8). Emanuel further contends that managed care organizations have systematically pursued drastic cost reductions by restructuring of delivery systems and investing in expensive and elaborate information systems. HMOs have bought out physician practices and have become involved in a number of related activities with no substantial evidence that a high quality of health care will be achieved at lower prices.

To date, this particular enactment of a patient's bill of rights and the issues of just or unjust cost-cutting activities of HMOs as described by Emanuel (2000) do, indeed, affect the role of the educator. These issues determine whether nurse educators can surmount the obstacles potentially blocking the patient education process. In the interest of cutting costs, HMOs have also succeeded in shortening lengths of hospital stays. This development, in turn, has had a tremendous effect on the delivery of education to the hospitalized patient and presents serious obstacles to the implementation of this mandate. Lack of time serves as a major barrier to the nurse in being able to provide sufficient information for self-care, and illness acuity level interferes with the patient's ability to process information necessary to meet his or her physical and emotional needs.

Clearly, professional nurses are mandated by organizational policy as well as by federal and state regulations to provide patient education. Thus, great care must be taken to ensure that the education justly due to the client will be addressed postdischarge, either in the ambulatory care setting, at home, or in the physician's office.

Legality of Patient Education and Information

The patient's right to adequate information regarding his or her physical condition, medications, risks, and access to information regarding alternative treatments is specifically spelled out in various renditions of the *Patient's Bill of Rights*

(AHA, 1992; President's Advisory Commission, 1998; ANA, 2001; Association of American Physicians and Surgeons, 1995). As noted earlier, many states have adopted these rights as part of their health code, thus rendering them legal and enforceable by law. Patients' rights to education and instruction are also regulated through standards promulgated by accrediting bodies such as the Joint Commission, formerly known as the Joint Commission on Accreditation of Healthcare Organizations (JCAHO). Although these standards are not enforceable in the same manner as law, lack of organizational conformity can lead to loss of accreditation, which in turn jeopardizes the facility's eligibility for third-party reimbursement, as well as loss of Medicare and Medicaid reimbursement. Lack of organizational conformity can also lead to loss of public confidence.

In addition, state regulations pertaining to patient education are published and enforced under threat of penalty (fine, citation, or both) by the department of health in many states. Federal regulations, enforceable as laws, also mandate patient education in those healthcare facilities receiving Medicare and Medicaid funding. And, as discussed earlier, the federal government also mandates full patient disclosure in cases of participation in biomedical research in any setting or for any federally funded project or experimental research involving human subjects.

Federal authorities have generally tended to hold physicians responsible and accountable for proper patient education. This is particularly true as it pertains to issues of informed consent, such as those highlighted in *Scalia v. St. Paul Fire and Marine Ins. Co.*, 1975 (Smith, 1987). It is a well-known fact—at least in hospitals—that patient education usually is carried out by the nurse or some other physician-appointed designee. Physicians' responsibility notwithstanding, from a professional and legal vantage point, nurses are fully legitimized in their role as patient educators by virtue of their respective nurse practice acts. The issue regarding patient education is not necessarily one of omission on anyone's part. Rather, the heart of the matter may be proper documentation (or the lack thereof) that provides evidence of written testimony that client education has indeed occurred.

Documentation

The 89th Congress enacted the Comprehensive Health Planning Act in 1965, Public Law 89-97, 1965 (Boyd, Gleit, Graham, & Whitman, 1998). The entitlements of Medicare and Medicaid—which revolutionized the provision of health care for the elderly and the poor—were established through this act. One acknowledgment in the act was the importance of the preventive and rehabilitative dimensions of health care. Thus, to qualify for Medicare and Medicaid reimbursement, "a hospital has to show evidence that patient education has been a part of patient care" (Boyd et al., 1998, p. 26).

For at least the past 20 years, the Joint Commission (formerly JCAHO) has reinforced the federal mandate by requiring evidence (documentation) of patient and/or family education in the patient record. Pertinent to this point is the doctrine of *respondeat superior,* or the master-servant rule. *Respondeat superior* provides that the employer may be held liable for negligence, assault and battery, false imprisonment, slander, libel, or any other tort committed by an employee (Lesnik & Anderson, 1962). The landmark case supporting the doctrine of *respondeat superior* in the healthcare field was the 1965 case of *Darling v. Charleston Memorial Hospital.* Although the Darling case dealt with negligence in the performance of professional duties of the physician, it brought out—possibly for the first time—the professional obligations or duties of nurses to ensure the well-being of the patient (Brown, 1976).

Casey (1995) points out that of all omissions in documentation, patient teaching has been identified as "probably the most undocumented skilled service because nurses do not recognize the scope and depth of the teaching they do" (p. 257). Lack of documentation also reflects negligence in adhering to the mandates of the particular nurse practice act. This laxity is unfortunate, because patient records can be subpoenaed for court evidence. Appropriate documentation can be the determining factor in the outcome of litigation. Pure and simple, if the instruction isn't documented, it didn't occur!

Furthermore, documentation is a vehicle of communication that provides critical information to other healthcare professionals involved with the patient's care. Failure to document not only renders other staff potentially liable, but also renders the facility liable and in jeopardy of losing its Joint Commission accreditation. Concomitantly, the institution is also in danger of losing its appropriations for Medicare and Medicaid reimbursement.

In any litigation where the doctrine of *respondeat superior* is applied, outcomes can hold the organization liable for damages (monetary retribution). Thus it behooves the nurse as both employee and professional not only to provide patient education, but also to document it appropriately and to be critically conscious of the legal and financial ramifications to the healthcare facility in which he or she is employed.

Snyder (1996) presents an invaluable description of an interdisciplinary method to document patient education. The method involves use of a flow sheet that fits into the client's chart. The flow sheet includes identification of client and family educational needs based on a number of variables; these include the following:

- Readiness to learn (based on admission assessment of the client)
- Obstacles to learning, which might include language, lack of vision, or other challenges
- Referrals, which might include a patient advocate, the library, or an ethics committee

The form provides documentation space for who was taught (e.g., client or family), what was taught (e.g., self-injection of insulin), when it was taught, what strategies of teaching were used (instructional methods and materials), and how the client responded to instruction (what outcomes were achieved).

Table 2–1 is a visual representation of the relationship of ethical principles to the laws and professional standards applicable to each principle. It should be noted that the AHA's 1975 original draft rendition of a *Patient's Bill of Rights*, along with all the later renditions of these rights, are linked to or associated with every ethical principle. The *Patient's Bill of Rights* (AHA, 1992) is rooted in the conditions of participation in Medicare set forth under federal standards established by the Center for Medicare and Medicaid Services (CMS). These standards are further emphasized by corresponding accreditation standards promulgated by the Joint Commission. All these laws and professional standards serve to ensure the fundamental rights of every person as a consumer of healthcare services.

Economic Factors of Patient Education: Justice and Duty Revisited

Some might consider the parameters of healthcare economics and finances as objective information that can be used for any number of purposes. Fiscal solvency and forecasting of economic growth of an organization are good examples of this phenomenon. Others would agree that in addition to the legal considerations that mandate adherence to regulations in health care regardless of the economics involved, there is also an ethical dimension that speaks certainly to quality of care and also to justice, which refers to the equal distribution of goods and services.

In the interest of patient care, the client as a human being has a right to quality care regardless of his or her economic status, national origin, race, and the like. Furthermore, health professionals have a duty to see to it that such services are provided. In like manner, the healthcare organization has the right to expect that it will receive its fair share of reimbursable revenues for services rendered.

Thus, as an employee of the provider organization, the nurse has a duty to carry out organizational policies and mandates by acting in an accountable and responsible manner. This duty includes assuming fiscal accountability for patient education activities, whether these are offered on an inpatient or ambulatory care basis or as a service to the larger community.

The principle of justice is a critical consideration within the discourse on patient education. The rapid changes and trends so evident in the contemporary healthcare arena are, for the most part, economically driven. Described as chaotic by some, the healthcare system in

Table 2–1 LINKAGES BETWEEN ETHICAL PRINCIPLES AND THE LAW

Ethical Principles	Legal Actions/Decisions and Standards of Practice
Autonomy (self-determination)	Cardozo decision regarding informed consent Institutional review boards Patient Self-Determination Act *Patient's Bill of Rights* Joint Commission/CMS standards
Veracity (truth telling)	Cardozo decision regarding informed consent *Patient's Bill of Rights* *Tuma* decision Joint Commission/CMS standards
Confidentiality (privileged information)	Privileged information *Patient's Bill of Rights* Joint Commission/CMS standards HIPAA
Nonmalfeasance (do no harm)	Malpractice/negligence rights and duties Nurse practice acts *Patient's Bill of Rights* *Darling v. Charleston Memorial Hospital* State health codes Joint Commission/CMS standards
Beneficence (doing good)	*Patient's Bill of Rights* State health codes Job descriptions Standards of practice Policy and procedure manuals Joint Commission/CMS standards
Justice (equal distribution of benefits and burdens)	*Patient's Bill of Rights* Antidiscrimination/affirmative action laws Americans with Disabilities Act Joint Commission/CMS standards

many ways defies the humanistic and charitable underpinnings that have characterized healthcare services in this country across the decades. Indeed, organizations that provide health care are caught between the proverbial horns of the dilemma of allocating scarce resources in a just yet economically feasible manner.

On the one hand, the realities of capitation and managed care result in shrinking revenues. This trend, in turn, dictates shorter patient stays in hospitals and doing more with less. Despite continued, severe shortages of healthcare personnel in most geographic areas of the country, healthcare facilities are concomitantly expanding their clinical expertise into satellite types of ambulatory and home care services. On the other hand, these same organizations are held to the exact standards of care that are underwritten by the *Patient's Bill of Rights* (AHA, 1992), which is regulated as a contingency of Medicare and Medicaid participation by the CMS and for agency accreditation by the Joint Commission. In turn, although there are some exceptions (e.g., home healthcare agencies), hospital accreditation in particular dictates eligibility for third-party reimbursement in both the public and private sectors.

Over and above the financial facts, these same charitable, not-for-profit organizations no longer enjoy the legal immunity that existed in yesteryear. The doctrine of *respondeat superior* is alive and well. In a Supreme Court decision stemming from *Abernathy v. Sisters of St. Mary's* in 1969, the court held that a "non-governmental charitable institution is liable for its own negligence and the negligence of its agents and employees acting within the scope of their employment" (Strader, 1985, p. 364). The court further declared that this ruling would apply to all future cases as of November 10, 1969. Thus the regulated right of clients to health education carries a corresponding duty of healthcare organizations to provide that service.

In an environment of shrinking healthcare dollars, continuous shortages of staff, and dramatically shortened lengths of stay yielding rapid patient turnover, the organization is challenged to ensure the competency of nursing staff

to provide educational services, and to do so in the most efficient and cost-effective manner possible. This is an interesting dilemma when considering the fact that patient education is invariably identified, directly or indirectly, as a legal responsibility of registered nurses in the respective nurse practice acts of all states. Unfortunately, few, if any, prelicensure education programs adequately prepare nursing students for this critical function.

Financial Terminology

Given the fact that the role of the nurse as educator is an essential aspect of care delivery, included is an overview of fiscal terminology that directly affects both staff and patient education. Such educational services are not provided without an accompanying cost of human and material resources. Thus, it is important to know that expenditures are essentially classified into two categories: direct and indirect costs.

Direct Costs

Direct costs are tangible, predictable expenditures, a substantial portion of which include personnel salaries, employment benefits, and equipment (Gift, 1994). This portion of an organizational budget is almost always the largest of the total budgetary outlay of any healthcare facility.

Because of the labor-intensive function of nursing care delivery, the costs of nurses' salaries and benefits usually account for at least 50%— if not more—of the total facility budget. Of course, the higher the educational level of nursing staff, the higher the salaries and benefits, and thus, the higher the institution's total direct costs.

Although the purpose of salary is to buy an employee's time and particular expertise, it is often difficult to predict how long it will take to plan, implement, and evaluate various educational programs being offered. For example, if planning and carrying out patient or staff education exceeds the allocated time and the nurse educator draws overtime pay, the extra cost may not have been anticipated in the budget planning process.

Time is also considered a direct cost and is a major factor included in a cost-benefit analysis. In other words, if the time it takes to prepare and offer patient or staff education programs is greater than the financial gain to the institution, the facility may seek other ways of providing this service, such as computerized programmed instruction or a patient television channel.

Also, equipment is classified as a direct cost. No organization can function without proper equipment and the need to replace it when necessary. Teaching requires audiovisual equipment and tools for instruction, such as overhead projectors, slide projectors, models, copy machines, computers, and closed-circuit televisions. Although renting or leasing equipment may sometimes be less expensive than purchasing it, rental and leasing costs are still categorized as direct costs.

Direct costs are divided into two types: fixed and variable. *Fixed costs* are those that are predictable, remain the same over time, and can be controlled. Salaries, for example, are fixed costs because they remain relatively stable and can also be manipulated. The facility usually makes annual decisions to give employee raises, to freeze salaries, or to cut positions, thereby influencing the budgeted amount for direct cost expenditures. In addition, mortgages, loan repayments, and the like are included as fixed costs.

Variable costs are those costs that, in the case of healthcare organizations, depend on volume. The number of meals prepared, for example, depends on the patient census. From an educational perspective, the demand for patient teaching depends on the number and diagnostic types of hospitalized patients. For example, if the volume of cardiac bypass surgical patients is low, educational costs may be high due to the fact that intensive one-to-one instruction would need to be offered to each patient admitted. Conversely, if the volume of bypass surgeries is high, it is less expensive to provide standardized programs of instruction via group teaching sessions for these cardiac clients. As another example, if demand or turnover of nursing staff increases, the number of orientation sessions for new employees would also increase in volume. Supplies, also a direct, variable cost, can change depending on the amount and type needed. Variable costs can become fixed costs when volume remains consistently high or low over time.

Indirect Costs

Indirect costs are those costs not directly related to the actual delivery of an educational program. These include, but are not limited to, institutional overhead such as heating and air conditioning, lighting, space, and support services of maintenance, housekeeping, and security. Such services are necessary and ongoing whether or not an educational session is in progress.

Hidden costs, a type of indirect cost, can neither be anticipated nor accounted for until after the fact. Low employee productivity can produce hidden costs. Organizational budgets are prepared on the basis of what is known and predictable, with projections for variability in patient census included. Personnel budgets are based on levels of staff needed (e.g., number of RNs, LPNs and nursing assistants) to accommodate the expected patient volume. This is determined by an annual projection of patient days and how many patients an employee can effectively care for on a daily basis. Low productivity of one or two personnel on a nursing unit, for example, can have a significant impact on the workload of others, which, in turn, leads to low morale and employee turnover. Turnover increases recruitment and new employee orientation costs. In this respect, the costs are appropriately identified as hidden.

In a classic description of understanding costs, Gift (1994) makes a point of distinguishing between costs—direct or indirect—and charges. As just described, direct and indirect costs are those expenses incurred by the facility. Charges are set by the provider, but they are billed to the recipient of the services. There may or may not be a balanced relationship between costs and charges. In the retail business, for example, if costs of raw materials are low, while charges for the items, goods, or services are high, the retailer yields a profit. In the healthcare arena, not-for-profit organizations are limited by federal law as to the amount they can charge a client in relation to the actual cost of a service. In many instances, particularly as it relates to pharmaceutical goods, the actual cost to the facility is what the client is charged. As such, the facility provides a service but realizes no financial profit (Kaiser Family Foundation, 2005).

Cost Savings, Cost Benefit, and Cost Recovery

Patient teaching is mandated by state laws, professional and institutional standards, accrediting body protocols, and regulations for participation in Medicare and Medicaid reimbursement programs. However, unless it is ordered by a physician, patient education costs are generally not recoverable under third-party reimbursement as a separate entity. Even though the costs of educational programs, for both patients and nursing staff, are a legitimate expense to the facility, these costs usually are subsumed under hospital room

rates and are, therefore, technically absorbed by the healthcare organization.

Hospitals realize *cost savings* when patient lengths of stay are shortened or fall within the allotted diagnostic related group (DRG) time frames. Patients who have fewer complications and use less expensive services will yield a cost savings for the institution. In an ambulatory care setting such as an HMO, cost savings are realized when patient education keeps people healthy and independent for a longer period of time, which prevents high utilization of expensive diagnostic testing or inpatient services. However, and perhaps most importantly, patient education becomes even more essential when a pattern of early discharge is detected, resulting in frequent re-admissions to an agency. The facility comes under scrutiny by HCFA/CMS and may be penalized either through citation or loss of payment—in which case, cost savings becomes a moot point.

Cost benefit occurs when there is increased patient satisfaction with an institution as a result of the services it renders, including educational programs it provides such as childbirth classes, weight and stress reduction sessions, and cardiac fitness and rehabilitation programs. This is an opportunity for an institution to capture a patient population for lifetime coverage. Patient satisfaction is critical to the individual's return for future healthcare services.

Cost recovery results when either the patient or insurer pays a fee for educational services that are provided. Cost recovery is realized through the marketing of health education programs offered for a fee.

Under Medicare and Medicaid guidelines, reimbursement may be made for programs "furnished by providers of services to the extent that the programs are appropriate, integral parts in the rendition of covered services which are reasonable and necessary for the treatment of the individual's illness or injury" (Kaiser Family Foundation, 2005). The key to success in obtaining third-party reimbursement is the ability to demonstrate that as a result of education, patients can manage self-care at home and consequently experience fewer hospitalizations.

To take advantage of cost recovery, hospitals and other healthcare agencies develop and market a cadre of health education programs that are open to all consumers in the community. No matter whether a client is charged in full or pays on a sliding scale for these services, the American mentality is "if it costs something, it must be worth something." Thus, fee-for-service programs usually are well attended and result in revenues for the institution. The critical element, of course, is not only the recovery of costs but also *revenue generation*. Revenue generation refers to income realized over and above program costs, which can also be regarded as profit.

To offset the dilemma of striving for cost containment and solvency in an environment of shrinking fiscal resources, healthcare organizations have developed alternative strategies for patient education to realize cost savings, cost benefit, cost recovery, or revenue generation. For example, a preoperative teaching program for surgical patients given prior to admission to the hospital has been found to lower patient anxiety, increase patient satisfaction, and decrease nursing hours during hospitalization (Wasson & Anderson, 1993).

Program Planning and Implementation

The key elements to consider when planning a patient education offering intended for generation of revenue include an accurate assessment of direct costs such as paper supplies, printing of program brochures, publicity, rental space, and time (based on an hourly rate) required of professional personnel to prepare and offer the service. If an hourly rate is unknown, a simple rule of thumb is to divide the annual base salary by 2080, which is the standard number of hours worked by most people in the course of 1 year.

If the program is to be offered on the premises of the facility, there may be no need to plan for a rental fee for space. However, indirect costs such as housekeeping and security should be prorated as a bona fide expense. Such a practice not only is good fiscal management, but also provides an accounting of the contributions of other departments to the educational efforts of the facility.

Fees for a program should be set at a level high enough to cover the aggregate costs of program preparation and delivery. If the intent of an education program is for cost savings to the facility, such as provision of education classes for diabetics in the community to reduce the number of costly hospital admissions, then the aim may be to break even on costs. The price is set by dividing the calculated cost by the number of anticipated attendees. If the goal is for cost benefit to the institution, success can be measured by increased patient satisfaction (as determined by questionnaires or evaluation forms) or by an increase in the use of the sponsor's services (as determined by record keeping). If the intent is to offer a series of classes for smoking cessation or childbirth to improve the wellness of the community and to generate income for the facility, then the fee is set higher than cost so as to realize a profit (cost recovery).

Over the course of a year, it is usually necessary for nurse educators to give an annual report to administration of time and money spent and whether such expenditures were profitable to the institution in terms of cost savings, cost benefit, or cost recovery.

Cost-Benefit Analysis and Cost-Effectiveness Analysis

In the majority of healthcare organizations, the education department bears the major responsibility for staff development, for in-service employee training, and for patient education programs that exceed the boundaries of bedside instruction. Total budget preparation for these departments is best explained by the experts in the field. Fisher, Hume, and Emerick (1998), for example, address the need for staff development departments to engage in responsibility-centered budgeting (RCB), which also is referred to as activity-based management (ABM). Given the shift away from providing at-will services and toward greater demand for cost accountability for educational programs, they propose a template for costing out programs that allows staff development departments to identify and recoup their true costs while responding to increased market competition.

There is no single best method for measuring the effectiveness of patient education programs. Most experts in the field tend to rely on determining actual costs or actual impact of programs in relationship to outcomes by employing one of two concepts: cost-benefit analysis or cost-effectiveness analysis (Abruzzese, 1992).

Cost-benefit analysis refers to measuring the relationship between costs and outcomes. Outcomes can be the actual amount of revenue generated as a result of an educational offering, or they can be expressed in terms of shorter patient stays or reduced hospitalizations for particular diagnostic groups of patients. If, under DRGs or capitation methods of reimbursement, the facility makes a profit, this can be expressed in monetary terms. If an analysis reveals that an educational program costs less than the revenue

it generates, that expense can be recovered by third-party reimbursement, or that savings are greater than costs to the facility, then the program is considered to be of cost benefit. The measurement of costs against monetary gains is commonly referred to as the *cost-benefit ratio*.

Cost-effectiveness analysis refers to the impact an educational offering has on patient behavior. If program objectives are achieved, as evidenced by positive and sustained changes in behavior of the participants over time, the program is said to be cost effective. Although behavioral changes are highly desirable, in many instances they are less observable, less tangible, and not easily measurable. For example, reduction in patient anxiety cannot be converted into a gain in real dollars. Therefore, it is wise to analyze the outcome of teaching interventions by comparing behavioral outcomes between two or more programs to identify the one that is most effective and efficient when actual costs cannot be determined.

As difficult as it may be from the standpoint of justice, the nurse educator must attempt to interpret the costs of behavioral changes (outcomes) to the institution by conducting a cost-effectiveness analysis between programs. This can be accomplished by first identifying and itemizing for each program all direct and indirect costs, including any identifiable hidden costs. Second, it is necessary to identify and itemize any benefits derived from the program offering, such as revenue gained or decreased readmission rates that can be expressed in monetary values. Results of these findings can then be recorded on a grid so that each program's cost effectiveness is visually apparent (see **Figure 2–1**).

Mitton and Donaldson (2004) suggest a nonvested team approach to an analysis of program effectiveness for the purpose of determining the allocation or reallocation of valuable resources

Figure 2–1 Cost effectiveness grid.

Program	I	II
Costs		
Direct	$	$
Indirect	$	$
Hidden	$	$
Benefits		
Decreased readmissions	$	$
Revenue generated	$	$
Total	$	$

between and among services or programs. This approach ensures the integrity of the total process of program evaluation. In addition to this recommendation, the International Council of Nurses (ICN) published a position statement in 2001 that, among other things, obligates nurses to demonstrate their value in promoting cost-effective, quality care by playing a leadership role in program planning and evaluation, in policy setting, and in interactive networking on cost-effectiveness research, cost-saving strategies, and best practice standards (Ghebrehiwet, 2005).

State of the Evidence

Practice that is driven by evidence is defined as being "practice that is based on research, clinical expertise, and patient preferences that guide decisions about the healthcare of individual patients" (HPNA Position Paper, 2004, p. 66). In this chapter, the six ethical principles have been explicated in terms of their relationship to patient education, in particular, and to health-care services, in general.

Comparatively speaking, the application of ethics (known as applied ethics) to health care is a relatively recent phenomenon. Much evidence suggests that the tried-and-true ethical principles as well as a wide variety of ethical theories play a highly significant role in shaping contemporary healthcare delivery practices and decision making. In our increasingly multicultural and pluralistic society, the challenge is to be able to address the vast array of biomedical ethics issues confronting healthcare practitioners on a daily basis in a way that preserves an individual's rights but also protects the well-being of other persons, groups, and communities. The complex and technological advances in health care have given rise to numerous questions about what is right or wrong, yet very few clear-cut or perfectly right answers have been forthcoming. Numerous case studies, books, and articles on how to deal with ethical dilemmas abound. They attempt to provide evidence for nursing practice, including patient education, about how to deliver care in the most equitable and beneficial manner possible.

Laws and standards that govern the role of the nurse as educator are firmly established and provide the legal foundations and professional expectations in practice for the delivery of quality patient care. Also well established is the importance of documenting nursing interventions, but more research that provides evidence of the frequency and amount of patient education nurses do daily on an informal basis that never gets recorded must be conducted. In addition, although strategies exist for analyzing cost effectiveness and cost benefits as a means to strengthen the value and accountability of the nurse educator to the client and to the employing agency, more research evidence is needed to substantiate the importance of the educator's role in influencing overall costs of care.

Further research needs to be conducted to determine, through comparative analysis, which types of patient education programs are the most equitable, beneficial, and cost effective for patients, nursing staff, the institution, and the communities served. Evidence is scarce on the economics associated with various approaches to education and the value of the nurse educator's role as it impacts on behavioral outcomes related to cost savings, cost benefit, and cost recovery.

Summary

Ethical and legal dimensions of human rights provide the justification for patient education, particularly as it relates to issues of self-determination and informed consent. These rights are enforced through federal and state regulations and through performance standards promulgated by accrediting bodies and professional organizations for implementation at the local level. The nurse's role as educator is legitimized through the definition of nursing practice as set forth by the prevailing nurse practice act in the state where the nurse is licensed and employed. In this respect, patient education is a nursing duty that is grounded in justice; that is, the nurse has a legal responsibility to provide patient education and, regardless of their culture, race, ethnicity, and so forth, all clients have a right to health education relevant to their physical and emotional needs. Justice also dictates that education programs should be designed to be consistent with organizational goals while meeting the needs of patients to be informed, self-directed, and in control of their own health, and ultimately of their own destiny.

REVIEW QUESTIONS

1. What are the definitions of the terms *ethical, moral,* and *legal,* and how are they distinct from one another?

2. Which national, state, professional, and private-sector organizations legislate, regulate, and provide standards to ensure the protection of human rights in matters of health care?

3. Which ethical viewpoint, deontological or teleological, refers to the decision-making approach that choices should be made for the common good of people?

4. With respect to ethical, moral, and legal obligations, how does the American Hospital Association's *Patient's Bill of Rights* compare to the American Nurses Association's *Code of Ethics for Nurses With Interpretive Statements*?

5. What are the six ethical principles that dictate the actions of healthcare providers in delivering services to clients?

6. Why are nurse practice acts so important to nurses in carrying out their roles and responsibilities to the public?

7. What is the difference between the terms *negligence* and *malpractice*?

8. When was informed consent established as a basic tenet of ethics and what is the nurse's role in situations involving informed consent?

9. What is meant by the legal term *respondeat superior*, and how does this term apply to professional nursing practice?

10. Why is documentation of professional nursing duties, particularly patient education, so important in the provision of care by nurses?

11. What are four examples of direct costs and five examples of indirect costs in the provision of patient/staff education?

12. What are the definitions of these terms: *fixed direct costs, variable direct costs, indirect costs, cost savings, cost benefit, cost recovery, cost-benefit analysis,* and *cost-effectiveness analysis*?

References

Abernathy v. Sisters of St. Mary's, 446 SW2d 559 (MO1969).

Abood, S. (2001). The Bush regulatory agenda. *American Journal of Nursing, 101*(8), 22.

Abruzzese, R. S. (1992). *Nursing staff development: Strategies for success.* St. Louis, MO: Mosby.

American Hospital Association. (1975). *Patient's bill of rights.* Chicago: Author.

American Hospital Association. (1992). *A patient's bill of rights.* Retrieved March 27, 2007, from http://www.patienttalk.info/AHA-Patient_Bill_of_Rights.htm

American Nurses Association. (1976). *Code of ethics for nurses with interpretative statements.* Kansas City, MO: Author.

American Nurses Association. (1978). *Model nurse practice act.* Washington, DC: Author.

American Nurses Association. (1985). *Code of ethics for nurses with interpretive statements*. Kansas City, MO: Author.

American Nurses Association. (2001). *Code of ethics for nurses with interpretative statements*. Washington, DC: American Nurses Publishing. Retrieved January 20, 2007, from http://nursingworld.org

Association of American Physicians and Surgeons. (1995). *Patients' bill of rights*. Retrieved March 27, 2007, from http://www.aapsonline.org/patients/billrts.htm

Boyd, M. D., Gleit, C. J., Graham, B. A., & Whitman, N. I. (1998). *Health teaching in nursing practice: A professional model* (3rd ed.). Stamford, CT: Appleton & Lange.

Brent, N. J. (2001). *Nurses and the law* (2nd ed.). Philadelphia: Saunders.

Brown, R. H. (1976). The pediatrician and malpractice. *Pediatrics, 57*, 392–401.

Casey, F. S. (1995). Documenting patient education: A literature review. *Journal of Continuing Education in Nursing, 26*(6), 257–260.

Centers for Disease Control and Prevention. (2005). *Tuskegee timeline*. Retrieved March 27, 2007, from http://www.cdc.gov/nchstp/od/tuskegee/time.htm

Cisar, N. S., & Bell, S. K. (1995). Informed consent: An ethical dilemma. *Nursing Forum, 30*(3), 20–28.

Creighton, H. (1986). Informed consent. *Nursing Management, 17*(10), 11–13.

Curtin, L. (1978). A proposed model for critical ethical analysis. *Nursing Forum, 17*(1), 13–17.

Darling v. Charleston Memorial Hospital, 211 NE2d253 (IL 1965).

Department of Health and Human Services (DHHS). (1983). Protection of human subjects: Reports of the president's commission for the study of ethical problems in medicine and biomedical and behavioral research. *Federal Register, 48*(146), 34408–34412.

Dickey, S. B. (2006). Informed consent: Ethical issues. In V. D. Lachman (Ed.), *Applied ethics in nursing*. New York: Springer Publishing Company.

Edward, P. (1967). Kant, Immanuel. In *Encyclopedia of philosophy*. New York, MacMillan Publishing.

Emanuel, E. J. (2000). Justice and managed care: Four principles for the just allocation of health care resources. *Hastings Center Report, 30*(3), 8–16.

Fisher, M. L., Hume, R., & Emerick, R. (1998). Costing nursing education programs: It's as easy as 1-2-3.

Journal for Nurses in Staff Development, 14(5), 227–285.

Ghebrehiwet, T. (2005). The ICN code of ethics for nurses. Helping nurses make ethical decisions. *Reflections on Nursing Leadership, 31*(3), 26–28. Retrieved January 18, 2007, from http://www.nursingsociety.org/RNL/3Q_2005/features/features6.html

Gift, A. G. (1994). Understanding costs. *Clinical Nurse Specialist, 8*(2), 90.

Hall, K. (1992). Cardozo, Benjamin N. In *The Oxford Companion to the Supreme Court of the United States,* (pp. 126–127). New York: Oxford University Press.

Hall, J. K. (1996). *Nursing Ethics and the Law*. Philadelphia: W. B. Saunders Company.

HPNA position paper. (2004). Value of the professional nurse in end-of-life care. *Journal of Hospice and Palliative Nursing, 6*(1), 65–66.

International Council of Nursing. (2001). *Position statement. Promoting the value and cost-effectiveness of nursing*. Retrieved February 15, 2007, from http://www.icn.ch/psvalue.htm

Kaiser Family Foundation. (2005). Navigating Medicare and Medicaid, 2005. Retrieved March 27, 2007, from http://kff.org/medicare/7240.cfm

Kohlenberg, E. M. (2006). Patients' rights and ethical issues. In V. D. Lachman (Ed.), *Applied Ethics in Nursing* (pp. 39–46). New York: Springer Publishing Company.

Legal Action Center. (2001). *HIV/AIDS. Testing, confidentiality, and discrimination*. Legal Action Center of the City of New York, Inc. New York.

Lesnick, M. J., & Anderson, B. E. (1962). *Nursing practice and the law*. Philadelphia: Lippincott.

Mezey, M., Evans, L. K., Golob, Z. D., Murphy, E., & White, G. B. (1994). The patient self-determination act: Sources of concern for nurses. *Nursing Outlook, 42*(1), 30–38.

Mikos, C. A. (2004). Inside the nurse practice act. *Nursing Management, 35*(9), 20, 22, 91.

Mitton, C., & Donaldson, C. (2004). Health care priority setting: Principles, practice and challenges. *Cost Effectiveness and Resource Allocation, 2*(3). Retrieved February 20, 2007, from http://www.resource-allocation.com/content/2/1/3

New York State Nurses Association. (1972). *New York state nurse practice act*. Retrieved March 4, 2007, from http://www.op.nysed.gov/article139.htm

New York State Nurses Association. (2001). Code of ethics for nurses with interpretative statements. *NYSNA Report, 32*(7), 5–7.

President's Advisory Commission on Consumer Protection and Quality in the Healthcare Industry. (1998). *Consumer bill of rights and responsibilities.* Retrieved January 20, 2007, from http://www.hcqualitycommission.gov/final/append_a.html

Rankin, S. H., & Stallings, K. D. (1990). *Patient education: Principles and practices.* Philadelphia: Lippincott.

Reising, D. L., & Allen, P. N. (2007). Protecting yourself from malpractice claims. *American Nurse Today, 2*(2), 39–44.

Rivera, G. (1972). *Willowbrook: A report on how it is and why it doesn't have to be that way.* New York: Vintage Books.

Schloendorff v. Society of New York Hospitals, 211NY, 125, 128, 105 N.E. 92,93 (1914).

Smith, C. E. (1987). *Patient education: Nurses in partnership with other health professionals.* Philadelphia: Saunders.

Snyder, B. (1996, March). An easy way to document patient ed. *RN,* 43–45.

Strader, M. K. (1985). Malpractice and nurse educators: Defining legal responsibilities. *Journal of Nursing Education, 24*(9), 363–367.

Thomas, S. B., & Quinn, S. C. (1991). The Tuskegee Syphilis Study, 1932 to 1972: Implications for HIV education and AIDS risk education programs in the black community. *American Journal of Public Health, 81*(11), 1498–1505. Retrieved March 27, 2007, from http://www.pubmedcentral.nih.gov/articlerender.fcgi?tool=pubmed+pubmedid=1951814

Tong, R. (2007). *New perspectives in health care ethics.* Upper Saddle River, NJ: Pearson Prentice Hall.

Ulrich, L. P. (1999). *The patient self-determination act: Meeting the challenges in patient care.* Washington, DC: Georgetown University Press.

Wasson, D., & Anderson, M. (1993). Hospital-patient education: Current status and future trends. *Journal of Nursing Staff Development, 10*(3), 147–151.

Weisbard, A. J., & Arras, J. D. (1984). Commissioning morality: An introduction to the symposium. *Cardozo Law Review, 6*(4), 223–241.

Yoder Wise, P. S. (1995). *Leading and managing in nursing.* St. Louis, MO: Mosby.

Zuckerman, J. (2001, August 3). Patient's bill of rights. *New York Times,* 1.

Chapter 3

Applying Learning Theories to Healthcare Practice

Margaret M. Braungart

Richard G. Braungart

CHAPTER HIGHLIGHTS

Applying Learning Theories
  Behaviorist Learning Theory
  Cognitive Learning Theory
  Social Learning Theory
  Psychodynamic Learning Theory
  Humanistic Learning Theory
Neuropsychology and Learning
Comparison of Learning Theories

Common Principles of Learning
  How Does Learning Occur?
  *What Kinds of Experiences Facilitate or
    Hinder the Learning Process?*
  *What Helps Ensure That Learning Becomes
    Relatively Permanent?*
State of the Evidence

KEY TERMS

- learning
- learning theory
- respondent conditioning
- systematic desensitization
- stimulus generalization
- discrimination learning
- spontaneous recovery
- operant conditioning
- escape conditioning
- avoidance conditioning
- metacognition
- gestalt perspective

- information processing
- cognitive development
- social constructivism
- social cognition
- cognitive-emotional perspective
- role modeling
- vicarious reinforcement
- defense mechanisms
- resistance
- transference
- hierarchy of needs
- therapeutic relationship

OBJECTIVES

After completing this chapter, the reader will be able to

1. Differentiate among the basic approaches to learning for each of the five learning theories.
2. Define the principal constructs of each learning theory.
3. Give an example applying each theory to changing the attitudes and behaviors of learners in a specific situation.
4. Discuss how neuroscience research has contributed to a better understanding of learning and learning theories.
5. Outline alternative strategies for learning in a given situation using at least two different learning theories.
6. Identify the differences and similarities in the learning theories specific to (a) the basic procedures of learning, (b) the assumptions made about the learning, (c) the task of the educator, (d) the sources of motivation, and (e) the way in which the transfer of learning is facilitated.

Learning is defined in this chapter as a relatively permanent change in mental processing, emotional functioning, and/or behavior as a result of experience. It is the lifelong, dynamic process by which individuals acquire new knowledge or skills and alter their thoughts, feelings, attitudes, and actions.

Learning enables individuals to adapt to demands and changing circumstances and is crucial in health care—whether for patients and families grappling with ways to improve their health and adjust to their medical conditions, for students acquiring the information and skills necessary to become a nurse, or for nurses and other healthcare staff devising and learning more effective approaches to educating and treating patients and each other in partnership. Despite the significance of learning to each individual's development, functioning, health and well-being, debate continues about how learn-

ing occurs, what kinds of experiences facilitate or hinder the learning process, and what ensures that learning becomes relatively permanent.

Until the late 19th century, most of the discussions and debates about learning were grounded in philosophy, school administration, and conventional wisdom (Hilgard, 1996). Around the dawn of the 20th century, the new field of educational psychology emerged and became a defining force for the scientific study of learning, teaching, and assessment (Woolfolk, 2001). As a science, educational psychology rests on the systematic gathering of evidence or data to test theories and hypotheses about learning.

A *learning theory* is a coherent framework of integrated constructs and principles that describe, explain, or predict how people learn. Rather than offering a single theory of learning, educational psychology provides alternative theories and perspectives on how learning occurs and what motivates people to learn and change (Hilgard & Bower, 1966; Ormrod, 2004; Snowman & Biehler, 2006).

The construction and testing of learning theories over the past century have contributed much to our understanding of how individuals acquire knowledge and change their ways of thinking, feeling, and behaving. Reflecting an evidence-based approach to learning, the accumulated body of research information can be used to guide the educational process and has challenged a number of popular notions and myths about learning (e.g., "Spare the rod and spoil the child," "Males are more intelligent than females," "You can't teach an old dog new tricks."). In addition, the major learning theories have wide applicability and form the foundation of not only the field of education but also psychological counseling, workplace organization and human resource management, and marketing and advertising.

Whether used singly or in combination, learning theories have much to offer the practice of health care. Increasingly, health professionals must demonstrate that they regularly employ sound methods and a clear rationale in their education efforts, patient and client interactions, staff management and training, and continuing education and health promotion programs (Ferguson & Day, 2005).

Given the current structure of health care in the United States, nurses, in particular, are often responsible for designing and implementing plans and procedures for improving health education and encouraging wellness. Beyond one's profession, however, knowledge of the learning process relates to nearly every aspect of daily life. Learning theories can be applied at the individual, group, and community levels not only to comprehend and teach new material, but also to solve problems, change unhealthy habits, build constructive relationships, manage emotions, and develop effective behavior.

This chapter reviews the principal psychological learning theories that are useful to health education and clinical practice. Behaviorist, cognitive, and social learning theories are most often applied to patient education as an aspect of professional nursing practice. It is argued in this chapter that emotions and feelings also need explicit focus in relation to learning in general (Goleman, 1995) and to health care in particular (Halpern, 2001). Why? Emotional reactions are often learned as a result of experience, they play a significant role in the learning process, and they are a vital consideration when dealing with health, disease, prevention, wellness, medical treatment, recovery, healing, and relapse prevention. To address this concern, psychodynamic and humanistic perspectives are treated as learning theories in this review because they encourage a patient-centered approach to care and add much to our understanding of human motivation and emotions in the learning process.

The chapter is organized as follows. First, the basic principles of learning advocated by behaviorist, cognitive, social learning, psychodynamic, and humanistic theories are summarized and illustrated with examples from psychology and nursing research. With the current upsurge and interest in neuroscience research, brief mention is made of the contributions of neuropsychology to understanding the dynamics of learning and sorting out the claims of learning theories. Next, the learning theories are compared with regard to:

- Their fundamental procedures for changing behavior

- The assumptions made about the learner
- The role of the educator in encouraging learning
- The sources of motivation for learning
- The ways in which learning is transferred to new situations and problems

Finally, the theories are compared and then synthesized by identifying their common features and addressing three questions: (1) How does learning occur? (2) What kinds of experiences facilitate or hinder the learning process? (3) What helps ensure that learning becomes relatively permanent? While surveying this chapter, readers are encouraged to think of ways to apply the learning theories to both their professional and personal lives.

The goals of this chapter are to provide a conceptual framework for subsequent chapters in this book and to offer a toolbox of approaches that can be used to enhance learning and change in patients, students, staff, and oneself. Although there is a trend toward integrating learning theories in education, it is argued that knowledge of each theory's basic principles, advantages, and shortcomings allows nurses and other health professionals to select, combine, and apply the most useful components of learning theories to specific patients and situations in health care. After completing the chapter, readers should be able to identify the essential principles of learning, describe various ways in which the learning process can be approached, and develop alternative strategies to change attitudes and behaviors in different settings.

Learning Theories

This section summarizes the basic principles and related concepts of the behaviorist, cognitive, social learning, psychodynamic, and humanistic learning theories. While reviewing

each theory, readers are asked to consider the following questions:

- How do the environment and the internal dynamics of the individual influence learning?
- Is the learner viewed as relatively passive or more active?
- What is the educator's task in the learning process?
- What motivates individuals to learn?
- What encourages the transfer of learning to new situations?
- What are the contributions and criticisms of each learning theory?

Behaviorist Learning Theory

Focusing mainly on what is directly observable, behaviorists view learning as the product of the stimulus conditions (S) and the responses (R) that follow—sometimes termed the S-R model of learning. Whether dealing with animals or people, the learning process is relatively simple. Generally ignoring what goes on inside the individual—which, of course, is always difficult to ascertain—behaviorists closely observe responses and then manipulate the environment to bring about the intended change. Currently in education and clinical psychology, behaviorist theories are more likely to be used in combination with other learning theories, especially cognitive theory (Bush, 2006; Dai & Sternberg, 2004). Behaviorist theory continues to be considered useful in nursing and health care.

To modify people's attitudes and responses, behaviorists either alter the stimulus conditions in the environment or change what happens after a response occurs. Motivation is explained as the desire to reduce some drive (drive reduction); hence, satisfied, complacent, or satiated individuals have little motivation to learn and change. Getting behavior to transfer from the initial learning situation to other settings is largely a matter of practice (strengthening habits). Transfer is aided by a similarity in the stimuli and responses in the learning situation relative to future situations where the response is to be performed. Much of behaviorist learning is based on respondent conditioning and operant conditioning procedures.

Respondent conditioning (also termed *classical* or *Pavlovian conditioning*) emphasizes the importance of stimulus conditions and the associations formed in the learning process (Ormrod, 2004). In this basic model of learning, a neutral stimulus (NS)—a stimulus that has no particular value or meaning to the learner—is paired with a naturally occurring unconditioned or unlearned stimulus (UCS) and unconditioned response (UCR) (**Figure 3–1**). After a few such pairings, the neutral stimulus alone, without the unconditioned stimulus, elicits the same unconditioned response. Thus, learning takes place when the newly conditioned stimulus (CS) becomes associated with the conditioned response (CR)—a process that may well occur without conscious thought or awareness.

Consider an example from health care. Someone without much experience with hospitals (NS) may visit a sick relative. While in the

Figure 3–1 Respondent conditioning model of learning.

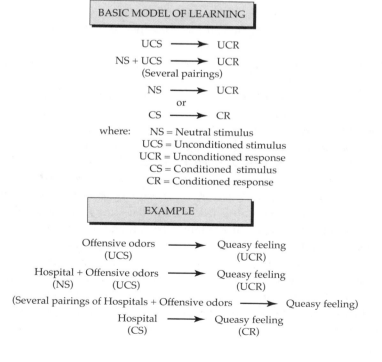

BASIC MODEL OF LEARNING

UCS ⟶ UCR

NS + UCS ⟶ UCR
(Several pairings)

NS ⟶ UCR

or

CS ⟶ CR

where: NS = Neutral stimulus
UCS = Unconditioned stimulus
UCR = Unconditioned response
CS = Conditioned stimulus
CR = Conditioned response

EXAMPLE

Offensive odors ⟶ Queasy feeling
(UCS)   (UCR)

Hospital + Offensive odors ⟶ Queasy feeling
(NS)   (UCS)   (UCR)

(Several pairings of Hospitals + Offensive odors ⟶ Queasy feeling)

Hospital ⟶ Queasy feeling
(CS)   (CR)

relative's room, the visitor may smell offensive odors (UCS) and feel queasy and light-headed (UCR). After this initial visit and later repeated visits, hospitals (now the CS) may become associated with feeling anxious and nauseated (CR), especially if the visitor smells odors similar to those encountered during the first experience (see Figure 3–1). Respondent conditioning highlights the importance of the atmosphere and its effects on staff morale in health care. Often without thinking or reflection, patients and visitors formulate these associations as a result of their hospital experiences, providing the basis for long-lasting attitudes toward medicine, healthcare facilities, and health professionals.

Besides influencing the acquisition of new responses to environmental stimuli, principles of respondent conditioning may be used to extinguish a previously learned response. Responses decrease if the presentation of the conditioned stimulus is not accompanied by the unconditioned stimulus over time. Thus, if the visitor who became dizzy in one hospital subsequently goes to other hospitals to see relatives or friends without smelling offensive odors, then her discomfort and anxiety about hospitals may lessen after several such experiences.

Systematic desensitization is a technique based on respondent conditioning that is used by psychologists to reduce fear and anxiety in their clients (Wolpe, 1982). The assumption is that fear of a particular stimulus or situation is learned, so it can, therefore, be unlearned or extinguished. Fearful individuals are first taught relaxation techniques. While they are in a state of relaxation, the fear-producing stimulus is gradually introduced at a nonthreatening level so that anxiety and emotions are not aroused. After repeated pairings of the stimulus under relaxed, nonfrightening conditions, the indi-

vidual learns that no harm will come to him or her from the once fear-inducing stimulus. Finally, the client is able to confront the stimulus without being anxious and afraid.

As examples from healthcare research, respondent conditioning has been used to extinguish chemotherapy patients' anticipatory nausea and vomiting (Stockhurst, Steingrueber, Enck, & Klosterhalfen, 2006), while systematic desensitization has been used to treat drug addiction (Piane, 2000), phobias (McCullough & Andrews, 2001), tension headaches (Deyl & Kaliappan, 1997), and to teach children with ADHD or autism to swallow pills (Beck, Cataldo, Slifer, Pulbrook, & Guhman, 2005). As another illustration, prescription drug advertisers regularly employ conditioning principles to encourage consumers to associate a brand name medication with happy and improved lifestyles; once conditioned, consumers will likely favor the advertised drug over the competitors' medications and the much less expensive generic form. As a third example, taking the time to help patients relax and reduce their stress when applying some medical intervention—even a painful procedure—lessens the likelihood that patients will build up negative and anxious associations about medicine and health care.

Certain respondent conditioning concepts are especially useful in the healthcare setting. *Stimulus generalization* is the tendency of initial learning experiences to be easily applied to other similar stimuli. For example, when listening to friends and relatives describe a hospital experience, it becomes apparent that a highly positive or negative personal encounter may color patients' evaluations of their hospital stays as well as their subsequent feelings about having to be hospitalized again. With more and varied experiences, individuals learn to differentiate among similar stimuli, and we say that *discrimination learning* has occurred. As an illustration, patients who have been hospitalized a number of times often have learned a lot about hospitalization. As a result of their experiences, they make sophisticated distinctions and can discriminate among stimuli (e.g., what the various noises mean and what the various health professionals do) that novice patients cannot. Much of professional education and clinical practice involves moving from being able to make generalizations to discrimination learning.

Spontaneous recovery is a useful respondent conditioning concept that needs to be given careful consideration in relapse prevention programs. The principle of the concept operates as follows: Although a response may appear to be extinguished, it may recover and reappear at any time (even years later), especially when stimulus conditions are similar to those in the initial learning experience. Spontaneous recovery helps us understand why it is so difficult to completely eliminate unhealthy habits and addictive behaviors such as smoking, alcoholism, or drug abuse.

Another widely recognized approach to learning is *operant conditioning*, which was developed largely by B. F. Skinner (1974, 1989). Operant conditioning focuses on the behavior of the organism and the reinforcement that occurs after the response. A reinforcer is a stimulus or event applied after a response that strengthens the probability that the response will be performed again. When specific responses are reinforced on the proper schedule, behaviors can be either increased or decreased.

Table 3–1 summarizes the principal ways to increase and decrease responses by applying the contingencies of operant conditioning. Understanding the dynamics of learning presented in this table can prove useful in assessing and identifying ways to change individuals' behaviors in the healthcare setting. The key is to carefully observe individuals' responses to specific stimuli and then decide the best reinforcement procedures to use to change a behavior.

Two methods to *increase* the probability of a response are to apply positive or negative reinforcement after a response occurs. According to Skinner (1974), giving positive reinforcement (i.e., reward) greatly enhances the likelihood that a response will be repeated in similar circumstances. As an illustration, although a patient moans and groans as he attempts to get up and walk for the first time after an operation, praise and encouragement (reward) for his efforts at walking (response) will improve the chances that he will continue struggling toward independence.

A second way to increase a behavior is by applying negative reinforcement after a response is made. This form of reinforcement involves the removal of an unpleasant stimulus through either escape conditioning or avoidance conditioning. The difference between the two types of negative reinforcement relates to timing.

In *escape conditioning*, as an unpleasant stimulus is being applied, the individual responds in some way that causes the uncomfortable stimulation to cease. Suppose, for example, that when a member of the healthcare team is being chastised in front of the group for being late and missing meetings, she says something humorous. The head of the team stops criticizing her and laughs. Because the use of humor has allowed the team member to escape an unpleasant situation, chances are that she will employ humor again to alleviate a stressful encounter and thereby deflect attention from her problem behavior.

In *avoidance conditioning*, the unpleasant stimulus is anticipated rather than being applied

---

Table 3–1 OPERANT CONDITIONING MODEL: CONTINGENCIES TO INCREASE
AND DECREASE THE PROBABILITY OF AN ORGANISM'S RESPONSE

I. To *increase* the probability of a response:

  A. *Positive reinforcement:* application of a pleasant stimulus

     Reward conditioning: a pleasant stimulus is applied following an organism's response

  B. *Negative reinforcement:* removal of an aversive or unpleasant stimulus

     Escape conditioning: as an aversive stimulus is applied, the organism makes a response that causes the unpleasant stimulus to cease

     Avoidance conditioning: an aversive stimulus is anticipated by the organism, which makes a response to avoid the unpleasant event

II. To *decrease* or extinguish the probability of a response:

  A. *Nonreinforcement:* an organism's conditioned response is not followed by any kind of reinforcement (positive, negative, or punishment)

  B. *Punishment:* following a response, an aversive stimulus that the organism cannot escape or avoid is applied

---

directly. Avoidance conditioning has been used to explain some people's tendency to become ill so as to avoid doing something they do not want to do. For example, a child fearing a teacher or test may tell his mother that he has a stomachache. If allowed to stay home from school, the child increasingly may complain of sickness to avoid unpleasant situations. Thus, when fearful events are anticipated, sickness, in this case, is the behavior that has been increased through negative reinforcement.

According to operant conditioning principles, behaviors also may be *decreased* through either nonreinforcement or punishment. Skinner (1974) maintained that the simplest way to extinguish a response is not to provide any kind of reinforcement for some action. For example, offensive jokes in the workplace may be handled by showing no reaction; after several such experiences, the joke teller, who more than likely wants attention—and negative attention is preferable to no attention—may curtail his or her use of offensive humor. Keep in mind, too, that desirable behavior that is ignored may lessen as well.

If nonreinforcement proves ineffective, then punishment may be employed as a way to decrease responses, although there are risks in using this approach. Under punishment conditions, the individual cannot escape or avoid an unpleasant stimulus. Suppose, for example, the healthcare team member's attempt at humor is met by the leader's curt remark, "You are continually a source of difficulty in this group, and if this continues, your job is in jeopardy," embarrassing her in front of her peers. The problem with using punishment as a technique for teaching is that the learner may become highly emotional and may well divert attention away from the behavior that needs to be changed. Some people who are being punished become so emotional (sad or angry) that they do not remember the behavior for which they are being punished. One of the cardinal rules of operant conditioning is to "punish the behavior, not the person."

If punishment is employed, it should be administered immediately after the response with no distractions or means of escape. Punishment must also be consistent and at the highest reasonable level (e.g., health professionals who apologize and smile as they admonish the behavior of a staff member or client are sending out mixed messages and are not likely to be taken seriously or to decrease the behavior they intend). Moreover, punishment should not be prolonged (bringing up old grievances or complaining about a misbehavior at every opportunity), but there should be a time-out following punishment to eliminate the opportunity for positive reinforcement. The purpose of punishment is not to do harm or to serve as a release for anger; rather, the goal is to decrease a specific behavior and to instill self-discipline.

The use of reinforcement is central to the success of operant conditioning procedures. For operant conditioning to be effective, it is necessary to assess what kinds of reinforcement are likely to increase or decrease behaviors for each individual. Not every client, for example, finds health practitioners' terms of endearment rewarding. Comments such as "Very nice job, dear," may be presumptuous or offensive to some clients. A second issue involves the timing of reinforcement. Through experimentation with animals and humans, it has been demonstrated that the success of operant conditioning procedures partially depends on the schedule of reinforcement. Initial learning requires a continuous schedule, reinforcing the behavior quickly every time it occurs. If the desired behavior does not occur, then responses that approximate or resemble it can be reinforced, gradually shaping behavior in the direction of the goal for learning. As an illustration, for geriatric patients who appear lethargic and unresponsive, nurses or physicians might begin by rewarding small gestures such as eye contact or a hand that reaches out, then build on these friendly behaviors toward greater human contact and connection with reality. Once a response is well established, however, it becomes ineffective and inefficient to continually reinforce the behavior; reinforcement then can be administered on a fixed (predictable) or variable (unpredictable) schedule after a given number of responses have been emitted or after the passage of time.

Operant conditioning techniques provide relatively quick and effective ways to change behavior. Carefully planned programs using behavior modification procedures can readily be applied to health care. For example, computerized instruction and tutorials for patients and staff rely heavily on operant conditioning principles in structuring learning programs. In the clinical setting, the families of chronic back pain patients have been taught to minimize their attention to the patients whenever they complain and behave in dependent, helpless ways, but to pay a lot of attention when the patients attempt to function independently, express a positive attitude, and try to live as normal a life as possible. Some patients respond so well to operant conditioning that they report experiencing less pain as they become more active and involved. Operant conditioning and behavior modification techniques also have been found to work well with some nursing home and long-term care residents, especially those who are losing their cognitive skills (Proctor, Burns, Powell, & Tarrier, 1999).

The behaviorist theory is simple and easy to use, and it encourages clear, objective analysis of observable environmental stimulus conditions, learner responses, and the effects of reinforcements on people's actions. There are, however, some criticisms and cautions to consider. First, this is a teacher-centered model in which learners are assumed to be relatively passive and easily manipulated, which raises a crucial ethical question: who is to decide what the desirable behavior should be? Too often the desired response is conformity and cooperation to make someone's job easier or more profitable. Second, the theory's emphasis on extrinsic rewards and external incentives reinforces and promotes materialism rather than self-initiative, a love of learning, and intrinsic satisfaction. Third, research evidence supporting behaviorist theory is often based on animal studies, the results of which may not be applicable to human behavior. A fourth shortcoming of behavior modification programs is that clients' changed behavior may deteriorate over time, especially once they are back in their former environment—an environment with a system of rewards and punishments that may have fostered their problems in the first place.

We now move from focusing on responses and behavior to the role of mental processes in learning.

Cognitive Learning Theory

While behaviorists generally ignore the internal dynamics of learning, cognitive learning theorists stress the importance of what goes on inside the learner. Cognitive theory is assumed to be comprised of a number of subtheories and is widely used in education and counseling. The key to learning and changing is the individual's cognition (perception, thought, memory, and ways of processing and structuring information). Cognitive learning, a highly active process largely directed by the individual, involves perceiving the information, interpreting it based on what is already known, and then reorganizing the information into new insights or understanding (Bandura, 2001; Hunt, Ellis, & Ellis, 2004).

Cognitive theorists, unlike behaviorists, maintain that reward is not necessary for learning. More important are learners' goals and expectations, which create disequilibrium, imbalance, and tension that motivate them to act. Educators trying to influence the learning process must recognize the variety of past experiences, perceptions, ways of incorporating and thinking about information, and diverse aspirations, expectations, and social influences that affect any learning situation. A learner's *metacognition*, or understanding of her way of learning, influences the process as well. To promote transfer of learning, the learner must mediate or act on the information in some way. Similar patterns in the initial learning situation and subsequent situations facilitate this transfer.

Cognitive learning theory includes several well-known perspectives, such as gestalt, information processing, human development, social constructivism, and social cognition theory. More recently, attempts have been made to incorporate considerations related to emotions within cognitive theory. Each of these perspectives emphasizes a particular feature of cognition, which, when pieced together, indicates much about what goes on inside the learner. As the various cognitive perspectives are briefly summarized here, readers are encouraged to think of their potential applications in the healthcare setting. In keeping with cognitive principles of learning, being mentally active with information encourages memory and retention.

One of the oldest psychological theories is the *gestalt perspective*, which emphasizes the importance of perception in learning and laid the groundwork for the various other cognitive perspectives that followed (Kohler, 1947, 1969; Murray, 1995). Rather than focusing on discrete stimuli, gestalt refers to the configuration or patterned organization of cognitive elements, reflecting the maxim that the whole is greater than the sum of the parts. A principal assumption is that each person perceives, interprets, and responds to any situation in his or her own way. While there are many gestalt principles worth knowing (Hilgard & Bower, 1966), several will be discussed here as they relate to health care.

A basic gestalt principle is that psychological organization is directed toward simplicity, equilibrium, and regularity. For example, study the bewildered faces of some patients listening to a complex, detailed explanation about their disease, when what they desire most is a simple, clear explanation that settles their uncertainty and relates directly to them and their familiar experiences.

Another central gestalt principle is that perception is selective, which has several ramifications. First, because no one can attend to all the surrounding stimuli at any given time, individuals orient themselves to certain features of an experience while screening out or ignoring other features. Patients in severe pain or worried about their hospital bills may not attend to well-intentioned patient education information. Second, what individuals pay attention to and what they ignore are influenced by a host of factors: past experiences, needs, personal motives and attitudes, reference groups, and the particular structure of the stimulus or situation (Sherif & Sherif, 1969). Assessing these internal and external dynamics has a direct bearing on how a health educator approaches any learning situation with an individual or group. Moreover, because individuals vary widely with regard to these and other characteristics, they will perceive, interpret, and respond to the same event in different ways, perhaps distorting reality to fit their goals and expectations. This tendency helps explain why an approach that is effective with one client may not work with another client. People with chronic illnesses—even different people with the same illness—are not alike, and helping any patient with disease or disability includes recognizing each person's unique perceptions and subjective experience (Imes, Clance, Gailis, & Atkeson, 2002).

Information processing is a cognitive perspective that emphasizes thinking processes: thought, reasoning, the way information is encountered and stored, and memory functioning (Gagné, 1985; Sternberg, 2006). How information is incorporated and retrieved is useful for health professionals to know, especially in relation to older people's learning (Hooyman & Kiyak, 2005; Kessels, 2003).

An information-processing model of memory functioning is illustrated in **Figure 3–2**. Tracking learning through the various stages is helpful in assessing what happens to information as it is perceived, interpreted, and remembered by each learner, which, in turn, may suggest ways of improving the structure of the learning situation as well as how to correct misconceptions, distortions, and errors in learning.

The first stage in the memory process involves paying attention to environmental

Figure 3–2 Information-processing model of memory.

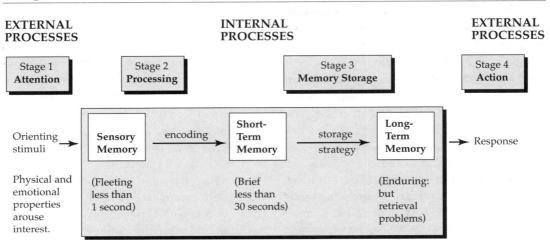

stimuli; attention, then, is the key to learning. Thus, if a client is not attending to what a nurse educator is saying, perhaps because the client is weary or distracted, it would be prudent to try the explanation at another time when he is more receptive and attentive.

In the second stage, the information is processed by the senses. Here it becomes important to consider the client's preferred mode of sensory processing (visual, auditory, or motor manipulation) and to ascertain whether there are sensory deficits.

In the third stage, the information is transformed and incorporated (encoded) briefly into short-term memory, after which it is either disregarded and forgotten or stored in long-term memory. Long-term memory involves the organization of information by using a preferred strategy for storage (e.g., imagery, association, rehearsal, or breaking the information into units). While long-term memories are enduring, a central problem is retrieving the stored information at a later time.

The last stage involves the action or response that the individual makes on the basis of how information was processed and stored. Education involves assessing how a learner attends to, processes, and stores the information that is presented as well as finding ways to encourage the retention and retrieval processes. Errors are corrected by helping learners reprocess what needs to be learned (Kessels, 2003).

In general, cognitive psychologists note that memory processing and the retrieval of information are enhanced by organizing information and making it meaningful. A widely used descriptive model has been provided by Robert Gagné (1985). Subsequently, Gagné and his colleagues outlined nine events and their corresponding cognitive processes that activate effective learning (Gagné, Briggs, & Wagner, 1992):

- Gain the learner's attention (reception)
- Inform the learner of the objectives and expectations (expectancy)

- Stimulate the learner's recall of prior learning (retrieval)
- Present information (selective perception)
- Provide guidance to facilitate the learner's understanding (semantic encoding)
- Have the learner demonstrate the information or skill (responding)
- Give feedback to the learner (reinforcement)
- Assess the learner's performance (retrieval)
- Work to enhance retention and transfer through application and varied practice (generalization)

In employing this model, instructors must carefully analyze the requirements of the activity, design and sequence the instructional events, and select appropriate media to achieve the outcomes.

Within the information-processing perspective, Sternberg (1996) reminds us to consider styles of thinking, which he defined as "a preference for using abilities in certain ways" (p. 347). Thinking styles concern differences, he noted, and not judgments of better or worse. In education, the instructor's task is to get in touch with the learner's way of processing information and thinking. Some implications for health care are the need to carefully match jobs with styles of thinking, to recognize that people may shift from preferring one style of thinking to another, and, most important, to appreciate and respect the different styles of thinking reflected among the many players in the healthcare setting (see Chapter 4 on learning styles). Yet striving for a match in styles is not always necessary or desirable. Tennant (2006) notes that adult learners may actually benefit from grappling with views

and styles of learning unlike their own, which may promote maturity, creativity, and a greater tolerance for differences. Since nurses are expected to instruct a variety of people with diverse styles of learning, Tennant's suggestion has interesting implications for nursing education programs.

The information-processing perspective is particularly helpful for assessing problems in acquiring, remembering, and recalling information. Some strategies include the following: (1) have learners indicate how they believe they learn (metacognition); (2) ask them to describe what they are thinking as they are learning; (3) evaluate learners' mistakes; and (4) give close attention to their inability to remember or demonstrate information. For example, forgetting or having difficulty in retrieving information from long-term memory is a major stumbling block in learning. This problem may occur because the information has faded from lack of use, other information interferes with its retrieval (what comes before or after a learning session may well confound storage and retrieval), or individuals are motivated to forget for a variety of conscious and unconscious reasons. This material on memory processing and functioning is highly pertinent to healthcare practice—whether in developing health education brochures, engaging in one-to-one patient education, delivering a staff development workshop, preparing community health lectures, or studying for one's courses and examinations. Focusing on attention, storage, and memory is essential in the patient education of older adults, including the identification of fatigue, medications, and anxieties that may interfere with learning and remembering (Kessels, 2003).

Heavily influenced by gestalt psychology, *cognitive development* is a third perspective on learning that focuses on qualitative changes in perceiving, thinking, and reasoning as individuals grow and mature (Santrock, 2006; Vander Zanden, Crandell, & Crandell, 2007). Cognitions are based on how external events are conceptualized, organized, and represented within each person's mental framework or schema, which is partially dependent on the individual's stage of development in perception, reasoning, and readiness to learn.

Much of the theory and research in this area has been concerned with identifying the characteristics and advances in the thought processes of children and adolescents. A principal assumption is that learning is a developmental, sequential, and active process that transpires as the child interacts with the environment, makes discoveries about how the world operates, and interprets these discoveries in keeping with what s/he knows (schema).

Jean Piaget is the best-known of the cognitive developmental theorists. His observations of children's perceptions and thought processes at different ages have contributed much to our recognition of the unique, changing abilities of youngsters to reason, conceptualize, communicate, and perform (Piaget & Inhelder, 1969). By watching, asking questions, and listening to children, Piaget identified and described four sequential stages of cognitive development (sensorimotor, preoperational, concrete operations, and formal operations). These stages become evident over the course of infancy, early childhood, middle childhood, and adolescence, respectively (see Chapter 5 on developmental stages). According to Piaget's theory of cognitive learning, children take in information as they interact with people and the environment. They either make their experiences fit with what they already know (assimilation) or change their perceptions and interpretations in keeping with the new information (accommodation).

Health professionals and family members need to determine what children are perceiving and thinking in a given situation. As an illustration, young children usually do not comprehend fully that death is final. They respond to the death of a loved one in their own way, perhaps asking God to give back the dead person or believing that if they act like a good person, the deceased loved one will return to them (Gardner, 1978).

Within the cognitive development perspective are some differences worth considering. For example, while Piaget stressed the importance of perception in learning and viewed children as little scientists exploring, interacting, and discovering the world in a relative solitary manner, Russian psychologist Lev Vygotsky (1986) emphasized the significance of language, social interaction, and adult guidance in the learning process. When teaching children, Vygotsky says the job of adults is to interpret, respond, and give meaning to children's actions. Rather than the discovery method favored by Piaget, Vygotsky advocated clear, well-designed instruction that is carefully structured to advance each person's thinking and learning.

In practice, some children may learn more effectively by discovering and putting pieces together on their own, whereas other children benefit from a more social and directive approach. It is the health educator's responsibility to identify the child's or teenager's stage of thinking, to provide experiences at an appropriate level for children to actively discover and participate in the learning process, and to determine whether a child learns best through language and social interaction or through perceiving and experimenting in his or her own way. Research suggests that young children's learning is often more solitary, whereas older children may learn more readily through social interaction (Palincsar, 1998).

What do cognitive developmental theorists say about adult learning? First, although the cognitive stages develop sequentially, some adults never reach the formal operations stage. These adults may learn better from explicitly concrete approaches to health education. Second, adult developmental psychologists and gerontologists have proposed advanced stages of reasoning in adulthood beyond formal operations. For example, it is not until the adult years that people become better able to deal with contradictions, synthesize information, and more effectively integrate what they have learned—characteristics that differentiate adult thought from adolescent thinking (Kramer, 1983). Third, older adults may demonstrate an advanced level of reasoning derived from their wisdom and life experiences, or they may reflect lower stages of thinking due to lack of education, disease, depression, extraordinary stress, or medications (Hooyman & Kiyak, 2005).

Research indicates that adults generally do better with self-directed learning (emphasizing learner control, autonomy, and initiative), an explicit rationale for learning, a problem-oriented rather than subject-oriented approach, and the opportunity to use their experiences and skills to help others (Tennant, 2006). Also, keep in mind that anxiety, the demands of adult life, and childhood experiences may interfere with learning in adulthood.

Because cognitive theory was criticized for neglecting the social context, the effects of social factors on perception, thought, and motivation are receiving increased attention. *Social constructivism* and *social cognition* are two increasingly popular perspectives within cognitive theory. Drawing heavily from gestalt psychology and developmental psychology, social constructivists take issue with some of the highly rational assumptions of the information-processing view and build on the works of John Dewey, Jean Piaget, and Lev Vygotsky (Palincsar, 1998). Social constructivists posit that individuals formulate or construct their own versions of reality and that learning and human development are richly colored by the social and cultural context in which people find themselves. A central tenet of this approach is that ethnicity, social class, gender, family life, past history, self-concept, and the learning situation itself all influence an individual's perceptions, thoughts, emotions, interpretations, and responses to information and experiences. A second principle is that effective learning occurs through social interaction, collaboration, and negotiation (Shapiro, 2002).

According to this view, the players in any healthcare setting may have differing perceptions of external reality, including distorted perceptions and interpretations. Every person operates on the basis of her or his unique representations and interpretations of a situation, all of which have been heavily influenced by that individual's social and cultural experiences. The impact of culture cannot be ignored, and learning is facilitated by sharing beliefs, by acknowledging and challenging differing conceptions, and by negotiating new levels of conceptual understanding (Marshall, 1998). Cooperative learning and self-help groups are examples of social constructivism in action. With America's rapidly changing age and ethnic composition, the social constructivist perspective has much to contribute to health education and health promotion efforts.

Rooted in social psychology, the social cognition perspective reflects a constructivist orientation and highlights the influence of social factors on perception, thought, and motivation. A host of scattered explanations can be found under the rubric of social cognition (Fiske & Taylor, 1991; Moskowitz, 2005), which, when applied to learning, emphasize the need for instructors to consider the dynamics of the social environment and groups on both interpersonal and intrapersonal behavior. As an illustration, attribution theory concerns the cause-and-effect relationships and explanations that individuals formulate to account for their own and others' behavior and the way in which the world operates. Many of these explanations are unique to the individual and tend to be strongly colored by cultural values and beliefs. For example, patients with certain religious views or a particular parental upbringing may believe that their disease is a punishment for their sins (internalizing blame); other patients may attribute their disease to the actions of others (externalizing blame). From this perspective, patients' attributions may or may not promote wellness and well-being. The route to changing health behaviors is to change distorted attributions. The medical staff's prejudices, biases (positive and negative), and attributions need to be considered as well in the healing process.

Cognitive theory has been criticized for neglecting emotions, and recent efforts have been made to incorporate considerations related to emotions within a cognitive framework, known as the *cognitive-emotional perspective*. As Eccles and Wigfield (2002) commented, " 'cold' cognitive models cannot adequately capture conceptual change; there is a need to consider affect as well" (p. 127).

Several slightly different cognitive orientations to emotions have been proposed and are briefly summarized in the following list:

- Empathy and the moral emotions (e.g., guilt, shame, distress, moral outrage) play a significant role in influencing

children's moral development and in motivating people's prosocial behavior and ethical responses (Hoffman, 2000).
- Memory storage and retrieval, as well as moral decision making, involve both cognitive and emotional brain processing, especially in response to situations that directly involve the self and are stressful (Greene, Sommerville, Nystrom, Darley, & Cohen, 2001).
- Emotional intelligence (EI) entails managing one's emotions, self-motivation, reading the emotions of others, and working effectively in interpersonal relationships, which some argue is more important to leadership, social judgment, and moral behavior than cognitive intelligence (Goleman, 1995).
- Self-regulation includes monitoring cognitive processes, emotions, and one's surroundings to achieve goals, which is considered a key factor to successful living and effective social behavior (Eccles & Wigfield, 2002).

The implications are that nursing and other health professional education programs would do well to exhibit and encourage empathy and emotional intelligence in working with patients, family, and staff and to attend to the dynamics of self-regulation as a way to promote positive personal growth and effective leadership. Research indicates that the development of these attributes in self and patients is associated with a greater likelihood of healthy behavior, psychological well-being, optimism, and meaningful social interactions (Brackett, Lopes, Ivcevic, Mayer, & Salovey, 2004).

A significant benefit of the cognitive theory to health care is its encouragement of recognizing and appreciating individuality and diversity in how people learn and process experiences. When applied to health care, cognitive theory has been useful in formulating exercise programs for breast cancer patients (Rogers, Matevey, Hopkins-Price, Shah, Dunnington, & Courneya, 2004), understanding individual differences in bereavement (Stroebe, Folkman, Hansson, & Schut, 2006), and dealing with adolescent depression in girls (Papadakis, Prince, Jones, & Strauman, 2006). Cognitive theory highlights the wide variation in how learners actively structure their perceptions; confront a learning situation; encode, process, store, and retrieve information; and manage their emotions, all of which are affected by social and cultural influences. The challenge to educators is to identify each learner's level of cognitive development and the social influences that affect learning, and then find ways to foster insight, creativity, and problem solving. Difficulties lie in ascertaining exactly what is transpiring inside the mind of each individual and in designing learning activities that encourage people to restructure their perceptions, reorganize their thinking, regulate their emotions, change their attributions and behavior, and create solutions.

The next learning theory to be discussed combines principles from both the behaviorist and cognitive theories.

Social Learning Theory

Social learning theory is largely the work of Albert Bandura (1977; 2001), who mapped out a perspective on learning that includes consideration of the personal characteristics of the learner, behavior patterns, and the environment. The theory has gone through several "paradigm shifts" (2001, p. 2). In early formulations, he emphasized behaviorist features and the imitation of role models; next the focus was on cognitive considerations, such as the attributes of the self and the internal processing of the learner. More recently, his attention turned to the impact of social factors and the social context within which learning and behavior occur. As the model has evolved, the learner has become viewed as central (what Bandura calls a "human agency"), which suggests the need to identify what learners are perceiving and how they are interpreting and responding to social situations. As such, careful consideration needs to be given to the healthcare environment as a social situation.

One of Bandura's early observations was that individuals need not have direct experiences to learn; considerable learning occurs by taking note of other people's behavior and what happens to them. Thus, learning is often a social process, and other individuals, especially significant others, provide compelling examples or role models for how to think, feel, and act. *Role modeling* is a central concept of the theory. As an example, a more experienced nurse who demonstrates desirable professional attitudes and behaviors sometimes is used as a mentor for a less experienced nurse. Research indicates that nurse managers' attitudes and actions—ensuring safety, integrating knowledge with practice, sharing feelings, challenging staff nurses and students, and their competence and willingness to provide guidance to others—influence the outcomes of the clinical supervision process (Berggren & Severinsson, 2006). How nurse mentors perceive their role is an important consideration in the leadership selection process (Neary, 2000).

Vicarious reinforcement is another concept from the social learning theory and involves determining whether role models are perceived as rewarded or punished for their behavior. Reward is not always necessary, however, and the behavior of a role model may be imitated even when no reward is involved for either the role model or the learner. In many cases, however, whether the model is viewed by the observer as rewarded or punished may have a direct influence on learning. This relationship may be one reason why it is difficult to attract health professionals to geriatric care. Although some highly impressive role models work in the field, geriatric health care is often accorded lower status with less pay in comparison to other specialty areas.

While social learning theory is based partially on behaviorist principles, the self-regulation and control that the individual exerts in the process of acquiring knowledge and changing behavior are considered more critical and are more reflective of cognitive principles. Bandura (1977) out-

lined a four-step, largely internal process that directs social learning, as can be seen in **Figure 3–3**. Although some components are similar to the information processing model described previously, a principal difference is the inclusion of a motivational component in the social learning theory model.

First is the attentional phase, a necessary condition for any learning to occur. Research indicates that role models with high status and competence are more likely to be observed, although the learner's own characteristics (needs, self-esteem, competence) may be the more significant determiner of attention. Second is the retention phase, which involves the storage and retrieval of what was observed. Third is the reproduction phase, where the learner copies the observed behavior. Mental rehearsal, immediate

Figure 3–3 Social learning theory.

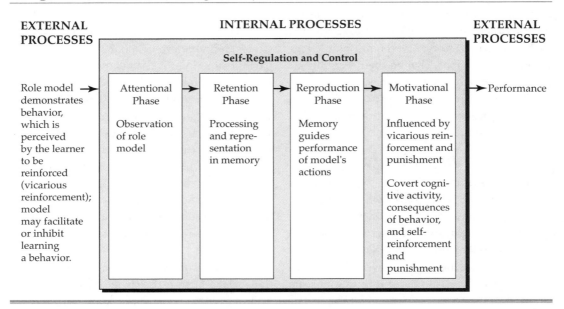

EXTERNAL PROCESSES	INTERNAL PROCESSES				EXTERNAL PROCESSES
	Self-Regulation and Control				
Role model demonstrates behavior, which is perceived by the learner to be reinforced (vicarious reinforcement); model may facilitate or inhibit learning a behavior.	Attentional Phase Observation of role model	Retention Phase Processing and representation in memory	Reproduction Phase Memory guides performance of model's actions	Motivational Phase Influenced by vicarious reinforcement and punishment Covert cognitive activity, consequences of behavior, and self-reinforcement and punishment	Performance

Source: Based on Bandura (1977).

enactment, and corrective feedback strengthen the reproduction of behavior. Fourth is the motivational phase, which focuses on whether the learner is motivated to perform a certain type of behavior. Reinforcement or punishment for a role model's behavior, the learning situation, and the appropriateness of subsequent situations where the behavior is to be displayed all affect a learner's performance (Bandura, 1977; Gage & Berliner, 1998). Well suited to conducting health education and staff development training, this organized approach to learning requires attention to the social environment, the behavior to be performed, and the individual learner (Bahn, 2001).

Reflecting a constructivist orientation, Bandura (2001) shifted his focus to sociocultural influences, viewing the learner as the agent through which learning experiences are filtered. As he argues, the human mind is not just reactive; it is generative, creative, and reflective. Essentially, the individual engages in a transactional relationship between the social environment and the self, where sociocultural factors are mediated by "psychological mechanisms of the self-system to produce behavioral effects" (p. 4). In his model, Bandura stressed the internal dynamics of personal selection, intentionality, self-regulation, self-efficacy, and self-evaluation in the learning process. Culture and self-efficacy play a key role, with Bandura noting that individualistic cultures interpret self-efficacy differently than group-oriented cultures. However defined, a low sense of self-efficacy in either kind of culture produces stress. This perspective applies particularly well to the acquisition of health behaviors and partially explains why some people select positive role models and effectively regulate their attitudes, emotions, and actions, whereas other people choose negative role models and engage in unhealthy and destructive behaviors. Healthcare professionals need to find ways to encourage patients' feelings of competency and to promote wellness rather than fostering dependency, helplessness, and feelings of low self-worth.

The social learning theory extends the learning process beyond the educator–learner relationship to the larger social world. The theory helps explain the socialization process as well as the breakdown of behavior in society. Responsibility is placed on the educator or leader to act as an exemplary role model and to choose socially healthy experiences for individuals to observe and repeat (requiring the careful evaluation of learning materials for stereotypes, mixed or hidden messages, and negative effects). Yet simple exposure to role models correctly performing a behavior that is rewarded (or performing some undesirable behavior that is punished) does not ensure learning. Attention to the learner's self-system and the dynamics of self-regulation may help sort out the varying effects of the social learning experience.

In health care, social learning theory has been applied to nursing education, to addressing psychosocial problems, and to maximizing the use of support groups. For example, research indicates that those managers who are aware of their roles and responsibilities in promoting a positive work environment enhance learning, competence, and satisfaction; dissatisfaction, of course, has a detrimental effect and is a significant cause of staff turnover (Kane-Urrabazo, 2006). Nurses have applied social learning principles successfully when working with teenage mothers (Stiles, 2005) and in addressing alcoholism among older adults (Akers, 1989). A major difficulty is that this theory is complex and not easily operationalized, measured, and assessed.

The final two theories to be reviewed in this chapter focus on the importance of emotions and feelings in the learning process.

Psychodynamic Learning Theory

Although not typically treated as a learning theory, some of the constructs from the psychodynamic theory (based on the work of Sigmund Freud and his followers) have significant implications for learning and changing behavior (Hilgard & Bower, 1966; Slipp, 2000). Largely a theory of motivation stressing emotions rather than cognition or responses, the psychodynamic perspective emphasizes the importance of conscious and unconscious forces in guiding behavior, personality conflicts, and the enduring effects of childhood experiences. As Pullen (2002) pointed out, negative emotions are important to recognize and assess in nurse–patient–doctor–family interactions, and the psychodynamic theory can be helpful in this regard.

A central principle of the theory is that behavior may be conscious or unconscious—that is, individuals may or may not be aware of their motivations and why they feel, think, and act as they do. According to the psychodynamic view, the most primitive source of motivation comes from the id and is based on libidinal energy (the basic instincts, impulses, and desires we are born with), which includes eros (the desire for pleasure and sex, sometimes called the "life force") and thanatos (aggressive and destructive impulses, or death wish). Patients who survive or die despite all predictions to the contrary provide illustrations of such primitive motivations. The id, according to Freud, operates on the basis of the pleasure principle—to seek pleasure and avoid pain. For example, dry, dull lectures given by nurse educators who go through the motions of the presentation without much enthusiasm or emotion inspire few people (patients, staff, or students) to listen to the information or heed the advice being given. This does not mean, however, that only pleasurable presentations will be acceptable.

The id (primitive drives) and superego (internalized societal values and standards, or the conscience) are mediated by the ego, which operates on the basis of the reality principle—rather than insisting on immediate gratification, people learn to take the long road to pleasure and to weigh the choices or dilemmas in the conflict between the id and superego. Healthy ego (self) development, as emphasized by Freud's followers, is an important consideration in the health fields. For example, patients with ego strength can cope with painful medical treatments because they recognize the long-term value of enduring discomfort and pain to achieve a positive outcome. Patients with weak ego development, in contrast, may miss their appointments and treatments or engage in short-term pleasurable activities that work against their healing and recovery. Helping patients develop ego strength and adjust realistically to a changed body image or lifestyle brought about by disease and medical interventions is a significant aspect of the learning and healing process. Nurses and other health professionals, too, require personal ego strength to cope with the numerous predicaments in the everyday practice of delivering care as they face conflicting values, ethics, and demands. Professional burnout, for example, is rooted in an overly idealized concept of the healthcare role and unrealistic expectations for the self in performing the role. Malach-Pines (2000) notes that burnout may stem from nurses' childhood experiences with lack of control.

When the ego is threatened, as can easily occur in the healthcare setting, *defense mechanisms* may be employed to protect the self. The short-term use of defense mechanisms is a way of coming to grips with reality. The danger comes in the overuse or long-term reliance on defense mechanisms, which allows individuals to avoid reality and may act as a barrier to learning and transfer. **Table 3–2** describes some of the more commonly used defense mechanisms. Because of the stresses involved in health care, knowledge of defense mechanisms is useful, whether nursing students are grappling with the challenges of nursing education, staff nurses are dealing with the strains of working in hospitals and long-term care facilities, or patients and their families are learning to cope with illness.

As an example of defense mechanisms in health care, Kübler-Ross (1969) pointed out that many terminally ill patients' initial reaction to being told they have a serious threat to their health and well-being is to employ the defense mechanism of denial. It is too overwhelming for patients to process the information that they are likely to die. While most patients gradually accept the reality of their illness, the dangers are that if they remain in a state of denial, they may not seek treatment and care, and if their illness is contagious, they may not protect others against infection. In turn, a common defense mechanism employed by healthcare staff is to intellectualize rather than deal realistically at an emotional level with the significance of disease and death. For example, one study reported that nurses may strive too quickly to classify terminally ill patients within a denial-acceptance framework and, as a result, may not listen to patients attempting to tell their stories and interpret their illness experiences (Telford, Kralik, & Koch, 2006). Protecting the self (ego)

Table 3–2 Ego Defense Mechanisms: Ways of Protecting the Self from Perceived Threat

Denial: ignoring or refusing to acknowledge the reality of a threat

Rationalization: excusing or explaining away a threat

Displacement: taking out hostility and aggression on other individuals rather than directing anger at the source of the threat

Depression: keeping unacceptable thoughts, feelings, or actions from conscious awareness

Regression: returning to an earlier (less mature, more primitive) stage of behavior as a way of coping with a threat

Intellectualization: minimizing anxiety by responding to a threat in a detached, abstract manner without feeling or emotion

Projection: seeing one's own unacceptable characteristics or desires in other people

Reaction formation: expressing or behaving the opposite of what is really felt

Sublimation: converting repressed feelings into socially acceptable action

Compensation: making up for weaknesses by excelling in other areas

by dehumanizing patients and treating them as diseases and body parts rather than as whole individuals (with spiritual, emotional, and physical needs) are occupational hazards for nurses and other health professionals.

Another central assumption of the psychodynamic theory is that personality development occurs in stages, with much of adult behavior derived from earlier childhood experiences and conflicts. One of the most widely used models of personality development is Erikson's (1968) eight stages of life, organized around a psychosocial crisis to be resolved at each stage (see Chapter 5). Treatment regimens, communication, and health education need to include considerations of the patient's stage of personality development. For example, in working with 4- and 5-year-old patients, where the crisis is initiative versus guilt, health professionals should encourage the children to offer their ideas and to make and do things themselves. Staff also must be careful not to make these children feel guilty for their illness or misfortune. As a second example, the adolescent's psychosocial developmental needs to have friends and to find an identity require special attention in health care. Adolescent patients may benefit from help and support in adjusting to a changed body image and in addressing their fears of weakness, lack of activity, and social isolation. One danger is that young people may treat their illness or impairment as a significant dimension of their identity and self-concept—well described in poet Lucy Grealy's personal account in *Anatomy of a Face* (1994).

According to the psychodynamic view, personal difficulties arise and learning is limited when individuals become fixated or stuck at an earlier stage of personality development. They then must work through their previously unresolved crises to develop and mature emotionally.

For example, some staff members and patients feel an inordinate need to control the self, other people, and certain social situations. This behavior may be rooted in their inability to resolve the crisis of trust versus mistrust at the earliest stage of life. In working with these individuals, it is essential to build a trusting relationship and to encourage them gradually to relinquish some control.

Past conflicts, especially during childhood, may interfere with the ability to learn or to transfer learning. What people resist talking about or learning, termed *resistance*, is an indicator of underlying emotional difficulties, which must be dealt with for them to move ahead emotionally and behaviorally. For instance, a young, pregnant teenager who refuses to engage in a serious conversation about sexuality (e.g., changes the subject, giggles, looks out into space, expresses anger) indicates underlying emotional conflicts that need to be addressed. One study explored psychodynamic sources of resistance among nursing students and how they engaged with or resisted the learning process. A number of factors requiring consideration surfaced, including childhood struggles, a history of overadaptation, self-image, and learning climate (Gilmartin, 2000).

Serious problems in miscommunication can occur in health care as a result of childhood learning experiences. For example, some physicians and nurses may have had the childhood experience of standing helplessly by watching someone they loved and once depended on endure disease, suffering, and death. Although they could do little as children to improve the situation, they may be compensating for their childhood feelings of helplessness and dependency as adults by devoting their careers to fending off and fighting disease and death. These motivations, however, may not serve them well as they attempt to cope, communicate, and educate dying patients and their families.

Emotional conflicts are not always due to internal forces; society exerts pressures on individuals that promote emotional difficulties as well. The reluctance of health professionals to be open and honest with a terminally ill patient partially may be derived from American culture, which encourages medical personnel to fix their patients and extend life. Staff members may or may not be conscious of these pressures, but either way they are likely to feel guilty and that they are failures when dealing with a dying patient.

The concept of transfer has special meaning to psychodynamic theorists. *Transference* occurs when individuals project their feelings, conflicts, and reactions—especially those developed during childhood with significant others such as parents—onto authority figures and other individuals in their lives. The danger is that the relationship between the health professional and the patient may become distorted and unrealistic because of the biases inherent in the transference reaction. For example, because patients are sick, they may feel helpless and dependent and then regress to an earlier stage in life when they relied on their parents for help and support. Their childhood feelings and relationship with a parent—for better or worse—may be transferred to a nurse or physician taking care of them. While sometimes flattering, the love and dependency that patients feel may operate against the autonomy and independence needed to get back on their feet. A particular patient may also remind a staff member of someone from her or his past, creating a situation of countertransference.

The psychodynamic approach reminds health professionals to pay attention to emotions, unconscious motivations, and the psychological growth and development of all those involved in health care and learning. Health care rests on both interpersonal and intrapersonal processes involved in the therapeutic use of the self in carrying out patient care (Gallop & O'Brien, 2003). Psychodynamic theory is well suited to understanding patient and family noncompliance (Menahern & Halasz, 2000), trauma and loss (Duberstein & Masling, 2000), palliative care and the deeply emotional issues of terminal illness (Chochinov & Breitbart, 2000), and the anxieties of working with long-term psychiatric residents (Goodwin & Gore, 2000). From a professional perspective, when examining the problems of bullying nurse managers or the failure of nurses to formally report incidents of violence and aggression, results indicated the need to consider childhood and adult experiences with abuse and violence, as well as guilt, low self-image, and cultural expectations about nurses (Ferns, 2006).

The psychodynamic approach has been criticized because much of the analysis is speculative and subjective, and the theory is difficult to operationalize and measure. Psychodynamic theory also can be used inappropriately; it is not the job of health professionals with little clinical psychology or psychiatric training to probe into the private lives and feelings of patients so as to uncover deep, unconscious conflicts. Another danger is that health professionals may depend on the many psychodynamic constructs as a way of intellectualizing or explaining away, rather than dealing with, people as individuals who need emotional care.

Humanistic Learning Theory

Underlying the humanistic perspective on learning is the assumption that each individual is unique and that all individuals have a desire to grow in a positive way. Unfortunately, positive psychological growth may be damaged by some of society's values and expectations (e.g., males are less emotional than females, some ethnic groups are inferior to others, making money is more important than caring for people) and by adults' mistreatment of their children and each other (e.g., inconsistent or harsh discipline, humiliation and belittling, abuse and neglect). Spontaneity, the importance of emotions and feelings, the right of individuals to make their own choices, and human creativity are the cornerstones of a humanistic approach to learning (Rogers, 1994; Snowman & Biehler, 2006). Humanistic theory is especially compatible with nursing's focus on caring and patient centeredness—an orientation that is increasingly challenged by the emphasis in medicine and health care on science, technology, cost efficiency, for-profit medicine, bureaucratic organization, and time pressures.

Like the psychodynamic theory, the humanistic perspective is largely a motivational theory. From a humanistic perspective, motivation is derived from each person's needs, subjective feelings about the self, and the desire to grow. The transfer of learning is facilitated by curiosity, a positive self-concept, and open situations in which people respect individuality and promote freedom of choice. Under such conditions, transfer is likely to be widespread, enhancing flexibility and creativity.

Maslow (1954, 1987), a major contributor to humanistic theory, is perhaps best known for identifying the *hierarchy of needs* (**Figure 3–4**), which he says plays an important role in human motivation. At the bottom of the hierarchy are physiological needs (food, warmth, sleep); then come safety needs; then the need for belonging and love; followed by self-esteem. At the top of the hierarchy are self-actualization needs (maximizing one's potential). Additional considerations include cognitive needs (to know and understand) and, for some individuals, aesthetic needs (the desire for beauty). An assumption is that basic-level needs must be met before individuals can be concerned with learning and self-actualizing. Thus, clients who are hungry, tired, and in pain will be motivated to get these biological needs met before being interested in learning about their medications, rules for self-care, and health education. While intuitively appealing, research has not been able to support Maslow's hierarchy of needs with much consistency. For example, although some people's basic needs may not be met, they may nonetheless engage in creative activities, extend themselves to other people, and enjoy learning (Pfeffer, 1985).

Besides personal needs, humanists contend that self-concept and self-esteem are necessary considerations in any learning situation. The therapist Carl Rogers (1961, 1994) argued that what people want is unconditional positive self-regard (the feeling of being loved without strings attached). Experiences that are threatening, coercive, and judgmental undermine the ability and enthusiasm of individuals to learn. It is essential that those in positions of authority convey a fundamental respect for the people with whom they work. If a health professional is prejudiced against AIDS patients, then little will be healing or therapeutic in her relationship with them until she is genuinely able to feel respect for the patient as an individual.

Rather than acting as an authority, say humanists, the role of any educator or leader is to be a facilitator (Rogers, 1994). Listening—rather than talking—is the skill needed. Because the uniqueness of the individual is fun-

Figure 3–4 Maslow's hierarchy of needs.

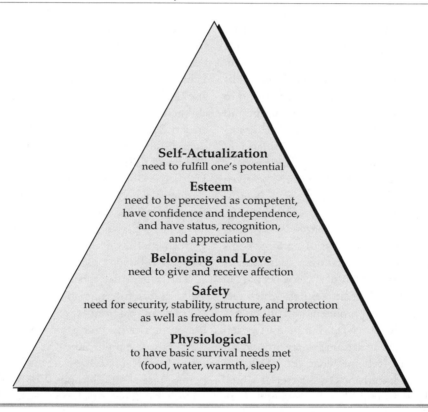

Self-Actualization
need to fulfill one's potential

Esteem
need to be perceived as competent,
have confidence and independence,
and have status, recognition,
and appreciation

Belonging and Love
need to give and receive affection

Safety
need for security, stability, structure, and protection
as well as freedom from fear

Physiological
to have basic survival needs met
(food, water, warmth, sleep)

Source: Adapted from Maslow (1987).

damental to the humanistic perspective, much of the learning experience requires a direct relationship between the educator and the learner, with instruction tailored to the needs, self-esteem, and positive growth of each learner. Learners, not educators, choose what is to be learned, and within this framework educators serve as resource persons whose job is to encourage learners to make wise choices. Because the central focus is on learners' perceptions, desires, and decision making, the humanistic orienta-

tion is referred to as a learner-directed approach (Snowman & Biehler, 2006).

Mastering information and facts is not the central purpose of the humanistic model of learning. Instead, fostering curiosity, enthusiasm, initiative, and responsibility is much more important and enduring and should be the primary goal of any educator. Rather than inserting health education videos into television sets for hospital patients to view or routinely distributing lots of pamphlets and pages of small-print instructions, the humanist perspective would suggest establishing rapport and becoming emotionally attuned to patients and their family members. In professional education, the goal is to provide psychologically safe classrooms and clinical environments, where humanistic principles can be taught through caring, role modeling, small-group discussion, case discussions, attention to self-awareness and feelings, role playing, and videotaping students in the clinical setting followed by feedback and reflection (Biderman, 2003). Providing time for student reflection is essential, and instructor feedback must be given sensitively and thoughtfully (Fryer-Edwards, Arnold, Baile, Tulsky, Petracca, & Back, 2006).

Humanistic psychology contends that feelings and emotions are the keys to learning, communication, and understanding. Humanists worry that in today's stressful society, people can easily lose touch with their feelings, which sets the stage for emotional problems and difficulties in learning (Rogers, 1961). To humanists, "tell me how you feel" is a much more important instruction than "tell me what you think," as thoughts and admonitions (the latter of which Rogers calls "the shoulds") may be at odds with true feelings. Consider the implications of the following statements: (1) a young person who says, "I know I should go to medical school and become a doctor because I am smart and that is what my parents want, but I don't feel comfortable with sick people—I don't even like them!" or (2) the dying patient who says, "I realize that I am going to die and should be brave, but I feel so sad that I am losing my family, my friends, and my self; frankly, I am afraid of dying—all the pain and suffering, being a burden—I'm scared!" In both cases, humanists would argue, the overriding factor that will affect the behavior of the young person and the dying patient is their feelings, not their cognitions.

The humanistic learning theory has modified the approach to education and changing behavior by giving primary focus to the subjective needs and feelings of the learner and by redefining the role of the educator. Humanistic principles have been a cornerstone of self-help groups, wellness programs, and palliative care. Humanistic theory has also been found to be well suited to working with children and young patients undergoing separation anxiety due to illness, surgery, and recovery (Holyoake, 1998) and for working in the areas of mental health and palliative care (Barnard, Hollingum, & Hartfiel, 2006). Similar to psychodynamic theory, a principal emphasis is on the healing nature of the *therapeutic relationship* (Pearson, 2006) and the need for nursing students and health professionals to grow emotionally from their healthcare experiences (Block & Billings, 1998).

The humanistic theory has its weaknesses as well. Research has not been able to substantiate some of its strongest claims, and the theory has been criticized for promoting self-centered learners who cannot take criticism or compromise their deeply felt positions. Charged with being more of a philosophy—or a cult—than a science, the touchy-feely approach of humanists makes some learners and educators feel truly uncomfortable. Moreover, information, facts, memorization, drill, practice, and the tedious work sometimes required to master knowledge, which humanists minimize and sometimes disdain, have been found to contribute to significant learning, knowledge building, and skill development (Gage & Berliner, 1992).

Neuropsychology and Learning

One of the newest and most rapidly growing areas of psychology research involves investigations into the physiological and neurological bases of thinking, learning, and behavior. Neuroscience research has implications for learning in several ways: (1) by documenting the dynamics of brain and central nervous system processing of information; (2) by understanding and working with children and adults who have neurological conditions, face mental health issues, or have learning disabilities; (3) by answering questions about the relationship between stress and learning; and (4) by providing evidence to support the assumptions of various learning theories or the integration of these theories.

Much of the information in these areas has been gained through advances in neuroimaging techniques such as functional magnetic resonance imaging (fMRI) and positron emission tomography (PET). Other methodologies include animal studies based on surgery, electrical recordings (EEG and ERP), and case studies of children and adults with head trauma, brain lesions, and neurological abnormalities (Byrnes, 2001). While the research findings highlight some of the underlying biological mechanisms of learning and provide evidence to support some of the principal constructs and dynamics of existing learning theories, there is as yet no coherent physiological or neuropsychological theory of learning.

In synthesizing neuropsychology research, some generalizations about learning can be made (Anderson, 1997; Gazzaniga, 2000; Page, 2006; Phelps, 2006; Shors, 2006; Silverstein & Uhlhaas, 2004). Each generalization, listed below, has implications for health education in the clinical setting, and readers are encouraged to formulate applications to nursing and health care.

- Emotions have been found to play a key role in Pavlovian conditioning, information processing, memory, and motivation. Emotions are considered to interact with cognitive factors in any learning situation, suggesting that they cannot be ignored when teaching, learning, reasoning, or making decisions.

- Neuropsychology studies of learning have confirmed a number of learning theories and constructs, including gestalt principles, constructivism, Piaget's notions of assimilation and accommodation, and Freud's conceptualization of conscious and unconscious processes. Neurological studies also have documented physiological arousal and tracked attention, perception, and the organization of experience while learning.

- Learning is a function of physiological and neurological developmental changes that are ongoing and dynamic; the brain is less fixed than once thought, and it changes with learning and experience (called "plasticity").

- Brain processing is different for each learner; thus, gaining the learner's attention, controlling the pace of learning, and identifying the specific mechanisms for enhancing learning are unique for each person.

- Learning is an active, multifaceted, complex process that involves preferred and interacting sensory modes, is colored by the past and present social context, and is regulated largely by the learner on the basis of his or her development, experiences, and sense of self.

- Meaningful practice strengthens learning connections, which may fade from lack of use; thus, one-shot patient education efforts are not likely to be effective in changing behavior.

- Stress can interfere with or stimulate learning, although the responses to stress may change with age and differ for males and females, or for those who have experienced traumatic events.

Neurophysiological aspects of learning become all the more germane for children and adults with physiological disorders; for those with mental, emotional, and behavioral problems; and for those facing the stresses of trauma, disease, disability, and socioeconomic hardship. Despite numerous neuroscientific studies related to learning, the research is in its early stages and remains fragmented, scattered, and lacking in integration. In addition, neuropsychological studies are often based on animal research or on highly specialized and restricted human samples, so few generalizations can be made about most people. Although addressing the various biological connections to learning is currently a popular and relatively well-funded area of research, there is a risk of reducing human behavior to mere biology while ignoring the individual as a person as well as the significance and complexity of psychological and social processes in any learning situation.

Comparison of Learning Theories

Table 3–3 provides a comparative summary of the five learning theories outlined in this chapter. Generalizations can be made about both the differences and the similarities in what the theories say about acquiring knowledge and changing feelings, attitudes, and behavior. With regard to some of the differences among the theories, each theory has its own assumptions, vocabulary, and way of conceptualizing the learning process. The theories differ in their emphasis on the relative influence of external or internal factors in learning, the view

of the learner as more passive or active, the task of the educator, the explanation of motivation, and the way in which the transfer of learning is accomplished.

A logical question is which of these five theories best describes or explains learning—which theory, in other words, would be the most helpful to health professionals interested in increasing knowledge or changing the behavior of patients, staff, or themselves? The answer to this question is that each theory contributes to understanding various aspects of the learning process and can be used singly or in combination to help practitioners acquire new information and alter existing thoughts, feelings, and behavior.

Each theory gives focus to important considerations in any learning situation, involving the consideration of external social factors and internal psychological processing. For example, behaviorists urge us to pay attention to and change stimulus conditions and to provide reinforcement to alter behavior. While criticized for being reductionistic, behaviorists' emphasis on manipulating the environment and reinforcements is admittedly simpler and easier than trying to undertake a massive overhaul of an individual's internal dynamics (perceptions, cognition, memory, feelings, and personality history and conflicts). Moreover, getting someone first to behave in a more appropriate way (abstaining from bad habits and engaging in healthy behavior) may not be as threatening or daunting to the learner as it would be to suggest the need for internal personality changes. Desired responses are modified and strengthened through practice; the new learned responses, in turn, may lead to more fundamental changes in attitudes and emotions. The social learning perspective is another relatively simple theory to use, stressing the importance of effective role models, who, by

Table 3–3 SUMMARY OF LEARNING THEORIES

Learning Procedures	Assumptions About the Learner	Educator's Task	Sources of Motivation	Transfer of Learning
Behaviorist				
Environmental stimulus conditions and reinforcement promote changes in responses. To change behavior, change the environment.	Passive, reactive learner responds to environmental conditions (stimuli and reinforcement).	Active educator manipulates stimuli and reinforcement to direct learning and change.	Drive reduction.	Practice; similarity in stimulus conditions and responses between learning and new situations.
Cognitive				
Internal perception and thought processing within context of human development promote learning and change. To change behavior, change cognitions.	Active learner determines patterning of experiences; is strongly influenced by attributions.	Active educator structures experiences (through organization and meaningfulness) to encourage the reorganization of cognitions.	Goals. Expectations. Disequilibrium.	Mental and physical activity. Common patterns. Understanding. Learning to learn.
Social Learning				
External role models and their perceived reinforcement along with learner's internal influences. To change behavior, change role models, perceived reinforcement, and the learner's self-regulating mechanisms.	Active learner observes others and regulates decision to reproduce behavior.	Active educator models behavior, encourages perception of reinforcement, carefully evaluates learning materials for social messages, and attempts to influence learner's self-regulation.	Socialization experiences, role models, and self-reactive influences (observe self, set goals, and reinforce performance).	Similarity of setting and role models' behavior.

continues

Table 3–3 SUMMARY OF LEARNING THEORIES (CONTINUED)

Learning Procedures	Assumptions About the Learner	Educator's Task	Sources of Motivation	Transfer of Learning
Psychodynamic				
Internal forces such as developmental stage, childhood experiences, emotional conflicts, and ego strength influence learning and change. To change behavior, change interpretations and make unconscious motivations conscious.	Active learner's lifestyle, past experiences, and current emotional conflicts influence what is learned and how it is remembered and performed.	Educator as a reflective interpreter makes sense of learner's personality and motivation by listening and posing questions to stimulate conscious awareness, insight, and ego strength.	Pleasure principle and reality principle. Imbalance. Conscious and unconscious influence of conflict, development, and defense mechanisms.	Personality conflict, resistance, and transference associated with learning situations may act as barrier.
Humanistic				
Internal feelings about self, ability to make wise choices, and needs affect learning and change. To change behavior, change feelings, self-concept, and needs.	Active learner attempts to actualize potential for positive self-growth and confirm self-concept; is spontaneous, creative, and playful.	Facilitative educator encourages positive self-growth, listens empathetically, allows freedom of choice, and respects learner.	Needs, desire for positive self-growth, and confirmation of self-concept.	Positive or negative feelings about self and freedom to learn promote or inhibit transfer.

their example, demonstrate exactly what behavior is expected.

Cognitive, social learning, psychodynamic, and humanistic theories remind us to consider internal factors—perceptions, thoughts, ways of processing information, feelings, and emotions. These factors cannot be ignored because, ultimately, it is the learner who controls and regulates learning: how information is perceived, interpreted, and remembered, and whether the new knowledge is expressed or performed.

In practice, learning theories should not be considered to be mutually exclusive but rather to operate together to change attitudes and behavior. For example, patients undergoing painful procedures are first taught systematic desensitization (behaviorist) and while experiencing pain or discomfort are encouraged to employ imagery, such as thinking about a favorite, beautiful place or imagining the healthy cells gobbling up the unhealthy cells (cognitive). Staff members are highly respectful, upbeat, and emotionally supportive of each patient (humanistic) and create the time and opportunity to listen to patients discuss some of their deepest fears and concerns (psychodynamic). Waiting rooms and lounge areas for patients and their families are designed to be comfortable, friendly, and pleasant to facilitate conversation and interaction, while support groups may help patients and family members learn from each other about how to cope with illness or disability and how to regulate their emotions so that their health is not further compromised (social learning).

Another generalization from this discussion is that some learning theories are better suited to certain kinds of individuals than to others. While theoretical assumptions about the learner range from passive to highly active, passive individuals may learn more effectively from behav-

iorist techniques, whereas curious, highly active, and self-directed persons may do better with cognitive and humanistic approaches. Also, keep in mind that some learners require external reinforcement and incentives, whereas other learners do not seem to need—and may even resent—attempts to manipulate and reinforce them.

Individuals who are well educated, verbal, and reflective may be better candidates for cognitive and psychodynamic approaches, whereas behaviorist approaches may be more suitable for persons whose cognitive processes are impaired or who are uncomfortable dealing with abstractions or scrutinizing and communicating their thoughts and emotions.

In addition, each individual's preferred modes of learning and processing may help determine the selection of suitable theoretical approaches. That is, while some individuals learn by acting and responding (behaviorist), the route to learning for others may be through perceptions and thoughts (cognitive) or through feelings and emotions (humanistic and psychodynamic). Most people appear to benefit from demonstration and example (social learning).

Common Principles of Learning

Taken together, the theories discussed in this chapter indicate that learning is a more complicated process than any one theory implies. Besides the distinct considerations for learning suggested by each theory, the similarities among the perspectives point to some core features of learning. The issues raised at the beginning of the chapter can be addressed by synthesizing the learning theories and identifying their common principles.

1. How Does Learning Occur?

Learning is an active process that takes place as individuals interact with their environment and incorporate new information or experiences with what they already know or have learned. Factors in the environment that affect learning include the society and culture, the structure or pattern of stimuli, the effectiveness of role models and reinforcements, feedback for correct and incorrect responses, and opportunities to process and apply learning to new situations.

Furthermore, the individual exerts significant control over learning, often involving considerations of his or her developmental stage, past history (habits, cultural conditioning, socialization, childhood experiences, and conflicts), cognitive style, dynamics of self-regulation, conscious and unconscious motivations, personality (stage, conflicts, and self-concept), and emotions. Also, learners often have a preferred mode for taking in information (visual, motor, auditory, or symbolic), and, while some individuals may learn best on their own, others will benefit from expert guidance, social interaction, and cooperative learning.

Learning is an individual matter. Neuropsychology research is beginning to document the uniqueness of each person's way of actively perceiving and processing information, his or her flexibility and reactions to stress, and the impact of culture and emotions on how and what is learned.

A critical influence on whether learning occurs is motivation (see Chapter 6 on motivation). The learning theories reviewed here suggest that to learn, the individual must want to gain something (receive rewards and pleasure, meet goals and needs, confirm expectations, grow in positive ways, or resolve conflicts), which, in turn, arouses the learner by creating tension (drives to be reduced, disequilibrium, and imbalance) and the propensity to act or change behavior.

The relative success or failure of the learner's performance may affect subsequent learning experiences. In some cases, an inappropriate, maladaptive, or harmful previously learned behavior may need to be extinguished and then replaced with a more positive response. It is, of course, easier to instill new learning than to correct faulty learning.

2. What Kinds of Experiences Facilitate or Hinder the Learning Process?

The educator exerts a critical influence on learning through role modeling, the selection of learning theories, and how the learning experience is structured for each learner. To be effective, educators must have knowledge (of the material to be learned, the learner, the social context, and educational psychology), and they must be competent (be imaginative, flexible, and able to employ teaching methods; display solid communication skills; and have the ability to motivate others).

All the learning theories discussed in this chapter acknowledge the need to recognize and relate the new information to the learner's past experiences (old habits, culture, familiar patterns, childhood memories, feelings about the self, and what is valued, normative, and perceived as successful or rewarded in society). The ultimate control over learning rests with the learner, but effective educators influence and guide the process so that learners advance in their knowledge, perceptions, thoughts, emotional maturity, and behavior.

Ignoring these considerations, of course, may hinder learning. Other impediments to learning may involve a lack of clarity and meaningfulness in what is to be learned, neglect or harsh punishment, fear, or negative or ineffective role models. Providing inappropriate materials for the individual's ability, readiness to learn, or stage of life-cycle development is another obstacle to learning. Moreover, individuals are unlikely to want to learn if they have had detrimental socialization experiences, are deprived of stimulating environments, and are without goals and realistic expectations for themselves.

3. What Helps Ensure That Learning Becomes Relatively Permanent?

Four considerations assist learning in becoming permanent. First, the likelihood of learning is enhanced by organizing the learning experience, making it meaningful and pleasurable, recognizing the role of emotions in learning, and by pacing the presentation in keeping with the learner's ability to process information. Second, practicing (mentally and physically) new knowledge or skills under varied conditions strengthens learning. The third issue concerns reinforcement. Although reinforcement may or may not be necessary, some theorists have argued that it may be helpful because it serves as a signal to the individual that learning has occurred.

A fourth consideration involves whether learning transfers beyond the initial educational setting. Learning cannot be assumed to be relatively lasting or permanent; it must be assessed and evaluated by the educator soon after the learning experience has occurred as well as by follow-up measurements at later times. Research skills, knowledge of evaluation procedures, and

the willingness and resources to engage in educational assessment are now considered essential responsibilities of the educator in carrying out the teaching/learning process. Evaluation feedback can then be used by the nurse educator to revamp and revitalize learning experiences.

State of the Evidence

The study of learning in educational psychology is based on evidence from research similar to that advocated in nursing, medicine, and health care. Rather than assuming the instructor knows best, we gather evidence and test learning theories, teaching methods, and what is believed to be true about learners, teachers, and the environment. The research results are then evaluated for the purpose of modifying the theories, methods, and assumptions about learning.

Ideally in health education, existing research in psychology, nursing, and medicine is used to design learning experiences for patients, families, and communities. The same is true for developing, implementing and evaluating teaching and learning experiences for nursing students and staff. On the basis of the research findings, what does not work is eliminated, modifications are made grounded in additional research, and new programs are attempted and assessed. Educational accountability is stressed, and decisions about how to educate must be justified on the basis of data and research.

The applications of the learning theories and principles discussed in this chapter are illustrated by a number of research studies in nursing, psychology, education, and health care. It is the research that has allowed us to gain some confidence about choosing the most appropriate theories and principles for each educational experience, and it is the research that has helped us hone our approach to teaching and learning in the healthcare setting. Educational research has confirmed many of the constructs and principles from the various learning perspectives. It also has provided evidence to dispute some of the conventional wisdom and myths about learning—helping us realize that punishment is not generally effective and may inhibit learning; males are not necessarily more intelligent than females; and when teaching people, there are a number of strongly held realities that may or may not be rational, which strongly influence each learner's processing of the educational experience. The research on learning in general and health care in particular clearly demonstrates there is no one-size-fits-all approach to educating patients, nursing students, or nursing staff. To be effective, educational experiences need to be refined and tailored to each individual learner.

Though many advancements have been made in understanding the learning process over the past century, much remains unknown and requires careful research, such as why some patients and nursing students are so much more eager to learn than others, what can be done to encourage reluctant learners to change their attitudes or behavior, how the various learning theories and principles can work together for every learner, and how the healthcare setting changes the teaching/learning situation. In the future, more interdisciplinary efforts between psychologists and nurses are needed to move us toward a more sophisticated level of research and understanding that can be applied to the healthcare setting.

Research is not a panacea, however. Critics charge that the widely promoted research-based evidence approach to education and health care is jargonistic, places the emphasis on outcomes rather than on the process of learning, and oversimplifies the complexity of learning in any attempt to measure and evaluate it. The challenges of measurement are immense and require a highly sophisticated knowledge of research methods and their weaknesses. Another problem is the lack of resources, support, and well-trained personnel needed to truly implement and sustain a research-based approach to teaching and learning (Ferguson & Day, 2005).

Summary

This chapter demonstrates that learning is complex. Readers may feel overwhelmed by the diverse theories, sets of learning principles, and cautions associated with employing the various approaches. Yet, like the blind men exploring the elephant, each theory highlights an important dimension that affects the overall learning process, and together the theories provide a wealth of complementary strategies and alternative options. There is, of course, no single best way to approach learning, although all the theories indicate the need to be sensitive to the unique characteristics and motivations of each learner. For additional sources of information about psychological theories of learning and health care, see **Table 3–4**.

Educators in the health professions cannot be expected to know everything about the teaching and learning process. More importantly, perhaps, is that they can determine what needs to be known, where to find the necessary information, and how to help individuals, groups, and themselves benefit directly from a learning situation. Psychology and nursing work well together. Psychology has much to contribute to healthcare practice, and nursing is in a strategic position to apply and test psychological principles, constructs, and theories in both the educational and clinical settings.

Table 3–4 PSYCHOLOGICAL THEORIES OF LEARNING AND HEALTHCARE: LINKS

Internet Educational Psychology resources (ERIC):
http://www.lib.muohio.edu/edpsych/internetresources.html

McMaster University: Evidence-based medicine links:
http://www.mlanet.org/education/telecon/ebhc/resource.html

U.S. Department of Education: Evidence-Based Education help desk:
http://www.whatworkshelpdesk.ed.gov

American Psychological Association (search for learning topics):
http://www.apa.org

National Institutes of Health (search for patient education topics):
http://www.nih.gov

Learning Theory Resources (Nova Southeastern University):
http://www.nova.edu/~burmeist/learning_theory.html

Learning Theory links (emTech.net):
http://www.emtech.net/learning_theories.htm

Nursing Patient Education resources (about.com):
http://nursing.about.com/od/patienteducation/Patient_Education_Tools_and_Information_for_Nurses.htm

REVIEW QUESTIONS

1. What are the five major learning theories discussed in this chapter?
2. What are the principal constructs and contributions of each of the five learning theories?
3. According to the concept of operant conditioning, what are three techniques to increase the probability of a response, and what are two techniques to decrease or extinguish the probability of a response?
4. What are some ways the behaviorist theory (which focuses on the environment and responses to it) and the cognitive perspective (which emphasizes the individual's internal processing) could be combined to facilitate knowledge acquisition or change a health behavior?
5. What is meant by the term *gestalt,* and to which major learning theory is it associated?
6. Which learning theory is a combination of the principles from both the behaviorist and cognitive perspectives?
7. Which perspective is based primarily on the theory of motivation and stresses emotions rather than cognition and stimulus-response connections?
8. How do the major learning theories compare to one another with regard to their similarities and differences?
9. How does motivation serve as the critical influence on whether learning occurs or not?
10. What types of experiences may facilitate or hinder the learning process?
11. What factors help ensure that learning becomes relatively permanent?
12. What are some ways that emotions might be given more explicit consideration in nurses' education and in patient education?
13. How has neuroscience research contributed to our understanding of learning and learning theories?

References

Akers, R. L. (1989). Social learning theory and alcohol behavior among the elderly. *Sociological Quarterly, 30,* 625–638.

Anderson, O. R. (1997). A neurocognitive perspective on current learning theory and science instructional strategies. *Science Education, 81,* 67–89.

Bahn, D. (2001). Social learning theory: Its application to the context of nurse education. *Nurse Education Today, 21,* 110–117.

Bandura, A. (1977). *Social learning theory.* Englewood Cliffs, NJ: Prentice-Hall.

Bandura, A. (2001). Social cognitive theory: An agentic perspective. *Annual Review of Psychology, 52,* 1–26.

Barnard, A., Hollingum, C., & Hartfiel, B. (2006). Going on a journey: Understanding palliative care nursing. *International Journal of Palliative Nursing, 12,* 6–12.

Beck, M. H., Cataldo, M., Slifer, K. J., Pulbrook, V., & Guhman, J. K. (2005). Teaching children with attention deficit hyperactivity disorder (ADHD) and autistic disorder (AD) how to swallow pills. *Clinical Pediatrics, 44,* 515–526.

Berggren, I., & Severinsson, E. (2006). The significance of nurse supervisors' different ethical decision-making styles. *Journal of Nursing Management, 14,* 637–643.

Biderman, A. (2003). Family medicine as a frame for humanized medicine in education and clinical practice. *Public Health Review, 31,* 23–26.

Block, S., & Billings, J. A. (1998). Nurturing humanism through teaching palliative care. *Academic Medicine, 73,* 763–765.

Brackett, M. A., Lopes, P. N., Ivcevic, Z., Mayer, J. D., & Salovey, P. (2004). Integrating emotion and cognition: The role of emotional intelligence. In D. Y. Dai & R. J. Sternberg (Eds.), *Motivation, emotion, and cognition: Integrative perspectives on intellectual functioning and development* (pp. 175–194). Mahwah, NJ: Lawrence Erlbaum.

Bush, G. (2006). Learning about learning: From theories to trends. *Teacher Librarian, 34,* 14–18.

Byrnes, J. P. (2001). *Minds, brains, and learning: Understanding the psychological and educational relevance of neuroscientific research.* New York: Guilford.

Chochinov, H. M., & Breitbart, W. (Eds.). (2000). *Handbook of psychiatry in palliative medicine.* New York: Oxford University Press.

Dai, D. Y., & Sternberg, R. J. (Eds.). (2004). *Motivation, emotion, and cognition: Integrative perspectives on intellectual functioning and development.* Mahwah, NJ: Lawrence Erlbaum.

Deyl, S. G., & Kaliappan, K. V. (1997). Improvement of psychosomatic disorders among tension headache subjects using behaviour therapy and somatic inkblot series. *Journal of Projective Psychology and Mental Health, 4,* 113–120.

Duberstein, P. R., & Masling, J. M. (Eds.). (2000). *Psychodynamic perspectives on sickness and health.* Washington, DC: American Psychological Association.

Eccles, J. S., & Wigfield, A. (2002). Motivational beliefs, values, and goals. *Annual Review of Psychology, 53,* 109–132.

Erikson, E. (1968). *Identity: Youth and crisis.* New York: Norton.

Ferguson, L., & Day, R. A. (2005). Evidence-based nursing education: Myth or reality? *Journal of Nursing Education, 44,* 107–115.

Ferns, T. (2006). Under-reporting of violent incidents against nursing staff. *Nursing Standard, 20,* 41–45.

Fiske, S. T., & Taylor, S. E. (1991). *Social cognition.* New York: McGraw-Hill.

Fryer-Edwards, K., Arnold, R. M., Baile, W., Tulsky, J. A., Petracca, F., & Back, A. (2006). Reflective teaching practices: An approach to teaching communication skills in a small-group setting. *Academic Medicine, 81,* 638–644.

Gage, N. L., & Berliner, D. C. (1992). *Educational psychology* (5th ed.). Boston: Houghton Mifflin.

Gage, N. L., & Berliner, D. C. (1998). *Educational psychology* (6th ed.). Boston: Houghton Mifflin.

Gagné, R. M. (1985). *The conditions of learning* (4th ed.). New York: Holt, Rinehart & Winston.

Gagné, R. M., Briggs, L. J., & Wagner, W. W. (1992). *Principles of instructional design* (4th ed.). Fort Worth, TX: HBJ College Publishers.

Gallop, R., & O'Brien, L. (2003). Re-establishing psychodynamic theory as foundational knowledge for psychiatric/mental health nursing. *Issues in Mental Health Nursing, 24,* 213–227.

Gardner, H. (1978). *Developmental psychology: An introduction.* Boston: Little, Brown.

Gazzaniga, M. S. (Ed.). (2000). *The new cognitive neurosciences* (2nd ed.). Cambridge, MA: MIT Press.

Gilmartin, J. (2000). Psychodynamic sources of resistance among student nurses: Some observations in a human relations context. *Journal of Advanced Nursing, 32,* 1533–1541.

Goleman, D. (1995). *Emotional intelligence.* New York: Bantam Books.

Goodwin, A. M., & Gore, V. (2000). Managing the stresses of nursing people with severe and enduring mental illness: A psychodynamic observation study of a long-stay psychiatric ward. *British Journal of Medical Psychology, 73,* 311–325.

Grealy, L. (1994). *Anatomy of a face.* Boston: Houghton Mifflin.

Greene, J. D., Sommerville, R. B., Nystrom, L. E., Darley, J. M., & Cohen, J. D. (2001). An fMRI investigation of emotional engagement in moral judgment. *Science, 293,* 2105–2108.

Halpern, J. (2001). *From detached concern to empathy: Humanizing medical practice.* New York: Oxford University Press.

Hilgard, E. R. (1996). History of educational psychology. In D. C. Berliner & R. C. Calfee (Eds.), *Handbook of educational psychology* (pp. 990–1004). New York: Simon & Schuster Macmillan.

Hilgard, E. R., & Bower, G. H. (1966). *Theories of learning* (3rd ed.). New York: Appleton-Century-Crofts.

Hoffman, M. L. (2000). *Empathy and moral development: Implications for caring and justice.* New York: Cambridge University Press.

Holyoake, D. D. (1998). A little lady called Pandora: An exploration of philosophical traditions of humanism and existentialism in nursing ill children. *Child Care, Health and Development, 24,* 325–336.

Hooyman, N., & Kiyak, H. A. (2005). *Social gerontology* (7th ed.). Boston: Allyn & Bacon.

Hunt, R. R., Ellis, H. C., & Ellis, H. (2004). *Fundamentals of cognitive psychology* (7th ed.). New York: McGraw-Hill.

Imes, S. A., Clance, P. R., Gailis, A. T., & Atkeson, E. (2002). Mind's response to the body's betrayal: Gestalt/existential therapy for clients with chronic or life-threatening illnesses. *Journal of Clinical Psychology, 58,* 1361–1373.

Kane-Urrabazo, C. (2006). Management's role in shaping organizational culture. *Journal of Nursing Management, 14,* 188–194.

Kessels, R. P. C. (2003). Patients' memory of medical information. *Journal of the Royal Society of Medicine, 96,* 219–222.

Kohler, W. (1947). *Gestalt psychology.* New York: Mentor Books.

Kohler, W. (1969). *The task of gestalt psychology.* Princeton, NJ: Princeton University Press.

Kramer, D. A. (1983). Post-formal operations? A need for further conceptualization. *Human Development, 26,* 91–105.

Kübler-Ross, E. (1969). *On death and dying.* New York: Macmillan.

Malach-Pines, A. (2000). Nurses' burnout: An existential psychodynamic perspective. *Journal of Psychosocial Nursing and Mental Health Services, 38,* 23–31.

Marshall, H. H. (1998). Teaching educational psychology: Learner-centered constructivist perspectives. In N. M. Lambert & B. L. McCombs (Eds.), *How students learn: Reforming schools through learner-centered education* (pp. 449–473). Washington, DC: American Psychological Association.

Maslow, A. (1954). *Motivation and personality.* New York: Harper & Row.

Maslow, A. (1987). *Motivation and personality* (3rd ed.). New York: Harper & Row.

McCullough, L., & Andrews, S. (2001). Assimilative integration: Short-term dynamic psychotherapy for treating affect phobias. *Clinical Psychology Science and Practice, 8,* 82–97.

Menahern, S., & Halasz, G. (2000). Parental noncompliance—a paediatric dilemma: A medical and psychodynamic perspective. *Child Care, Health and Development, 26,* 61–72.

Moskowitz, G. B. (2005). *Social cognition: Understanding self and others.* New York: Guilford.

Murray, D. J. (1995). *Gestalt psychology and the cognitive revolution.* New York: Harvester Wheatsheaf.

Neary, M. (2000). Supporting students' learning and professional development through the process of continuous assessment and mentorship. *Nurse Education Today, 20,* 463–474.

Ormrod, J. E. (2004). *Human learning* (4th ed.). Upper Saddle River, NJ: Prentice-Hall.

Page, M. P. A. (2006). What can't functional neuroimaging tell the cognitive psychologist? *Cortex, 42,* 428–443.

Palincsar, A. S. (1998). Social constructivist perspectives on teaching and learning. *Annual Review of Psychology, 49,* 345–375.

Papadakis, A. A., Prince, R. P. O., Jones, N. P., & Strauman, T. J. (2006). Self-regulation, rumination, and vulnerability to depression in adolescent girls. *Developmental Psychopathology, 18,* 815–829.

Pearson, A. (2006). Powerful caring. *Nursing Standard, 20*(48), 20–22.

Pfeffer, J. (1985). Organizations and organizational theory. In G. Lindzey & E. Aronson (Eds.), *Handbook of social psychology: Vol. 1. Theory and method* (3rd ed., pp. 379–440). New York: Random House.

Phelps, E. Z. (2006). Emotion and cognition: Insights from studies of the human amygdala. *Annual Review of Psychology, 57,* 27–53.

Piaget, J., & Inhelder, B. (1969). *The psychology of the child* (H. Weaver, Trans.). New York: Basic Books.

Piane, G. (2000). Contingency contracting and systematic desensitization for heroin addicts in methadone maintenance programs. *Journal of Psychoactive Drugs, 32,* 311–319.

Proctor, R., Burns, A., Powell, H. S., & Tarrier, N. (1999). Behavioural management in nursing and residential homes: A randomized controlled trial. *Lancet, 354,* 26–29.

Pullen, M. L. (2002). Joe's story: Reflection on a difficult interaction between a nurse and a patient's wife. *International Journal of Palliative Nursing, 8,* 481–488.

Rogers, C. (1961). *On becoming a person.* Boston: Houghton Mifflin.

Rogers, C. (1994). *Freedom to learn* (3rd ed.). New York: Merrill.

Rogers, L. Q., Matevey, C., Hopkins-Price, P., Shah, P., Dunnington, G., & Courneya, K. S. (2004). Exploring social cognitive theory constructs for promoting exercise among breast cancer patients. *Cancer Nursing, 27,* 462–473.

Santrock, J. W. (2006). *Life-span development* (10th ed.). Boston: McGraw-Hill.

Shapiro, A. (2002). The latest dope on research (about constructivism): Part I: Different approaches to constructivism—What it's all about. *International Journal of Education Reform, 12,* 62–77.

Sherif, M., & Sherif, C. W. (1969). *Social psychology.* New York: Harper & Row.

Shors, T. J. (2006). Stressful experience and learning across the lifespan. *Annual Review of Psychology, 57,* 55–85.

Silverstein, S. M., & Uhlhaas, P. J. (2004). Gestalt psychology: The forgotten paradigm in abnormal psychology. *American Journal of Psychology, 117,* 259–277.

Skinner, B. F. (1974). *About behaviorism.* New York: Vintage Books.

Skinner, B. F. (1989). *Recent issues in the analysis of behavior.* Columbus, OH: Merrill.

Slipp, S. (2000). Subliminal stimulation research and its implications for psychoanalytic theory and treatment. *Journal of the American Academy of Psychoanalysis, 28,* 305–320.

Snowman, J., & Biehler, R. (2006). *Psychology applied to teaching* (11th ed.). Boston: Houghton Mifflin.

Sternberg, R. J. (1996). Styles of thinking. In P. B. Baltes & U. M. Staudinger (Eds.), *Interactive minds: Life-span perspectives on the social foundation of cognition* (pp. 347–365). New York: Cambridge University Press.

Sternberg, R. J. (2006). *Cognitive psychology* (4th ed.). Belmont, CA: Thomson/Wadsworth.

Stiles, A. S. (2005). Parenting needs, goals, & strategies of adolescent mothers. *MCN American Journal of Maternal/Child Nursing, 30,* 327–333.

Stockhurst, U., Steingrueber, H. J., Enck, P., & Klosterhalfen, S. (2006). Pavlovian conditioning of nausea and vomiting. *Autonomic Neuroscience, 129,* 50–57.

Stroebe, M. S., Folkman, S., Hansson, R. O., & Schut, H. (2006). The prediction of bereavement outcome: Development of an integrative risk factor framework. *Social Science and Medicine, 63,* 2440–2451.

Telford, K., Kralik, D., & Koch, T. (2006). Acceptance and denial: Implications for people adapting to chronic illness. Literature review. *Journal of Advanced Nursing, 55,* 457–464.

Tennant, M. (2006). *Psychology and adult learning* (3rd ed.). New York: Routledge.

Vander Zanden, J. W., Crandell, T. L., & Crandell, C. H. (2007). *Human development* (8th ed.). Boston: McGraw-Hill.

Vygotsky, L. S. (1986). *Thought and language.* Cambridge, MA: MIT Press.

Wolpe, J. (1982). *The practice of behavior therapy* (3rd ed.). New York: Pergamon.

Woolfolk, A. E. (2001). *Educational psychology.* Boston: Allyn & Bacon.

Part Two

Characteristics of the Learner

Chapter 4

Determinants of Learning

Sharon Kitchie

CHAPTER HIGHLIGHTS

KEY TERMS

- ❏ determinants of learning
- ❏ learning needs
- ❏ readiness to learn
- ❏ learning styles

OBJECTIVES

After completing this chapter, the reader will be able to

1. State the nurse educator's role in the learning process.

2. Identify the three components of what is known as *determinants of learning*.

3. Describe the steps involved in the assessment of learning needs.

4. Explain methods that can be used to assess learner needs.

5. Discuss the factors that need to be assessed in each of the four types of readiness to learn.

6. Describe what is meant by learning styles.

7. Discriminate between the major learning style models and instruments identified.

8. Discuss ways to assess learning styles.

9. Identify the evidence that supports assessment of learning needs, readiness to learn, and learning styles.

In a variety of settings, nurses are responsible for the education of patients, families, nursing staff, and nursing students. Numerous factors make the nurse educator's role particularly challenging in meeting the information needs of these various groups of learners. For example, same-day surgery has compressed patient and family contact with the nurse. Often the teachable moment is hard to capture because of shortened hospital stays. In the case of staff, their educational and experiential levels differ widely and time constraints are ever present in the practice arena. Staffing patterns such as 10- or 12-hour shifts, part-time employment, and various job functions can put the educator's ability to complete an accurate education assessment of staff to the test. Also, the ethnic and racial composition of nursing students has been changing in recent years (Heller, Oros, & Durney-Crowley, 2000). In addition, students are entering schools of nursing at an older age, bringing with them diverse life experiences and the demands of working and raising families while furthering their education. These and other changing healthcare trends and population demographics mean that the nurse educator must constantly assess the determinants of learning for the varied audience of learners whom they have the responsibility to teach.

To meet these challenges, the nurse educator must beware of what factors influence how well an individual learns. The three *determinants of learning* that require assessment are (1) the needs of the learner, (2) the state of readiness to learn, and (3) the preferred learning styles for processing information. This chapter will address these three determinants of learning as they impact on the effective and efficient delivery of patient, student, and staff education.

The Educator's Role in Learning

The role of educating others is one of the most essential interventions that a nurse performs. To do it well, the nurse must identify the information learners need as well as consider their readiness to learn and their styles of learning. The learner, not the teacher, is the single most important person in the education process. Learning can be greatly enhanced by the educator serving as a facilitator in helping the learner become aware of what needs to be known, the value of knowing, and how to be actively involved in acquiring information (Musinski, 1999). Just providing information to the learner, however, does not ensure that learning will occur. There is no guarantee that the learner will learn the information given, although there is more of an opportunity to learn if the educator assesses the determinants of learning.

Assessment permits the nurse educator to facilitate the process of learning by arranging experiences within the environment that assist the learner to find the purpose, the will, and the most suitable approaches for learning. An assessment of the three determinants enables the educator to identify information and present it in a variety of ways, which a learner cannot do alone. Manipulating the environment allows learners to experience meaningful parts and wholes to reach their individual potentials.

The educator plays a crucial role in the learning process by:

- Assessing problems or deficits.
- Providing important information and presenting it in unique and appropriate ways.
- Identifying progress being made.
- Giving feedback and follow-up.
- Reinforcing learning in the acquisition of new knowledge, skills, and attitudes.
- Evaluating learners' abilities.

The educator is vital in giving support, encouragement, and direction during the process of learning. Learners may make self-choices without the assistance of an educator, but these choices may be limited or inappropriate. For example, the nurse facilitates necessary changes in the home environment, such as minimizing distractions by having family members turn off the television, to provide a quiet environment conducive for concentrating on a learning activity. The educator assists in identifying optimal learning approaches and activities that can both support and challenge the learner based on his or her individual learning needs, readiness to learn, and learning style.

Assessment of the Learner

Nursing assessment of learners' needs, readiness, and styles of learning is the first and most important step in instructional design—but it is also the step most likely to be neglected. The importance of assessment of the learner may seem self-evident, yet often only lip service is given to this initial phase of the educational process. Frequently, the nurse delves into teaching before addressing all of the determinants of learning. It is not unusual that patients with the same condition are taught with the same materials in the same way (Haggard, 1989). The result is that information given to the patient is neither individualized nor based on an adequate educational assessment. Recent evidence suggests, however, that individualizing teaching based on prior assessment improves patient outcomes (Corbett, 2003; Kim et al., 2004; Miaskowski et al., 2004). For example, Corbett's research demonstrates that providing individualized education to home care patients with diabetes significantly improves their foot care practices.

For years nurses have been taught that any nursing intervention should be preceded by an assessment. Few would deny that this is the correct approach, no matter whether planning for giving direct physical care, meeting the psychosocial needs of a patient, or teaching someone to be independent in self-care or in the delivery of care. The effectiveness of nursing care clearly depends on the scope, accuracy, and comprehensiveness of assessment prior to interventions.

What is it about assessment that is so significant and fundamental to the educational process? This initial step in the process validates the need for learning and the approaches to be used in designing learning experiences. Patients who desire or require information to maintain optimal health or staff nurses who must have a greater scope or depth of knowledge to deliver quality care to patients deserve to have an assessment done by the educator so that their needs as learners are appropriately addressed.

Assessments do more than simply identify and prioritize information for purposes of setting behavioral goals and objectives, planning instructional interventions, and being able to evaluate in the long run whether the learner has achieved the desired goals and objectives. Good assessments ensure that optimal learning will occur with the least amount of stress and anxiety for the learner. Assessment prevents needless repetition of known material, saves time and energy on the part of both the learner and the educator, and helps to establish rapport between the two parties (Haggard, 1989). Furthermore, it increases the motivation to learn by focusing on what the patient or staff member feels is most important to know or to be able to do.

Why, then, is this first step in the education process so overlooked or only partially carried out? Lack of time is the number one reason for nurse educators to shortchange the assessment phase. Such factors as shortened hospital stays and limited contact in other settings with patients and families as well as tighter schedules of nursing staff as a result of increased practice demands have reduced the amount of time available for instruction. Because time constraints are a major concern when carrying out patient or staff education, nurses must become skilled in accurately conducting assessments of the three determinants of learning so as to have reserve time for actual teaching. In addition, many nurses, although expected and required by their nurse practice acts to instruct others, are unfamiliar with the principles of teaching and learning. The nurse in the role of educator must become more acquainted and comfortable with all the elements of instructional design, but particularly with the assessment phase, since it provides the foundation for the rest of the educational process.

Assessment of the learner includes attending to the following three determinants (Haggard, 1989):

1. Learning needs—what the learner needs and wants to learn.
2. Readiness to learn—when the learner is receptive to learning.
3. Learning style—how the learner best learns.

Assessing Learning Needs

Learning needs are defined as gaps in knowledge that exist between a desired level of performance and the actual level of performance (Healthcare Education Association, 1985). A learning need is the gap between what someone knows and what someone needs or wants to know. Such gaps exist because of a lack of knowledge, attitude, or skill.

Of the three determinants, learning needs must be identified first so that an instructional plan can be designed to address any deficits in the cognitive, affective, or psychomotor domains. Once it is discovered what needs to be taught, a determination can be made about when and how learning can most optimally occur.

Not every individual perceives a need for education. Often, learners are not aware of what they don't know or want to know. Consequently, it is up to the educator to assist them in identifying, clarifying, and prioritizing their needs and interests. Once this is determined, the information gathered can, in turn, be used to set objectives and plan appropriate and effective teaching and learning approaches for education to begin at a point suitable to the learner rather than from an unknown or inappropriate place.

Significant differences have been found to exist between the perception of needs identified by patients versus the needs identified by nurses caring for them. In one early study, there was only a 20% nurse–patient agreement score with respect to congruency on needs/problems identified (Roberts, 1982). Mordiffi, Tan, and Wong (2003) cite more recent evidence from their research that the preoperative information provided by nurses and doctors was considered insufficient by the majority (66.7%) of patients who rated knowledge about anesthesia before scheduled surgery to be very or extremely important to them. Other authors also substantiate comparative incongruence in the perception of learning needs by patients and providers (Carlson, Ivnik, Dierkhising, O'Byrne, & Vickers, 2006; Kiesler & Auerbach, 2006; Suhonen, Nenonen, Laukka, & Valimaki, 2005; Timmins, 2005).

According to the estimates of many cognitive experts in behavior and social sciences (Bloom, 1968; Bruner, 1966; Carroll, 1963; Kessels, 2003; Ley, 1979; Skinner, 1954) most learners—90–95% of them, can master a subject with a high degree of success if given sufficient time and appropriate support. It is the task of the educator to facilitate the determination of what exactly needs to be learned and identify approaches for presenting information in a way that will be best understood by the learner.

The following are important steps in the assessment of learning needs:

1. *Identify the learner.* Who is the audience? If the audience is one individual, is there a single need or do many needs have to be fulfilled? Is there more than one learner? If so, are their needs congruent or diverse? The development of formal and informal education programs for patients and their families, nursing staff, or students must be based on accurate identification of the learner. For example, an educator may believe that all postpartum mothers need a formal class on safety issues for the newborn. This perception may be based on the educator's interaction with a few patients and may not be true of all postpartum

mothers. Or the manager of a healthcare agency might request an in-service workshop for all staff on documentation of infection control because of an isolated incident involving one staff member's failing to appropriately follow established infection control techniques. This break in protocol may or may not indicate that everyone needs to have an update on policies and procedures.

2. *Choose the right setting.* Establishing a trusting environment will help learners feel a sense of security in confiding information, believe their concerns are taken seriously and considered important, and feel respected. Assuring privacy and confidentiality is recognized as essential to establishing a trusting relationship.

3. *Collect data about the learner.* Once the learner is identified, the educator can determine characteristic needs of the population by exploring typical health problems or issues of interest to that population. Subsequently, a literature search can assist in identifying the type and extent of content to be included in teaching sessions as well as the educational strategies for teaching a specific population based on the analysis of needs. For example, Bibb (2001) collected data about a targeted patient population at one military treatment facility and found that education programs did not provide adequate support for the growing number of older, more chronically ill participants. Rutten, Arora, Bakos, Aziz, and Rowland (2005) studied cancer patients to determine the characteristic learning needs of that population.

4. *Collect data from the learner.* Learners are usually the most important source of needs assessment data about themselves. Allow the patient and/or family members to identify what is important to them, what they perceive their needs to be, what types of social support systems are available, and what assistance these supports can provide. If the audience for teaching consists of staff members or students, solicit them for information as to those areas of practice in which they feel they need new or additional information. Actively engaging learners in defining their own problems and needs motivates them to learn because they have an investment in planning for a program specifically tailored to their unique circumstances. Also, the learner is important to include as a source of information since, as noted previously, the educator may not always perceive the same learning needs as the learner.

5. *Involve members of the healthcare team.* Other healthcare professionals will likely have insight into patient or family needs or the educational needs of the nursing staff or students as a result of their frequent contacts with consumers as well as caregivers. Nurses are not the sole teachers, and they must remember to collaborate with other members of the healthcare team for a richer assessment of learning needs. In addition, associations such as the American Heart Association, the American Diabetes Association, and the American Cancer Society are examples of organizations that are excellent sources of health-related information.

6. *Prioritize needs.* A list of identified needs can become endless and seemingly impossible to accomplish. Maslow's (1970) hierarchy of human needs may help the educator with prioritizing (**Figure** 4–1) so that the learner's basic needs are attended to first and foremost before higher needs can be met. For example, learning about a low-sodium diet will not occur if a patient faces problems with basic physiological needs such as pain and discomfort. These latter needs must be addressed before any other higher order learning can occur.

Setting priorities for learning is often difficult when the nurse educator is faced with many learning needs in several areas. An effort to prioritize the identified needs will help the patient or nursing staff to set realistic and achievable learning goals. Choosing what information to cover is imperative, and choices must be made deliberately. Learning needs must be prioritized based on the criteria in **Table** 4–1 (Healthcare Education Association, 1985, p. 23) to foster maximum learning.

Not all learners need to know everything, and good assessment skills can help to discriminate the need to know from the nice to know information. If patients want to know the pathophysiology of their disease, that curiosity is

Figure 4–1 Maslow's hierarchy of needs.

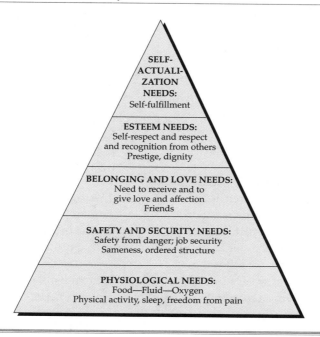

SELF-ACTUALI-ZATION NEEDS:
Self-fulfillment

ESTEEM NEEDS:
Self-respect and respect and recognition from others
Prestige, dignity

BELONGING AND LOVE NEEDS:
Need to receive and to give love and affection
Friends

SAFETY AND SECURITY NEEDS:
Safety from danger; job security
Sameness, ordered structure

PHYSIOLOGICAL NEEDS:
Food—Fluid—Oxygen
Physical activity, sleep, freedom from pain

Source: Reprinted from Lafleur-Brooks, M. (1979). *Health unit coordinating.* Philadelphia: W.B. Saunders, p. 48.

Table 4–1   CRITERIA FOR PRIORITIZING LEARNING NEEDS

Mandatory: Needs that must be learned for survival or situations in which the learner's life or safety is threatened. Learning needs in this category must be met immediately. For example, a patient who has experienced a recent heart attack needs to know the signs and symptoms and when to get immediate help. The nurse who works in a hospital must learn how to do cardiopulmonary resuscitation or be able to carry out correct isolation techniques for self-protection.

Desirable: Needs that are not life dependent but are related to well-being or the overall ability to provide quality care in situations involving changes in institutional procedure. For example, it is important for patients who have cardiovascular disease to

understand the effects of a high-fat diet on their condition. It is desirable for nurses to update their knowledge by attending an in-service program when hospital management decides to focus more attention on the appropriateness of patient education materials in relation to the patient populations being served.

Possible: Needs for information that are nice to know but not essential or required or situations in which the learning need is not directly related to daily activities. The patient who is newly diagnosed as having diabetes mellitus most likely does not need to know about traveling across time zones or staying in a foreign country because this information does not relate to the patient's everyday activities.

---

fine, but it is not fundamental to learning how to carry out self-care activities that are essential for discharge from the hospital. A helpful analogy to remember is, "One does not have to know how an engine works to be able to drive a car." Often, highly technical information will serve only to confuse and distract patients from learning what they need to know to comply with their regimen (Hansen & Fisher, 1998; Kessels, 2003).

Education in and of itself is not always the answer to a problem. Often, healthcare providers believe that more education is necessary when something goes wrong, when something is not being done, when a patient is not following a prescribed regimen, or when a staff member does not adhere to a protocol. In such instances, always look for other nonlearning needs. For example, the nurse may discover that the patient is not taking his

medication and may begin a teaching plan without adequate assessment. The patient may already understand the importance of taking a prescribed medication, know how to administer it, and be willing to follow regimen, but he may not have the finances necessary to purchase the medication. In this case, the patient does not have a learning need but rather requires social or financial support to obtain the medication.

7. *Determine availability of educational resources.* A need may be identified, but it may be useless to proceed with interventions if the proper educational resources are not available, are unrealistic to obtain, or do not match the learner's needs. In this case, it may be better to focus on other identified needs. For example, a patient who has asthma needs to learn how to use an

inhaler and peak-flow meter. The nurse educator may determine that this patient learns best if the nurse first gives a demonstration on the use of the inhaler and peak-flow meter and then allows the patient the opportunity to do a return demonstration. If the proper equipment is not available for demonstration/return demonstration at that moment, it might be better for the nurse educator to concentrate on teaching the signs and symptoms the patient might experience when having poor air exchange than to cancel the encounter altogether. Thereafter, the educator would work immediately on obtaining the necessary equipment for future encounters.

8. *Assess demands of the organization.* This assessment will yield information that reflects the climate of the organization. What are the organization's philosophy, mission, strategic plan, and goals? The educator should be familiar with standards of performance required in various employee categories, along with job descriptions and hospital, professional, and agency regulations. If, for example, the organization is focused on health promotion versus trauma care, then there likely will be a different educational focus or emphasis that dictates learning needs of both consumers and employees.

9. *Take time-management issues into account.* Because time constraints are a major impediment to the assessment process, Rankin and Stallings (2005) suggest the educator should emphasize the following important points with respect to time-management issues:

- Although close observation and active listening take time, it is much more efficient and effective to do a good initial assessment than to waste time going back to discover the obstacles to learning that prevented progress in the first place.

- Learners must be given time to offer their own perceptions of their learning needs if the educator expects them to take charge and become actively involved in the learning process.

- Assessment can be made anytime and anywhere the educator has formal or informal contact with learners. Data collection does not have to be restricted to a specific, predetermined schedule. With patients, many potential opportunities arise, such as when giving a bath, serving a meal, making rounds, distributing medications, and so forth. For staff, assessments can be made when stopping to talk in the hallway or while enjoying lunch or break time together.

- Informing someone ahead of time that the educator wishes to spend time discussing problems or needs gives the person advanced notice to sort out his or her thoughts and feelings.

- Minimizing interruptions and distractions during planned assessment interviews maximizes productivity such that the educator might accomplish in 15 minutes what otherwise might have taken an hour in less directed, more frequently interrupted circumstances.

Methods to Assess Learning Needs

The nurse in the role of educator must obtain objective data about the learner as well as subjective data from the learner. The following are various methods that can be used to assess learner needs and should be used in conjunction with one another to yield the most reliable information (Haggard, 1989).

Informal Conversations

Often learning needs will be discovered during impromptu conversations that take place with other healthcare team members involved in the care of the client, and between the nurse and the patient or his or her family. The nurse educator must rely on active listening. Nursing staff can provide valuable input about what they perceive to be their learning. Posing open-ended questions will encourage learners to reveal information about what they perceive their learning needs to be.

Structured Interviews

The structured interview is perhaps the most common form of needs assessment to solicit the learner's point of view. The nurse asks the learner direct and often predetermined questions to gather information about learning needs. As with the gathering of any information from a learner in the assessment phase, the nurse should strive to establish a trusting environment, use open-ended questions, choose a setting that is free of distractions, and allow the learner to state what are believed to be the learning needs.

It is important to remain nonjudgmental when collecting information about the learner's strengths, beliefs, and motivations. Notes should be taken with the learner's permission, so important information is not lost. The telephone is a good tool to use for an interview if it is impossible to ask questions in person. The major drawback of a telephone interview, however, is the inability on the part of the nurse educator to perceive nonverbal cues from the learner.

Interviews yield answers that may reveal uncertainties, conflicts, inconsistencies, unexpected problems, anxieties, fears, and present knowledge base. Examples of questions that could be asked of a patient as learner are as follows:

- What do you think caused your problem?
- How severe is your illness?
- What does your illness/health mean to you?
- What do you do to stay healthy?
- What results do you hope to obtain from treatments?
- What are your strengths and weaknesses?

If the learner is a staff member or student, the following questions could be asked:

- What do you think are your biggest challenges to learning?
- Which skill(s) do you need help in performing?
- What obstacles have you encountered in the past when you were learning new information?
- What do you see as your strengths and weaknesses as a learner?

These types of questions help to determine the needs of the learner and serve as a foundation for beginning to plan for an educational intervention.

Focus Groups

Focus groups involve getting together a small number (4 to 12) of potential learners (Breitrose, 1988) to determine areas of educational need by using group discussion to identify points of view or knowledge about a certain topic. A facilitator leads the discussion by asking questions that are open ended to encourage detailed discussion. These groups of potential learners in most cases should be homogeneous with similar characteristics such as age, gender, and past experience with the topic under discussion. However, if the purpose of the focus group is to solicit attitudes about a particular subject or to discuss ethical issues, for example, it may not be necessary nor recommended to have a homogeneous group. Focus groups are ideal during the initial stage of information gathering to provide qualitative data for a complete assessment of learning needs.

Self-Administered Questionnaires

The learner's written responses to questions about learning needs can be obtained by survey instruments. Checklists are one of the most common forms of questionnaires. They are easy to administer, provide more privacy than interviews, and yield easy-to-tabulate data. Learners seldom object to this method of obtaining information about their learning needs. Sometimes learners may have difficulty rating themselves and may need the educator to clarify terms or provide additional information to help them understand what is being assessed. The educator's role is to encourage learners to make as honest a self-assessment as possible. Because checklists usually reflect what the nurse educa-

tor perceives as needs, there should also be a space for the learner to add any other items of interest or concern.

One example of a highly reliable and valid self-assessment tool is the patient learning needs scale (Redman, 2003). This instrument is designed to measure patients' perceptions of learning needs to manage their health care at home following a medical or surgical illness (Bubela et al., 2000).

Tests

Giving written pretests before teaching is planned can help identify the knowledge levels of potential learners regarding a particular subject and assist in identifying their specific learning needs. Also, this approach prevents the educator from repeating already known material in the teaching plan. Furthermore, pretest results are useful to the educator after the completion of teaching to determine whether learning has taken place by comparing pretest scores to posttest scores.

The diabetes knowledge test is an example of a tool available to assess learning needs for self-management of diabetes (Panja, Starr, & Colleran, 2005). These researchers compared patients' diabetes knowledge with their glycemic control. Their findings demonstrate that an inverse linear relationship exists between performance on this diabetes test and HbA1c values. This test is available at the Michigan Diabetes Research and Training Center (http://www.med.umich.edu/mdrtc/survey/index.html). Redman (2003) describes this and many other measurement instruments for patient education that measure knowledge and learning assessment/design/delivery.

The educator must always consider the reported characteristics of the self-administered questionnaire or test before using it. The criteria to consider are: for what the tool was designed (i.e., if it is relevant to what the nurse educator is now wanting to assess), whether the results will be meaningful, whether each of the measured constructs is well defined, if adequate testing of the instrument has been conducted, whether the instrument has been used in a similar setting, and if the instrument has been used with a population similar to the educator's. The educator needs to consider the purpose, conceptual basis, development, and psychometric properties when evaluating the adequacy of any questionnaire or test (Waltz, Strickland, & Lenz, 2005).

Observations

Observing health behaviors in several different time periods can help to determine conclusions about established patterns of behavior that cannot and should not be drawn from a single observation. Actually watching the learner perform a skill more than once is an excellent way of assessing a psychomotor need. Are all steps performed correctly? Is there any difficulty with manipulating various equipment? Does the learner require prompting? Learners may believe they can accurately perform a skill or task (e.g., walking with crutches, changing a dressing, giving an injection), but the educator can best determine if additional learning may be needed by observing the skill performance.

Learners who observe themselves performing a skill that is videotaped can more easily identify their learning needs. This process is known as reflection on action (Grant, 2002). The learner identifies what was done well and what could have been done better in his or her actual performance. Evidence to support this method of assessing learning needs is suggested in a study by Landry, Smith, and Swank (2006), who conducted an experimental intervention measuring

mothers' critique of their own videotaped responsive behaviors in the home setting that would facilitate their infants' development.

Patient Charts

Physicians' progress notes, nursing care plans, nurses' notes, and discharge planning forms can provide information on the learning needs of clients. The nurse educator needs to follow a consistent format from chart to chart so that each chart is reviewed in the same manner to identify learning needs based on the same information. Also, documentation by other members of the healthcare team, such as physical therapists, social workers, respiratory therapists, and nutritionists, can yield valuable insights with respect to the needs of the learner.

Assessing Learning Needs of Nursing Staff

Williams (1998) specifically addressed the importance of identifying the learning needs of staff nurses using the following methods:

WRITTEN JOB DESCRIPTIONS

A written description of what is required to effectively carry out job responsibilities can reflect the potential learning needs of staff. This information forms the basis of establishing content in an orientation program for new staff or of designing continuing education opportunities for seasoned nurses.

FORMAL AND INFORMAL REQUESTS

Often staff will be asked for ideas for educational programs, which reflect what they perceive as needs. When conducting a formal educational program, the educator must verify that these requests are congruent with the needs of other staff members.

QUALITY ASSURANCE REPORTS

Trends found in incident reports indicating safety violations or errors in procedures are a source for establishing learning needs of staff that education can address.

CHART AUDITS

Trends in practice can be identified through chart auditing. Does the staff have a learning need in terms of the actual charting? Is a new intervention being implemented? Does the record indicate some inconsistency with implementation of an intervention?

RULES AND REGULATIONS

A thorough knowledge of hospital, professional, and healthcare requirements helps to identify possible learning needs of staff. The educator should monitor new rules of practice arising from changes occurring within an institution or external to the organization that may have implications for the delivery of care.

FOUR-STEP APPRAISAL OF NEEDS

Panno (1992), expanding on Knox's (1974, 1977, 1986) interest in teaching related to adult development and learning, described a systematic approach for assessing learning needs of caregivers and the organizations in which they practice. Knox's interpretation of how adults learn has led to information for the development and coordination of education programs that would be responsive to the backgrounds and aspirations of various adult learners. Panno's four steps in assessing learning needs include:

1. Defining the target population.
2. Analyzing learner and organizational needs.
3. Analyzing the perceived needs of the learner and comparing these to the actual needs.

4. Using data to prioritize learning needs identified.

This organizing framework can be used to assess multiple caregiver levels, from registered nurse to the nursing assistant, which are typically the target audiences for in-service programs within an institution. Panno (1992) pointed out that often plans for educational activities are based on personal preference, mandates from administration, intuition, or trends in the profession, which may meet the sponsor's needs but not the needs of the learner. This systematic approach is useful because it benefits all involved and is a process that justifies the resources required for the assessment process.

Readiness to Learn

Once learning needs have been identified, the next step is to determine the learner's readiness to receive information. *Readiness to learn* can be defined as the time when the learner demonstrates an interest in learning the information necessary to maintain optimal health or to become more skillful in a job. Often, educators have noted that when a patient or staff member asks a question, the time is prime for learning. Readiness to learn occurs when the learner is receptive, willing, and able to participate in the learning process. Rarely is someone not ready to learn. It is the responsibility of the educator to discover through assessment exactly when patients or staff are ready to learn, what they need or want to learn, and adapt the content to fit each learner.

Assessing readiness to learn requires the educator to first understand what needs to be taught, then collect and validate that information, and then apply the same methods that were used to assess learning needs, such as making observations, conducting interviews, gathering information from the learner as well as other healthcare team members, and reviewing written data in charts. This must be done prior to the time when actual learning is to occur.

No matter how important the information is or how much the educator feels the recipient of teaching needs the information, if the learner is not ready, the information will not be absorbed. The educator, in conjunction with the learner, must determine what needs to be learned and what the learning objectives should be to establish which domain and at what level these objectives should be classified. Otherwise both the educator's and the learner's time could very well be wasted, because the established objectives may be beyond the readiness of the learner.

Timing—that is, the point at which teaching should take place—is very important. Anything that affects physical or psychological comfort can affect a learner's ability and willingness to learn. A learner who is not receptive to information at one time may be more receptive to the same information at another time. Because the nurse often has limited contact with patients and family members due to short hospital stays or a one-hour visit in the outpatient setting, teaching must be brief and basic. Timing also is an important factor with the nursing staff. Readiness to learn is based on current demands of practice and needs to correspond to the ever constant changes in health care. Adults, whether patients, family, nursing staff, or students, are eager to learn when the subject of teaching is relevant and applicable to their everyday concerns.

Before teaching can begin, the educator must find the time to first take a PEEK (Lichtenthal, 1990) at the four types of readiness to learn— physical readiness, emotional readiness, experiential readiness, and knowledge readiness. These four types of readiness to learn, which may be obstacles or enhancers to learning, must be taken into consideration (**Table 4–2**).

Physical Readiness

Five major components to physical readiness— measures of ability, complexity of task, environ-

---

Table 4–2 TAKE TIME TO TAKE A PEEK AT THE FOUR TYPES OF READINESS TO LEARN

P = PHYSICAL READINESS
- Measures of ability
- Complexity of task
- Environmental effects
- Health status
- Gender

E = EMOTIONAL READINESS
- Anxiety level
- Support system
- Motivation
- Risk-taking behavior
- Frame of mind
- Developmental stage

E = EXPERIENTIAL READINESS
- Level of aspiration
- Past coping mechanisms
- Cultural background
- Locus of control
- Orientation

K = KNOWLEDGE READINESS
- Present knowledge base
- Cognitive ability
- Learning disabilities
- Learning styles

Source: From Lichtenthal, C. (1990, August). *A self-study model on readiness to learn.* Reprinted with permission from Cheryl Lichtenthal Harding. Unpublished manuscript.

mental effects, health status, and gender—must be considered by the educator because they impact on the degree or extent to which learning will occur.

MEASURES OF ABILITY

Ability to perform a task requires fine and/or gross motor movements, sensory acuity, adequate strength, flexibility, coordination, and endurance. Each developmental stage in life is characterized by physical and sensory abilities or is affected by individual disabilities. For example, walking on crutches is a psychomotor skill for which a patient must have the physical ability to be ready to learn. If a person has a visual deficit, eyeglasses or a magnifying glass should be available to allow the patient, for example, to see the lines on an insulin syringe. If the educator is conducting an in-service workshop on lifting and transfer activities, staff must have the endurance level required to return demonstrate this skill. Creating a stimulating and accepting environment by using instructional tools to match learners' physical and sensory abilities will encourage readiness to learn.

COMPLEXITY OF TASK

Variations in the complexity of the task will affect the extent to which behavioral changes in the cognitive, affective, and psychomotor domains can be mastered by the learner. The more complex the task, the more difficult it is to achieve. Psychomotor skills, once acquired, are usually retained better and longer than learning in the other domains (Greer, Hitt, Sitterly, & Slebodnick, 1972). Once ingrained, psychomotor, cognitive, and affective behaviors become habitual and may be difficult to alter. For example, if the learner has been performing a psychomotor skill over a long period of time and

then the procedural steps of the task change, the learner will need to unlearn those steps and relearn a new way. This requirement may increase the complexity of the task and put additional physical demands on the learner as a result of lengthening the time needed to adjust to doing something in a new way. Older adults, in particular, have developed elaborate cognitive schemas over the years, and when they are faced with information contrary to their preexisting knowledge and beliefs, they will find the effort to change both difficult, confusing, and time consuming (Kessels, 2003).

ENVIRONMENTAL EFFECTS

An environment conducive to learning will help to keep the learner's attention and stimulate interest in learning. Unfavorable conditions, such as extremely high levels of noise or frequent interruptions, can interfere with the accuracy and precision in performing cognitive and manual dexterity tasks. Intermittent noise tends to have greater disruptive effects on learning than the more rapidly habituated steady-state noise. McDonald, Wiczorek, and Walker (2004) examined background noise and interruption for these effects on college students to learn health information. The results of their research suggest that distraction, including noise, during health teaching adversely affects readiness to learn.

The older adult, in particular, needs more time to react and respond to stimuli. The increased inability to receive, process, and transmit information is a characteristic of aging. Environmental demands requiring older persons to feel rushed or to perform tasks within a short time frame can overwhelm them. When an activity is self-paced, the older learner will respond more favorably.

HEALTH STATUS

The amount of energy available, as well as an individual's present comfort level, are factors significantly influencing that individual's readiness to learn. Energy-reducing demands caused by the body's response to illness require the learner to expend large amounts of physical and psychic energy, with little reserve left for actual learning. A person's health status, whether well, acutely ill, or chronically ill, must be taken into serious consideration when assessing for readiness.

Healthy learners have energy available for learning. Readiness to learn about health-promoting behaviors is based on their perception of self-responsibility (See Chapter 6 on Health Belief and Health Promotion Models). The extent to which an illness is perceived to potentially affect future well-being influences someone's desire to learn both preventive and promotion measures. If learners perceive a threat to their quality of life, more information likely will be sought in an attempt to control the negative effects of an illness (Bubela & Galloway, 1990).

Learners who are acutely ill tend to focus their energies on the physiological and psychological demands of their illness. Learning is at a minimum because most of these individuals' energy is needed for the demands of the illness and gaining immediate relief. Any learning that may occur should be related to treatments, tests, and minimizing pain or other discomforts. As these patients improve and the acute phase of illness diminishes, they can then focus on learning follow-up management and the avoidance of complications.

The educator must assess an acutely ill person's readiness to learn by observing his or her energy levels and comfort status. Improvement in physical status usually results in more receptivity to learning. However, medications that induce side effects such as drowsiness, mental depression, impaired depth perception, decreased ability to concentrate, and learner fatigue will also reduce task-handling capacity. For example, giving a patient a sedative prior to a learning experience may result in less apprehension, but cognitive and psychomotor abilities may be impaired. Thus, physical safety is a major concern, and mastery of a skill requires a longer time, more physical output, and more frustration for the learner (Greer et al., 1972).

Chronic illness, on the other hand, has no time limits and is of long-term duration. Models of how people deal with chronic illness also are useful as frameworks for understanding readiness to learn (Lubkin & Larsen, 2006). The physiological and psychological demands vary in chronic illness and are not always predictable. Patients go through different stages in dealing with their illness similar to the adjustment stages for a person experiencing a loss (Boyd, Gleit, Graham, & Whitman, 1998). If the learner is in the avoidance stage, readiness to learn will be limited to simple explanations, because the patient's energy is concentrated on denial. Energy levels will stabilize and become redirected as awareness of the realities of the situation increase. Readiness to learn may be indicated by the questions the patient asks. Burton (2000) describes the Corbin and Strauss (1991) chronic illness trajectory framework. This framework reflects the continual nature of adaptation required in living with chronic illness.

Unlike the Corbin and Strauss model, Patterson (2001) describes a shifting perspectives model that suggests living with chronic illness is an ongoing and continually dynamic process. This model provides an explanation of chronically ill persons' variations in their attention to symptoms over time. The individual's perspective shifts in the degree to which illness is in the foreground or background of their world. Understanding this cycle is important when assessing readiness to learn, as the nurse educator cannot assume that an approach that worked at one time will be just as effective at another time. A chronically ill person's receptivity to learning and practicing self-care measures is not static and will fluctuate over time.

GENDER

Research indicates that women are generally more receptive to medical care and take fewer risks to their health than men (Ashton, 1999; Bertakis, Rahman, Helms, Callahan, & Robbins, 2000; Stein & Nyamathi, 2000). This difference may arise because women traditionally have taken the role of caregivers and therefore are more open to health promotion teaching. In addition, they have more frequent contacts with health providers while bearing and raising children. Men, on the other hand, tend to be less receptive to healthcare interventions and are more likely to be risk takers. A good deal of this behavior is thought to be socially induced; changes are beginning to be seen in the health-seeking behavior of men and women due to the increased attention paid to healthier lifestyles and the blending of gender roles in the home and workplace.

Emotional Readiness

The learner must be emotionally ready to learn. Like physical readiness, emotional readiness includes several factors that need to be assessed. These factors will be discussed in the following pages.

ANXIETY LEVEL

Anxiety is a factor that influences the ability to perform at cognitive, affective, and psychomotor levels. Anxiety impacts on the patients' ability to concentrate and retain information (Kessels, 2003; Stephenson, 2006). Depending on the level of anxiety, it may or may not be a hindrance to the learning of new skills. Some degree of anxiety is a motivator to learn, but too low or too high anxiety will interfere with readiness to learn. On either end of the continuum, mild or severe anxiety may lead to inaction on the part of the learner. If anxiety is low, the individual is not driven to take steps to promote his or her health or prevent diseases. Moderate anxiety, on the other hand, drives someone to take action. As the level of anxiety begins to increase, emotional readiness peaks and then begins to decrease in an inversely U-shaped curvilinear manner based on the Yerkes-Dodson law (Ley, 1979), as shown in **Figure 4–2**. A moderate level of anxiety is best for success in learning and is considered the optimal time for teaching.

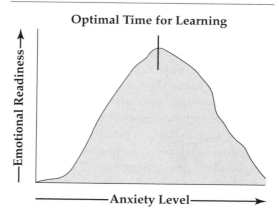

Figure 4–2 Effect of anxiety on emotional readiness to learn.

Optimal Time for Learning

Emotional Readiness →

←Anxiety Level→

Fear is a major contributor to anxiety and thus negatively affects readiness to learn in any of the learning domains. The performance of a task in and of itself may be fear inducing to a patient because of its very nature or meaning. For example, having to learn self-administration of a medication by injection may produce fear for the patient because of the necessity of inflicting pain on oneself and the perceived danger of the needle breaking off into the skin. A staff member or nursing student, on the other hand, may have real difficulty mastering a skill because of the fear of harming a patient or of failing to do a procedure correctly.

Fear may also lead patients to deny their illness, which interferes with their ability to learn. If a situation is life threatening or overwhelming, anxiety will be high, and readiness to learn will be diminished. While teaching may be imperative for survival, learning usually can take place only if instructions are simple and are repeated over and over again. In such circumstances, families and support persons also should be educated to reinforce information and assist with caregiving responsibilities. In later stages of adaptation, acceptance of illness will allow the individual to be more receptive to learning because anxiety levels will be less acute.

Discovering what stressful events or major life changes the learner is experiencing will give the educator clues as to that person's emotional readiness to learn. The nurse must first identify the source and level of anxiety. If stress levels are high, they can be moderated by participation in such activities as support groups and by the use of relaxation techniques such as imagery or yoga (Stephenson, 2006). Education is an excellent intervention to spur someone to take action when anxiety levels have been moderated or anxiety has been lessened when a patient is dealing with a stressful life event.

SUPPORT SYSTEM

The availability and strength of a support system also influence emotional readiness and are closely tied to how anxious someone might feel. If members of the patient's support system are available to assist with self-care activities at home, then they should be present during at least some of the teaching sessions to learn how to help the patient if the need arises. Kitchie's (2003) descriptive correlational study suggests that families and friends are important for medication adherence among the elderly who experience chronic illness. Although the educator should not draw any conclusions about causal relationships from this type of study, the educator's assessment will benefit from incorporating questions about the learner's social network. Social support is important in buffering the effects of stressful events (Gavan, 2003; Kitchie, 2003). A strong positive support system can decrease anxiety, while the lack of one can increase anxiety levels.

Beddoe (1999) describes the unique opportunity that nurses have to provide emotional support to patients. She labels this opportunity as the reachable moment—the time when a nurse truly connects with clients by directly meeting them on mutual terms. The reachable moment allows for the mutual exchange of concerns and a sharing of possible intervention options without the nurse being inhibited by prejudice or bias. When the client feels emotionally supported, the stage is set for the teachable moment, when the client will be most receptive to learning.

MOTIVATION

Emotional readiness is strongly associated with motivation, which is a willingness to take action. Knowing the motivational level of the learner assists the educator in determining when someone is ready to learn. Assessment of emotional readiness involves ascertaining the level of motivation, not necessarily the reasons for the motivation. There are many reasons why a learner may be motivated to learn, and almost any reason to learn is a valid one.

The level of motivation is related to what learners perceive as an expectation of themselves or others. Interest in informal or formal teacher–learner interactions is a cue to motivation. The learner who is ready to learn shows an interest in what the nurse educator is doing by demonstrating a willingness to participate or to ask questions. Prior learning experiences, whether they be past accomplishments or failures, will be reflected in the current level of motivation demonstrated by the learner for accomplishing the task at hand (see Chapter 6).

RISK-TAKING BEHAVIOR

Taking risks is intrinsic in the activities people perform daily. Many activities are done without thinking about the outcome. According to Joseph (1993), some patients, by the very nature of their personalities, will take more risks than others. The educator can assist patients to develop strategies that help reduce the risk of their choices. If patients participate in activities that may shorten their life spans, rather than complying with a recommended treatment plan, the educator must be willing to teach these patients how to recognize certain body symptoms and then what to do if they have them.

Understanding how much risk-taking behaviors staff nurses have or do not have will help the nurse educator understand why some learners may be hesitant to try new approaches to delivering care. Wolfe (1994) stated that taking risks can be threatening when the outcomes are not guaranteed. Educators can, however, help individuals learn how to take risks. First, the decision has to be made to take the risk. The next step is to develop strategies to minimize the risk. Then the learner needs to develop a worst, best, and most probable case scenario. Lastly, the learner must decide whether the worst-case scenario developed is acceptable.

FRAME OF MIND

Frame of mind involves concern about the here and now versus the future. If survival is of primary concern, then readiness to learn will be focused on the present to meet basic human needs. According to Maslow (1970), physical needs such as food, warmth, comfort, and safety as well as psychosocial needs of feeling accepted and secure must be met before someone can focus on higher order learning. People from lower socioeconomic levels tend to concentrate on immediate, current concerns because they are trying to satisfy everyday needs. Ramanadhan and Viswanath (2006) used national data from the 2003 Health Information National Trends survey to examine informational seeking behaviors of adults. They found that a significant percentage of those diagnosed with a serious disease, such as cancer, report that they do not seek or receive health information beyond that given by health care providers. Furthermore, compared to seekers of health information, nonseeker patients were more likely to come from the lowest income and education groups and were less attentive about getting health information from the media. These findings have implications for educators when deciding on the best method for reaching various segments of the population.

Children regard life in the here and now because they are developmentally focused on what makes them happy and satisfied. In addition, their thinking is concrete rather than abstract. Adults who have reached self-actualization and those whose basic needs are met are more ready to learn health promotion tasks and are said to have a more futuristic orientation.

DEVELOPMENTAL STAGE

Each task associated with human development produces a peak time for readiness to learn, known as a teachable moment (Hansen & Fisher, 1998; Hotelling, 2005; Tanner, 1989; Wagner & Ash, 1998). Unlike children, adults can build on meaningful past experiences and are strongly driven to learn information that will help them to cope better with real-life tasks. They see learning as relevant when they can apply new knowledge to help them solve immediate problems. Children, on the other hand, desire to learn for learning's sake and actively seek out experiences that give them pleasure and comfort. Erickson's well-accepted theory on the eight stages of psychosocial learning is most relevant to an individual's emotional readiness (see Chapter 5).

Experiential Readiness

Experiential readiness refers to the learner's past experiences with learning and includes five elements. The educator should assess whether previous learning experiences have been positive or negative in overcoming problems or accomplishing new tasks. Someone who has had negative experiences with learning is not likely to be motivated or willing to take a risk to change behavior or acquire new behaviors.

LEVEL OF ASPIRATION

The extent to which someone is driven to achieve is related to the type of short- and long-term goals established—not by the educator, but by the learner. Previous failures and past successes influence what goals learners set for themselves. Early successes are important moti-

vators in learning subsequent skills. Satisfaction, once achieved, elevates the level of aspiration, which, in turn, increases the probability of continued performance output in undertaking future endeavors to change behavior.

PAST COPING MECHANISMS

The coping mechanisms someone has been using must be explored to understand how the learner has dealt with previous problems. Once these mechanisms are identified, the educator must determine if past coping strategies have been effective and, if so, whether they work well under the present learning situation.

CULTURAL BACKGROUND

Knowledge on the part of the educator about other cultures and being sensitive to behavioral differences between cultures are important to avoid teaching in opposition to cultural beliefs (see Chapter 8). Assessment of what an illness means to the patient from the patient's cultural perspective is imperative in determining readiness to learn. Remaining sensitive to cultural influences allows the teacher to bridge the gap, when necessary, between the medical healthcare culture and the patient's culture. Building on the learner's knowledge base or belief system (unless it is dangerous to well-being), rather than attempting to change it or claim it is wrong, will encourage rather than dampen readiness to learn.

Language is also a part of culture and may prove to be a significant obstacle to learning if the educator and the learner do not fluently speak the same language. Assessing whether the learner understands English well enough to be able to express himself so others will understand is the first step. A qualified interpreter will be necessary if the learner and caregiver do not fluently speak the same language. Enlisting the help of someone other than a trained interpreter to bridge language differences may negatively influence learning. This effect will depend on such issues as the sensitivity of the topic and the need for privacy. In some instances, the patient may not want family members or associates to know about a health concern or illness.

Remember, also, that medical terminology in and of itself may be a foreign language to many patients, whether or not they are from another culture or their primary language is the same or different than that of the educator. In addition, sometimes a native language does not have an equivalent word to describe the terms that are being used in the teaching situation. Differences in language compound the cultural barrier. Teaching should not be started unless you have determined that the learner understands you and that you have an understanding of the learner's culture (see Chapter 8).

LOCUS OF CONTROL

Whether readiness to learn comes from internal or external stimuli can be determined by ascertaining the learner's previous life patterns of responsibility and assertiveness. When patients are internally motivated to learn, they have what is known as an internal locus of control. They are ready to learn when they feel a need to know about something. This drive to learn comes from within the learner. Usually, this type of learner will indicate a need to know by asking questions. Remember that when someone asks a question, the time is prime for learning. If patients have an external locus of control—that is, they are externally motivated—then someone other than themselves must encourage a feeling of wanting to know something. The responsibility often falls on the educator's shoulders to motivate them to want to learn.

ORIENTATION

The tendency to adhere to a parochial or cosmopolitan point of view is known as orientation. Patients with a parochial orientation tend to be more close minded in their thinking, are more conservative in their approach to situations, are less willing to learn new material, and place the most trust in traditional authority figures such as the physician. This type of orientation is seen most often in people who have been raised in a small-town atmosphere or who come from cohesive neighborhoods or protective family environments. Conversely, people who exhibit a cosmopolitan orientation most likely have a more worldly perspective on life due to broader experiences outside their immediate spheres of influence. These individuals are more likely to be receptive to new ideas and to opportunities to learn new ways of doing things. One must be careful not to unfairly stereotype individuals, but learners usually possess representative characteristics of one or the other of these two opposing types of orientation.

Knowledge Readiness

Knowledge readiness refers to the learner's present knowledge base, the level of learning capability, and the preferred style of learning. These components must be assessed to determine readiness to learn, and teaching should be planned accordingly.

PRESENT KNOWLEDGE BASE

How much someone already knows about a particular subject or how proficient that person is at performing a task is an important factor to determine before designing and implementing instruction. If the educator makes the mistake of teaching subject material that has already been learned, then he or she risks, at the very least, creating boredom and disinterest in the learner, or, at the extreme, causing insult to the learner, which could produce resistance to further learning. The nurse educator must always find out what the learner knows prior to teaching and build on this knowledge base to encourage readiness to learn. In teaching patients, the educator also must consider how much information the patient wants to receive. Some patients want to know the details to make informed decisions about their care, whereas others prefer a more general and less in-depth approach and can be overwhelmed with too much information.

COGNITIVE ABILITY

The extent to which information can be processed is indicative of the learner's capabilities. The educator must match the level of behavioral objectives to the cognitive ability of the learner. The learner who is capable of understanding, memorizing, recalling, or recognizing subject material is functioning at a lower level in the cognitive domain than the learner who demonstrates problem solving, concept formation, or application of information. For example, nursing staff or students who are able to answer questions about cardiopulmonary resuscitation (CPR) on a written test demonstrate an understanding of the subject, but this does not necessarily mean that they can transfer this knowledge to perform CPR in the clinical setting. Patients who are able to identify risk factors of hypertension (a low level of functioning in the cognitive domain) may struggle with generalizing this information to incorporate a low-salt diet into their lifestyle.

Individuals with cognitive impairment due to mental retardation present a special challenge to the educator and will require simple explanations and step-by-step instruction with frequent repetition. Be sure to make information meaningful to those with cognitive impairments by teaching at their level and communicating in ways that the learner will be able to understand (see Chapter 9, Special Populations). Enlisting the help of members of the patient's support system by teaching them requisite skills will allow them to positively contribute to the reinforcement of self-care activities.

LEARNING AND READING DISABILITIES

Learning disabilities, which may be accompanied by low-level reading skills, are not necessarily indicative of an individual's intellectual abilities but will require special or innovative approaches to instruction to sustain or bolster readiness to learn. Individuals with low-literacy skills and learning disabilities become easily discouraged unless the teacher recognizes their special needs and seeks ways to help them accommodate or overcome their problems with encoding words and comprehending information (see Chapters 7 and 9).

LEARNING STYLES

A variety of preferred styles of learning exist, and assessing how someone learns best and likes to learn will help the educator to select teaching approaches accordingly. Knowing the teaching methods and materials with which a learner is most comfortable or, conversely, those that the learner does not tolerate well will help the educator to tailor teaching to meet the needs of individuals with different styles of learning, thereby increasing their readiness to learn. For more information on learning styles, see the following discussion.

Learning Styles

Learning styles refers to the ways in which, and conditions under which, learners most efficiently and most effectively perceive, process, store, and recall what they are attempting to learn (James & Gardner, 1995) and how they prefer to approach different learning tasks (Cassidy, 2004). Keefe (1979) defines learning style as the way the learners learn, taking into account cognitive, affective, and physiological factors that affect how learners perceive, interact with, and respond to the learning environment.

Learning style models are based on the premise that certain characteristics of style are biological in origin, whereas others are sociologically developed as a result of environmental influences. Recognizing that people have different approaches to learning helps the nurse educator to understand the differences in educational interests and needs of diverse populations. Accepting diversity of style can help educators create an atmosphere for learning that offers experiences that encourage each individual to reach his or her full potential. Understanding learning style also can help educators to make deliberate decisions about program development and instructional design (Arndt & Underwood, 1990; Coffield, Moseley, Hall, & Ecclestone, 2004; Morse, Oberer, Dobbins, & Mitchell, 1998). In addition, consideration given to matching the learning style of nursing staff orientees with the training style of clinical nurse preceptors may provide the opportunity to maximize learning outcomes during staff orientation to clinical sites (Anderson, 1998).

No learning style is either better or worse than another. Given the same content, most learners can assimilate information with equal success, but how they go about mastering the content is determined by their individual style. The more flexible the educator is in using teaching methodologies and tools related to individual learning styles, the greater the likelihood that learning will occur.

Six Learning Style Principles

Six principles have emerged from research about learning styles. To develop these six principles, Friedman and Alley (1984) reviewed an enormous volume of literature, which included more than 30 different learning style instruments. The six principles still remain valid and are summarized below:

1. *Both the style by which the educator prefers to teach and the style by which the learner prefers to learn can be identified.* Identification of different styles offers specific clues as to the way a person learns. By understanding one's own learning style, the educator can appreciate why it may be easier to help one style of learner to master information but more difficult to work with another learner who needs an entirely different approach to learning.

2. *Educators need to guard against relying on teaching methods and tools that match their own preferred learning styles.* Nurse educators need to realize that just because they gravitate to learning a certain way, it does not mean that everyone else can or wants to learn this way. It is much easier for an educator to change teaching approaches than for learners to adapt to the educator's style.

3. *Educators are most helpful when they assist learners in identifying and learning through their own style preferences.* Each learner is unique and complex, with a distinct learning style preference that distinguishes him from another learner. Making learners aware of their individual style preferences will lead to an understanding of which teaching–learning approaches work best for them. Also, an awareness of their preference

for a particular learning style sensitizes learners to the fact that whatever style is most comfortable for them may not be the best approach for others.

4. *Learners should have the opportunity to learn through their preferred style.* The nurse educator can provide the means by which each learner can experience successful learning. Visual learners, for example, should be given reading materials, videos, computer simulations, models, and diagrams from which to learn rather than insisting that they listen to a lecture or audiotape or become involved in role playing. As another example, concrete thinkers need facts, whereas abstract thinkers need theories to capitalize on their strengths.

5. *Learners should be encouraged to diversify their style preferences.* Today, learners are constantly faced with learning situations in which one approach to learning will not suffice if they are to reach their fullest potential. Without encouragement, learners tend to automatically gravitate to using their preferred style of learning. The more frequently learners are exposed to different methods of learning, the less stressful those methods will be in future learning situations.

6. *Educators can develop specific learning activities that reinforce each modality or style.* Awareness of various methods and materials available is the key to addressing and augmenting different learning styles. Using only a limited number of educational strategies will selectively exclude many learners.

Three mechanisms to determine learning style are observation, interviews, and administration of learning style instruments. By observing the learner in action, the educator can ascertain how the learner grasps information and problem solves. For example, when doing a math calculation, does the learner write every step down or only the answer? In an interview, the educator can ask the learner about preferred ways of learning as well as the environment most comfortable for learning. Is group discussion or self-instruction more preferable? Is a warm or cold room more conducive to concentration? Simply asking the question, "How do you learn best?" will give the educator valuable information. Finally, the educator can administer learning style instruments, like those described in the next section.

All three techniques should be used to determine learning style. Assessment is foremost in the educational process. Once data are gathered through interview, observation, and instrument administration, then learning style can be validated, and methods and materials for instruction can be chosen by the educator to match learner preferences and to direct patients, nursing students, or staff toward those ways they best can learn.

Using the learning style approach to instruction has enormous and exciting implications. Educational experiences that are adapted to coincide with learning styles increases the likelihood that learning will take place. Understanding and recognizing various styles can influence decision making about planning, implementing, and evaluating educational programs.

Learning Style Models and Instruments

The identification and application of information about learning styles continues to be an emerging movement, but it is just beginning to be applied to the health education field. To date, researchers have defined learning styles differently, although the concepts in each definition are often overlapping. No single framework for instructional design is forthcoming, yet each proposed framework provides the educator with a more profound view of the learner than previously known (Knowles, 1990; Morse et al., 1998; Villejo & Meyers, 1991).

This chapter does not attempt to include all the instruments that are available, but rather highlights those commonly cited in recent reviews and in health sciences research literature that refer to the psychometric properties of each. These instruments are believed to be the most useful to nurse educators for assessment purposes.

Before using any learning style instrument, it is important to determine its reliability and validity and to realize that a totally inclusive instrument that measures all domains of learning—cognitive, affective, and psychomotor—does not exist. Therefore, it is best to use more than one measurement tool for assessment. Also, the educator should not rely heavily on these instruments because they are intended not for diagnosis but rather to validate what the learner perceives in comparison to what the educator perceives. These instruments will help the nurse in developing a more personalized form of instruction.

Right-Brain/Left-Brain and Whole-Brain Thinking

Although not technically a model, right-brain/left-brain thinking along with whole-brain thinking adds to our understanding of brain functions that are associated with learning. Over 30 years ago, Dr. Roger Sperry and his research team established that the brain operates in many ways as two brains (Herrmann, 1988; Sperry, 1977), with each hemisphere having separate and complementary functions. The left hemisphere of the brain was found to be the vocal and analytical side, which is used for verbalization and for reality-based and logical thinking. The right hemisphere was found to be the emotional, visual-spatial, and nonverbal side, with thinking processes that are intuitive, subjective, relational, holistic, and time free. Sperry and his colleagues discovered that learners are able to use both sides of the brain because of a connector between the two hemispheres called the corpus callosum.

There is no correct or wrong side of the brain. Each hemisphere gathers in the same sensory information but handles the information in different ways. One hemisphere may take over and inhibit the other in processing information, or the task may be divided between the two sides, with each handling the part best suited to its way of processing information. Recognizing that one side of the brain is better equipped for certain kinds of tasks than for others, educators can find the most effective way to present information to learners who may have a dominant brain hemisphere (**Table 4–3**). Brain hemisphericity is linked to cognitive learning style or the way individuals perceive and gather information to problem solve, complete assigned tasks, relate to others, and meet the daily challenges of life.

Neuroimaging methods, such as positron emission tomography (PET) and functional magnetic resonance imaging (fMRI), provide the educator with knowledge on how the brain works. This information adds to the relevance of learning styles and brain hemispherical performance. McIntosh (1998) proposed a general hypothesis that learning and memory are emergent

---

Table 4–3 EXAMPLES OF HEMISPHERE FUNCTIONS

Left-Hemisphere Functions	Right-Hemisphere Functions
Thinking is critical, logical, convergent, focal	Thinking is creative, intuitive, divergent, diffuse
Analytical	Synthesizing
Prefers talking and writing	Prefers drawing and manipulating objects
Responds to verbal instructions and explanations	Responds to written instructions and explanations
Recognizes/remembers names	Recognizes/remembers faces
Relies on language in thinking and remembering	Relies on images in thinking and remembering
Solves problems by breaking them into parts, then approaches the problem sequentially, using logic	Solves problems by looking at the whole, the configurations, then approaches the problem through patterns, using hunches
Good organizational skills, neat	Loose organizational skills, sloppy
Likes stability, willing to adhere to rules	Likes change, uncertainty
Conscious of time and schedules	Frequently loses contact with time and schedules
Algebra is the preferred math	Geometry is the preferred math
Not as good at interpreting body language	Good at interpreting body language
Controls emotions	Free with emotions

---

properties of network interactions. Sylvester (1995, 1998) reported on the research that has led to a better understanding of the functions of the brain and individual learning differences. Iaccino (1993) provided more detailed accounts of the clinical evidence that has contributed to the left–right dichotomy of the brain. These advances in technology have confirmed many of the assumptions about the functioning of the brain, which can be applied by educators to assessing learning styles, choosing education techniques (Caulfield, Kidd, & Kocher, 2000; Stover, 2001), and identifying strengths and weaknesses in their own teaching approaches.

Most individuals have a dominant side of the brain. Gondringer (1989) reported that most learners have left-brain dominance and that only approximately 30% have right-brain dominance. This may be because the Western world is geared toward rewarding left-brain skills to

the extent that right-brain skills go undeveloped. However, teaching methods that enable the learner to use both sides of the brain need to be employed. For example, to stimulate the development of left-brain thinking, the nurse educator should provide a structured environment by relying on specific objectives and a course outline. To stimulate the development of the right brain, the nurse educator should provide a more unstructured, free-flowing environment that allows for creative opportunities. By employing teaching strategies aimed at helping the learner use both brain hemispheres, the educator will facilitate more effective and efficient learning. Whole-brain thinking allows the learner to get the best of both worlds in developing his or her thought processes. Duality of thinking is what educators should strive to teach to encourage learners to reach their full learning potentials.

As Gardner (1999a) pointed out, the brain does not exist in isolation but rather is connected to the entire body. He argued that for the brain to be more than an organ, consideration must be given to a number of variables, such as mental processes, feelings, desires, and cultural influences that are important in the development and expression of one's learning style. What learners choose to learn is influenced by the set of values both educators and learners bring to the teaching–learning situation.

INSTRUMENTS TO MEASURE RIGHT-BRAIN/ LEFT-BRAIN AND WHOLE-BRAIN THINKING

Two instruments are used to measure right and left brain dominance. The first is called the brain preference indicator (BPI). It consists of a set of questions used to determine hemispheric functioning. The BPI instrument reveals a general style of thought that results in a consistent pattern of behavior in all areas of the individual's life. Although there is no reported reliability or validity of this instrument, it does provide a starting point for the educator to understand his or her own right- or left-brain preferences. More information about the BPI can be found in *Whole-Brain Thinking* by Wonder and Donovan (1984).

The other instrument available with widespread commercial use is the Herrmann brain dominance instrument (HBDI). Herrmann's (1988) model incorporates theories on growth and development and considers learning styles as learned patterns of behavior. The HBDI classifies learners in terms of the following four different modes, with each quadrant corresponding to a brain structure and different preferences for thinking:

Quadrant A (left brain, cerebral)— Logical, analytical, quantitative, factual, critical

Quadrant B (left brain, limbic)— Sequential, organized, planned, detailed, structured

Quadrant C (right brain, limbic)— Emotional, interpersonal, sensory, kinesthetic, symbolic

Quadrant D (right brain, cerebral)— Visual, holistic, innovative

The author suggests that his HBDI is psychometrically sound, although there are very few independent studies of its reliability and validity (Coffield et al., 2004). The HBDI mostly has been used in the business world with minimal validation in the health sciences. More information about the model is available at Herrmann International's Web site, www.hbdi.com.

Field-Independent/ Field-Dependent Perception

An extensive series of studies by Witkin, Oltman, Raskin, and Karp (1971b) identified two styles of learning in the cognitive domain, which are based on the bipolar distribution of characteristics of how learners process and structure information in their environment. They hypothesized that learners have preference styles for certain environmental cues. A field-independent person perceives items as separate or differentiated from the surrounding field; a field-dependent person's perception is influenced by or immersed in the surrounding field.

Field-independent individuals have internalized frames of reference such that they experience themselves as separate or differentiated from others and the environment. They are less sensitive to social cues, are not affected by criticism, favor an active participant role, and are eager to test out their ideas or opinions in a group.

Field-dependent individuals, on the other hand, are more externally focused and as such are socially oriented, more aware of social cues, able to reveal their feelings, and are more dependent on others for reinforcement. They have a need for extrinsic motivation and externally defined objectives and learn better if the material has a social context. They are more easily affected by criticism, take a passive, spectator role, and change their opinions in the face of peer pressure.

Field independence/dependence is thought to be related to hemispheric brain processes (Chall & Mirsky, 1978). The studies in *Sex and the Brain* (Durden-Smith & deSimone, 1983) reveal that the right hemisphere in males tends to be more dominant than their left hemisphere; the opposite is true for females. Males tend to have better visual-spatial abilities, and females tend to have better linguistic skills. Although females generally do not do as well as males on tests of spatial ability, men should be measured only against other men, and women against women, to reduce the differential test effect on the sexes. To date, sex-related differences in behavior have been documented in the literature (Speck, Ernst, Braun, Koch, Miller, & Chang, 2000), but the neuroanatomic processes remain unclear (Gur et al., 1999) and significance of these research findings for the educator is difficult to gauge. Garity (1985) suggested that these individual differences in characteristics and interpersonal behavior can be used as a basis for understanding different learning styles and can facilitate the way educators work with learners, structure the learning task, and structure the environment (**Table 4–4**).

INSTRUMENT TO MEASURE FIELD INDEPENDENCE/FIELD DEPENDENCE

Witkin, Oltman, Raskin, and Karp (1971a) devised a tool called the group embedded figures test (GEFT) to measure field independence/dependence—how a person's perception of an item is influenced by the context in which it appears. Bonham (1988) noted that the GEFT,

---

Table 4–4 CHARACTERISTICS OF FIELD-INDEPENDENT AND FIELD-DEPENDENT LEARNERS

Field-Independent Learners	Field-Dependent Learners
Are not affected by criticism	Are easily affected by criticism
Will not conform to peer pressure	Will conform to peer pressure
Are less influenced by external feedback	Are influenced by feedback (grades and evaluations)
Learn best by organizing their own material	Learn best when material is organized
Have an impersonal orientation to the world	Have a social orientation to the world
Place emphasis on applying principles	Place emphasis on facts
Are interested in new ideas or concepts for own sake	Prefer learning to be relevant to own experience
Provide self-directed goals, objectives, and reinforcement	Need external goals, objectives, and reinforcements
Prefer lecture method	Prefer discussion method

which takes approximately 30 minutes to complete, is designed to determine a person's ability to find simple geometric figures within complex drawings. Witkin's work is based on 35 years of psychological research on more than 2,000 individuals. Educators must keep in mind that the GEFT is based on psychological research when they attempt to broadly apply findings to the educational setting (Witkin, Moore, & Oltman, 1977). Bonham (1988) pointed out in her analysis of learning style instruments that the GEFT measures the ability to do something, not the manner (style) in which it is done. There is no way to tell whether a person could choose which style is most effective in a given situation (Shipman & Shipman, 1985; Witkin & Goodenough, 1981). Older adults generally do not do well on tests in which speed is important (Botwinick, 1978), but this assessment tool is a timed test so age bias is a concern (Santrock, 2006).

The best time to use the GEFT seems to be when the educator wants to measure field independence, not field dependence, in determining the extent to which learners are able to ignore distractions from other persons who may offer incorrect information or ideas. The results could help individuals understand why they may have trouble with a particular learning experience (Bonham, 1988). For example, Deture (2004) designed a study to identify those learner attributes that may be used to predict student success in Web-based, distance education courses. He administered the GEFT and the online technologies self-efficacy scale (OTSES) to community college students to determine their entry level confidence with computer skills for online learning. His findings showed a significant positive correlation between the GEFT and the OTSES scores, supporting the notion that field-independent students tend to be more confident

with online technologies. Thus field-dependent students may need more assistance with Web-based courses, and the educator may need to find other methods of instruction for their learning to be more successful and less anxiety producing.

Flynn and associates (1999) found a significant association between the number of interruptions and distractions in an ambulatory care pharmacy and dispensing errors (incorrect label information). As the distractions (field background elements) increased, more errors occurred. Field-dependent pharmacists tended to get more distracted and to fill prescriptions inaccurately. Consideration of field independence/dependence can be useful for the educator who is involved with teaching in a clinical setting characterized by constant distractions.

Also, the educator can use this instrument to determine whether a learner sees the whole first (global, field independent) and then the individual parts (specific, field dependent), or vice versa. The field-independent person will want to know the end result of teaching and learning prior to concentrating on the individual parts of the process, whereas the field-dependent person will want to know the individual parts in sequence prior to looking at the expected overall outcome of teaching–learning efforts. The GEFT has been reasonably well validated in predicting academic performance (Oltman, Raskin, Witkin, & Karp, 1978). This instrument is available for purchase at Mind Garden, Inc., which can be accessed at http://www.mindgarden.com.

Dunn and Dunn Learning Styles

In 1967, Rita and Kenneth Dunn set out to develop a user-friendly model that would assist educators in identifying those characteristics that allow individuals to learn in different ways (Dunn and Dunn, 1978). The model includes motivational factors, social interaction, and physiological and environmental elements. These researchers identified the following five basic stimuli (as shown in **Figure 4–3**) that affect a person's ability to learn:

1. Environmental elements (such as sound, light, temperature, and design), which are biological in nature.
2. Emotional elements (such as motivation, persistence, responsibility, and structure), which are developmental and emerge over time as an outgrowth of experiences that have happened at home, school, play, or work.

3. Sociological patterns (such as the desire to work alone or in groups or a combination of these two approaches), which are thought to be socioculturally based.
4. Physical elements (such as perceptual strength, intake, time of day, and mobility), which are also biological in nature and relate to the way learners function physically.
5. Psychological elements (such as the way learners process and react to information), which are also biological in nature.

Figure 4–3 Dunn and Dunn's learning style elements.

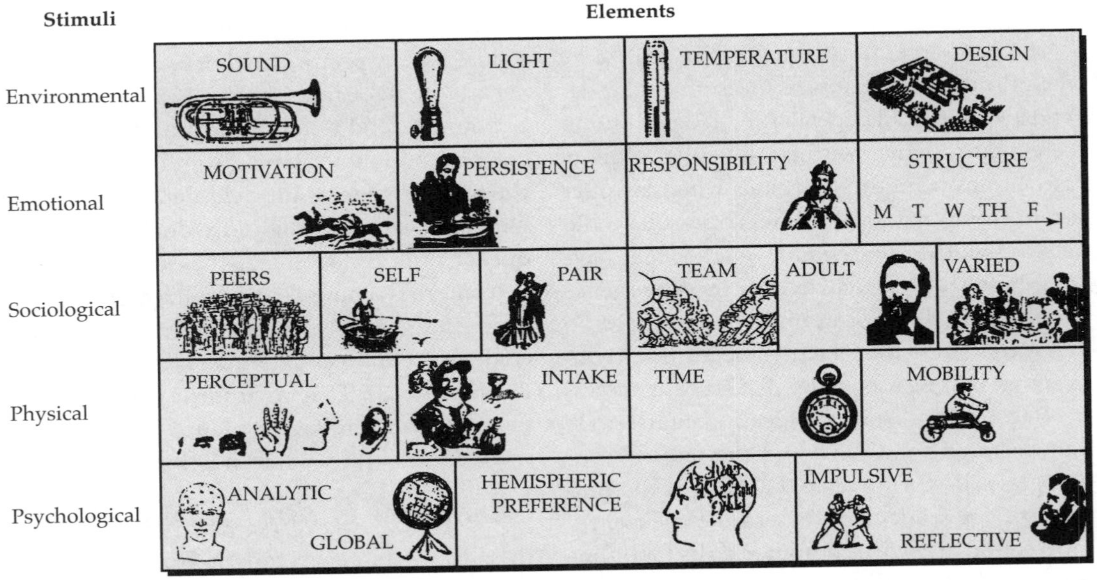

Source: Dunn, R. (1983). Can students identify their own learning styles? *Educational Leadership, 40*(5), 61. Reprinted by permission of the Association for Supervision and Curriculum Development. All rights reserved.

THE ENVIRONMENTAL ELEMENTS

Sound Individuals react to sound in different ways. Some need complete silence, others are able to block out sounds around them, and still others require sound in their environment for learning. Cognizant of the effect of sound on learning, the educator should permit learners to study either in silent areas or with music from headsets to prevent interfering with those who need quiet.

Light Some learners work best under bright lights, whereas others need dim or low lighting. The educator should provide lighting conducive to learning by moving furniture around to establish both well- and dimly lit areas and permitting learners to sit where they are most comfortable.

Temperature Some learners have difficulty thinking or concentrating if a room is too hot or, conversely, if it is too cold. The educator needs to make learners aware of the temperature of the environment and encourage them to wear lighter or heavier clothing. If windows are available, they should be opened to permit variable degrees of temperature in the room to accommodate different comfort levels.

Design Dunn and Dunn established that when learners are seated on wooden, steel, or plastic chairs, 75% of the total body weight is supported on only four square inches of bone. This results in fatigue, discomfort, and the need for frequent body position changes (Dunn & Dunn, 1987). Also, some learners are more relaxed and can learn better in an informal environment by being able to position themselves in a lounge chair, on the floor, on pillows, or on carpeting. Others cannot learn in an informal environment because it makes them drowsy. If possible, the educator should vary the furniture in the classroom to allow some to sit more formally or informally while learning.

THE EMOTIONAL ELEMENTS

Motivation Motivation, or the desire to achieve, increases when learning success increases. Unmotivated learners need short learning assignments that enhance their strengths. Motivated learners, by comparison, are eager to learn and should be told exactly what they are required to do, with resources available so they can self-pace their learning.

Persistence Learners differ in their preference to complete tasks in one sitting or to take periodic breaks and return to the task at a later time. By giving learners objectives and a time interval for completion of a task ahead of time, those with long attention spans can get the job done in a block of time, while those whose attention span is short can take the opportunity for breaks without feeling guilty or rushed.

Responsibility Responsibility involves the desire to do what the learner thinks is expected. It is related to the concept of conformity or following through on what an educator asks or tells the learner to do. Learners with low responsibility scores usually are nonconforming. They do not like to do something because someone asks them to do it. Knowing this, the educator should give them choices and allow learners to select different ways to complete the assignment. When given appropriate choices, the nonconformist will likely be more willing to meet expectations set forth.

Structure   Structure refers to either the preference for specific directions, guidance, or rules prior to carrying out an assignment or the preference for doing an assignment without structure in the learner's own way. Structure should vary in the amount and kind that is provided, depending on the learner's ability to make responsible decisions and the requirements of the task.

THE SOCIOLOGICAL ELEMENTS

Learning Alone   Some learners prefer to study by themselves, whereas others prefer to learn with a friend or colleague. When learners prefer to be with others, group discussion and role playing may facilitate learning. For learners who do not do well learning with others because they tend to socialize or are unable to concentrate, self-instruction, one-to-one interaction, or lecture-type methods are the best approaches.

Presence of an Authority Figure   Some learners feel more comfortable when someone with authority or recognized expertise is present during learning. Others become nervous, feel stifled, and have trouble concentrating. Depending on the style of the learner, either one-to-one interaction or self-study may be the appropriate approach.

Variety of Ways   Some learners are flexible and can learn as well alone as they can with authority figures and peer groups. These learners are versatile in their style of learning and would benefit from having different opportunities as opposed to routine approaches.

THE PHYSICAL ELEMENTS

Perceptual Strengths   Four types of learners are distinguished in this category: (1) those with auditory preferences, who learn best while listening to verbal instruction; (2) those with visual preferences, who learn best from reading or observation; (3) those with tactile preferences, who learn best when they can underline as they read, take notes when they listen, and otherwise keep their hands busy; and (4) those with kinesthetic preferences, who absorb and retain information best when allowed to perform whole-body movement or participate in simulated or real-life experiences.

Auditory learners should be introduced to new information first by hearing about it, followed by verbal feedback for reinforcement of the information. Lecture and group discussion are instructional methods best suited to their style. Visual learners learn more easily by viewing, watching, and observing. Simulation and demonstration methods of instruction are therefore most beneficial to their learning. Tactile learners learn through touching, manipulating, and handling objects, so they remember more when they write, doodle, draw, or move their fingers. The use of models and computer-assisted instruction is most suitable for their learning style. Kinesthetic learners learn more easily by doing and experiencing. They profit most from opportunities for field trips, role-playing, interviewing, and participating in return demonstration.

Intake   Some learners need to eat, drink, chew, or bite objects while concentrating. Others prefer no intake until after they have finished studying. A list of rules needs to be established to satisfy the oral needs of those who prefer intake while learning so that their behavior does not disturb others nor interfere with building rules and regulations of the agency.

Time of Day   Some learners perform better at one time of day than another. The four time-of-day preferences are on a continuum, and the educator needs to identify these preferences with an effort toward structuring teaching and learning to occur during the times that are most suitable for the learner:

> Early-morning learners—Their ability to concentrate and focus energies on learning is high in the early hours of the day and wanes as the day progresses.
>
> Late-morning learners—Their concentration and energy curve peaks around noontime, when their ability to perform is at its height.
>
> Afternoon learners—Their concentration and energy curve is highest in the mid- to late afternoon, when performance is at its peak.
>
> Evening learners—Their ability to concentrate and focus energies is greatest at the end of day.

Dunn (1995) contends that among adults, the majority fall on the two extremes of the continuum: 55% are morning people and 28% work best in the evening. Many adults experience energy lows in the afternoon. School-aged children, on the other hand, have high energy levels in the late morning and early afternoon. About 13% of high school students work best in the evening. This time sensitivity means that it may be easier or more difficult for a person to learn a new skill or behavior at certain times of the day than at other times. To enhance learning potential, the educator should try to schedule teaching during the learner's best time of day.

Mobility   Mobility refers to how still the learner can sit and for how long a period of time.

Some learners need to move about, whereas others can sit for hours engaged in learning. For those who require mobility, it is necessary to provide opportunity for movement by assigning them to less restrictive sections of the room. During workshops or any type of group learning, nurse educators should give frequent 30- to 60-second breaks during which participants can stand. This is a good time to have the participants turn to one another and share one thing that they have learned during that time.

The Psychological Elements

Global Versus Analytic   Some learners are global in their thinking and learn best by obtaining meaning from a broad, overall concept before focusing on the details in the surrounding environment. Other learners are analytic in their thinking and learn sequentially in a step-by-step process.

Hemispheric Preference   Learners who possess right-brain preference tend to learn best in environments that have low illumination, background music, casual seating, and tactile instructional resources. Learners with left-brain preference require an opposite environment of bright lighting, quiet setting, formal seating, and visual or auditory instructional resources.

Impulsivity Versus Reflectivity   Impulsive learners prefer opportunities to participate verbally in groups and tend to answer questions spontaneously and without consciously processing their thinking. Reflective learners seldom volunteer information unless they are asked to do so, prefer to contemplate information, and tend to be uncomfortable participating in group discussions (Dunn, 1984).

INSTRUMENT TO MEASURE THE DUNN AND DUNN LEARNING STYLE INVENTORY

The Dunn and Dunn learning style inventory is a self-reporting instrument that is widely used in the identification of how individuals prefer to function, learn, concentrate, and perform in their educational activities. It is available in three different forms: for grades 3–5; for grades 6–12; and in an adult version, called the productivity environmental preference survey (PEPS). Dunn and Dunn stress that the PEPS is not intended to be used as an indicator of underlying psychological factors, value systems, or the quality of attitudes. This instrument yields information concerned with the patterns through which learning occurs but does not assess the finer aspects of an individual's skills, such as the ability to outline procedures and to organize, classify, or analyze new material. It indicates how people prefer to learn, not the abilities they possess.

What has evolved since the model was first developed is a highly tested and continuously revised instrument that is valid and reliable as reported by those who like and use the instrument (Dunn & Griggs, 2003). However, others highlight major problems with the design and reliability of the instrument (Coffield et al., 2004).

Jung and Myers-Briggs Typology

Carl G. Jung (1921/1971), a Swiss psychiatrist, developed a theory that explains personality similarities and differences by identifying attitudes of people (*extraverts* and *introverts*) along with opposite mental functions, which are the ways people perceive or prefer to take in and make use of information from the world around them. Jung proposed that people are likely to operate in a variety of ways depending on the circumstances. Despite these situational adaptations, each individual will tend to develop comfortable patterns, which dictate behavior in certain predictable ways. Jung used the word *type* to identify these styles of personality.

Jung said that everyone uses these opposing perceptions to some degree when dealing with people and situations, but each person has a preference for one way of looking at the world. Individuals become more skilled in arriving at a decision in either a thinking or feeling way and can function as extraverts at one time and as introverts at another time, but they tend to develop patterns that are most typical and comfortable.

Isabel Myers and her mother, Katherine Briggs, became convinced that Jung's theories had an application for increasing human understanding (Myers, 1980). In addition to Jung's dichotomies, Myers and Briggs discovered another dichotomy (Myers, 1987) and thus made explicit one underdeveloped aspect of Jung's model (**Figure 4–4**). According to Myers and Briggs an individual comes to a conclusion about or becomes aware of something through a preference of judging or perceiving.

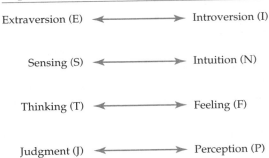

Figure 4–4 Myers-Briggs dichotomous dimensions or preferences.

Extraversion (E) ⟷ Introversion (I)

Sensing (S) ⟷ Intuition (N)

Thinking (T) ⟷ Feeling (F)

Judgment (J) ⟷ Perception (P)

By combining the different preferences, Myers and Briggs identified 16 personality types, each with its own strengths and interests (**Figure 4–5**). People can be classified into the 16 personality types by using the following four constructs:

1. *Extraversion-introversion (E-I)* reflects an orientation to either the outside world of people and things or to the inner world of concepts and ideas. This pair of opposite preferences describes the extent to which our behavior is determined by our attitudes toward the world. Jung invented the terms from Latin words meaning outward turning (extraversion) or inward turning (introversion).

   Individuals who prefer extraversion operate comfortably and successfully by interacting with things external to themselves, such as other people, experiences, and situations. They like to clarify thoughts and ideas through talking and doing. Those who operate more comfortably in an extraverted way think aloud.

   Those with a preference for introversion, on the other hand, are more interested in the internal world of their minds, hearts, and souls. They like to brew over thoughts and actions, reflecting on them until they become more personally meaningful. Those who operate more comfortably in an introverted way are often thoughtful, reflective, and slow to act because they need time to translate internal thoughts to the external world. Their thoughts are well formulated before they are willing to share them with others.

2. *Sensing-intuition (S-N)* describes perception as coming directly through the five senses or indirectly by way of the unconscious. This pair of opposite preferences explains how people understand what is experienced. People who prefer sensing experience the world through their senses—vision, hearing, touch, taste, and smell. They observe what is real, what is factual, and what is actually happening. Seeing or experiencing is believing. These sensory functions allow the individual to observe carefully, gather facts, and focus on practical actions.

   Conversely, those people who prefer intuition tend to read between the lines, focus on meaning, and attend to what might be. Those with intuition preferences view the world through possibilities and relationships and are tuned into subtleties of body language and tones of

Figure 4–5 Myers-Briggs types.

ISTJ	ISFJ	INFJ	INTJ
ISTP	ISFP	INFP	INTP
ESTP	ESFP	ENFP	ENTP
ESTJ	ESFJ	ENFJ	ENTJ

Source: Modified and reproduced by special permission of the publisher. Myers, I. B. (1998). *Introduction to type.* Palo Alto, CA: Consulting Psychologists Press, Inc. All rights reserved. Further reproduction is prohibited without the publisher's written consent.

voice. This kind of perception leads them to examine problems and issues in creative and original ways.

3. *Thinking-feeling (T-F)* is the approach used by individuals to arrive at judgments through objective versus subjective processes. Thinking types analyze information, data, situations, and people and make decisions based on logic. They are careful and slow in the analysis of the data, because accuracy and thoroughness are important to them. They trust objectivity and put faith in logical predictions and rational arguments. Thinking types explore and weigh all alternatives, and the final decision is reached impersonally, unemotionally, and carefully.

In the feeling preference, on the other hand, the approach to decision making takes place through a subjective, perceptive, empathetic, and emotional perspective. Individuals who prefer feeling search for the effect of a decision on themselves and others. They consider alternatives and examine evidence to develop a personal reaction and commitment. They believe the decision-making process is complex and not totally objective. Circumstantial evidence is extremely important, and these individuals see the world as gray rather than black and white.

4. *Judging-perceiving (J-P)* According to Myers and Briggs, an individual comes to a conclusion about or becomes aware of something (Figure 4–4) through a preference of judging, which is the desire to regulate and bring closure to circumstances in life or through their

preference of perceiving, which is the desire to be open minded and understanding.

INSTRUMENT TO MEASURE THE MYERS-BRIGGS PERSONALITY TYPES

Myers and Briggs developed an instrument called the Myers-Briggs Type Indicator (MBTI) that would permit people to learn about their own type of behavior and thus understand themselves better with respect to the way in which they interact with others. Although the MBTI is not a learning style instrument per se, it does measure differences in personality types, which are combinations of the four dichotomous preferences. The MBTI is a forced-choice, self-report inventory.

The Myers-Briggs Type Indicator can be useful for the educator to understand the many different ways in which learners perceive and judge information and how they prefer to learn. Logical, detailed individuals (Sensing-Thinking type) may have difficulty communicating with those who are more holistically oriented (Intuitive-Feeling type). What each party values and believes most and the ways to go about learning or dealing with information will be different and may lead to misunderstandings and conflicts (Bargar & Hoover, 1984). Another example of how these two preferences function is that the Sensing-Thinking learner's preferred learning style emphasizes hands-on experience, demonstration, and application of concepts, whereas Intuition-Feeling learners prefer emphasis on the theoretical concerns before they can concentrate on the practical applications. Examples are listed in **Table 4–5.**

Since its development in the 1920s, this instrument has undergone several revisions, with mixed reviews on its reliability and valid-

Table 4–5 MYERS-BRIGGS TYPES: EXAMPLES OF LEARNING

Extraversion	Introversion
Likes group work	Likes quiet space
Dislikes slow-paced learning	Dislikes interruptions
Likes action and to experience things so as to learn	Likes learning that deals with thoughts, ideas
Offers opinions without being asked	Offers opinions only when asked
Asks questions to check on the expectations of educator	Asks questions to allow understanding of learning activity
Sensing	**Intuition**
Practical	Always likes something new
Realistic	Imaginative
Observant	Sees possibilities
Learns from orderly sequence of details	Prefers the whole concept versus details
Thinking	**Feeling**
Low need for harmony	Values harmony
Finds ideas and things more interesting than people	More interested in people than things or ideas
Analytical	Sympathetic
Fair	Accepting
Judging	**Perceiving**
Organized	Open ended
Methodical	Flexible
Work oriented	Play oriented
Controls the environment	Adapts to the environment

ity (Capraro & Capraro, 2002; Coffield et al., 2004). Schoessler, Conedera, Bell, Marshall, and Gilson (1993) discussed the use of the MBTI to develop a continuing education department for nursing, and Hardy and Smith (2001) explained how they restructured their orientation program to match preceptor and orientee relative to teaching and learning and teaching traits as a result of individual MBTI scores. The MBTI instrument and MBTI products are available at CPP, Inc., which can be accessed at www.cpp.com/products/mbti/index.asp

Kolb's Experiential Learning Model

David Kolb (1984) developed his learning style model in the early 1970s as a management expert from Case Western Reserve University. He believed that knowledge is acquired through a transformational process, which is continuously created and recreated. The learner is not a blank slate, but he or she approaches a topic to be learned with preconceived ideas. Kolb's theory on learning style is that it is a cumulative result of past experiences, heredity, and the demands of the present environment. These factors combine to produce different individual orientations to learning.

Kolb's model, known as the cycle of learning, includes four modes of learning that reflect two major dimensions: perception and processing. He hypothesized that learning results from the way learners perceive as well as how they process what they perceive. The dimension of perception involves two opposite perceptual viewpoints. Some learners perceive through concrete experience (CE mode), whereas others perceive through abstract conceptualization (AC mode).

At the CE stage of the learning cycle, learners tend to rely more on feelings than on a systematic approach to problems and situations. Learners who fall into this category like relating with people, benefit from specific experiences, and are sensitive to others. They learn from feeling.

At the AC stage, on the other hand, learners rely on logic and ideas rather than on feelings to deal with problems or situations. People who fall into this category use systematic planning and logical analysis to solve problems. They learn by thinking.

The process dimension also has two opposing orientations. Some learners process information through reflective observation (RO mode), whereas others process information through active experimentation (AE mode).

At the RO stage of the learning cycle, learners rely on objectivity, careful judgment, personal thoughts, and feelings to form opinions. People who fall into this category look for the meaning of things by viewing them from different perspectives. They learn by watching and listening.

At the AE stage of the learning cycle, learning is active, and learners like to experiment to get things done. They prefer to influence or change situations and see the results of their actions. They enjoy involvement and are risk takers. They learn by doing.

Kolb described each learning style as a combination of the four basic learning modes (CE, AC, RO, and AE), identifying separate learning style types that best define the strengths and weaknesses of a learner. The learner predominantly demonstrates characteristics of one of four style types: (1) diverger, (2) assimilator, (3) converger, or (4) accommodator, which are discussed as they appear in clockwise order in **Figure 4–6**, starting with the diverger.

The *diverger* combines the learning modes of CE and RO. People with this learning style are good at viewing concrete situations from many points of view. They like to observe, gather information, and gain insights rather than take action. Working in groups to generate ideas appeals to them. They place a high value on understanding for knowledge's sake and like to personalize learning by connecting information with something familiar in their experiences. They have active imaginations, enjoy being involved, and are sensitive to feelings. Divergent thinkers learn best, for example, through group discussions and participating in brainstorming sessions.

The *assimilator* combines the learning modes of RO and AC. People with this learning style demonstrate the ability to understand large amounts of information by putting it into concise and logical form. They are less interested in people and more focused on abstract ideas and concepts. They are good at inductive reasoning, value theory over practical application of ideas, and need time to reflect on what has been learned and how information can be integrated into their past experiences. They rely on knowledge from

Figure 4–6 Kolb's learning style inventory.

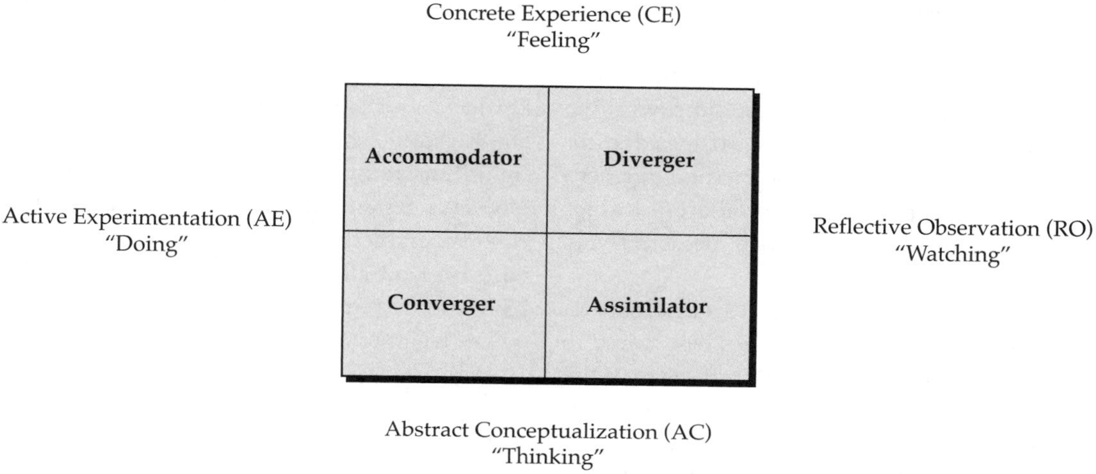

Concrete Experience (CE)
"Feeling"

Accommodator	**Diverger**
Converger	**Assimilator**

Active Experimentation (AE)
"Doing"

Reflective Observation (RO)
"Watching"

Abstract Conceptualization (AC)
"Thinking"

Source: Kolb, D. (1984). *Experiential learning: Experience as a source of learning and development.* Upper Saddle River, NJ: Prentice-Hall, Inc. Figures 3.1, 4.2. Reprinted by permission.

experts. Assimilative thinkers learn best, for example, through lecture, one-to-one instruction, and self-instruction methods with ample reading materials to support their learning.

The *converger* combines the learning modes of AC and AE. People with this learning style type find practical application for ideas and theories and have the ability to use deductive reasoning to solve problems. They like structure and factual information, and they look for specific solutions to problems. Learners with this style prefer technical tasks rather than dealing with social and interpersonal issues. Kolb postulates that individuals with this learning style have skills that are important for specialist and technology careers. The convergent thinker learns best, for example, through demonstration/return demonstration methods of teaching accompanied by handouts and diagrams.

The *accommodator* combines the learning modes of AE and CE. People with this learning style learn best by hands-on experience and enjoy new and challenging situations. They act on intuition and gut feelings rather than on logic. These risk takers like to explore all possibilities and learn by experimenting with materials and objects. Accommodative thinkers are perhaps the most challenging to educators because they demand new and exciting experiences and are willing to take risks that might endanger their safety. Role playing, gaming, and computer simulations, for example, are methods of teaching most preferred by this style of learner.

For every group of learners, about 25% will fall into each of the four categories. Kolb believes that understanding a person's learning style, including its strengths and weaknesses, represents a major step toward increasing learning power and helping learners to get the most from their learning experiences. By using different teaching strategies to address these four learning styles, particular modes of learning can be matched, at least some of the time, with the educator's methods of teaching. If the educator predominantly uses only one method of teaching, such as the lecture to promote learning, then 75% of all learners will be selectively excluded.

When teaching groups of learners, instruction should begin with activities best suited to the divergent thinker and progress sequentially to include activities for the assimilator, converger, and accommodator, respectively (Arndt & Underwood, 1990). This pattern works because learners must first have foundational knowledge of a subject before they can test out information. Otherwise, they will be operating from a level of ignorance. They must first have familiarity with facts and ideas before they can explore and test concepts.

INSTRUMENT TO MEASURE KOLB'S EXPERIENTIAL LEARNING STYLE

The learning style inventory (LSI) is a self-report questionnaire that requires respondents on each of the 12 items to rank four sentence endings corresponding to each of the four learning styles. A scoring process reduces the ranking evidence to four mode scores (CE, RO, AC, and AE) which are further reduced to two dimension scores (concrete-abstract and reflective-active). Two combinations of dimensions scores measure the learner's preference for abstractness versus concreteness (AC-CE) and for action versus reflection (AE-RO). The predominant score indicates the learner's style (diverger, assimilator, converger, or accommodator).

The Kolb model is popular in the healthcare field and has been the subject of many studies. Some scholars believe that the model's validity has not been demonstrated (Coffield et al., 2004). Kolb argues otherwise and states that the LSI has considerable construct validity (Delahoussaye, 2002). The latest LSI (version 3) has significantly improved psychometric properties, especially test-retest reliability (Castro, 2006). A considerable body of research positively reports on Kolb's learning style instrument. The LSI can be obtained from Hay Resources Direct (www.haygroup.com/TL/).

4MAT System

McCarthy (1981) developed a model based on previous research on learning styles and brain functioning. In particular, she used Kolb's model combined with right-brain/left-brain research findings to create the 4MAT system (**Figure 4–7**). McCarthy's model describes four types of learners:

> Type 1/Imaginative: Learners who demand to know why. These learners like to listen, speak, interact, and brainstorm.
>
> Type 2/Analytic: Learners who want to know what to learn. These learners are most comfortable observing, analyzing, classifying, and theorizing.
>
> Type 3/Common sense: Learners who want to know how to apply the new learning. These learners are happiest when experimenting, manipulating, improving, and tinkering.
>
> Type 4/Dynamic: Learners who ask, what if? These learners enjoy modifying, adapting, taking risks, and creating.

McCarthy defines the learning process as a natural sequence from Type 1 to Type 4. Edu-

Figure 4–7 McCarthy's 4MAT system.

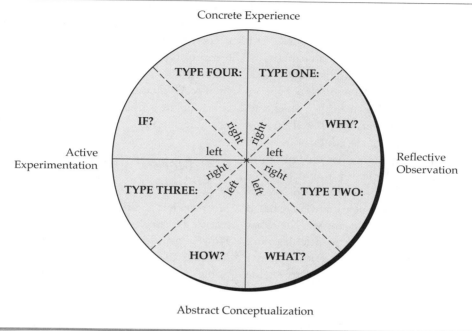

Source: From Guild, P. B., & Garger, S. (1998). *Marching to different drummers.* Alexandria, VA: Association for Supervision and Curriculum Development.

cators can address all four learning styles by teaching sequentially, thus attending to all types of learners. Learners are then able to work with their own strongest learning style, while at the same time developing the ability through exposure to work in the other quadrants.

To use this sequence, learners begin in the first quadrant, known as Type 1, and engage the right brain by sensing and feeling their way through an experience. Eventually, they move to the left brain to analyze what they have experienced. They ask, "Why is this important? Why should I try to learn this?"

The next quadrant is Type 2, in which learning also begins with the right brain to make observations and integrate data with present knowledge. Learners then engage the left brain to think about new theories and concepts relative to these observations. They ask, "What is it I am supposed to be learning? What is the relationship?"

In the third quadrant, Type 3 learners begin with the left brain by working with defined concepts, then shift to the right brain to experiment with what has to be learned. They ask, "How does this work? How can I figure this out?"

Finally, Type 4 learners also begin with the left brain by analyzing the practicality of what has been learned. They then move to the right brain to show mastery through application and the sharing of findings with others. They ask, "If I learn this, what can I do with it? Can I apply it?"

The learning sequence is circular and cyclic, beginning at Type 1 and moving to Type 4, which is characteristic of a higher level and greater complexity of learning. Based on this model, it is important for the educator to begin Type 1 learning by including personal meaning for the learner to make the learning experience relevant and to answer the why question. Next, it is essential to introduce new knowledge based on accurate information to answer the what question. The third step in sequential learning is to deal with reality in a practical manner through application of knowledge to enable learners to answer the how question. Finally, in the fourth step, the learning experience must allow the learner to be innovative and inspiring and to create new dynamic possibilities so the if question is answered.

By using this sequential approach to learning, the educator can instill personal meaning and motivation for what is to be learned (Type 1), assist the learner in the acquisition of the new knowledge and concepts (Type 2), allow for active experimentation (Type 3), and provide the opportunity for more complex synthesis and extension through practical application (Type 4). Through use of the 4MAT system, each learning style will then have an opportunity to exert itself at least part of the time.

INSTRUMENT TO MEASURE THE 4MAT SYSTEM

McCarthy's consulting and publishing company has its own Web site at www.aboutlearning.com.

The 4MAT instructional design and the learning type measure instrument is a 26-point, self-report questionnaire. Although there is little published information on the psychometric properties of the 4MAT system, including the learning type measure, it appears to have face validity. There seems to be no direct criticism of the 4MAT model, and it is accepted by many educators as a useful approach for presenting new information.

Gardner's Eight Types of Intelligence

Most models and measurement instruments on learning style focus on the adult as learner. However, children also have their own way of learning that can be assessed from the standpoint of each individual's unique pattern of growth and neurological functioning. Psychologist Howard Gardner (1983) developed a theory focused on seven kinds of intelligence in children. Gardner based his theory on findings from brain research, developmental work, and psychological testing. He identified seven kinds of intelligence located in different parts of the brain: (1) linguistic, (2) logical-mathematical, (3) spatial, (4) musical, (5) bodily kinesthetic, (6) interpersonal, and (7) intrapersonal. Also, Gardner (1999b) identified an eighth kind of intelligence called naturalistic. Each learner has all the eight kinds of intelligence but in different proportions.

Linguistic intelligence seems to be in the Broca's area of the left side of the brain. Children with a preference for this type of intelligence have highly developed auditory skills and think in words. They like writing, telling stories, spelling words, and reading, and they can recall names, places, and dates. These children learn best by verbalizing, hearing, or seeing words. Word games or crossword puzzles are an excellent method for helping these children to learn new material.

Logical-mathematical intelligence involves both sides of the brain. The right side deals with concepts, and the left side remembers symbols. The children who are strong in this intelligence explore patterns, categories, and relationships. In the adolescent years, they have the ability for logical thinking with a high degree of abstraction. As learners, they question many things and ask where, what, and when. A question such a learner might ask is, "If people are always supposed to be good to each other, then why do people always say they are sorry?" They can do arithmetic problems quickly in their heads, like to learn by computers, and do experiments to test concepts they do not understand. They enjoy strategy board games such as chess or checkers.

Spatial intelligence is related to the right side of the brain. Children with high spatial intelligence learn by images and pictures. They enjoy such things as building blocks, jigsaw puzzles, and daydreaming. They like to draw or do other art activities, can read charts and diagrams, and learn with visual methods such as videos or photographs.

Musical intelligence is also related to the right side of the brain. Musically intelligent children can be found singing a tune, telling you when a note is off key, playing musical instruments with ease, dancing to music, and keeping time rhythmically. They are also sensitive to sounds in the environment, such as the sound of walking on snow on a cold winter morning. Often, musically intelligent children learn best with music playing in the background.

Bodily kinesthetic intelligence includes the basal ganglia and cerebellum of the brain in addition to other brain structures. Children with this type of intelligence learn by processing knowledge through bodily sensations, such as moving around or acting things out. It is difficult for these learners to sit still for long periods of time. They are good at athletic sports and have highly developed fine-motor coordination. Use of body language to communicate and copying people's behaviors or movements come easily for this group of learners.

Interpersonal intelligence involves the prefrontal lobes of the brain. Children with high interpersonal intelligence understand people, are able to notice others' feelings, tend to have many friends, and are gifted in social skills. They learn best in groups and gravitate toward activities that involve others in problem solving.

Intrapersonal intelligence also involves the prefrontal lobes of the brain. Children with this type of intelligence have strong personalities, prefer the inner world of feelings and ideas, and like being alone. They are very private individuals, desire a quiet area to learn, and prefer to be by themselves to learn. They tend to be self-directed and self-confident. They learn well with independent, self-paced instruction.

Naturalistic intelligence refers to sensing abilities in making patterns and connections to elements in nature. Children with high naturalistic intelligence can distinguish and categorize objects or phenomena in nature. They enjoy subjects, shows, and stories that deal with animals or naturally occurring phenomena and are keenly aware of their surroundings and subtle changes in their environment.

Educators should always approach children from the perspective of these different intelligences (Armstrong, 1987). Often it can be difficult to assess the preferred learning style of a child when he or she is facing an illness or surgery.

Asking some key questions of the child or parents may give the educator some clues. What subjects does the child excel in or like best? What kinds of hobbies does the child have? What excites this child? What kinds of toys does the child play with? What inner qualities does the child possess, such as courage, playfulness, curiosity, friendliness, or creativity? What talents does the child possess?

By using Gardner's theory of the eight intelligences, the educator can assess each child's style of learning and tailor teaching accordingly. For example, if the educator wants to assist a child in learning about a kidney disorder, then one of these following eight different approaches can be used, depending on the child's style of learning:

Linguistic—Practice quizzing the child orally on the different parts of the kidney, the disease itself, and ways to take care of oneself.

Spatial—Have a diagram or chart that allows the child to associate different colors or shapes with concepts. Storytelling illustrating a child with the same chronic illness can be used.

Kinesthetic—Have a kidney model available that can be felt, taken apart, and manipulated. Have the child identify tactile features of the kidney or act out appropriate behavior.

Logical-mathematical—Group concepts into categories, starting with simple generalizations or health behaviors. Reasoning works well in showing the child the consequences of actions.

Musical—Teach self-care or the material to be learned by putting information into a song. Soft music also serves as a relaxing influence on the child.

Interpersonal—Have a group of children play a card game such as a version of Old Maid that matches information with medical pictures or pictures of healthcare activities and procedures.

Intrapersonal—Suggest that the child become active by writing to friends, family, or local and state government officials to advocate for kidney disease research. Such learners need to research the facts and then convey these findings to others.

Naturalist—Provide pet therapy, allow the child to engage in an outside activity such as gardening or nature walks, or offer videos where nature, science, or animals are featured.

Although this theory on multiple intelligences was originally designed for use with children, several recent articles address its application with adults. For example, this theory was implemented with nursing students for classroom learning (Amerson, 2006). Many educators see the theory as simple common sense—that children (and adults) have varied talents and learn in different ways even though there is no empirical evidence supporting multiple intelligences theory (Gardner, 2004; Waterhouse, 2006). Additional information about Gardner's theory is available for purchase at his Web site (www.howardgardner.com).

VARK Learning Styles

Fleming and Mills (1992) suggested four categories or preferences—visual, aural, read/write, and kinesthetic—that seem to reflect learning style experiences of their students. VARK is technically about a person's preference for taking in and putting out information. According to Fleming and Mills, an individual learns most effectively and comfortably by one of the following ways:

> *Visual learners* Like graphical representations such as flowcharts with step-by-step directions.
>
> *Aural learners* Enjoy listening to lectures, often need directions read aloud, and prefer to discuss topics and form study groups.
>
> *Read/write learners* Like the written word by reading or writing with references to additional sources of information.
>
> *Kinesthetic learners* Enjoy doing hands-on activities, such as role playing and return demonstration.

INSTRUMENT TO MEASURE THE VARK

The VARK questionnaire provides users with a profile of their learning preferences for taking in and giving out information. VARK's modalities are a part of the Myers-Briggs personality type indicator and Gardner's multiple intelligences theory.

The VARK consists of 16 questions with four options, and the learner can select more than one option for each question. This instrument, recently updated, is free either as an online or printable version (www.vark-learn.com). Although psychometrics on this instrument are not available, the educator may find it to be an excellent tool to help open a dialogue with learners on the differences that exist in the way individuals prefer to learn. The VARK questionnaire is easy to use and can be applied in the healthcare setting.

Interpretation of the Use of Learning Style Models and Instruments

Learning style is an important concept but caution must be exercised in assessing styles so as not to ignore other factors that are equally important to teaching and learning, such as readiness and capabilities to learn, educational background, and rates of learning. Styles, which vary from person to person, also differ from capabilities. The style by which someone learns describes how that individual processes stimuli as opposed to capabilities that define how much and how well the information is processed (Thompson & Crutchlow, 1993).

Many learning theorists advocate that learning style be matched with a similar teaching style for learners to attain an optimal level of achievement. However, research in this area is clouded by inconsistent findings. It may be that learning occurs not so much as a result of matching teacher and learner styles, but that when the educator uses a variety of teaching approaches rather than relying on just one, learners feel less stressed. As a result, they will be more satisfied overall with their learning experience and hence be more motivated to learn. Nevertheless, using teaching methods that coincide with the dominant learning style of individuals is usually considered the best way to promote the greatest levels of achievement (deTornay & Thompson, 1987). Application of learning style theory to facilitate the education process allows the educator to approach each learner holistically by recognizing that not all learners process information in the same way (Arndt & Underwood, 1990).

Research indicates that learning style preferences prevail over time, although they may fluctuate depending on the context in which learners are operating at any given moment. The concept of matching styles implies that individuals are static, which contradicts the purpose of education. Learners need to experience some discomfort before they can grow. Educators need to generate dynamic disequilibrium rather than creating an environment that is too harmonious (Joyce, 1984).

When selecting a learning style instrument, the educator must first evaluate the instrument for validity, reliability, and the population for which it is intended. In addition, the ease of administering the instrument as well as analyzing the results needs to be taken into consideration. Also, copyright laws must be adhered to, which means that the instrument must be bought or the author's permission must be obtained before implementing the tool.

For purposes of assessment, the nurse educator is encouraged to use two or more learning style models and instruments. If the educator focuses on only one, then the possibility arises of trying to make learners fit into a particular style type that does not accurately suit them— a forced choice with no options. Given the teaching–learning situation, the educator may find certain learning style models and instruments to be more appropriate than others in providing strategies for dealing with needs, problems, or unique circumstances.

Of course, it may not always be practical to administer learning style instruments due to cost, time, accessibility, or appropriateness for a specific population. Therefore, educators should follow the general guidelines listed below when assessing individual learning styles:

- Become familiar with the different models and instruments available and the various ways in which styles are classified so that they are easier to recognize.
- Identify key elements of an individual's learning style by observing and asking questions to verify observations. Then match instructional methods and materials to those unique qualities. For example, the following questions could elicit valuable information: Do you prefer to attend lectures or group discussions? Which do you like best, reading or viewing a film? Would you like me to demonstrate this skill first, or would you rather learn by doing while I talk you through the procedure?
- Always allow learners the opportunity to say when a teaching method or instructional material is not working for them.
- Encourage learners to become aware of their learning styles as a way to increase understanding both from the educator's and the learner's perspectives. Everyone should realize that a variety of learning modalities exist and that no one style is better than another.
- Be cautious about saying that certain instructional methods are always more effective for certain styles. Remember that everyone is unique, circumstances may alter preferences, and there are many different ways to influence learning.
- Prompt learners to expand their style ranges rather than to seek only comfortable experiences.
- Provide learning choices that enable learners to operate, at least some of the time, in the style by which they prefer to learn.

- Use a team of educators who have varied teaching styles to present new and complex information in different ways for the mastery of information.

Caution must be exercised when using any of these instruments to assess learning style. The educator must remember not to place too much emphasis or reliance on these tools to categorize learners. The goal should not be to stereotype learners as to style but rather to ensure that each individual learner is given an equal opportunity to learn the best or most comfortable way. Understanding how someone prefers to learn assists the educator in choosing diverse teaching methods and materials to meet the needs of that learner and all learners.

State of the Evidence

Interwoven into each section of this chapter are examples of specific published research about the determinants of learning. This chapter's framework for assessing the evidence to be included in support of the three determinants of learning is based on the framework suggested by Lohr (2004). She cites four dimensions of evidence that need to be considered when making a decision about the available evidence, which are:

1. Level of evidence (study design)
2. Quality of evidence (concern with bias)
3. Relevance of evidence (implying applicability)
4. Strength of evidence (precision, reproducibility, and attributability)

Using this framework was helpful in deciding what is considered appropriate evidence, where the evidence comes from (refereed journals as opposed to Internet commercial sites),

and whether all the evidence counts (or counts in the same way when there are several articles from which to choose). Most of the literature about the determinants of learning is descriptive in nature or expert opinion and many lack the scientific rigor needed as evidence of strength. These studies were not included in this chapter.

The research included in this chapter gives support to the importance of conducting an educational assessment. However, a deficit of evidence on the process and criteria for assessment is striking when compared to the number of studies that provide evidence for the effectiveness of different teaching methodologies. Many of the current scientifically designed studies do not take into account all the determinants of learning before examining the benefits of various teaching interventions. Every learner has different learning needs, readiness to learn, and learning styles, which may account for the paucity of experimental research. Even though very few systemic reviews that pertained to learning styles were found, the evidence suggests that learning style instruments should be used with caution.

The lack of research-based evidence about the three determinants of learning suggests that educational assessment is not an easy area in which to conduct research. It is essential to acknowledge this limitation and to remember that nursing research in comparison to other sciences is still young. In addition, nursing research is supported by a much smaller number of investigators.

Even though much more evidence is needed, the available evidence on conducting an education assessment does substantiate its importance and does provide direction for the nurse as educator. Conducting a needs assessment on all three determinants is essential before any educational intervention is performed.

Summary

This chapter stressed the importance of the assessment phase of learning, because the educator must be aware of and know how to determine learning needs, readiness to learn, and individual learning styles prior to planning for any educational encounter.

Learning is a complex concept that is not directly seen but can be inferred from permanent changes that occur in the learner's behavior in the cognitive, psychomotor, and affective domains. Behavioral objectives for these three domains should not be set until the educator establishes what the needs of the learner are, when the learner is ready to learn, and how the learner best learns. Based on the findings from assessment of these determinants, the educator is able to choose the teaching approaches and learning activities most suited for each individual.

Identifying and prioritizing learning needs requires discovering what the learner feels is important and the educator knows to be important. Once needs are established and agreed upon, the educator must assess the learner's readiness to learn based on the physical, emotional, experiential, and knowledge components particular to each learner. Assessing learning styles by way of interviewing, observing, and instrument measurement can reveal how individuals best learn as well as how they prefer to learn.

By accepting the diversity of needs, readiness levels, and styles among learners, the educator can create a versatile atmosphere and facilitate optimal experiences that encourage all learners to reach their full potential. Whoever the audience may be, teaching interventions and learning activities most beneficial for the learner should be selected on the basis of the three determinants of learning.

REVIEW QUESTIONS

1. How would you define the term *determinants of learning*?
2. What are four of the seven methods to assess patient learning needs?
3. What is meant by the term *readiness to learn*?
4. What are the four types of readiness to learn?
5. What are the components of each type of readiness to learn?
6. What is the definition of the term *learning style*?
7. What are the six learning style principles that should guide the nurse educator in teaching any audience of learners?
8. Which models and instruments are available to determine someone's learning style?
9. What does each of the eight learning style models and instruments measure?
10. What evidence is available to support the determinants of learning?

References

Amerson, R. (2006). Energizing the nursing lecture: Application of the theory of multiple intelligence learning. *Nursing Education Perspectives, 27*(4), 194–196.

Anderson, J. K. (1998). Orientation with style: Matching teaching/learning style. *Journal for Nurses in Staff Development, 14*(4), 192–197.

Armstrong, T. (1987). *In their own way*. New York: St. Martin's Press.

Arndt, M. J., & Underwood, B. (1990). Learning style theory and patient understanding. *Journal of Continuing Education in Nursing, 21*(1), 28–31.

Ashton, K. C. (1999). How men and women with heart disease seek care: The delay experience. *Progress in Cardiovascular Nursing, 14*(2), 53–60.

Bargar, R., & Hoover, R. (1984). Psychological type and the matching of cognitive styles. *Theory into Practice, 23*(1), 56–63.

Beddoe, S. S. (1999). Reachable moment. *Image: Journal of Nursing Scholarship, 31*(3), 248.

Bertakis, K. D., Rahman, A., Helms, L. J., Callahan, E. J., & Robbins, J. A. (2000). Gender differences in the utilization of health care services. *Journal of Family Practice, 49*(2), 147–152.

Bibb, S. C. (2001). Population based needs assessment in the design of patient education programs. *Military Medicine, 166*(4), 297–300.

Bloom, B. (1968). *Learning for mastery*. Instruction and Curriculum, Topical Papers and Reprints No. 1. Durham, NC: National Laboratory for Higher Education.

Bonham, L. A. (1988). Learning style instruments: Let the buyer beware. *Lifelong Learning, 11*(6), 14–17.

Botwinick, J. (1978). *Aging and behavior* (2nd ed.). New York: Springer.

Boyd, M. D., Gleit, C. J., Graham, B. A., & Whitman, N. I. (1998). *Health teaching in nursing practice: A professional model* (3rd ed.). Stamford, CT: Appleton & Lange.

Breitrose, P. (1988). *Focus groups—When and how to use them: A practical guide*. Palo Alto, CA: Health Promotion Resource.

Bruner, J. (1966). *Toward a theory of instruction*. Cambridge, MA: Harvard University Press.

Bubela, N., & Galloway, S. (1990). Factors influencing patients' informational needs at time of hospital discharge. *Patient Education and Counseling, 16,* 21–28.

Bubela, N., Galloway, S., McCay, E., McKibbon, A., Nagle, L., Pringle, D., et al. (2000). Patient learning needs scale. Informational needs of surgical patients following discharge. *Applied Nursing Research, 13,* 12–18.

Burton, C. (2000). Re-thinking stroke rehabilitation: The Corbin and Strauss chronic illness trajectory framework. *Journal of Advanced Nursing, 32*(3), 595–602.

Capraro, R. M., & Capraro, M. M. (2002). Myers-Briggs Type Indicator score reliability across studies: A meta-analytic approach. *Educational and Psychological Measurement, 62,* 590–602.

Carlson, M. L., Ivnik, M. A., Dierkhising, R. A., O'Byrne, M. M., & Vickers, K. S. (2006). A learning needs assessment of patients with COPD. *MEDSURG Nursing, 15*(4), 204–212.

Carroll, I. (1963). A model of school learning. *Teachers College Record, 64,* 723–733.

Cassidy, S. (2004). Learning styles: An overview of theories, models, and measures. *Educational Psychology, 24*(4), 419–444.

Castro, O. (2006). Learning styles—How making too many "wrong mistakes" is the right thing to do: A response to Sparks. *Foreign Language Annals, 39*(3), 529–535.

Caulfield, J., Kidd, S., & Kocher, T. (2000). Brain-based instruction in action. *Educational Leadership, 58*(3), 62–65.

Chall, J., & Mirsky, A. (eds.). (1978). *Education and the brain. Seventy-seventh yearbook of the National Society for the Study of Education* [Part 2]. Chicago: University of Chicago Press.

Coffield, F., Moseley, D., Hall, E., & Ecclestone, K. (2004). *Should we be using learning styles? What research has to say about practice*. Available at http://www.lsrc.ac.uk/publications/index.asp

Corbett, C. F. (2003). A randomized pilot study of improving foot care in home health patients with diabetes. *Diabetes Educator, 29*(2), 273–282.

Corbin, J. M., & Strauss, A. (1991). A nursing model for chronic illness management based upon the trajectory framework. *Scholarly Inquiry for Nursing Practice: An International Journal, 5*(3), 155–174.

Delahoussaye, M. (2002). The perfect learner: An expert debate on learning styles. *Training, 39*(5), 28–36.

deTornay, R., & Thompson, M. A. (1987). *Strategies for teaching nursing* (3rd ed.). Albany, NY: Delmar.

Deture, M. L. (2004). Investigating the predictive value of cognitive style and online technologies self-efficacy in predicting student success in online distance education courses. *Dissertation Abstracts International Section A: Humanities and Social Sciences, 64*(8-A), 2761.

Dunn, R. (1984). Learning style: State of the science. *Theory into Practice, 23*(1), 10–19.

Dunn, R. (1995). *Strategies for educating diverse learners.* Bloomington, IN: Phi Delta Kappa Educational Foundation.

Dunn, K., & Dunn, R. (1987). Dispelling outmoded beliefs about student learning. *Educational Leadership, 44*(6), 55–62.

Dunn, R., & Dunn, K. (1978). *Teaching students through their individual learning styles: A practical approach.* Reston, VA: National Association of Secondary School Principals.

Dunn, R., & Griggs, S. (2003). *Synthesis of the Dunn and Dunn learning styles model research: Who, what, when, where and so what: The Dunn and Dunn learning styles model and its theoretical cornerstone.* New York: St. John's University.

Durden-Smith, J., & deSimone, D. (1983). *Sex and the brain.* New York: Arbor House.

Fleming, N. D., & Mills, C. (1992). Not another inventory, rather a catalyst for reflection. *To Improve the Academy, 11*, 137–144.

Flynn, E. A., Barker, K. N., Gibson, J. T., Pearson, R. E., Berger, B. A., & Smith, L. A. (1999). Impact of interruptions and distractions on dispensing errors in an ambulatory care pharmacy. *American Journal of Health-System Pharmacy, 56*(13), 1319–1325.

Friedman, P., & Alley, R. (1984). Learning/teaching styles: Applying the principles. *Theory into Practice, 23*(1), 77–81.

Gardner, H. (1983). *Frames of mind.* New York: Basic Books.

Gardner, H. (1999a). *The disciplined mind: What all students should understand.* New York: Simon and Schuster.

Gardner, H. (1999b). *Intelligence reframed: Multiple intelligences for the 21st century.* New York: Basic Books.

Gardner, H. (2004). *Changing minds: The art and science of changing our own and other people's minds.* Boston: Harvard Business School Press.

Garity, J. (1985). Learning styles: Basis for creative teaching and learning. *Nurse Educator, 10*(2), 1216.

Gavan, C. S. (2003). Successful aging families—a challenge for nurses. *Holistic Nursing Practice, 17*(1), 11–18.

Gondringer, N. (1989). Whole brain thinking: A potential link to successful learning. *Journal of the American Association of Nurse Anesthetists, 57*(3), 217–219.

Grant, J. (2002). Learning needs assessment: Assessing the need. *British Medical Journal, 324*, 156–159.

Greer, G., Hitt, J. D., Sitterly, T. E., & Slebodnick, E. B. (1972). An examination of four factors impacting on psychomotor performance effectiveness. In D. P. Ely (Ed.), *Psychomotor domain: A resource book for media specialists.* Washington, DC: Gryphon House.

Gur, R. C., Turetsky, B. I., Matsui, M., Yan, M., Bilker, W., Hughett, P., et al. (1999). Sex differences in brain gray and white matter in healthy young adults: Correlations with cognitive performance. *Journal of Neuroscience, 19*(10), 4065–4072.

Haggard, A. (1989). *Handbook of patient education.* Rockland, MD: Aspen.

Hansen, M., & Fisher, J. C. (1998). Patient-centered teaching: From theory to practice. *American Journal of Nursing, 98*(1), 56–60.

Hardy, R., & Smith, R. (2001). Enhancing staff development with a structured preceptor program. *Journal of Nursing Quality Assurance, 15*(2), 9–17.

Healthcare Education Association. (1985). *Managing Hospital Education.* Laguna Niguel, CA: Healthcare Education Associates.

Heller, B. T., Oros, M. T., & Durney-Crowley, J. (2000). The future of nursing education: Ten trends to watch. *Nursing and Health Care Perspectives, 21*(1), 9–13.

Herrmann, N. (1988). *The creative brain.* Lake Lure, NC: Brain Books.

Hotelling, B. A. (2005). Promoting wellness in Lamaze classes. *Journal of Perinatal Education, 14*(3), 45–50.

Iaccino, J. F. (1993). *Left-brain–right-brain differences: Inquiries, evidence and new approaches.* Hillsdale, NJ: Lawrence Erlbaum Associates.

James, W. B., & Gardner, D. L. (1995). Learning styles: Implications for distance learning. *New Directions for Adult and Continuing Education, 67*(1), 19–32.

Joseph, D. H. (1993). Risk: A concept worthy of attention. *Nursing Forum, 28*(1), 12–16.

Joyce, B. (1984). Dynamic disequilibrium: The intelligence of growth. *Theory into Practice, 23*(1), 26–34.

Jung, C. G. (1971). Psychological types. In *Collected works* (Vol. 6, R. F. C. Hull, Trans.). Princeton, NJ: Princeton University Press. (Originally published in German as *Psychologische Typen*, Zurich: Rasher Verlag, 1921).

Keefe, J. W. (1979). *Student learning styles: Diagnosing and prescribing programs.* Reston, VA: National Association of Secondary School Principals.

Kessels, R. P. C. (2003). Patients' memory for medical information. *Journal of the Royal Society of Medicine, 96*(5), 219–222.

Kiesler, D. J., & Auerbach, S. M. (2006). Optimal matches of patient preferences for information, decision making and interpersonal behavior: Evidence, models and interventions. *Patient Education and Counseling, 61*(3), 319–341.

Kim, J., Dodd, M., West, C., Paul, S., Facione, N., Schumacher, K., et al. (2004). The PRO-SELF Pain Control Program improves patients' knowledge of cancer pain management. *Oncology Nursing Forum, 31*(6), 1137–1143.

Kitchie, S. (2003). Rural elders with chronic disease: Place of residence, social network, social support, and medication adherence. (Doctoral dissertation, Binghamton University, 2003). *Dissertation Abstracts International–B* [Online], *64*(08), 3745. (UMI No. 3102848).

Knowles, M. (1990). The application of brain dominance technology to the training profession. In M. Knowles, *The adult learner: A neglected species* (4th ed.). Houston, TX: Gulf Publishing Company.

Knox, A. B. (1974). *Life-long self-directed education.* San Francisco: Jossey-Bass.

Knox, A. B. (1977). *Adult development and learning.* San Francisco: Jossey-Bass.

Knox, A. B. (1986). *Helping adults learn.* San Francisco: Jossey-Bass.

Kolb, D. A. (1984). *Experiential learning: Experience as the source of learning and development.* Englewood Cliffs, NJ: Prentice-Hall.

Landry, S. H., Smith, K. E., & Swank, P. R. (2006). Responsive parenting: Establishing early foundations for social, communication, and independent problem-solving skills. *Developmental Psychology, 42*(4), 627–642.

Ley, P. (1979). Memory for medical information. *British Journal of Social & Clinical Psychology, 18*(2), 245–255.

Lichtenthal, C. (1990). *A self-study model on readiness to learn.* Unpublished manuscript.

Lohr, N. K. (2004). Rating the strength of scientific evidence: Relevance for quality improvement programs. *International Journal for Quality in Health Care, 16*(1), 9–18.

Lubkin, I. M., & Larsen, P. D. (2006). *Chronic illness: Impact and interventions* (6th ed.). Sudbury, MA: Jones and Bartlett.

Maslow, A. (1970). *Motivation and personality.* New York: Harper & Row.

McCarthy, B. (1981). *The 4MAT system: Teaching to learning styles with right/left mode techniques.* Barrington, IL: Excel.

McDonald, D. D., Wiczorek, M., & Walker, C. (2004). Factors affecting learning during health education sessions. *Clinical Nursing Research, 132,* 156–167.

McIntosh, A. R. (1998). Understanding neural interactions in learning and memory using functional neuroimaging. *Annals of the New York Academy of Sciences. Olfaction and Taste XII: An International Symposium, 855,* 556–571.

Miaskowski, C., Dodd, M., West, C., Schumacher, K., Paul, S. M., Tripathy, D., et al. (2004). Randomized clinical trial of the effectiveness of a self-care intervention to improve cancer pain management. *Journal of Clinical Oncology, 22*(9), 1713–1720.

Mordiffi, S. Z., Tan, S. P., & Wong, M. K. (2003). Information provided to surgical patients versus information needed. *Association of Operating Room Nurses, 77*(3), 546–562.

Morse, J. S., Oberer, J., Dobbins, J. A., & Mitchell, D. (1998). Understanding learning styles. Implications for staff development educators. *Journal of Nursing Staff Development, 14*(1), 41–46.

Musinski, B. (1999). The educator as facilitator: A new kind of leadership. *Nursing Forum, 34*(1), 23–29.

Myers, I. B. (1980). *Gifts differing*. Palo Alto, CA: Consulting Psychologists Press.

Myers, I. B. (1987). *Introduction to type*. Palo Alto, CA: Consulting Psychologists Press, Inc.

Oltman, P. K., Raskin, E., Witkin, H. A., & Karp, S. A. (1978). Group embedded figures test. In O. K. Buros (Ed.), *The eighth mental measurements yearbook* (Vol. 1). Lincoln: University of Nebraska Press.

Panja, S., Starr, B., & Colleran, K. M. (2005). Patient knowledge improves glycemic control: Is it time to go back to the classroom? *Journal of Investigative Medicine, 53*(5), 264–266.

Panno, J. M. (1992). A systematic approach for assessing learning needs. *Journal of Nursing Staff Development, 8*(6), 267–273.

Patterson, B. L. (2001). The shifting perspectives model of chronic illness. *Journal of Nursing Scholarship, 33*(1), 21–26.

Ramanadhan, S., & Viswanath, K. (2006). Health and the information nonseeker: A profile. *Health Communication, 20*(2), 131–139.

Rankin, S. H., & Stallings, L. D. (2005). *Patient education in health and illness* (5th ed.). Philadelphia: Lippincott, Williams & Wilkins.

Redman, B. K. (2003). *Measurement tools in patient education*. New York: Springer Publishing Company, Inc.

Roberts, C. (1982). Identifying the real patient problems. *Nursing Clinics of North America, 17*(3), 484–485.

Rutten, L. J., Arora, N. K., Bakos, A. D., Aziz, N., & Rowland, J. (2005). Information needs and sources of information among cancer patients: A systematic review of research (1980–2003). *Patient Education and Counseling, 57*(3), 250–261.

Santrock, J. W. (2006). *Life-span development* (10th ed.). Boston: McGraw-Hill.

Schoessler, M., Conedera, F., Bell, L. F., Marshall, D., & Gilson, M. (1993). Use of the Myers-Briggs type indicator to develop a continuing education department. *Journal of Nursing Staff Development, 9*(1), 8–13.

Shipman, S., & Shipman, V. C. (1985). Cognitive styles: Some conceptual, methodological, and applied issues. In E. W. Gordon (Ed.), *Review of research in education* (12th ed.). Washington, DC: American Educational Research Associates.

Skinner, B. F. (1954). The science of learning and the art of teaching. *Harvard Educational Review, 24*, 86–97.

Speck, O., Ernst, T., Braun, J., Koch, C., Miller, E., & Chang, L. (2000). Gender differences in the functional organization of the brain for working memory. *Neuroreport, 11*(11), 2581–2585.

Sperry, R. W. (1977). Bridging science and values: A unifying view of mind and brain. *American Psychologist, 32*(4), 237–245.

Stein, J. A., & Nyamathi, A. (2000). Gender differences in behavioural and psychosocial predictors of HIV testing and return for test results in a high-risk population. *AIDS Care, 12*(3), 343–356.

Stephenson, P. L. (2006). Before the teaching begins: Managing patient anxiety prior to providing education. *Clinical Journal of Oncology Nursing, 10*(2), 241–245.

Stover, D. (2001). Applying brain research in the classroom is not a no-brainer. *Education Digest, 66*(8), 26–29.

Suhonen, R., Nenonen, A., Laukka, A., & Valimaki, M. (2005). Patients' informational needs and information received do not correspond in hospital. *Journal of Clinical Nursing, 14*, 1167–1176.

Sylvester, R. (1995). *A celebration of neurons: An educator's guide to the human brain*. Alexandria, VA: Association for Supervision and Curriculum Development.

Sylvester, R. (1998). The brain revolution. *School Administrator, 55*(1), 6.

Tanner, G. (1989). A need to know. *Nursing Times, 85*(31), 54–56.

Thompson, C., & Crutchlow, E. (1993). Learning style research: A critical review of the literature and implications for nursing education. *Journal of Professional Nursing, 9*(1), 34–40.

Timmins, F. (2005). A review of the information needs of patients with acute coronary syndromes. *Nursing in Critical Care, 10*(4), 174–183.

Villejo, L., & Meyers, C. (1991). Brain function, learning styles, and cancer patient education. *Seminars in Oncology Nursing, 7*(2), 97–104.

Wagner, P. S., & Ash, K. L. (1998). Creating the teachable moment. *Journal of Nursing Education, 37*(6), 278–280.

Waltz, C. F., Strickland, O. L., & Lenz, E. L. (2005). *Measurement in nursing and health research* (3rd ed.). New York: Springer Publishing Company.

Waterhouse, L. (2006). Multiple intelligences, the Mozart effect, and emotional intelligence: A critical review. *Educational Psychologist, 41*(4), 207–225.

Williams, M. L. (1998). Making the most of learning needs assessments. *Journal for Nurses in Staff Development, 14*(3), 137–142.

Witkin, H., & Goodenough, D. R. (1981). *Cognitive styles: Essence and origins*. New York: International Universities Press.

Witkin, H., Moore, C. A., & Oltman, P. K. (1977). Cognitive styles and their educational implications. *Review of Educational Research, 47*, 1–64.

Witkin, H., Oltman, P. K., Raskin, E., & Karp, S. (1971a). *Group embedded figures test*. Palo Alto, CA: Consulting Psychologists Press.

Witkin, H., Oltman, P. K., Raskin, E., & Karp, S. (1971b). *A manual for the embedded figures test*. Palo Alto, CA: Consulting Psychologists Press.

Wolfe, P. (1994). Risk taking: Nursing's comfort zone. *Holistic Nurse Practice, 8*(2), 43–52.

Wonder, J., & Donovan, M. (1984). *Whole-brain thinking*. New York: Ballantine.

Chapter 5

Developmental Stages of the Learner

Susan B. Bastable

Michelle A. Dart

CHAPTER HIGHLIGHTS

Developmental Characteristics
The Developmental Stages of Childhood
  Infancy (First 12 Months of Life) and Toddlerhood (1–2 Years of Age)
  Early Childhood (3–5 Years of Age)
  Middle and Late Childhood (6–11 Years of Age)
  Adolescence (12–19 Years of Age)

The Developmental Stages of Adulthood
  Young Adulthood (20–40 Years of Age)
  Middle-Aged Adulthood (41–64 Years of Age)
  Older Adulthood (65 Years of Age and Older)
The Role of the Family in Patient Education
State of the Evidence

KEY TERMS

❑ pedagogy
❑ object permanence
❑ causality
❑ animistic thinking
❑ syllogistical reasoning
❑ conservation
❑ imaginary audience

❑ personal fable
❑ andragogy
❑ dialectical thinking
❑ ageism
❑ gerogogy
❑ crystallized intelligence
❑ fluid intelligence

OBJECTIVES

After completing this chapter, the reader will be able to

1. Identify the physical, cognitive, and psychosocial characteristics of learners that influence learning at various stages of growth and development.
2. Recognize the role of the nurse as educator in assessing stage-specific learner needs according to maturational levels.
3. Determine the role of the family in patient education.
4. Discuss appropriate teaching strategies effective for learners at different developmental stages.

When planning, designing, and implementing an educational program, the nurse as educator must carefully consider the characteristics of learners with respect to their developmental stage in life. The more heterogeneous the target audience, the more complex the development of an educational program to meet the diverse needs of the population. Conversely, the more homogeneous the population of learners, the more straightforward the approach to teaching.

An individual's developmental stage significantly influences the ability to learn. Pedagogy, andragogy, and gerogogy are three different orientations to learning in childhood, young and middle adulthood, and older adulthood, respectively. To meet the health-related educational needs of learners, a developmental approach must be used. Three major stage-range factors associated with learner readiness—physical, cognitive, and psychosocial maturation—must be taken into account at each developmental period throughout the life cycle.

Developmental psychologists have for years explored the various patterns of behavior particular to stages of development. Educators, more than ever before, acknowledge the effects of growth and development on an individual's willingness and ability to make use of instruction.

This chapter has specific implications for staff nurses and staff development and in-service nurse educators because of the recent mandates by the Joint Commission (formerly known as JCAHO—the Joint Commission on Accreditation of Healthcare Organizations). For healthcare agencies to meet Joint Commission accreditation requirements, teaching plans must address stage-specific competencies of the learner. In this chapter, the distinct life stages of learners are examined from the perspective of physical, cognitive, and psychosocial development; the role of the nurse in assessment of stage-specific learner needs; the role of the family in the teaching–learning process; and the teaching strategies specific to meeting the needs of learners at various developmental stages of life.

A deliberate attempt has been made to minimize reference to age as the criterion for categorization of learners. Research on life-span development shows that chronological age per se is not the only predictor of learning ability (Santrock, 2006; Vander Zanden, Crandell, &

Crandell, 2007; Whitener, Cox, & Maglich, 1998). At any given age, one finds a wide variation in the acquisition of abilities related to the three fundamental domains of development: physical (biological), cognitive, and psychosocial (emotional-social) maturation. Age ranges, included after each developmental stage heading in this chapter, are intended only to be used as approximate age-strata reference points or general guidelines; they do not imply that chronological ages necessarily correspond perfectly to the various stages of development. Thus, the term developmental stage will be the perspective used based on the confirmation by psychologists that human growth and development are sequential but not always specifically age related.

Recently it has become clear that development is contextual. Even though the passage of time has traditionally been synonymous with chronological age, social and behavioral psychologists have begun to consider the many other changes occurring over time that affect the dynamic relationship between a human being's biological makeup and the environment. It is now understood that three important contextual influences act on and interact with the individual to produce development (Santrock, 2006; Vander Zanden et al., 2007):

1. **Normative age-graded influences** are strongly related to chronological age and are similar for individuals in a particular age group, such as the biological processes of puberty and menopause, and the sociocultural processes of transitioning to different levels of formal education or to retirement.
2. **Normative history-graded influences** are common to people in a particular age cohort or generation because they have been uniquely exposed to similar historical circumstances, such as the Vietnam War, the age of computers, or the terrorist event of September 11, 2001.
3. **Normative life events** are the unusual or unique circumstances, positive or negative, that are turning points in someone's life that cause them to change direction, such as a house fire, serious injury in an accident, winning the lottery, divorce, or an unexpected career opportunity.

Although this chapter focuses on the patient as the learner throughout the life span, the stage-specific characteristics of adulthood and the associated principles of adult learning presented herein can be applied to any audience of young, middle, or older adult learners, whether the nurse is instructing the general public in the community, preparing students in a nursing education program, or teaching continuing education to staff nurses.

Developmental Characteristics

As noted, actual chronological age is only a relative indicator of someone's physical, cognitive, and psychosocial stage of development. Unique as each individual is, however, some typical developmental trends have been identified as milestones of normal progression through the life cycle. When dealing with the teaching–learning process, it is imperative to examine the developmental phases as individuals progress from infancy to senescence so as to fully appreciate the behavioral changes that occur in the cognitive, affective, and psychomotor domains.

As influential as age can be to learning readiness, it should never be examined in isolation.

Growth and development interact with experiential background, physical and emotional health status, and personal motivation, as well as numerous environmental factors such as stress, the surrounding conditions, and the available support systems, to affect a person's ability and readiness to learn.

Musinski (1999) describes three phases of learning: dependence, independence, and interdependence. These passages of learning ability from childhood to adulthood, labeled by Covey (1990) as the "maturity continuum," are identified as follows:

- *Dependence* is characteristic of the infant and young child, who are totally dependent on others for direction, support, and nurturance from a physical, emotional, and intellectual standpoint (unfortunately, some adults are considered to be stuck in this stage if they demonstrate manipulative behavior, do not listen, are insecure, or do not accept responsibility for their own actions).
- *Independence* occurs when a child develops the ability to physically, intellectually, and emotionally care for himself and make his own choices, including taking responsibility for learning.
- *Interdependence* occurs when an individual has advanced in maturity to achieve self-reliance, a sense of self-esteem, the ability to give and receive, and when that individual demonstrates a level of respect for others. Full physical maturity does not guarantee simultaneous emotional and intellectual maturity.

If the nurse as educator is to encourage learners to take responsibility for their own health, then learners must be recognized as an important source of data regarding their health status. Before any learning can occur, the nurse must assess how much knowledge the learner already possesses with respect to the topic to be taught. With the child as client, for example, new content should be introduced at appropriate stages of development and should build on the child's previous knowledge base and experiences.

The major question underlying the planning for educational experiences is: When is the most appropriate or best time to teach the learner? The answer is when the learner is ready—the teachable moment as defined by Havighurst (1976)—that point in time when the learner is most receptive to a teaching situation. It is important to remember that the nurse as educator does not always have to wait for teachable moments to occur; the teacher can create these opportunities by taking an interest in and attending to the needs of the learner. When assessing readiness to learn, the nurse educator must determine not only if an interpersonal relationship has been established, if prerequisite knowledge and skills have been mastered, and if the learner exhibits motivation, but also if the plan for teaching matches the developmental level of the learner (Polan & Taylor, 2003; Leifer & Hartston, 2004; Santrock, 2006; Vander Zanden et al., 2007).

The Developmental Stages of Childhood

Pedagogy is the art and science of helping children to learn (Knowles, 1990). The different stages of childhood are divided according to what developmental theorists and educational psychologists define as specific patterns of behavior seen in particular phases of growth and development. One common attribute through-out all phases of childhood is that learning is subject centered. The following is a review of the developmental characteristics in the four stages of childhood and the teaching strategies to be used in relation to the physical, cognitive, and psychosocial maturational levels indicative of learner readiness (see **Table 5–1**).

Infancy (First 12 Months of Life) and Toddlerhood (1–2 Years of Age)

The field of growth and development is highly complex, and at no other time is physical, cognitive, and psychosocial maturation so change-able as during the very early years of childhood. Because of the dependency of this age group, the main focus of instruction for health maintenance of children is geared toward the parents, who are considered to be the primary learners rather than the very young child (Palfrey, Hauser-Cram, Bronson, Warfield, Sirin, & Chan, 2005; Richmond & Kotelchuck, 1984; Santrock, 2006; Vander Zanden et al., 2007). However, the older toddler should not be excluded from healthcare teaching and can participate to some extent in the education process.

PHYSICAL, COGNITIVE, AND PSYCHOSOCIAL DEVELOPMENT

At no other time in life is physical maturation so rapid as during the period of development from infancy to toddlerhood (London, Ladewig, Ball, & Bindler, 2003). Exploration of self and the environment becomes paramount and a stimulant for further physical development (Vander Zanden et al., 2007). Patient education must focus on teaching the parents of very young children the importance of stimulation, nutrition,

the practice of safety measures to prevent illness and injury, and health promotion (Polan & Taylor, 2003; Richmond & Kotelchuck, 1984).

Piaget (1951, 1952, 1976), the noted expert in defining the key milestones in the cognitive development of children, labeled the stage of infancy to toddlerhood as the *sensorimotor period*. This period refers to the coordination and integration of motor activities with sensory perceptions. As children mature from infancy to toddlerhood, learning is enhanced through sensory experiences and through movement and manipulation of objects in the environment. Toward the end of the second year of life, the very young child begins to develop *object permanence*, that is, realizing that objects and events exist even when they cannot be seen, heard, or touched (Santrock, 2006). Motor activities promote their understanding of the world and an awareness of themselves as well as others' reactions in response to their own actions. Encouraging parents to create a safe environment will allow their child to develop with a decreased risk for injury.

The toddler has the rudimentary capacity for basic reasoning, understands object permanence, has the beginnings of memory, and begins to develop an elementary concept of *causality*, which refers to the ability to grasp a cause-and-effect relationship between two paired, successive events (Vander Zanden et al., 2007). With limited ability to recall past happenings or anticipate future events, the toddler is oriented primarily to the here and now and has little tolerance for delayed gratification. The child who has lived with strict routines and plenty of structure will have more of a grasp of time than the child who lives in an unstructured environment.

Children at this stage have short attention spans, are easily distracted, are egocentric in their thinking, and are not amenable to correction of

Table 5–1 STAGE-APPROPRIATE TEACHING STRATEGIES

Learner	General Characteristics	Teaching Strategies	Nursing Interventions
INFANCY–TODDLERHOOD			
Approximate age: Birth–2 years Cognitive stage: Sensorimotor Psychosocial stage: Trust vs. mistrust (Birth–12 mo) Autonomy vs. shame and doubt (1–2 yr)	Dependent on environment Needs security Explores self and environment Natural curiosity	Orient teaching to caregiver Use repetition and imitation of information Stimulate all senses Provide physical safety and emotional security Allow play and manipulation of objects	Welcome active involvement Forge alliances Encourage physical closeness Provide detailed information Answer questions and concerns Ask for information on child's strengths/limitations and likes/dislikes
EARLY CHILDHOOD			
Approximate age: 3–5 years Cognitive stage: Preoperational Psychosocial stage: Initiative vs. guilt	Egocentric Thinking precausal, concrete, literal Believes illness self-caused and punitive Limited sense of time Fears bodily injury Cannot generalize Animistic thinking (objects possess life or human characteristics) Centration (focus is on one characteristic of an object) Separation anxiety Motivated by curiosity Active imagination, prone to fears Play is his/her work	Use warm, calm approach Build trust Use repetition of information Allow manipulation of objects and equipment Give care with explanation Reassure not to blame self Explain procedures simply and briefly Provide safe, secure environment Use positive reinforcement Encourage questions to reveal perceptions/feelings Use simple drawings and stories Use play therapy, with dolls and puppets Stimulate senses: visual, auditory, tactile, motor	Welcome active involvement Forge alliances Encourage physical closeness Provide detailed information Answer questions and concerns Ask for information on child's strengths/limitations and likes/dislikes

MIDDLE AND LATE CHILDHOOD

	General Characteristics	Teaching Strategies	Nursing Interventions
Approximate age: 6–11 years Cognitive stage: Concrete operations Psychosocial stage: Industry vs. inferiority	More realistic and objective Understands cause and effect Deductive/inductive reasoning Wants concrete information Able to compare objects and events Variable rates of physical growth Reasons syllogistically Understands seriousness and consequences of actions Subject-centered focus Immediate orientation	Encourage independence and active participation Be honest, allay fears Use logical explanation Allow time to ask questions Use analogies to make invisible processes real Establish role models Relate care to other children's experiences; compare procedures Use subject-centered focus Use play therapy Provide group activities Use drawings, models, dolls, painting, audio- and video tapes	Welcome active involvement Forge alliances Encourage physical closeness Provide detailed information Answer questions and concerns Ask for information on child's strengths/limitations and likes/dislikes

ADOLESCENCE

	General Characteristics	Teaching Strategies	Nursing Interventions
Approximate age: 12–19 years Cognitive stage: Formal operations Psychosocial stage: Identity vs. role confusion	Abstract, hypothetical thinking Can build on past learning Reasons by logic and understands scientific principles Future orientation Motivated by desire for social acceptance Peer group important Intense personal preoccupation, appearance extremely important (imaginary audience) Feels invulnerable, invincible/immune to natural laws (personal fable)	Establish trust, authenticity Know their agenda Address fears/concerns about outcomes of illness Identify control focus Include in plan of care Use peers for support and influence Negotiate changes Focus on details Make information meaningful to life Ensure confidentiality and privacy Arrange group sessions Use audiovisuals, role play, contracts, reading materials Provide for experimentation and flexibility	Explore emotional and financial support Determine goals and expectations Assess stress levels Respect values and norms Determine role responsibilities and relationships Engage in 1:1 teaching without parents present, but with adolescent's permission inform family of content covered

(continues)

Table 5–1 STAGE-APPROPRIATE TEACHING STRATEGIES (CONTINUED)

Learner	General Characteristics	Teaching Strategies	Nursing Interventions
YOUNG ADULTHOOD			
Approximate age: 20–40 years Cognitive stage: Formal operations Psychosocial stage: Intimacy vs. isolation	Autonomous Self-directed Uses personal experiences to enhance or interfere with learning Intrinsic motivation Able to analyze critically Makes decisions about personal, occupational, and social roles Competency-based learner	Use problem-centered focus Draw on meaningful experiences Focus on immediacy of application Encourage active participation Allow to set own pace, be self-directed Organize material Recognize social role Apply new knowledge through role-playing and hands-on practice	Explore emotional, financial, and physical support system Assess motivational level for involvement Identify potential obstacles and stressors
MIDDLE-AGED ADULTHOOD			
Approximate age: 41–64 years Cognitive stage: Formal operations Psychosocial stage: Generativity vs. self-absorption and stagnation	Sense of self well-developed Concerned with physical changes At peak in career Explores alternative lifestyles Reflects on contributions to family and society Reexamines goals and values Questions achievements and successes Has confidence in abilities Desires to modify unsatisfactory aspects of life	Focus on maintaining independence and reestablishing normal life patterns Assess positive and negative past experiences with learning Assess potential sources of stress due to midlife crisis issues Provide information to coincide with life concerns and problems	Explore emotional, financial, and physical support system Assess motivational level for involvement Identify potential obstacles and stressors

OLDER ADULTHOOD

Approximate age: 65 years and over
Cognitive stage: Formal operations
Psychosocial stage: Ego integrity vs. despair

Cognitive changes

Decreased ability to think abstractly, process information
Decreased short-term memory
Increased reaction time
Increased test anxiety
Stimulus persistence (afterimage)
Focuses on past life experiences

Use concrete examples
Build on past life experiences
Make information relevant and meaningful
Present one concept at a time
Allow time for processing/response (slow pace)
Use repetition and reinforcement of information
Avoid written exams
Use verbal exchange and coaching
Establish retrieval plan (use one or several clues)
Encourage active involvement
Keep explanations brief
Use analogies to illustrate abstract information

Involve principal caregivers
Encourage participation
Provide resources for support (respite care)
Assess coping mechanisms
Provide written instructions for reinforcement
Provide anticipatory problem solving (what happens if . . .)

Sensory/motor deficits

Auditory changes
Hearing loss, especially high-pitched tones, consonants (S, Z, T, F, and G), and rapid speech
Visual changes
Farsighted (needs glasses to read)
Lenses become opaque (glare problem)
Smaller pupil size (decreased visual adaptation to darkness)
Decreased peripheral perception

Speak slowly, distinctly
Use low-pitched tones
Face client when speaking
Minimize distractions
Avoid shouting
Use visual aids to supplement verbal instruction
Avoid glares, use soft white light
Provide sufficient light
Use white backgrounds and black print
Use large letters and well-spaced print
Avoid color coding with pastel blues, greens, purples, and yellows
Increase safety precautions/provide safe environment

(continues)

Table 5–1 Stage-Appropriate Teaching Strategies (CONTINUED)

Learner	General Characteristics	Teaching Strategies	Nursing Interventions
OLDER ADULTHOOD (continued)	Yellowing of lenses (distorts low-tone colors: blue, green, violet) Distorted depth perception Fatigue/decreased energy levels Pathophysiology (chronic illness) **Psychosocial changes** Decreased risk taking Selective learning Intimidated by formal learning	Ensure accessibility and fit of prostheses (i.e., glasses, hearing aid) Keep sessions short Provide for frequent rest periods Allow for extra time to perform Establish realistic short-term goals Give time to reminisce Identify and present pertinent material Use informal teaching sessions Demonstrate relevance of information to daily life Assess resources Make learning positive Identify past positive experiences Integrate new behaviors with formerly established ones	

their own ideas. Unquestionably, they believe their own perceptions to be reality. Asking questions is the hallmark of this age group, and curiosity abounds as they explore places and things. They can respond to simple, step-by-step commands and obey such directives as "give Grandpa a kiss" or "go get your teddy bear" (Santrock, 2006).

Language skills are acquired rapidly during this period, and parents should be encouraged to foster this aspect of development by talking with and listening to their child. As they progress through this phase, children begin to engage in fantasizing and make-believe play. Because they are unable to distinguish fact from fiction and have limited cognitive capacity for understanding cause and effect, children may feel that illness and hospitalization are a punishment for something they did wrong (London et al., 2003). Children attributing the cause of illness to the consequences of their own transgressions is known as egocentric causation (Richmond & Kotelchuck, 1984).

According to Erikson (1963), the noted authority on psychosocial development, the period of infancy is one of *trust versus mistrust*. During this time, children must work through their first major dilemma of developing a sense of trust with their primary caretaker. As the infant matures into toddlerhood, *autonomy versus shame and doubt* emerges as the central issue. During this period of psychosocial growth, toddlers must learn to balance feelings of love and hate and learn to cooperate and control willful desires (see **Table 5–2**).

Children progress sequentially through accomplishing the tasks of developing basic trust in their environment to reaching increasing levels of independence and self-assertion. Their newly discovered sense of independence often is

expressed by demonstrations of negativism. Children may have difficulty in making up their minds, and, aggravated by personal and external limits, their level of frustration and feelings of ambivalence may be expressed in words and behaviors, such as in exhibiting temper tantrums to release tensions (Falvo, 1994). With peers, play is a parallel activity, and it is not unusual for them to end up in tears because they have not yet learned about tact, fairness, or rules of sharing (Babcock & Miller, 1994; Polan & Taylor, 2003).

Toddlers like routines because they give these children a sense of security, and they gravitate toward ritualistic ceremonial-like exercises when carrying out activities of daily living. Separation anxiety is also characteristic of this stage of development and is particularly apparent when children are hospitalized and feel insecure in an unfamiliar environment. This anxiety is often compounded when they are subjected to medical procedures and other healthcare interventions performed by people who are strangers to them (London et al., 2003).

TEACHING STRATEGIES

Patient education for infancy through toddlerhood need not be illness related. Usually less time is devoted to teaching parents about illness care, and considerably more time is spent teaching aspects of normal development, safety, health promotion, and disease prevention. When the child is ill, the first priority for teaching interventions would be to assess the parents' and child's anxiety levels and to help them cope with their feelings of stress related to uncertainty and guilt about the cause of the illness. Anxiety on the part of the child and parents can adversely affect their readiness to learn.

Although teaching activities primarily are directed to the main caregiver(s), children at this

Table 5–2 ERICKSON'S EIGHT STAGES OF PSYCHOSOCIAL DEVELOPMENT

Developmental Stages	Psychosocial Crises	Strengths
Infancy	Trust vs. mistrust	Hope
Toddlerhood	Autonomy vs. shame and doubt	Will
Early childhood	Initiative vs. guilt	Purpose
Middle and late childhood	Industry vs. inferiority	Competence
Adolescence	Identity vs. role confusion	Fidelity
Young adulthood	Intimacy vs. isolation	Love
Middle-aged adulthood	Generativity vs. self-absorption and stagnation	Care
Older adulthood	Ego integrity vs. despair	Wisdom

Source: Adapted from Ahroni, J. H. (1996). Strategies for teaching elders from a human development perspective. *Diabetes Educator, 22*(1), 48.

developmental stage in life have a great capacity for learning. Toddlers are capable of some degree of understanding procedures that they may experience. Because of the young child's natural tendency to be intimidated by unfamiliar people, it is imperative that a primary nurse be assigned to establish a relationship with the child and parents. This approach will not only provide consistency in the teaching–learning process but also help to reduce the child's fear of strangers. Parents should be present whenever possible during formal and informal teaching and learning activities to allay stress, which could be compounded by separation anxiety (London et al., 2003).

Ideally, health teaching should take place in an environment familiar to the child, such as the home or day-care center. When the child is hospitalized, the environment selected for teaching and learning sessions should be as safe and secure as possible, such as the child's bed or the playroom, to increase the child's sense of feeling protected.

Movement is an important mechanism by which toddlers communicate. Immobility due to illness or hospital confinement tends to increase children's anxiety by restricting activity. Nursing interventions that promote children's use of gross motor abilities and that stimulate their visual, auditory, and tactile senses should be chosen.

Developing a rapport with children through simple teaching will help to elicit their cooperation and active involvement. The approach to children should be warm, honest, calm, accepting, and matter-of-fact. A smile, a warm tone of voice, a gesture of encouragement, or a word of praise goes a long way in attracting children's attention and helping them adjust to new circumstances. Fundamental to the child's response is how the parents respond to healthcare personnel and medical interventions.

The following teaching strategies are suggested to convey information to members of this age group. These strategies feed into children's natural tendency for play and their need for active participation and sensory experiences.

FOR SHORT-TERM LEARNING

- Read simple stories from books with lots of pictures.
- Use dolls and puppets to act out feelings and behaviors.
- Use simple audiotapes with music and videotapes with cartoon characters.
- Role-play to bring the child's imagination closer to reality.
- Give simple, concrete, nonthreatening explanations to accompany visual and tactile experiences.
- Perform procedures on a teddy bear or doll first to help the child anticipate what an experience will be like.
- Allow the child something to do—squeeze your hand, hold a Band-Aid, cry if it hurts—to channel their responses to an unpleasant experience.
- Keep teaching sessions brief (no longer than about 5 minutes each) because of the child's short attention span.
- Cluster teaching sessions close together so that children can remember what they learned from one instructional encounter to another.
- Avoid analogies and explain things in straightforward and simple terms because children take their world literally and concretely.
- Individualize the pace of teaching according to the child's responses and level of attention.

FOR LONG-TERM LEARNING

- Focus on rituals, imitation, and repetition of information in the form of words and actions to hold the child's attention.

For example, practice washing hands before and after eating and toileting.

- Use reinforcement as an opportunity for children to achieve permanence of learning through practice.
- Employ the teaching methods of gaming and modeling as a means by which children can learn about the world and test their ideas over time.
- Encourage parents to act as role models because their values and beliefs serve to reinforce healthy behaviors and significantly influence the child's development of attitudes and behaviors.

Early Childhood (3–5 Years of Age)

Children in the preschool years continue with development of skills learned in the earlier years of growth. Their sense of identity becomes clearer, and their world expands to encompass involvement with others external to the family unit. Children in this developmental category acquire new behaviors that give them more independence from their parents and allow them to care for themselves more autonomously. Learning during this time period occurs through interactions with others and through mimicking or modeling the behaviors of playmates and adults (Richmond & Kotelchuck, 1984; Whitener et al., 1998).

PHYSICAL, COGNITIVE, AND PSYCHOSOCIAL DEVELOPMENT

The physical maturation during early childhood is an extension of the child's prior growth. Fine and gross motor skills become increasingly more refined and coordinated so that children are able to carry out activities of daily living with greater independence (Santrock, 2006; Vander Zanden et al., 2007). Although their efforts are more coordinated, supervision of activities is still required because they lack judgment in carrying out the skills they have developed.

The early childhood stage of cognitive development is labeled by Piaget (1951, 1952, 1976) as the *preoperational period*. This stage emphasizes the child's inability to think things through logically without acting it out and it is the transitional period when the child starts to use symbols (letters and numbers) to represent something (Santrock, 2006; Snowman & Biehler, 2006; Vander Zanden et al., 2007).

Children in the preschool years begin to develop the capacity to recall past experiences and anticipate future events. They can classify objects into groups and categories, but have only a vague understanding of their relationships. The young child continues to be egocentric and is essentially unaware of others' thoughts or the existence of others' points of view. Thinking remains literal and concrete—they believe what is seen and heard. Precausal thinking allows young children to understand that people can make things happen, but they are unaware of causation as the result of invisible physical and mechanical forces. They often believe that they can influence natural phenomena, and their beliefs reflect *animistic thinking*—the tendency to endow inanimate objects with life and consciousness (Pidgeon, 1977; Santrock, 2006).

Preschool children are very curious, can think intuitively, and pose questions about almost anything. They want to know the reasons, cause, and purpose for everything (the why) but are unconcerned at this point with the process (the how). Fantasy and reality are not well differentiated. Children in this cognitive stage mix fact and fiction, tend to generalize, think magically, develop imaginary playmates, and believe they can control events with their thoughts. At the same time, they do possess self-awareness and realize that they are vulnerable to outside influences (Santrock, 2006; Vander Zanden et al., 2007).

The young child also continues to have a limited sense of time. For children of this age, being made to wait 15 minutes before they can do something can feel like an eternity. They do, however, understand the timing of familiar events in their daily lives, such as when breakfast or dinner is eaten and when they can play or watch their favorite television program. Their attention span (ability to focus) begins to lengthen such that they can usually remain quiet long enough to listen to a song or hear a short story read (Santrock, 2006).

In the preschool stage, children begin to develop sexual identity and curiosity, an interest that may cause considerable discomfort for their parents. Cognitive understanding of their bodies related to structure, function, health, and illness becomes more specific and differentiated. They can name external body parts but have only an ill-defined concept of the size and shape of internal organs and the function of body parts (Kotchabhakdi, 1985).

Explanations of the purpose and reasons for a procedure remain beyond the young child's level of reasoning, so explanations have to be kept very simple and matter-of-fact (Pidgeon, 1985). Children at this stage have a fear of body mutilation and pain, which not only stems from their lack of understanding of the body but also is compounded by their active imagination. Their ideas regarding illness also are primitive with respect to cause and effect; illness is seen as a punishment for something they did wrong, either through omission or commission (Richmond & Kotelchuck, 1984). Health, on the other hand, may be identified with doing things right. Health allows them to play with friends and participate in desired activities; illness prevents them from doing so (Hussey & Hirsh, 1983).

Erikson (1963) has labeled the psychosocial maturation level in early childhood as the period of *initiative versus guilt*. Children take on tasks for the sake of being involved and on the move (see Table 5–2). Excess energy and a desire to dominate may lead to frustration and anger on their part. They show evidence of expanding imagination and creativity, are impulsive in their actions, and are curious about almost everything they see and do. Their growing imagination can lead to many fears—of separation, disapproval, pain, punishment, and aggression from others. Loss of body integrity is the preschool child's greatest threat, which significantly affects his or her willingness to interact with healthcare personnel (Poster, 1983; Vulcan, 1984).

In this phase of development, children begin interacting with playmates rather than just playing alongside one another. Appropriate social behaviors demand that they learn to wait for others, give others a turn, and recognize the needs of others. Play in the mind of a child is equivalent to the work performed by adults. Play can be as equally productive as adult work and is a means for self-education of the physical and social world (Whitener et al., 1998). It helps the child act out feelings and experiences to master fears, develop role skills, and express joys, sorrows, and hostilities. Through play, children in the preschool years also begin to share ideas and imitate parents of the same sex. Role-playing is typical of this age as the child attempts to learn the responsibilities of family members and others in society (Santrock, 2006).

TEACHING STRATEGIES

The nurse's interactions with preschool children and their parents are often sporadic, usually occurring during occasional well-child visits to the pediatrician's office or when minor medical problems arise. During these interactions, the nurse should take every opportunity to teach parents about health promotion and disease prevention measures, to provide guidance regarding normal growth and development, and to offer instruction about medical recommendations when illnesses do arise. Parents can be a great asset to the nurse in working with children in this developmental phase, and they should be included in all aspects of the educational plan and the actual teaching experience. Parents can serve as the primary resource to answer questions about children's disabilities, their idiosyncrasies, and their favorite toys—all of which may affect their ability to learn (Hussey & Hirsh, 1983; Ryberg & Merrifield, 1984; Woodring, 2000).

Children's fear of pain and bodily harm is uppermost in their minds, whether they are well or ill. Because young children have fantasies and active imaginations, it is most important for the nurse to reassure them and allow them to express themselves openly about their fears (Heiney, 1991). Choose your words carefully when describing procedures. Preschool children are familiar with many words, but using terms like "cut" or "knife" is frightening to them. Instead, use less threatening words like "fix," "sew," or "cover up the hole." "Band-Aids" rather than "dressings" is a much more understandable term, and bandages are often thought by children to have magical healing powers (Babcock & Miller, 1994).

Although still dependent on family, the young child has begun to have increasing contact with the outside world and is usually able to interact more comfortably with others. Nevertheless, significant adults in a child's life should be included as participants during teaching sessions. They can provide support to the child, substitute as the teacher if their child is reluctant to interact with the nurse, and reinforce teaching at a later point in time. The primary caretakers, usually the mother and father, are the recipients of the majority of the nurse's teaching efforts. They will be the learners to assist the child in achieving desired health outcomes (Hussey & Hirsh, 1983; Kennedy & Riddle, 1989; Whitener et al., 1998).

The following specific teaching strategies are recommended:

For Short-Term Learning

- Provide physical and visual stimuli because language ability is still limited, both for expressing ideas and for comprehending verbal instructions.
- Keep teaching sessions short (no more than 15 minutes) and scheduled sequentially at close intervals so that information is not forgotten.
- Relate information needs to activities and experiences familiar to the child. For example, ask the child to pretend to blow out candles on a birthday cake to practice deep breathing.
- Encourage the child to participate in selecting between a limited number of teaching–learning options, such as playing with dolls or reading a story, which promotes active involvement and helps to establish nurse–client rapport.
- Arrange small group sessions with peers as a way to make teaching less threatening and more fun.
- Give praise and approval, through both verbal expressions and nonverbal gestures, which are real motivators for learning.

- Give tangible rewards, such as badges or small toys, immediately following a successful learning experience as reinforcers in the mastery of cognitive and psychomotor skills.
- Allow the child to manipulate equipment and play with replicas or dolls to learn about body parts. Special kidney dolls, ostomy dolls with stomas, or orthopedic dolls with splints and tractions provide opportunity for hands-on experience.
- Use storybooks to emphasize the humanity of healthcare personnel; to depict relationships between the child, parents, and others; and to assist with helping the child identify with particular situations.

For Long-Term Learning

- Enlist the help of parents, who can play a vital role in modeling a variety of healthy habits, such as practicing safety measures and eating a balanced diet.
- Reinforce positive health behaviors and the acquisition of specific skills.

Middle and Late Childhood (6–11 Years of Age)

In middle and late childhood, children have progressed in their physical, cognitive, and psychosocial skills to the point where most begin formal training in structured school systems. They approach learning with enthusiastic anticipation, and their minds are open to new and varied ideas.

Children at this developmental level are motivated to learn because of their natural curiosity and their desire to understand more about themselves, their bodies, their world, and the influence that different things in the world have on them (Whitener et al., 1998). This stage is a period of great change for them, when attitudes, values, and perceptions of themselves, their society, and the world are shaped and expanded. Visions of their own environment and the cultures of others take on more depth and breadth (Santrock, 2006).

Physical, Cognitive, and Psychosocial Development

The gross- and fine-motor abilities of school-aged children are increasingly more coordinated so that they are able to control their movements with much greater dexterity than ever before. Involvement in all kinds of curricular and extracurricular activities helps them to fine-tune their psychomotor skills. Physical growth during this phase is highly variable, with the rate of development differing from child to child. Toward the end of this developmental period, girls more so than boys on the average begin to experience prepubescent bodily changes and tend to exceed the boys in physical maturation. Growth charts, which monitor the rate of growth, are a more sensitive indicator of health or disability than actual size (Burkett, 1989; Santrock, 2006; Vander Zanden et al., 2007).

Piaget (1951, 1952, 1976) has labeled the cognitive development in middle and late childhood as the period of *concrete operations*. During this time, logical, rational thought processes and the ability to reason inductively and deductively develop. Children in this stage are able to think more objectively, are willing to listen to others, and will selectively use questioning to find answers to the unknown. At this stage, they begin to use *syllogistical reasoning*—that is, they can consider two premises and draw a logical conclusion from them (Elkind, 1984). For example, they comprehend that mammals are warm-blooded, whales are mammals, so whales must be warm-blooded.

Also, they are intellectually able to understand cause and effect in a concrete way. Concepts such as *conservation*, which is the ability to recognize that the properties of an object stay the same even though its appearance and position may change, are beginning to be mastered. For example, they realize that a certain quantity of liquid is the same amount whether it is poured into a tall, thin glass or into a short, squat one (Snowman & Biehler, 2006). Fiction and fantasy are separate from fact and reality. The skills of memory, decision making, insight, and problem solving are all more fully developed (Protheroe, 2007).

Children in this developmental phase are capable of engaging in systematic thought through inductive reasoning. They are able to classify objects and systems, express concrete ideas about relationships and people, and carry out mathematical operations. Also, they begin to understand and use sarcasm as well as to employ well-developed language skills for telling jokes, conveying complex stories, and communicating increasingly more sophisticated thoughts (Snowman & Biehler, 2006).

Nevertheless, thinking remains quite literal, with only a vague understanding of abstractions. Early on in this phase, children are reluctant to do away with magical thinking in exchange for reality thinking. They cling to cherished beliefs, such as the existence of Santa Claus or the tooth fairy, for the fun and excitement that the fantasy provides them, even when they have information that proves contrary to their beliefs.

Children passing through elementary and middle schools have developed the ability to concentrate for extended periods, can tolerate delayed gratification, are responsible for independently carrying out activities of daily living, have a good understanding of the environment as a whole, and can generalize from experience (Vander Zanden et al., 2007). They understand time, can predict time intervals, are oriented to the past and present, have some grasp and interest in the future, and have a vague appreciation for how immediate actions can have implications over the course of time. Special interests in topics of their choice begin to emerge, and they can pursue subjects and activities with devotion to increase their talents in particular areas.

Children at this cognitive stage can make decisions and act in accordance with how events are interpreted, but they understand only to a limited extent the seriousness or consequences of their choices. Children in the early period of this developmental phase know the functions and names of many common body parts, whereas older children have a more specific knowledge of anatomy and can differentiate between external and internal organs with a beginning understanding of their complex functions (Kotchabhakdi, 1985).

In the shift from precausal to causal thinking, the child begins to incorporate the idea that illness is related to cause and effect and can recognize that germs create disease. Illness is thought of in terms of social consequences and role alterations, such as the realization that they will miss school and outside activities, people will feel sorry for them, and they will be unable to maintain their usual routines (Banks, 1990).

Research indicates, however, that systematic differences exist in children's reasoning skills with respect to understanding body functioning and the cause of illness as a result of their experiences with illness. Children suffering from chronic diseases have been found to have more sophisticated conceptualization of illness causality and body functioning than do their healthy peers. Piaget (1976) postulated that experience with a phenomenon catalyzes a better understanding of it.

On the other hand, the stress and anxiety resulting from having to live with a chronic illness can interfere with a child's general cognitive performance. Chronically ill children have a less refined understanding of the physical world than healthy children do, and the former often are unable to generalize what they learned about a specific illness to a broader understanding of illness causality (Perrin, Sayer, & Willett, 1991). Thus, illness may act as an intrusive factor in overall cognitive development (Palfrey et al., 2005).

Erikson (1963) characterized school-aged children's psychosocial stage of life as *industry versus inferiority*. During this period, children begin to gain an awareness of their unique talents and special qualities that distinguish them from one another (see Table 5–2). They begin to establish their self-concept as members of a social group larger than their own nuclear family and start to compare family values with those of the outside world.

The school environment, in particular, facilitates their gaining a sense of responsibility and reliability. With less dependency on family, they extend their intimacy to include special friends and social groups (Santrock, 2006). Relationships with peers and adults external to the home environment become important influences in their development of self-esteem and their susceptibility to social forces outside the family unit. School-aged children fear failure and being left out of groups. They worry about their inabilities and become self-critical as they compare their own accomplishments to those of their peers. They also fear illness and disability that could significantly disrupt their academic progress, interfere with social contacts, decrease their independence, and result in loss of control over body functioning.

TEACHING STRATEGIES

In today's healthcare environment, those in middle to late childhood and their families must be taught in an efficient, cost-effective manner how to maintain health and manage illness. Woodring (2000) emphasizes the importance of following sound educational principles with the child and family, such as identifying individual learning styles, determining readiness to learn, and accommodating particular learning needs and abilities to achieve positive health outcomes.

With their increased ability to comprehend information and their desire for active involvement and control of their lives, it is very important to include school-aged children in patient education efforts. The nurse in the role of educator should explain illness, treatment plans, and procedures in simple, logical terms in accordance with the child's level of understanding and reasoning. Although children at this stage of development are able to think logically, their ability for abstract thought remains limited. Therefore, teaching should be presented in concrete terms with step-by-step instructions (Pidgeon, 1985; Whitener et al., 1998). It is imperative that the nurse observe children's reactions and listen to their verbal feedback to confirm that information shared has not been misinterpreted or confused.

To the extent feasible, parents should be informed of what their child is being taught. Teaching parents directly is encouraged so that they may be involved in fostering their child's independence, providing emotional support and physical assistance, and giving guidance regarding the correct techniques or regimens in self-care management. Siblings and peers should also be considered as sources of support. In attempting to master self-care skills, children thrive on praise from others who are important in their lives as rewards for their accomplishments and successes (Hussey & Hirsh, 1983; Santrock, 2006).

Education for health promotion and health maintenance is most likely to occur in the school system through the school nurse, but the parents as well as the nurse outside the school setting should be told what content is being addressed. Information then can be reinforced and expanded on when in contact with the child in other care settings. Numerous opportunities for nurses to teach the individual child or groups of children about health promotion and disease and injury prevention are available in schools, physicians' offices, community centers, outpatient clinics, or hospitals. Health education for children of this age can be very fragmented because of the many encounters they have with nurses in a variety of settings.

The school nurse, in particular, is in an excellent position to coordinate the efforts of all other providers so as to avoid duplication of teaching content or the giving of conflicting information as well as to provide reinforcement of learning. According to *Healthy People 2010* (U.S. Department of Health and Human Services, 2000), health promotion regarding healthy eating, exercise, and prevention of injuries, as well as avoidance of tobacco, alcohol, and drug use, are just a few examples of goals set forth to improve the health of America's children. The school nurse plays a vital role in providing this education to the school-aged child to meet these goals (Leifer & Hartston, 2004). The school nurse has the opportunity to educate children in a group when teaching a class and on a one-to-one basis when encountering an individual child in the nurse's office for a particular problem or need.

The specific conditions that may come to the attention of the nurse in caring for children at this phase of development include problems such as behavioral disorders, hyperactivity, learning disorders, obesity, diabetes, asthma, and enuresis. Extensive teaching may be needed to help children and parents understand a particular condition and learn how to overcome or deal with it.

The need to sustain or bolster their self-image, self-concept, and self-esteem requires that children be invited to participate, to the extent possible, in planning for and carrying out learning activities (Snowman & Biehler, 2006). For children newly diagnosed with diabetes, for example, it is beneficial to allow them to administer an injection to a stuffed animal or another person. This strategy allows them to participate and will decrease their fear. Because of children's fears of falling behind in school, being separated from peer groups, and being left out of social activities, teaching must be geared toward fostering normal development despite any limitations that may be imposed by illness (Falvo, 1994; Leifer & Hartston, 2004).

Because children in middle and late childhood are used to the structured, direct, and formal learning in the school environment, they are receptive to a similar teaching–learning approach when hospitalized or confined at home. The following teaching strategies are suggested when caring for children in this developmental stage of life:

FOR SHORT-TERM LEARNING

- Allow school-aged children to take responsibility for their own health care because they are not only willing but

also capable of manipulating equipment with accuracy. Because of their adeptness in relation to manual dexterity, mathematical operations, and logical thought processes, they can be taught, for example, to calculate and administer their own insulin or use an asthma inhaler as prescribed.

- Teaching sessions can be extended to last as long as 30 minutes each because the increased cognitive abilities of school-aged children aids in the retention of information. However, lessons should be spread apart to allow for comprehension of large amounts of content and to provide opportunity for the practice of newly acquired skills between sessions.

- Use diagrams, models, pictures, videotapes, printed materials, and computers as adjuncts to various teaching methods because an increased facility with language (both spoken and written) as well as with mathematical concepts allows for these children to work with more complex instructional tools.

- Choose audiovisual and printed materials that show peers undergoing similar procedures or facing similar situations.

- Clarify any scientific terminology and medical jargon used.

- Use analogies as an effective means of providing information in meaningful terms, such as "Having a chest X-ray is like having your picture taken" or "White blood cells are like police cells that can attack and destroy infection."

- Use one-to-one teaching sessions as a method to individualize learning relevant to the child's own experiences and as a means to interpret the results of nursing interventions particular to the child's own condition.

- Provide time for clarification, validation, and reinforcement of what is being learned.
- Select individual instructional techniques that provide opportunity for privacy, an increasingly important concern for this group of learners, who often feel quite self-conscious and modest when learning about bodily functions.
- Employ group teaching sessions with others of similar age and with similar problems or needs to help children avoid feelings of isolation and to assist them in identifying with their own peers.
- Prepare children for procedures well in advance to allow them time to cope with their feelings and fears, to anticipate events, and to understand what the purpose of each procedure is, how it relates to their condition, and how much time it will take.
- Encourage participation in planning for procedures and events because active involvement will help the child to assimilate information more readily.
- Provide much-needed nurturance and support, always keeping in mind that young children are not just small adults. Praise and rewards will help motivate and reinforce learning.

FOR LONG-TERM LEARNING

- Help school-aged children acquire skills that they can use to assume self-care responsibility for carrying out therapeutic treatment regimens on an ongoing basis with minimal assistance.

- Assist them in learning to maintain their own well-being and prevent illnesses from occurring.

Research suggests that lifelong health attitudes and behaviors begin in the early childhood phase of development and remain intrapersonally consistent throughout the stage of middle to late childhood. The development of cognitive understanding of health and illness has been shown to follow a systematic progression parallel to the stage of general cognitive development (Santrock, 2006). As the child matures, beliefs about health and illness become less concrete and more abstract, less egocentric, and increasingly differentiated and consistent.

Motivation, self-esteem, and positive self-perception are personal characteristics that influence health behavior. Research has shown that the higher the grade level of the child, the greater the understanding of illness and an awareness of body cues. Thus, children become more actively involved in their own health care as they progress developmentally (Farrand & Cox, 1993; Whitener et al., 1998). Teaching should be directed at assisting them to incorporate positive health actions into their daily lives. Because of the importance of peer influence, group activities are an effective method of teaching health behaviors, attitudes, and values.

Adolescence (12–19 Years of Age)

The stage of adolescence marks the transition from childhood to adulthood. During this prolonged and very change-filled period of time, many adolescents and their families experience much turmoil. How adolescents think about themselves and the world significantly influences many healthcare issues facing them, from anorexia to diabetes. Teenage thought and behavior give insight into the etiology of some of the major health problems of this group of learners (Elkind, 1984). Adolescents are known to be among the nation's most at-risk populations (American Association of Colleges of Nursing, 1994). For patient education to be effective, an understanding of the characteristics of the adolescent phase of development is crucial (Ackard & Neumark-Sztainer, 2001; Girod, Pardales, Cavanaugh, & Wadsworth, 2005; Michaud, Stronski, Fonseca, & MacFarlane, 2004).

PHYSICAL, COGNITIVE, AND PSYCHOSOCIAL DEVELOPMENT

Adolescents vary greatly in their biological, psychological, social, and cognitive development. From a physical maturation standpoint, they must adapt to rapid, dramatic, and significant bodily changes, which can temporarily result in clumsiness and poorly coordinated movement. Alterations in physical size, shape, and function of their bodies, along with the appearance and development of secondary sex characteristics, bring about a significant preoccupation with their appearance and a strong desire to express sexual urges (Santrock, 2006; Vander Zanden et al., 2007).

Piaget (1951, 1952, 1976) termed this stage of cognitive development as the period of *formal operations*. Adolescents have attained a new, higher-order level of reasoning superior to earlier childhood thoughts. They are capable of abstract thought and complex logical reasoning described as propositional as opposed to syllogistic. Their reasoning is both inductive and deductive, and they are able to hypothesize and apply the principles of logic to situations never encountered before. Adolescents can conceptu-

alize and internalize ideas, debate various points of view, understand cause and effect, comprehend complex explanations, imagine possibilities, make sense out of new data, discern relationships among objects and events, and respond appropriately to multiple-step directions (Aronowitz, 2006; Vander Zanden et al., 2007).

Formal operational thought enables adolescents to conceptualize invisible processes and make determinations about what others say and how they behave. With this capacity, teenagers can become obsessed with what they think as well as what others are thinking, a characteristic known as adolescent egocentrism. They begin to believe that everyone is focusing on the same things they are—namely, themselves and their activities. Elkind (1984) labeled this belief as the *imaginary audience*, a type of social thinking that has considerable influence over an adolescent's behavior. The imaginary audience explains the pervasive self-consciousness of adolescents, who, on the one hand, may feel embarrassed because they believe everyone is looking at them and, on the other hand, desire to be looked at and thought about because this attention confirms their sense of being special and unique (Santrock, 2006; Snowman & Biehler, 2006; Vander Zanden et al., 2007).

Adolescents are able to understand the concept of health and illness, the multiple causes of diseases, the influence of variables on health status, and the ideas associated with health promotion and disease prevention. Parents and healthcare providers are their most frequent sources of health-related information (Ackard & Neumark-Sztainer, 2001). They recognize that illness is a process resulting from a dysfunction or nonfunction of a part or parts of the body and can comprehend the outcomes or prognosis of an illness. They can also identify health behaviors but may reject practicing them or begin to engage in risk-taking behaviors because of the social pressures they receive from peers as well as their feelings of invincibility (Girod et al., 2005). Elkind (1984) has labeled this second type of social thinking as the *personal fable*. The personal fable leads adolescents to believe that they are invulnerable—other people grow old and die, but not them; other people may not realize their personal ambitions, but they will.

This personal fable has value in that it allows individuals to carry on with their lives even in the face of all kinds of dangers. Unfortunately, it also leads teenagers to believe they are cloaked in an invisible shield that will protect them from bodily harm despite any risks to which they may subject themselves. They can understand implications of future outcomes, but their immediate concern is with the present.

Recent research, however, reveals that adolescents 15 years of age and older are not as susceptible to the personal fable as once thought (Cauffman & Steinberg, 2000). Although children in the mid- to late-adolescent period appear to be aware of the risks they take, it is important, nevertheless, to recognize that this population continues to need support and guidance (Brown, Teufel, & Birch, 2007).

Erikson (1968) has identified the psychosocial dilemma adolescents face as one of *identity versus role confusion*. These children indulge in comparing their self-image with an ideal image (see Table 5–2). Adolescents find themselves in a struggle to establish their own identity, match their skills with career choices, and determine their self. They work to emancipate themselves from their parents, seeking independence and autonomy so that they can emerge as more distinct individual personalities.

Teenagers have a strong need for belonging to a group, friendship, peer acceptance, and peer support. They tend to rebel against any actions or recommendations by adults whom they consider authoritarian. Their concern over personal appearance and their need to look and act like their peers drive them to conform to the dress and behavior of this age group, which is usually contradictory, nonconformist, and in opposition to the models, codes, and values of their parents' generation. Conflict, toleration, stereotyping, or alienation characterizes the relationship between adolescents and their parents and other authority figures (Hines & Paulson, 2006). Adolescents seek to develop new and trusting relationships outside the home but remain vulnerable to the opinions of those they emulate (Santrock, 2006).

Adolescents demand personal space, control, privacy, and confidentiality. To them, illness, injury, and hospitalization means dependency, loss of identity, a change in body image and functioning, bodily embarrassment, confinement, separation from peers, and possible death. The provision of knowledge alone is, therefore, not sufficient for this population. Due to the many issues apparent during the adolescent period, the need for coping skills is profound and can influence the successful completion of this stage of development (Grey, Kanner, & Lacey, 1999).

TEACHING STRATEGIES

Although the majority of individuals at this phase of development remain relatively healthy, an estimated 20% of the United States' teenagers have at least one serious health problem, such as asthma, learning disabilities, eating disorders (e.g., obesity, anorexia, or bulimia), diabetes, a range of disabilities as a result of injury, or psychological problems as a result of depression or physical and/or emotional maltreatment. In addition, adolescents are considered at high risk for teen pregnancy, the effects of poverty, drug or alcohol abuse, and sexually transmitted diseases such as venereal disease and AIDS. The three leading causes of death in this age group are accidents, homicide, and suicide (London et al., 2003). More than 50% of all adolescent deaths are a result of accidents and most involve motor vehicles (Santrock, 2006).

Despite all of these potential threats to their well-being, adolescents use medical services the least frequently of all age groups. Compounding this problem is the realization that adolescent health has not been a national priority and their health issues have been largely ignored by the healthcare system (American Association of Colleges of Nursing, 1994; Michaud et al., 2004). Thus, the educational needs of adolescents are broad and varied. The potential topics for teaching are numerous, ranging from sexual adjustment, contraception, and venereal disease to accident prevention, nutrition, and substance abuse.

Healthy teens have difficulty imagining themselves as sick or injured. Those with an illness or disability often comply poorly with medical regimens and continue to indulge in risk-taking behaviors. Because of their preoccupation with body image and functioning and the perceived importance of peer acceptance and support, they view health recommendations as a threat to their autonomy and sense of control.

Probably the greatest challenge to the nurse responsible for teaching the adolescent, whether healthy or ill, is to be able to develop a mutually respectful, trusting relationship (Brown et al., 2007). Adolescents, because of their well-developed cognitive and language abilities, are able to participate fully in all aspects of learning, but they need privacy, understanding, an hon-

est and straightforward approach, and unqualified acceptance in the face of their fears of embarrassment, losing independence, identity, and self-control (Ackard & Neumark-Sztainer, 2001). The Society of Adolescent Medicine cites availability, visibility, quality, confidentiality, affordability, flexibility, and coordination to be important factors in providing education effectively to the adolescent population (Leifer & Hartston, 2004; Girod et al., 2005).

The existence of an imaginary audience and personal fable can contribute to the exacerbation of existing problems or cause new ones. Adolescents with disfiguring handicaps, who as young children exhibited a great deal of spirit and strength, may now show signs of depression and lack of will. For the first time, they look at themselves from the standpoint of others and reinterpret behavior once seen as friendly as actually condescending. Teenagers may fail to use contraceptives because the fable tells them that other people will get pregnant or get venereal disease, but not them. Teenagers with chronic illnesses may stop taking prescribed medications because they feel they can manage without them to prove to others that they are well and free of medical constraints; other people with similar diseases need to follow therapeutic regimens, but not them.

Adolescents' language skills and ability to conceptualize and think abstractly give the nurse as educator a wide range of teaching methods and instructional tools from which to choose (Brown et al., 2007). The following teaching strategies are suggested when caring for adolescents:

For Short-Term Learning

- Use one-to-one instruction to ensure confidentiality of sensitive information.

- Choose peer group discussion sessions as an effective approach to deal with health topics as smoking, alcohol and drug use, safety measures, and teenage sexuality. Adolescents benefit from being exposed to others who have the same concerns or who have successfully dealt with problems similar to theirs.
- Use face-to-face or computer group discussion, role-playing, and gaming as methods to clarify values and problem solve, which feed into the teenager's need to belong and to be actively involved. Getting groups of peers together in person or via technology can be very effective in helping teens confront health challenges and learn how to significantly change behavior (Snowman & Biehler, 2006).
- Employ adjunct instructional tools, such as complex models, diagrams, and specific, detailed written materials, which can be used competently by many adolescents. Audiovisual materials in the form of computers, audiotapes, videotapes, simulated games, and interactive discs using the hardware of TV, audiocassette players, and computers usually are a comfortable approach to learning for adolescents, who generally have facility with technological equipment after years of academic and personal experience with telecommunications in the home and at school.
- Clarify any scientific terminology and medical jargon used.
- Share decision making whenever possible because control is an important issue for adolescents.
- Include them in formulating teaching plans related to teaching strategies, expected outcomes, and determining what needs to be learned and how it can best be achieved to meet their needs for autonomy.
- Suggest options so that they feel they have a choice about courses of action.
- Give a rationale for all that is said and done to help adolescents feel a sense of control.
- Approach them with respect, tact, openness, and flexibility to elicit their attention and encourage their responsiveness to teaching–learning situations.
- Expect negative responses, which are common when their self-image and self-integrity are threatened.
- Avoid confrontation and acting like an authority figure. Instead of directly contradicting their opinions and beliefs, acknowledge their thoughts and then casually suggest an alternative viewpoint or choices, such as "Yes, I can see your point, but what about the possibility of . . . ?"

For Long-Term Learning

- Accept adolescents' personal fable and imaginary audience as valid, rather than challenging their feelings of uniqueness and invincibility.
- Acknowledge that their feelings are very real because denying them their opinions simply will not work.
- Allow them the opportunity to test their own convictions. Let them know, for example, that while some other special people may get away without taking medication, others cannot. Suggest, if medically feasible, setting up a trial

period with medications scheduled farther apart or in lowered dosages to determine how they can manage.

Although much of patient education should be done directly with adolescents to respect their right to individuality, privacy, and confidentiality, teaching effectiveness may be enhanced by including their families to some extent (Brown et al., 2007). The nurse as educator can give guidance and support to families, helping them to better understand adolescent behavior (Hines & Paulson, 2006). Parents should be taught how to set realistic limits and at the same time foster the adolescent's sense of independence. Through prior assessment of potential sources of stress, teaching both the parents and the adolescent (as well as siblings) can be enhanced. Because of the ambivalence the adolescent feels while in this transition stage from childhood to adulthood, healthcare teaching, to be effective, must consider the learning needs of the adolescent as well as the parents (Ackard & Neumark-Sztainer, 2001; Falvo, 1994).

The Developmental Stages of Adulthood

Andragogy, the term coined by Knowles (1990) to describe his theory of adult learning, is the art and science of teaching adults. Education within this framework is more learner centered and less teacher centered; that is, instead of one party imparting knowledge on another, the power relationship between the educator and the adult learner is much more horizontal (Milligan, 1997). The concept of andragogy has served for years as a useful framework in guiding instruction for patient teaching and for continuing education of staff. Recently, based on emerging

research and theory from a variety of disciplines, Knowles, Holton, and Swanson (1998) discussed new perspectives on andragogy that have refined and strengthened the core adult learning principles Knowles originally proposed.

The following basic assumptions about Knowles's framework have major implications for planning, implementing, and evaluating teaching programs for adults as the individual matures:

1. His or her self-concept moves from one of being a dependent personality to being an independent, self-directed human being.
2. He or she accumulates a growing reservoir of previous experience that serves as a rich resource for learning.
3. Readiness to learn becomes increasingly oriented to the developmental tasks of social roles.
4. The perspective of time changes from one of postponed application of knowledge to one of immediate application; there is a shift in orientation of learning to being problem centered rather than subject centered.

A limitation of Knowles's assumptions about child versus adult learners is that they are derived from studies conducted on healthy people. It is important to keep in mind, however, that illness and injury have the potential for significantly changing cognitive and psychological processes used for learning (Best, 2001).

The period of adulthood constitutes three major developmental stages—the young adult stage, the middle-aged adult stage, and the older adult stage (see Table 5–1). Although adulthood, like childhood, can be divided into various developmental phases, the focus for learning is quite different. Whereas a child's readiness to learn depends on physical, cognitive, and psychosocial development, adults have essentially reached the peak of their physical and cognitive capacities.

The emphasis for adult learning revolves around differentiation of life tasks and social roles with respect to employment, family, and other activities beyond the responsibilities of home and career (Boyd, Gleit, Graham, & Whitman, 1998). In contrast to childhood learning, which is subject centered, adult learning is problem centered. The prime motivator to learn in adulthood is to be able to apply knowledge and skills for the solution of immediate problems. Unlike children, who enjoy learning for the sake of gaining an understanding of themselves and the world, adults must clearly perceive the relevancy in acquiring new behaviors or changing old ones for them to be willing and eager to learn. In the beginning of any teaching–learning encounter, therefore, adults want to know the benefit they will derive from their efforts at learning (Knowles et al., 1998).

In contrast to the child learner, who is dependent on authority figures for learning, the adult is much more self-directed and independent in seeking information. For adults, past experiences are internalized and form the basis for further learning. Adults already have a rich resource of stored information on which to build a further understanding of relationships between ideas and concepts. They are quicker than children at grasping relationships, and they do not tolerate learning isolated facts as well as children do (see Table 5–3).

Table 5–3 SUMMARY OF ADULT LEARNING PRINCIPLES

Adults learn best when:

Principle No. 1	Learning is related to an immediate need, problem, or deficit.
Principle No. 2	Learning is voluntary and self-initiated.
Principle No. 3	Learning is person centered and problem centered.
Principle No. 4	Learning is self-controlled and self-directed.
Principle No. 5	The role of the teacher is one of facilitator.
Principle No. 6	Information and assignments are pertinent.
Principle No. 7	New material draws on past experiences and is related to something the learner already knows.
Principle No. 8	The threat to self is reduced to a minimum in the educational situation.
Principle No. 9	The learner is able to participate actively in the learning process.
Principle No. 10	The learner is able to learn in a group.
Principle No. 11	The nature of the learning activity changes frequently.
Principle No. 12	Learning is reinforced by application and prompt feedback.

Source: Adapted from Burgireno, J. (1985). Maximizing learning in the adult with SCI. *Rehabilitation Nursing, 10*(5), 20–21.

Because adults already have established ideas, values, and attitudes, they also tend to be more resistant to change. In addition, adults must overcome obstacles to learning to a greater extent than children. For example, they have the burden of family, work, and social responsibilities, which can diminish their time, energy, and concentration for learning. Also, their need for self-direction may present problems because various stages of illness, as well as the healthcare setting in which they may find themselves, can force dependency. Anxiety, too, may negatively affect their motivation and ability to learn (Kessels, 2003). Furthermore, they may feel too old or too out of touch with the formal learning of the school years, and if past experiences with learning were not positive, they may shy away from assuming the role of learner for fear of the risk of failure (Boyd et al., 1998).

Although we accept adult learners as autonomous, self-directed, and independent, these individuals often want and need structure, clear and concise specifics, and direct guidance. As such, Taylor, Marienau, and Fiddler (2000) label adults as "paradoxical" learners.

Only recently has it been recognized that learning is a lifelong process that begins at birth and does not cease until the end of life. Growth and development are a process of becoming, and learning is inextricably a part of that process. As a person matures, learning is a significant and continuous task to maintain and enhance oneself (Knowles, 1990; Knowles et al., 1998). Social scientists now recognize that adulthood "is not a single monolithic stage, not an undifferentiated phase of life between adolescence and old age" (Vander Zanden et al., 2007, p. 443).

A variety of reasons explain why adults pursue learning throughout their lives. Basically, three categories describe the general orientation

of adults toward continuing education (Babcock & Miller, 1994):

1. *Goal-oriented learners* engage in educational endeavors to accomplish clear and identifiable objectives. Continuing education for them is episodic and occurs as a recurring pattern throughout their lives as they realize the need for or an interest in expanding their knowledge and skills. Adults who attend night courses or professional workshops do so to build their expertise in a particular subject or for advancement in their professional or personal lives.

2. *Activity-oriented learners* select educational activities primarily to meet social needs. The learning of content is secondary to their need for human contact. While they may choose to participate in support groups, special-interest groups, or self-help groups, or attend academic classes because of an interest in a particular topic being offered, they join essentially out of their desire to be around others and converse with people in similar circumstances—retirement, parenting, divorce, or widowhood. Their drive is to alleviate social isolation or loneliness.

3. *Learning-oriented learners* view themselves as perpetual students who seek knowledge for knowledge's sake. They are active learners all of their lives and tend to join groups, classes, or organizations with the anticipation that the experience will be educational and personally rewarding.

In most cases, all three types of learners initiate the learning experience for themselves. In planning educational activities for adults, it is important to determine their motives for wanting to be involved. That is, it is advantageous for the nurse educator to understand the purpose and expectations of the individuals who participate in continuing education programs. In that way, the nurse educator can best serve learners in the role as facilitator for referral or resource information, thus embracing the adults' state of independence and interdependence (Musinski, 1999).

Obviously, there are many differences between child and adult learners (see Table 5–1). As the following discussion will clearly reveal, there also are differences in the characteristics of adult learners within the three developmental stages of adulthood.

Young Adulthood (20–40 Years of Age)

The transition from adolescence to becoming a young adult has recently been termed *emerging adulthood*. Early adulthood comprises the cohort currently between 20–24 years of age who belong to the millennial or Net generation (Prensky, 2001) and the cohort currently aged 25–40, who are known as Generation X. Both generations exhibit their own characteristic traits and present different challenges to the nurse educator (Billings & Kowalski, 2004). These two age ranges of people constitute about 80 million Americans (Vander Zanden et al., 2007).

Young adulthood is a time for establishing long-term, intimate relationships with other people, choosing a lifestyle and adjusting to it, deciding on an occupation, and managing a home and family. All of these decisions lead to changes in the lives of young adults that can be a potential source of stress for them. It is a time when intimacy and courtship are pursued and

spousal and/or parental roles are developed (Santrock, 2006).

PHYSICAL, COGNITIVE, AND PSYCHOSOCIAL DEVELOPMENT

During this period, physical abilities for most young adults are at their peak, and the body is at its optimal functioning capacity (Vander Zanden et al., 2007). The vast majority of individuals at this stage can master, if they so desire, almost any psychomotor skill they undertake to accomplish (Santrock, 2006).

The cognitive capacity of young adults is fully developed, but with maturation, they continue to accumulate new knowledge and skills from an expanding reservoir of formal and informal experiences. Young adults continue in the *formal operations* stage of cognitive development (Piaget, 1951, 1952, 1976). These experiences add to their perceptions, allow them to generalize to new situations, and improve their abilities to critically analyze, problem solve, and make decisions about their personal, occupational, and social roles. Their interests for learning are oriented toward those experiences that are relevant for immediate application to problems and tasks in their daily lives. Young adults are motivated to learn about the possible implications of various lifestyle choices (Vander Zanden et al., 2007).

Erikson (1963) describes the young adult's stage of psychosocial development as the period of *intimacy versus isolation*. During this time, individuals work to establish a trusting, satisfying, and permanent relationship with others (see Table 5–2). They strive to establish commitment to others in their personal, occupational, and social lives. They are now working to maintain the independence and self-sufficiency they worked to obtain in adolescence.

Young adults face many challenges as they take steps to control their lives. Many of the events they experience are happy and growth promoting from an emotional and social perspective, but they also can prove disappointing and psychologically draining. The new experiences and multiple decisions they must make regarding choices for a career, marriage, parenthood, and higher education can be quite stressful. Young adults realize that the avenues they pursue will affect their lives for years to come (Santrock, 2006).

TEACHING STRATEGIES

Based on the paucity of literature on health teaching of individuals who belong specifically to this age cohort, young adulthood is considered to be the life-span period that has received the least attention by nurse educators. At this developmental stage, prior to the emergence of the chronic diseases that characterize the middle-age and older years, young adults are generally very healthy and tend to have limited exposure to health professionals. Their contact with the healthcare system is usually for preemployment, college, or presport physicals; for a minor episodic complaint; or for pregnancy and contraceptive care (Orshan, 2008). At the same time, young adulthood is a crucial period for the establishment of behaviors that help individuals to lead healthy lives, both physically and emotionally. Many of the choices young adults make, if not positive ones, will be difficult to modify later. As Havighurst pointed out, this stage is full of teachable moment opportunities, but it is the most devoid of efforts by health providers to teach (Johnson-Saylor, 1980).

Health promotion is the most neglected aspect of healthcare teaching at this stage of life. Adults aged 20–24 are the most likely group to lack health insurance coverage (Vander Zanden et al., 2007). Yet, many of the health issues related to risk factors and stress management are important to deal with to help young adults establish positive health practices for preventing problems with illness in the future. The major factors associated with increased risk of death in later life, such as high blood pressure, elevated cholesterol, obesity, smoking, overuse of alcohol and drugs, and pertinent family history of major illnesses such as cancer and heart disease all need to be addressed (Santrock, 2006).

The nurse as educator must find a way of reaching and communicating with this audience about health promotion and disease prevention measures. Readiness to learn does not always require the nurse educator to wait for it to develop. Rather, such readiness can be fostered through experiences the nurse creates. Knowledge of the individual's lifestyle can provide cues to concentrate on when determining specific aspects of education for the young adult. For example, if the individual is planning marriage, then teaching about family planning, contraception, and parenthood are potential topics to address (Orshan, 2008). The motivation for adults to learn comes in response to internal drives, such as need for self-esteem, a better quality of life, or job satisfaction, and in response to external motivators, such as job promotion, more money, or more time to pursue outside activities (Babcock & Miller, 1994; Vander Zanden et al., 2007).

When young adults are faced with acute or chronic illnesses, many of which may significantly alter their lifestyles, they are stimulated to learn so as to maintain their independence and return to normal life patterns. It is likely they will view an illness or disability as a serious setback to achieving their immediate or future life goals.

Because adults typically desire active participation in the educational process, it is important for the nurse as educator to allow them the opportunity for mutual collaboration in health education decision making. They should be encouraged to select what to learn (objectives), how they want material to be presented (instructional methods and tools), and which indicators will be used to determine the achievement of learning goals (evaluation) (Knowles, 1990). Also, it must be remembered that adults bring a variety of experiences that can serve as a foundation on which to build new learning to the teaching–learning situation. Consequently, it is important to draw on their experiences to make learning relevant, useful, and motivating. Young adults tend to be reluctant to expend the resources of time, money, and energy to learn new information, skills, and attitudes if they do not see the content of instruction as relevant to their current lives or anticipated problems (Collins, 2004).

Teaching strategies must be directed at encouraging young adults to seek information that expands their knowledge base, helps them control their lives, and bolsters their self-esteem. Whether they are well or ill, young adults need to know about the opportunities available for learning. Making them aware of health issues and learning opportunities can occur in a variety of settings, such as physicians' offices, community clinics, outpatient departments, or hospitals. In all cases, these educational opportunities must be convenient and accessible to them in terms of their lifestyle with respect to work and family responsibilities. Relevant, applicable, and practical information is what adults desire and value—they want to know "what's in it for me" (WIIFM), according to Collins (2004).

Because they tend to be very self-directed in their approach to learning, young adults do well with written patient education materials and audiovisual tools, including computer-assisted instruction, that allow them to independently self-pace their learning. Group discussion is an attractive method for teaching and learning because it provides young adults with the opportunity to interact with others of similar age and situation, such as parenting groups, prenatal classes, or marital adjustment sessions. Although assessment prior to teaching will help to determine the level at which to begin teaching, no matter what the content, the enduring axiom is to make learning easy and relevant. To facilitate learning, present concepts logically from simple to complex and to establish conceptual relationships through specific application of information (Collins, 2004; Musinski, 1999).

Middle-Aged Adulthood (41–64 Years of Age)

Just as adolescence is the link between childhood and adulthood, midlife is the transition period between young adulthood and older adulthood. Middle-aged Americans make up about one fifth of the population, and this current cohort has typically been labeled the baby-boom generation. Although this was once one of the most neglected age periods, baby boomers, who now make up this cohort, are receiving increasingly more attention by developmental psychologists and healthcare providers. This is because not only do they constitute the largest cohort of any current generation, but because current middle-aged adults are the best educated, most affluent in history, and they have the potential for a healthier life than ever before due to medical discoveries that can stave off the aging process. In just one century, the average life expectancy has increased by 30 years (Vander Zanden et al., 2007).

Thus, the concept of what has been thought of as middle age is being nudged upward. As more people live longer, middle age is now coming later in life than ever before. Adults are no longer considered to be over the hill when they celebrate their 40th birthday. Middle age for many healthy adults is starting later and lasting longer. Remember, chronological age is one factor, but biological, psychological, and social age also must be taken into account (Santrock, 2006).

During middle age, many individuals are highly accomplished in their careers, their sense of who they are is well developed, their children are grown, and they have time to share their talents, serve as mentors for others, and pursue new or latent interests. It is a time for them to reflect on the contributions they have made to family and society, relish in their achievements, and reexamine their goals and values.

PHYSICAL, COGNITIVE, AND PSYCHOSOCIAL DEVELOPMENT

During this stage of maturation, a number of physiological changes begin to take place. Skin and muscle tone decreases, metabolism slows down, body weight tends to increase, endurance and energy levels lessen, hormonal changes bring about a variety of symptoms, and hearing and visual acuity start to diminish. All these physical changes and others affect middle-aged adults' self-image, ability to learn, and motivation for learning about health promotion, disease prevention, and maintenance of health (Vander Zanden et al., 2007).

The ability to learn from a cognitive standpoint remains at a steady state for middle-aged adults as they continue in what Piaget (1951,

1952, 1976) labeled the *formal operations* stage of cognitive development. He maintained that cognitive development stopped with this stage (the ability to perform abstract thinking) that was achieved during adolescence. However, over the years critics of Piaget's theory have begun to assert the existence of *postformal operations*. That is, adult thought processes go beyond logical problem solving to include what is known as *dialectical thinking*. This is defined as the ability to search for complex and changing understandings to find a variety of solutions to any given situation or problem. In other words, adults are able to see the bigger picture (Vander Zanden et al., 2007).

For many adults, the accumulation of life experiences and their proven record of accomplishments often allow them to come to the teaching–learning situation with confidence in their abilities as learners. However, if their past experiences with learning were minimal or not positive, their motivation likely will not be at a high enough level to easily facilitate learning. Physical changes, especially with respect to hearing and vision, may impede learning as well (Santrock, 2006).

Erikson (1963) labeled this psychosocial stage of adulthood as *generativity versus self-absorption and stagnation*. Midlife marks a point at which adults realize that half of their potential life has been spent. This realization may cause them to question their level of achievement and success. Middle-aged adults, in fact, may choose to modify aspects of their lives that they perceive as unsatisfactory or adopt a new lifestyle as a solution to dissatisfaction.

Developing concern for the lives of their grown children, recognizing the physical changes in themselves, dealing with the new role of being a grandparent, and taking responsibility for their own parents whose health may be failing—all are factors that may cause them to become aware of their own mortality (see Table 5–2). At this time, middle-aged adults may either feel greater motivation to follow health recommendations more closely or, just the opposite, may deny illnesses or abandon healthy practices altogether (Falvo, 1994).

The later years of middle adulthood are the phase in which productivity and contributions to society are valued. They offer an opportunity to feel a real sense of accomplishment from having cared for others—children, spouse, friends, parents, and colleagues for whom they have served as mentor. During this time, individuals often become oriented away from self and family to the larger community. New social interests and leisure activities are pursued as they find more free time from family responsibilities and career demands. As they move toward their retirement years, individuals begin to plan for what they want to do after culminating their career. This transition sparks their interest in learning about financial planning, alternative lifestyles, and ways to remain healthy as they approach the later years (Vander Zanden et al., 2007).

TEACHING STRATEGIES

Depending on individual situations, middle-aged adults may be facing either a more relaxed lifestyle or an increase in stress level due to midlife crisis issues such as menopause, obvious physical changes in their bodies, responsibility for their own parents' declining health status, or concern about how finite their life really is. They may have regrets and feel they did not achieve the goals or live up to the values they had set for themselves in young adulthood or the expectations others had of them as young adults.

Santrock (2006) cites research that indicates that this stage in life is not so much seen as a crisis, but as a period of midlife consciousness.

When teaching members of this age group, the nurse must be aware of their potential sources of stress, the health risk factors associated with this stage of life, and the concerns typical of midlife. Misconceptions regarding physical changes such as menopause are common. Stress may interfere with their ability to learn or may be a motivational force for learning (Leifer & Hartston, 2004). Those who have lived healthy and productive lives are often motivated to make contact with health professionals to ensure maintenance of their healthy status. It is an opportune time on the part of the nurse educator to reach out to assist these middle-aged adults in coping with stress and maintaining optimal health status. Many need and want information related to chronic illnesses that can arise at this phase of life (Orshan, 2008).

Adult learners need to be reassured or complimented on their learning competencies. Reinforcement for learning is internalized and serves to reward them for their efforts. Teaching strategies for learning are similar to those instructional methods and tools used for the young adult learner, but the content is different to coincide with the concerns and problems specific to this group of learners.

Older Adulthood (65 Years of Age and Older)

The percentage of middle-aged adults in the United States has tripled since 1900, and by 2011, the first wave of baby boomers will reach 65 years of age. Older persons constitute approximately 12% of the U.S. population, but in the next 30 years, the ratio over age 65 will increase to one out of five (20%), or 70 million Americans. Those aged 85 and older make up the fastest-growing segment of the population in our country today, and that segment is expected to double by 2030. Some developmentalists, as Santrock (2006) points out, distinguish three categories of older adults: the young-old (65–74 years of age), the old-old (75–84 years of age), and the oldest-old (85 years and greater). With over 40% of the 2006 federal budget allocated for Medicare, Medicaid, and Social Security, a considerable portion of this country's fiscal resources are used for programs that support those 65 years and older (Vander Zanden et al., 2007).

Most older people suffer from at least one chronic condition, and many have multiple conditions. On the average, they are hospitalized longer than persons in other age categories and require more teaching overall to broaden their knowledge of self-care. In addition, it is approximated that as of 2001, 46% of Black Americans, 63% of those of Asian descent, and 74% of Caucasians over 65 years of age have a high school education. However, only 16% have a college degree at the bachelor's level or higher (Leifer & Hartston, 2004). Low educational levels, sensory impairments, the disuse of literacy skills once learned, and cognitive changes in the older adult population may contribute to these individuals' decreased ability to read and comprehend written materials (Best, 2001).

For these reasons, their patient education needs are generally greater and more complex than those for persons in any of the other developmental stages. Numerous studies have documented that older adults can benefit from health education programs. Their compliance, if they are given specific health directions, can be quite high. In light of considerable healthcare expenditures for older people, education programs to improve their health status would be a cost-effective measure (Best, 2001; Jackson, Davis, Murphy, Bairnsfather, & George, 1994; Pearson & Wessman, 1996).

Ageism describes prejudice against the older adult. This discrimination based on age, which exists in most segments of the American society, perpetuates the negative stereotype of aging as a period of decline (Gavan, 2003). Ageism, in many respects, is similar to the discriminatory attitudes of racism and sexism (Vander Zanden et al., 2007).

Because our society values physical strength, beauty, social networking, productivity, and integrity of body and mind, we fear the natural losses that accompany the aging process. Growing older is a normal event, yet the inevitable continuation of human development that results in biological, psychological, and social changes with the passage of time is a reminder of our own mortality. We must recognize that many older persons respond to these changes as challenges rather than defeats. Many aspects of older adulthood can be pleasurable, such as becoming a grandparent and experiencing retirement that gives one time to pursue lifelong interests, as well as freedom to explore new avenues of endeavor (Santrock, 2006).

Ageism, which interferes with interactions between the older adult and younger age groups, must be counteracted because it "prevents older people from living lives as actively and happily as they might" (Ahroni, 1996, p. 48). Given that the aging process is universal, eventually everyone is potentially subjected to this type of prejudice. New research that focuses on healthy development and positive lifestyle adaptations, rather than on illnesses and impairments in the older adult, can serve to reverse the stereotypical images of aging. Education to inform people of the significant variations that occur in the way that individuals age and education to help the older adult learn to cope with irreversible losses can combat the prejudice of ageism as well (Vander Zanden et al., 2007).

The teaching of older persons, known as *gerogogy*, is different from teaching younger adults (andragogy) and children (pedagogy). For teaching to be effective, gerogogy must accommodate the normal physical, cognitive, and psychosocial changes that occur at this phase of growth and development (Best, 2001). Until recently, little has been written about the special learning needs of older adults that acknowledge the physiological and psychological aging changes that affect their ability to learn.

Age changes, which begin in young and middle adulthood, progress significantly at this older adult stage of life. These changes often create barriers to learning unless nurses understand them and can adapt appropriate teaching interventions to meet the older person's needs. The following discussion of physical, cognitive, and psychosocial maturation is based on findings reported by numerous authors (Ahroni, 1996; Best, 2001; Gavan, 2003; Matsuda & Saito, 1998; Pearson & Wessman, 1996; Santrock, 2006; Theis & Merritt, 1994; Vander Zanden et al., 2007; Weinrich & Boyd, 1992).

PHYSICAL, COGNITIVE, AND PSYCHOSOCIAL DEVELOPMENT

With advancing age, so many physical changes occur that it becomes difficult to establish normal boundaries. As a person grows older, natural physiological changes in all systems of the body are universal, progressive, decremental, and intrinsic. Alterations in physiological functioning can lead secondarily to changes in learning ability. The senses of sight, hearing, touch, taste, and smell are usually the first areas of decreased functioning noticed by adults.

The sensory perceptive abilities that relate most closely to learning capacity are visual and auditory changes. Hearing loss, which is very common beginning in the late forties and fifties, includes diminished ability to discriminate high-pitched, high frequency sounds. Visual changes such as cataracts, macular degeneration, reduced pupil size, decline in depth perception, and presbyopia prevent older persons from being able to see small print, read words printed on glossy paper, or drive a car. Yellowing of the ocular lens produces color distortions and diminished color perceptions.

Other physiological changes affect organ functioning and result in decreased cardiac output, lung performance, and metabolic rate; these changes reduce energy levels and lessen the ability to cope with stress. Nerve conduction velocity also is thought to decline by as much as 15%, influencing reflex times and muscle response rates. The interrelatedness of each body system has a total negative cumulative effect on individuals as they grow older.

Aging affects the mind as well as the body. Cognitive ability changes with age as permanent cellular alterations invariably occur in the brain itself, resulting in an actual loss of neurons, which have no regenerative powers. Physiological research has demonstrated that people have two kinds of intellectual ability—crystallized and fluid intelligence. *Crystallized intelligence* is the intelligence absorbed over a lifetime, such as vocabulary, general information, understanding social interactions, arithmetic reasoning, and ability to evaluate experiences. This kind of intelligence actually increases with experience as people age. However, it is important to understand that crystallized intelligence can be impaired by disease states, such as the dementia seen in Alzheimer's disease. *Fluid intelligence* is the capacity to perceive relationships, to reason, and to perform abstract thinking. This kind of intelligence declines as degenerative changes occur.

The decline in fluid intelligence results in the following specific changes:

1. *Slower processing and reaction time*: Older persons need more time to process and react to information, especially as measured in terms of relationships between actions and results. However, if the factor of speed is removed from IQ tests, for example, older people can perform as well as younger people. In performance of activities of daily living when speed is not a factor, older adults can demonstrate their true abilities to function well and independently (Kray & Lindenberger, 2000).

2. *Persistence of stimulus (afterimage)*: Older adults can confuse a previous symbol or word with a new word or symbol just introduced.

3. *Decreased short-term memory*: Older adults sometimes have difficulty remembering events or conversations that occurred just hours or days before. However, long-term memory often remains strong, such as the ability to clearly and accurately remember something from their youth.

4. *Increased test anxiety*: People in the older adult years are especially anxious about making mistakes when performing; when they do make an error, they become easily frustrated. Because of their anxiety, they may take an inordinate amount of time to respond to questions, particularly on tests that are written rather than verbal.

5. *Altered time perception*: For older persons, life becomes more finite and compressed. Issues of the here and now tend to be more important, and some adhere to the philosophy, "I'll worry about that tomorrow." This way of thinking can be detrimental when applied to health issues because it serves as a vehicle for denial or delay in taking action.

Despite the changes in cognition as a result of aging, most research supports the premise that the ability of older adults to learn and remember is virtually as good as ever if special care is taken to slow the pace of presenting information, to ensure relevance of material, and to give appropriate feedback when teaching (see **Figure 5–1**).

Erikson (1963) labeled the major psychosocial developmental task at this stage in life as *ego integrity versus despair*. This phase of older adulthood includes dealing with the reality of aging, the acceptance of the inevitability that we all will die, the reconciling of past failures with present and future concerns, and developing a sense of growth and purpose for those years remaining (see Table 5–2). The most common psychosocial tasks of aging involve changes in lifestyle and social status as a result of

- Retirement (often mandatory at 70 years in this country)
- Illness or death of spouse, relatives, and friends
- The moving away of children, grandchildren, and friends
- Relocation to an unfamiliar environment such as an extended care facility or senior residential living center

Figure 5–1 (a) Elderly client variables influencing learning.
(b) Gerontological teaching strategies to optimize learning.

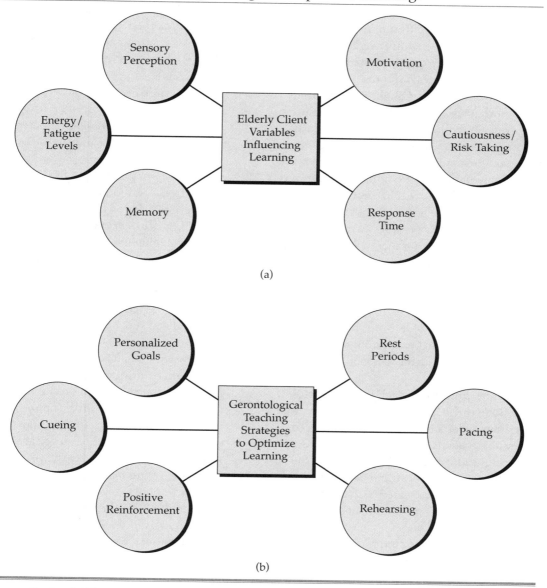

(a)

(b)

Source: Reprinted with permission from Rendon, D. C., David, D. K., Gioiella, E. C., & Tranzillo, M. J. (1986). The right to know, the right to be taught. *Journal of Gerontological Nursing, 12*(12), 34.

Depression, grief, loneliness, and isolation, once thought to be common traits among older adults, have now been found by researchers to vary from less frequent to no more frequent than the incidence rate found in middle adulthood. This is because older adults overall have fewer economic hardships and increased religiosity. However, depressive symptoms do increase in the oldest-old and are thought to be associated with more physical disability, more cognitive impairment, and lower socioeconomic status.

For those who experience major depression (the "common cold" of mental disorders), the most likely predictors are multiple losses over a short period of time with respect to a previous support network of home, friends, family, and job (Santrock, 2006). These losses, which signify a threat to one's own autonomy, independence, and decision making, result in isolation, financial insecurity, diminished coping mechanisms, and a decreased sense of identity, personal value, and societal worth. With aging, some individuals, particularly the oldest-old, begin to question their perception of a meaningful life—that is, the potential for further enjoyment, pleasure, and satisfaction.

Separate from biological aging but closely related are the many sociocultural factors that affect how older adults see themselves as competent individuals (Leifer & Hartston, 2004; Santrock, 2006; Vander Zanden et al., 2007). The following traits regarding personal goals in life and the values associated with them are significantly related to motivation and learning:

1. *Independence*: The ability to provide for one's needs is the most important aim of the majority of older persons, regardless of their state of health. Independence gives them a sense of self-respect, pride, and self-functioning so as not to be a burden to others. Health teaching is the tool to help them maintain or regain independence.

2. *Social acceptability*: The approval from others is a common goal of many older adults. It is derived from health, a sense of vigor, and feeling and thinking young. Despite declining physical attributes, the older adult often has residual fitness and functioning potentials. Health teaching can help to channel these potentials.

3. *Adequacy of personal resources*: Resources, both external and internal, are important considerations when assessing the older adult's current status. Life patterns, which include habits, physical and mental strengths, and economic situation, should be assessed to determine how to incorporate teaching to complement existing regimens and resources (financial and support system) with new required behaviors.

4. *Coping mechanisms*: The ability to cope with change during the aging process is indicative of the person's readiness for health teaching. Positive coping mechanisms allow for self-change as older persons draw on life experiences and knowledge gained over the years. Negative coping mechanisms indicate one's focus on losses and show that one's thinking is immersed in the past. The emphasis in teaching is on exploring alternatives, determining realistic goals, and supporting large and small accomplishments.

5. *Meaning of life*: For well-adapted older persons, having realistic goals allows

them the opportunity to enjoy the smaller pleasures in life, whereas less well-adapted individuals may be frustrated and dissatisfied with personal inadequacies. Health teaching must be directed at ways older adults can maintain optimal health so that they can derive pleasure from their leisure years.

TEACHING STRATEGIES

Learning in older adults can be affected by such sociological, psychological, and cognitive factors as retirement, economics, mental status, and information processing abilities (Santrock, 2006; Vander Zanden et al., 2007). Understanding older persons' developmental tasks will allow nurses to alter how they approach both well and ill individuals in terms of counseling, teaching, and establishing a therapeutic relationship. Nurses must be aware of the fact that older patients may delay medical attention. Decreased cognitive functioning, sensory deficits, lower energy levels, and other factors may prevent early disease detection and intervention. A decline in psychomotor performance affects the older adults' reflex responses and their ability to handle stress. Coping with simple tasks becomes more difficult. Chronic illnesses, depression, and literacy levels, particularly among the oldest-old, have implications with respect to how they care for themselves (eating, dressing, and taking medications) as well as the extent to which they understand the nature of their illnesses (Best, 2001; Katz, 1997; Phillips, 1999).

In working with older adults, reminiscing is a beneficial approach to use to establish a therapeutic relationship. Memories can be quite powerful. Talking with older persons about their experiences—marriage, children, grandchildren, jobs, community involvement, and the like—can be very stimulating. Furthermore, their answers

will give the nurse an insight into their humanness, their abilities, and their concerns.

Too many times nurses and other health professionals believe the adage, "You can't teach an old dog new tricks." Gavan (2003) warns that it is easy to fall into the habit of believing the myths associated with the intelligence, personality traits, motivation, and social relations of older adults. She outlined the following prevalent false stereotypes that must be dispelled to prevent harmful outcomes in the older adult when these myths are assumed to be true:

MYTH NO. 1: SENILITY   Intelligence test scores indicate that many older adults maintain their cognitive functioning well into their 80s and 90s and mental decline is not always due to the aging process itself but to disease processes, medication interactions, sensory deficits, dehydration, and malnutrition.

MYTH NO. 2: RIGID PERSONALITIES Personality traits, such as agreeableness, satisfaction, and extraversion, remain stable throughout the older adult years. Although diversity in personality traits among individuals in the older population exists as it does in all other stages of life, labeling older adults as cranky, stubborn, and inflexible does a disservice to them.

MYTH NO. 3: LONELINESS   As mentioned earlier, the belief that older adults are more frequently vulnerable to depression, isolation, and feelings of being lonely has not been upheld by research, which indicates that their satisfaction with life continues at a steady level throughout the period of adulthood.

MYTH NO. 4: ABANDONMENT   It is untrue that older adults are abandoned by their children, siblings, or good friends. The amount of contact older adults have with significant others remains constant over time. Successful aging depends on an extended family support network.

Also, Vander Zanden et al. (2007) point out that our American culture is preoccupied with youthfulness and has distorted notions about late adulthood that perpetuate negative views of this generation. There is no typical older adult—not all of them are unhealthy, unhappy, fearful, institutionalized, disengaged, dwell on their own mortality, or find themselves in financial straits.

Nurse educators may not even be aware of their stereotypical attitudes toward older adults. Furthermore, healthcare providers make assumptions about older clients that can cause them to overlook problems that could be treatable (Gavan, 2003). To check yourself, think about the last time you gave instruction to an older patient, and ask yourself:

- Did I talk to the family and ignore the patient when I described some aspect of care or discharge planning?
- Did I tell the older person not to worry when he or she asked a question? Did I say, "Just leave everything up to the doctors and nurses?"
- Did I eliminate information that I normally would have given a younger patient?
- Did I attribute a decline in cognitive functioning to the aging process without considering common underlying causes in mental deterioration, such as effects of medication interactions, fluid imbalances, poor nutrition, or sensory impairments?

Remember, older people can learn, but their abilities and needs differ from those of younger persons. The process of teaching and learning is much more rewarding and successful for both the nurse and the patient if it is tailored to fit the older adult's physical, cognitive, motivational, and social differences.

Because changes as a result of aging vary considerably from one individual to another, it is essential to assess each learner's physical, cognitive, and psychosocial functioning levels before developing and implementing any teaching plan. It is important to keep in mind that older adults have an overall lower educational level of formal schooling than the population as a whole. Also, they were raised in an era when consumerism and health education were practically nonexistent. As a result, older people may feel uncomfortable in the teaching–learning situation and may be reluctant to ask questions. In the future, as the older population becomes more educated and in tune with consumer activism in the health field, these individuals will likely have an increased desire to participate more in decision making and demand more detailed and sophisticated information. The proliferation of self-help literature and today's expectations for patients and families to take responsibility for self-care result in the present-day need for nurse educators to involve clients more fully in decisions affecting their health (Morra, 1991).

Health education for older persons should be directed at promoting their involvement and changing their attitudes toward learning (Ahroni, 1996; Weinrich & Boyd, 1992). A climate of mutual respect in which they are made to feel important for what they once were as well as for what they are today should be cultivated. Interaction needs to be supportive, not judgmental.

Interventions work best when they take place in a casual, informal atmosphere. In the primary care setting, where time is often limited, it may be beneficial to schedule additional time to allow for a more relaxed environment. Individual and situational variables such as motivation, life experiences, educational background, socioeconomic status, health or illness status, and motor, cognitive, and language skills may all influence the ability of the older adult to learn.

Some of the more common aging changes that affect learning and the teaching strategies specific to meeting the needs of the older adult are summarized in Table 5–1. When teaching older persons, abiding by the following specific tips can create an environment for learning that takes into account major changes in their physical, cognitive, and psychosocial functioning (Best, 2001; Doak, Doak, & Root, 1996; Fisher, 1999; Katz, 1997; Kessels, 2003; Phillips, 1999; Santrock, 2006; Vander Zanden et al., 2007; Weinrich & Boyd, 1992):

PHYSICAL NEEDS

1. To compensate for visual changes, teaching should be done in an environment that is brightly lit but without glare. Visual aids should include large print, well-spaced letters, and the use of primary colors. Bright colors and a visible name tag should be worn by the educator. Use white or off-white, flat matte paper and black print for posters, diagrams, and other written materials.

   Because of older persons' difficulty in discriminating certain shades of color, avoid blue, blue-green, and violet hues. Keep in mind that tasks that require recognizing different shades of color, such as test strips measuring the presence of sugar in the urine, may present learning difficulties for older patients. Color distortions can have an especially devastat-

ing effect on learning if, for example, the type of pills are referred to by color in guiding patients to take medications as prescribed. Green, blue, and yellow pills may all appear gray to older persons. Additional accommodations should be made to meet physical needs, such as arranging seats so that the learner is reasonably close to the instructor and to any visual aids that may be used. For patients who wear glasses, be sure they are readily accessible, lenses are clean, and frames are properly fitted.

2. To compensate for hearing losses, eliminate extraneous noise, avoid covering your mouth when speaking, directly face the learner, and speak slowly. Female instructors should wear bright lipstick, and male teachers can wear lip gloss. These techniques will assist the learner who may be seeking visual confirmation of what is being said.

   Low-pitched voices are heard best, but be careful not to drop your voice at the end of words or phrases. Do not shout, because it distorts sounds and the decibel level is usually not a problem for hearing-impaired persons. The intensity of sound seems to be less important than the pitch and rate of auditory stimuli.

   Word speed should not exceed 140 words spoken per minute. If the learner uses hearing aids, be sure they have working batteries. Ask for feedback from the learner to determine whether you are speaking too softly, too fast, or not distinctly enough. When addressing a group, microphones are useful aids. Be alert to nonverbal cues from the audience. Participants who are having difficulty with hearing your message may try to compensate by leaning forward, turning the good ear to the speaker, or cupping their hands to their ears. Ask older persons to repeat verbal instructions to be sure the entire message was heard and interpreted correctly.

3. To compensate for musculoskeletal problems, decreased efficiency of the cardiovascular system, and reduced kidney function, keep sessions short, schedule frequent breaks to allow for use of bathroom facilities, and allow time for stretching to relieve painful, stiff joints and to stimulate circulation. Provide pain medication and encourage the learner to follow his or her usual pain management routine. Also, provide comfortable seating.

4. To compensate for any decline in central nervous system functioning and decreased metabolic rates, set aside more time for the giving and receiving of information and for the practice of psychomotor skills. Also, do not assume that older persons have the psychomotor skills necessary to handle technological equipment for self-paced learning, such as tape recorders, computers, and videocassettes. In addition, they may have difficulty with independently applying prostheses or changing dressings because of decreased strength and coordination. Be careful not to misinterpret the loss of energy and motor skills as a lack of motivation.

COGNITIVE NEEDS

1. To compensate for a decrease in fluid intelligence, provide older persons with more opportunities to process and react to information and to see relationships between concepts. Research has shown that older adults can learn anything if new information is tied to familiar concepts drawn from relevant past experiences.

When teaching, avoid presenting long lists by dividing a series of directions for action into short, discrete, step-by-step messages and then waiting for a response after each one. For instance, if you want to give directions about following different menus depending on exercise levels, use an active voice to personalize the message. For example, instead of saying, "Use menu A if not active; use menu B if fairly active; use menu C if very active," you should say, "You should use menu A if you are not active." Then wait for the learner's response, which might be, "That's what I should eat if I'm not very active?" Follow up with the response, "That's right. And if you are fairly active, you should . . ."

Older persons also tend to confuse previous words and symbols with a new word or symbol being introduced. Again, wait for a response before introducing a new concept or word definition. For decreased short-term memory, coaching and repetition are very useful strategies that assist with recall. Memory can also be enhanced by involving the learner in devising ways to remember how or when to perform a procedure. Because many older adults experience test anxiety, try to explain procedures simply and thoroughly, reassure them, and, if possible, give verbal rather than written tests.

2. Be aware of the effects of medications and energy levels on concentration, alert-

ness, and coordination. Try to schedule teaching sessions before or well after medications are taken and when the person is rested. For example, the patient who has just returned from physical therapy or a diagnostic procedure will likely be too fatigued to attend to learning.

3. Be certain to ask what an individual already knows about a healthcare issue or technique before explaining it. Repetition for reinforcement of learning is one thing; repeating information already known may seem patronizing. You should never assume that because someone has been exposed to information before that they, in fact, learned it. Confirm their level of knowledge before beginning to teach. Basic information should be understood before progressing to more complex information.

4. Convincing older persons of the usefulness of what you are teaching is only half the battle in getting them motivated. You may also have to convince them that the information or technique you are teaching is correct. Anything that is entirely strange or that upsets established habits is likely to be far more difficult for them to learn. Information that confirms existing beliefs (cognitive schema) is better remembered than that which contradicts these beliefs. Patients with chronic illnesses frequently have established schemas about their medical conditions that they have embraced for years.

   As perception slows, the older person's mind has more trouble accommodating to new ways than does the mind of a younger person. Find out about older persons' health habits and beliefs before

trying to change their ways or teach something new. For example, many were taught as children that a bowel movement every day is necessary to prevent constipation. You need to identify this belief before trying to teach them to change their dependency on laxatives.

5. Arrange for brief teaching sessions, because a shortened attention span (attentional narrowing) requires scheduling a series of sessions to provide for sufficient time for learning. In addition, if the material is relevant and focused on the here and now, older persons are more likely to be attentive to the information being presented. If procedures or treatments are perceived as stressful or emotionally threatening, attentional narrowing occurs.

6. Take into account that the process of conceptualizing and the ability to think abstractly become more difficult with aging. Conclude each teaching session with a summary of the information presented and allow for a question and answer period to correct any misconceptions (see **Figure 5–2** for strategies to meet cognitive needs of older adults).

Psychosocial Needs

1. Assess family relationships to determine how dependent the older person is on other members for financial and emotional support. In turn, explore the level of involvement by family members in reinforcing the lessons you are teaching and in giving assistance with self-care measures. Do they help the older person to function independently, or do they foster dependency? With permission of the patient, include family members in teaching sessions and enlist their support.

Figure 5–2 A basic gerontological teaching–learning model for nursing.

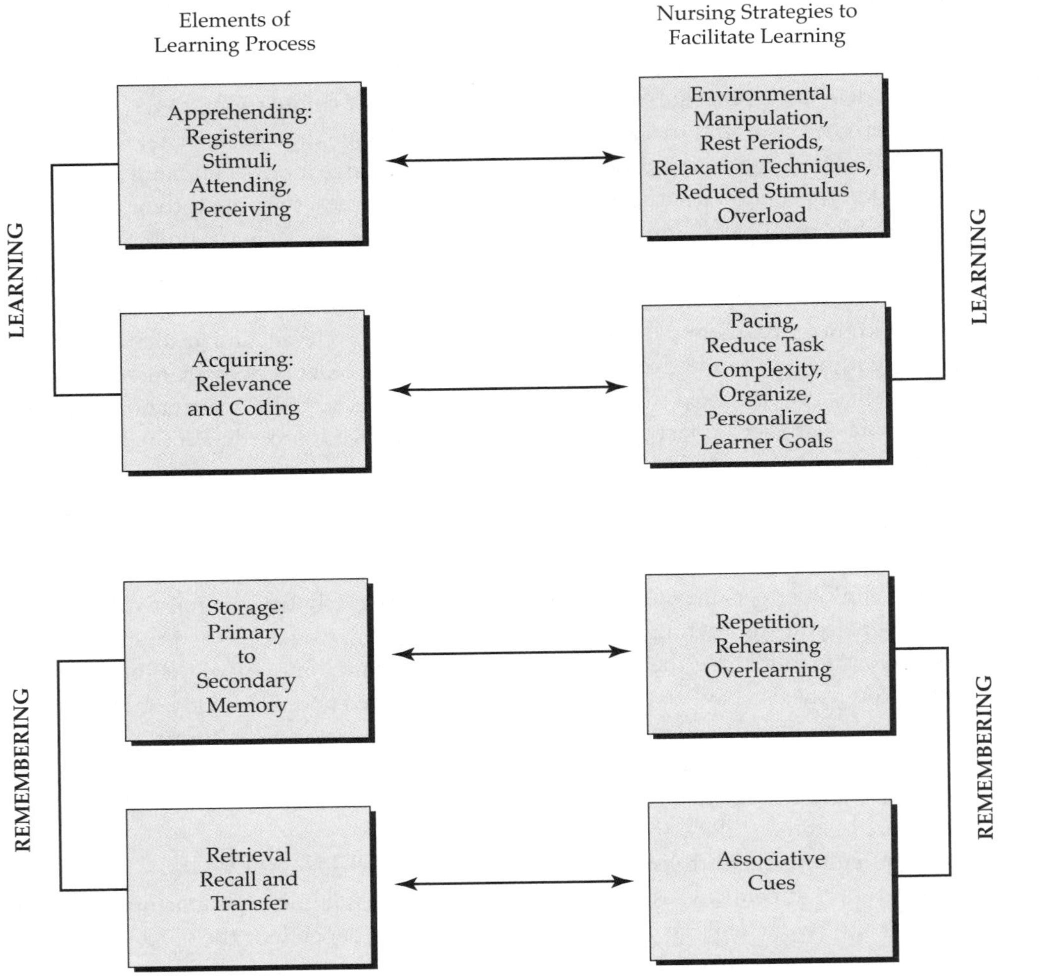

Elements of
Learning Process

Nursing Strategies to
Facilitate Learning

LEARNING

Apprehending:
Registering
Stimuli,
Attending,
Perceiving

Environmental
Manipulation,
Rest Periods,
Relaxation Techniques,
Reduced Stimulus
Overload

Acquiring:
Relevance
and Coding

Pacing,
Reduce Task
Complexity,
Organize,
Personalized
Learner Goals

LEARNING

REMEMBERING

Storage:
Primary
to
Secondary
Memory

Repetition,
Rehearsing
Overlearning

Retrieval
Recall and
Transfer

Associative
Cues

REMEMBERING

Source: Reprinted with permission from Rendon, D. C., Davis, D. K., Gioiella, E. C., & Tranzillo, M. J. (1986). The right to know, the right to be taught. *Journal of Gerontological Nursing, 12*(12), 36.

2. Determine availability of resources. A lack of resources can sabotage any teaching plan, especially if your recommendations include expecting older adults to carry out something they cannot afford or lack the means to do, such as buying or renting equipment, having transportation to get to therapy or teaching sessions, purchasing medications, and the like.

3. Encourage active involvement of older adults to improve their self-esteem and to stimulate them both mentally and socially. Teaching must be directed at helping them find meaningful ways to use talents acquired over their lifetime. Establishing a rapport based on trust can provide them contact with others as a means to bolster their sense of self-worth.

4. Identify coping mechanisms. No other time in the life cycle carries with it the number of developmental tasks associated with adaptation to loss of roles, social and family contacts, and physical and cognitive capacities that this time does. Teaching must include offering constructive methods of coping.

The older person's ability to learn may be affected by the methods and materials chosen for teaching. One-to-one instruction provides a nonthreatening environment for older adults in which to meet their individual needs and goals. This teaching approach helps them to compensate for their special deficits and promotes their active participation in learning. Group teaching also can be a beneficial approach for fostering social skills and maintaining contact with others through shared experiences.

Self-paced instructional tools may be very appropriate, but it is important to know the client's previous learning techniques, mental and physical abilities, and comfort levels with certain approaches before assigning any such tools. Many older adults grew up in a time when audiovisual aids did not exist to the extent they do today, and those who have always learned by reading and discussion may not like mediated devices. Introducing new teaching methods and tools, such as the use of computer and interactive video formats with-

out adequate instructions on how to operate these technical devices, may inhibit learning by increasing anxiety and frustration levels and may adversely affect self-esteem.

Games, role-playing, demonstration, and return demonstration can be used to rehearse problem solving and psychomotor skills as long as these methods, and the tools used to complement them, are designed appropriately to accommodate the various developmental characteristics of this age group. For example, speed or competition should not be factors in the games chosen and plenty of time should be reserved for return demonstrations. These teaching methods stimulate learning and can offer active learning opportunities to put knowledge into practice. Written materials, with attention being paid to appropriateness in terms of literacy level and visual impairments in the older adult, are excellent adjuncts to augment, supplement, and reinforce verbal instructions (see Chapters 7, 11, and 12 for specific information on literacy and the design and use of instructional methods and materials).

The Role of the Family in Patient Education

The role of the family is considered one of the key variables influencing positive patient care outcomes. The primary motives in patient education for involving family members in the care delivery and decision-making process are to decrease the stress of hospitalization, reduce costs of care, and effectively prepare the client for self-care management outside the healthcare setting. Family caregivers provide critical emotional, physical, and social support to the patient (Gavan, 2003; Reeber, 1992).

Under the most recent Joint Commission accreditation standards, new demands have been placed on healthcare organizations to show evidence that the family is included in patient education efforts. The standards mandate that the instruction of patients and significant others be considered an essential part in the healthcare team approach to providing care. Providers are responsible for assisting both patients and their family members to gain the knowledge and skills necessary to meet ongoing healthcare goals, particularly the first of the *Healthy People 2010* initiatives to increase the quality and years of a healthy life (U.S. Department of Health and Human Services, 2000). Interdisciplinary collaboration is a major resource for ensuring continuity of client teaching about healthy lifestyles in and across healthcare settings.

Including the family members in the teaching–learning process helps to ensure a win-win situation for both the client and the nurse educator. Family role enhancement and increased knowledge on the part of the family have positive benefits for the learner as well as the teacher. Clients derive increased satisfaction and greater independence in self-care, and nurses experience increased job satisfaction and personal gratification in helping clients to reach their potentials and achieve successful outcomes (Barnes, 1995; Gavan, 2003).

Numerous nursing, life-span development, and educational psychology theories provide the conceptual frameworks for understanding the dynamics and importance of family relationships as influential in achieving teaching–learning outcomes. Although a great deal of attention has been given to the ways in which young and adolescent families function, unfortunately minimal attention has been paid to the dynamics of the complex interactions that characterize the aging family (Gavan, 2003).

In patient education, the nurse may be tempted to teach as many family members as possible. In reality, it is difficult to coordinate the instruction of so many different people. The more individuals involved, the greater the potential for misunderstanding of instruction. The family must make the deliberate decision as to who is the most appropriate person to take the primary responsibility as the caregiver.

The nurse educator must determine how caregivers feel about the role of providing supportive care, about learning the necessary information, and what their learning style preferences, cognitive abilities, fears and concerns, and current knowledge of the situation are. Perceptions of the problem by both the family and the healthcare team must be determined to identify similarities and differences so that effective teaching can be provided (Leifer & Hartston, 2004). The caregiver needs information similar to what the patient is given to provide support, feedback, and reinforcement of self-care consistent with prescribed regimens of care.

Sometimes the family members need more information than the patient to compensate for any sensory deficits or cognitive limitations the patient may have. Anticipatory teaching with family caregivers can reduce their anxiety, uncertainty, and lack of confidence. What the family is to *do* is important, but what the family is to *expect* also is essential information to be shared during the teaching–learning process (Haggard, 1989). The greatest challenge for caregivers is to develop confidence in their ability to do what is right for the patient. Education is the means to help them confront this challenge.

The family can be the educator's greatest ally in preparing the patient for discharge and in helping the patient to become independent in self-care. The patient's family is perhaps the single most significant determinant of the success or failure of the education plan and achievement of successful aging (Gavan, 2003; Haggard, 1989). Rankin and Stallings's 2001 model for patient and family education serves as a foundation for assessing the family profile to determine the family members' understanding of the actual or potential health problem(s), the resources available to them, their ways of functioning, and their educational backgrounds, lifestyles, and beliefs.

Education is truly the most powerful tool nurse educators have to ensure safe discharge and the transfer of power to the patient–family dyad. It is imperative that attention be focused on both the assumed and the expected responsibilities of family caregivers. The role of the family has been stressed in each developmental section in this chapter. Table 5–1 outlines the appropriate nursing interventions with the family at different stages in the life cycle.

State of the Evidence

In an extensive review of the literature, a number of studies from primary and secondary sources by nurses and other healthcare professionals were found to support the application of teaching and learning principles to the education of middle-aged and older adult clients in various healthcare settings. However, current nursing research focusing specifically on patient education approaches to the age cohorts of children, adolescents, and the young adult population, as well as instructional needs of family members as caregivers was lacking. For example, the article by Richmond and Kotelchuck (1984) was an excellent and thorough examination of health maintenance in children, including children's cognitive understanding of health and disease, their psychological control over health, parental and media influences on health behaviors, the impact of school health education, and the role of health professionals in the management of childhood illness and health services for children, but it was written more than 2 decades ago. Present knowledge of new approaches to foster child health is sorely needed.

To bolster our general understanding of the physical, cognitive, and psychosocial (emotional) traits of human development across the life span, plenty of excellent resources, well-grounded by research evidence, exist from the fields of psychology in general and educational psychology in particular. However, much of the educational psychology literature focuses extensively on the application of teaching and learning principles only to preschool and K–12 classrooms. Understandably so, life-span developmental scientists do not give specific consideration to health education of well individuals with respect to disease prevention, risk reduction, and health promotion efforts nor the health promotion, maintenance, and rehabilitation measures for those who are acutely and chronically ill. The application and translation of developmental characteristics to the teaching and learning aspects of healthcare delivery is the responsibility of nurses and other professional providers. Much more investigation needs to be done to demonstrate how to effectively teach clients of different developmental stages based on their learning needs, learning styles, and readiness to learn for the achievement of the most positive client-centered outcomes possible.

Malcolm Knowles's original 1973 theory about adult learning and his subsequent modifications and clarifications of his theory (Knowles, 1990; Knowles et al., 1998) seem to be well accepted and have stood the test of time. Piaget's theory on cognitive development also has been accepted and extensively applied over the years, but recent critics of Piaget have challenged the assumptions underlying his theory with respect to the last stage of development (formal operations). Now a number of psychologists speculate that a fifth and qualitatively higher level of thinking follows adolescence and is postulated as the postformal operations period of adulthood. Vygotsky's sociocultural theory adds another dimension to understanding cognitive development (Santrock, 2006; Vander Zanden et al., 2007) that was not addressed by Piaget.

Erickson's theory of eight stages of psychosocial development, whereby individuals are faced with unique stage-related tasks (crises that must be resolved to reduce one's vulnerability and enhance one's potentials) are still recognized as the unique turning points in life that require successful completion for healthy, normal development to occur. Erickson's theory continues to be widely applied to the field of life-span development.

Recently, increased attention has been paid to the appropriateness of instructional methods and materials (especially as they relate to multimedia technology) for college-aged students and adult learners to meet their expectations for lifelong learning. Given the fact that our population is steadily aging, nurses are caring for an increasingly older audience of learners. Many of the current nursing students are somewhat older than the traditional college-aged students and nursing staff are adult continuing education learners. It is gratifying to witness the acknowledgement of these population changes with an emphasis on studying generational differences on learner preferences, modes of information processing, and on memory and recall with

respect to the impact of standard versus newer technological methods and tools for the effective delivery of instruction. Articles, such as those written by Billings and Kowalski (2004), Lewis (2003), Oblinger (2003), and Prensky (2001), are beginning to highlight the different experiences, values, beliefs, and needs of learners from varied generational backgrounds.

Although there has been an upsurge of interest in educational strategies and techniques for teaching and learning as it applies to certain population groups in the broad healthcare arena, much more research needs to be done as it relates to the creative leadership role of the nurse educator functioning as facilitator rather than teacher of patients and family members (at all stages of development) and of nursing students and staff (Donner, Levonian, & Slutsky, 2005). Research has only begun to scratch the surface on how teaching and learning are affected by situational variables, such as chronic illness, acute illness, or wellness; by personality traits, such as motivation and learning styles; by temperament responses, such as anxiety and attention span; and by sociocultural influences, such as gender, economic status, and educational background.

Another area requiring further exploration is the importance of the role of family and other support systems on the success of educational endeavors to help Americans of all ages maintain and improve their health status. There is a paucity of research evidence on family structure and the many changing relationships in our society that promote or hinder teaching and learning of clients in various healthcare settings.

The national initiatives of *Healthy People 2010* as well as pending policy goals at local and state levels will not be realized unless a better understanding is gained on the impact of physical, cognitive, psychological/emotional, and sociocultural changes that occur across the life course to serve as guidelines for teaching and learning in nursing practice.

Summary

It is important to understand the specific and varied tasks associated with each developmental stage to individualize the approach to education in meeting the needs and desires of patients and their families. Assessment of physical, cognitive, and psychosocial maturation within each developmental period is crucial in determining the strategies to be used to facilitate the teaching–learning process. The younger learner is, in many ways, very different from the adult learner. Issues of dependency, extent of participation, rate of and capacity for learning, and situational and emotional obstacles to learning vary significantly across the various phases of development.

Readiness to learn in children is very subject centered and highly influenced by their physical, cognitive, and psychosocial maturation. Motivation to learn in the adult is very problem centered and more oriented to psychosocial tasks related to roles and expectations of work, family, and community activities.

For patient education to be effective, the nurse in the role of educator must create an environment conducive to learning by presenting information at the learner's level, inviting participation and feedback, and identifying whether parental and/or peer involvement is appropriate or necessary. Nurses are the main source of health education. In concert with the client, they must facilitate the teaching–learning process by determining what needs to be taught, when to teach, how to teach, and who should be the focus of teaching in light of the developmental stage of the learner.

When nursing students and staff are the audience of learners, the educator also is responsible for assuming the leadership role as facilitator of the learning process. In conjunction with these adult learners, objectives can be established, and learner-centered approaches that challenge the educator's creativity can be used to foster self-direction, motivation, interest, and active participation for independence and interdependence in learning.

REVIEW QUESTIONS

1. What are the seven stages of development?
2. What are the definitions of *pedagogy*, *andragogy*, and *gerogogy*?
3. Who is the expert in cognitive development? What are the terms or labels used by this expert to identify the key cognitive milestones?
4. Who is the expert in psychosocial development? What are the terms or labels used by this expert to identify the key psychosocial milestones?
5. What are the salient characteristics at each stage of development that influence the ability to learn?
6. What are three main teaching strategies for each stage of development?
7. How do people you know in each stage of development compare with what you have learned about physical, cognitive, and psychosocial characteristics at the various developmental stages?
8. What is the role of the family in the teaching and learning process in each stage of development?
9. How does the role of the nurse as facilitator vary when teaching individuals at different stages of development?

References

Ackard, D. M., & Neumark-Sztainer, D. (2001). Health care information sources for adolescents: Age and gender differences on use, concerns, and needs. *Journal of Adolescent Health, 29*(3), 170–176.

Ahroni, J. H. (1996). Strategies for teaching elders from a human development perspective. *Diabetes Educator, 22*(1), 47–52.

American Association of Colleges of Nursing. (1994). *AACN Issue Bulletin.* Washington, DC: American Association of Colleges of Nursing.

Aronowitz, T. (2006). Teaching adolescents about adolescence: Experiences from an interdisciplinary adolescent health course. *Nurse Educator, 31*(2), 84–87.

Babcock, D. E., & Miller, M. A. (1994). *Client education: Theory & practice.* St. Louis, MO: Mosby–Year Book.

Banks, E. (1990). Concepts of health and sickness of preschool- and school-aged children. *Children's Health, 19*(1), 43–48.

Barnes, L. P. (1995). Finding the "win/win" in patient/family teaching. *MCN: American Journal of Maternal Child Nursing, 20*(4), 229.

Best, J. T. (2001). Effective teaching for the elderly: Back to basics. *Orthopedic Nursing, 20*(3), 46–52.

Billings, D., & Kowalski, K. (2004). Teaching learners from varied generations. *The Journal of Continuing Education, 35*(3), 104–105.

Boyd, M. D., Gleit, C. J., Graham, B. A., & Whitman, N. I. (1998). *Health teaching in nursing practice: A professional model* (3rd ed.). Norwalk, CT: Appleton & Lange.

Brown, S. L., Teufel, J. A., & Birch, D. A. (2007). Early adolescents' perceptions of health and health literacy. *Journal of School Health, 77*(1), 7–15.

Burkett, K. W. (1989). Trends in pediatric rehabilitation. *Nursing Clinics of North America, 24*(1), 239–255.

Cauffman, E., & Steinberg, L. (2000). (Im)maturity of judgment in adolescence: Why adolescents may be less culpable than adults. *Behavioral Science Law, 18,* 741–760.

Collins, J. (2004). Education techniques for lifelong learners. *RadioGraphics, 24*(5), 1483–1489.

Covey, S. (1990). *The seven habits of highly effective people.* New York: Simon & Schuster.

Doak, C. C., Doak, L. G., & Root, J. H. (1996). *Teaching patients with low literacy skills* (2nd ed.). Philadelphia: Lippincott.

Donner, C. L., Levonian, C., & Slutsky, P. (2005). Move to the head of the class: Developing staff nurses as teachers. *Journal for Nurses in Staff Development, 21*(6), 277–283.

Elkind, D. (1984). Teenage thinking: Implications for health care. *Pediatric Nursing, 10*(6), 383–385.

Erikson, E. H. (1963). *Childhood and society* (2nd ed.). New York: Norton.

Erikson, E. H. (1968). *Identity: Youth and crisis.* New York: Norton.

Falvo, D. R. (1994). *Effective patient education: A guide to increased compliance* (2nd ed.). Gaithersburg, MD: Aspen.

Farrand, L. L., & Cox, C. L. (1993). Determinants of positive health behavior in middle childhood. *Nursing Research, 42*(4), 208–213.

Fisher, E. (1999). Low literacy levels in adults: Implications for patient education. *The Journal of Continuing Education in Nursing, 30*(2), 56–61.

Gavan, C. S. (2003). Successful aging families: A challenge for nurses. *Holistic Nursing Practice, 17*(1), 11–18.

Girod, M., Pardales, M., Cavanaugh, S., & Wadsworth, P. (2005). By teens, for teachers: A descriptive study of adolescence. *American Secondary Education, 33*(2), 4–19.

Grey, M., Kanner, S., & Lacey, K. O. (1999). Characteristics of the learner: Children and adolescents. *Diabetes Educator, 25*(6), 25–33.

Haggard, A. (1989). *Handbook of patient education.* Rockville, MD: Aspen.

Havighurst, R. (1976). Human characteristics and school learning: Essay review. *Elementary School Journal, 77,* 101–109.

Heiney, S. P. (1991). Helping children through painful procedures. *American Journal of Nursing, 91*(11), 20–24.

Hines, A. R., & Paulson, S. E. (2006). Parents' and teachers' perceptions of adolescent storm and stress: Relations with parenting and teaching styles. *Adolescence, 41*(164), 597–614.

Hussey, C. G., & Hirsh, A. M. (1983). Health education for children. *Topics in Clinical Nursing, 5*(1), 22–28.

Jackson, R. H., Davis, T. C., Murphy, P., Bairnsfather, L. E., & George, R. B. (1994). Reading deficiencies in older patients. *American Journal of the Medical Sciences, 308*(2), 79–82.

Johnson-Saylor, M. T. (1980). Seize the moment: Health promotion for the young adult. *Topics in Clinical Nursing, 2*(2), 9–19.

Katz, J. R. (1997). Back to basics: Providing effective patient education. *American Journal of Nursing, 97*(5), 33–36.

Kennedy, C. M., & Riddle, I. I. (1989). The influence of the timing of preparation on the anxiety of preschool children experiencing surgery. *Maternal-Child Nursing Journal, 18*(2), 117–132.

Kessels, R. P. C. (2003). Patients' memory for medical information. *Journal of the Royal Society of Medicine, 96,* 219–222.

Knowles, M. (1990). *The adult learner: A neglected species* (4th ed.). Houston: Gulf.

Knowles, M. S., Holton, E. F., & Swanson, R. A. (1998). *The adult learner: The definitive classic in adult education and human resource development* (5th ed.). Houston: Gulf Publishing.

Kotchabhakdi, P. (1985). School-age children's conceptions of the heart and its function. Monograph 15. *Maternal-Child Nursing Journal, 14*(4), 203–261.

Kray, J., & Lindenberger, U. (2000). Adult age differences in task switching. *Psychology and Aging, 15*(1), 126–147.

Leifer, G., & Hartston, H. (2004). *Growth and development across the lifespan: A health promotion focus.* St. Louis, MO: Saunders.

Lewis, D. (2003). Computers in patient education. *Computer Informatics in Nursing, 21*(2), 88–96.

London, M. C., Ladewig, P. W., Ball, J. W., & Bindler, R. C. (2003). *Maternal-newborn & child nursing: Family-centered care.* Upper Saddle River, NJ: Prentice Hall.

Matsuda, O., & Saito, M. (1998). Crystallized and fluid intelligence in elderly patients with mild dementia of the Alzheimer type. *International Psychogeriatrics, 10*(2), 147–154.

Michaud, P.-A., Stronski, S., Fonseca, H., & MacFarlane, A. (2004). The development and pilot-testing of a training curriculum in adolescent medicine and health. *Journal of Adolescent Health, 35*(1), 51–57.

Milligan, F. (1997). In defense of andragogy. Part 2: An educational process consistent with modern nursing's aims. *Nurse Education Today, 17*, 487–493.

Morra, M. E. (1991). Future trends in patient education. *Seminars in Oncology Nursing, 7*(2), 143–145.

Musinski, B. (1999). The educator as facilitator: A new kind of leadership. *Nursing Forum, 34*(1), 23–29.

Oblinger, D. (2003, July/August). Boomers, Gen-Xers & millennials: Understanding the new students. *Educause*, 37–45.

Orshan, S. A. (2008). *Maternity, newborn, and woman's health nursing: Comprehensive care across the lifespan.* Philadelphia: Lippincott Williams & Wilkins.

Palfrey, J. S., Hauser-Cram, P., Bronson, M. B., Warfield, M. E., Sirin, S., & Chan, E. (2005). The Brookline early education project: A 25-year follow-up study of family-centered early health and development intervention. *Pediatrics, 116*(1), 144–152.

Pearson, M., & Wessman, J. (1996). Gerogogy. *Home Healthcare Nurse, 14*(8), 631–636.

Perrin, E. C., Sayer, A. G., & Willett, J. B. (1991). Sticks and stones may break my bones . . . Reasoning about illness causality and body functioning in children who have a chronic illness. *Pediatrics, 88*(3), 608–619.

Phillips, L. D. (1999). Patient education: Understanding the process to maximize time and outcomes. *Journal of Intravenous Nursing, 22*(1), 19–35.

Piaget, J. (1951). *Judgement and reasoning in the child.* London: Routledge and Kegan Paul.

Piaget, J. (1952). *The origins of intelligence in children.* New York: International Universities Press.

Piaget, J. (1976). *The grasp of consciousness: Action and concept in the young child.* (S. Wedgwood, Trans.). Cambridge, MA: Harvard University Press.

Pidgeon, V. A. (1977). Characteristics of children's thinking and implications for health teaching. *Maternal-Child Nursing Journal, 6*(1), 1–8.

Pidgeon, V. (1985). Children's concepts of illness: Implications for health teaching. *Maternal-Child Nursing Journal, 14*(1), 23–35.

Polan, E., & Taylor, D. (2003). *Journey across the lifespan: Human development and health promotion* (2nd ed.). Philadelphia: F. A. Davis.

Poster, E. C. (1983). Stress immunization: Techniques to help children cope with hospitalization. *Maternal-Child Nursing Journal, 12*(2), 119–134.

Prensky, M. (2001). Digital natives, digital immigrants. *On the Horizon, 9*(5), 1–6.

Protheroe, N. (2007). How children learn. *Principal, 86*(5), 40–44.

Rankin, S. H., & Stallings, K. D. (2001). *Patient education: Principles and practices* (4th ed.). Philadelphia: Lippincott.

Reeber, B. J. (1992). Evaluating the effects of a family education intervention. *Rehabilitation Nursing, 17*(6), 332–336.

Richmond, J. B., & Kotelchuck, M. (1984). Personal health maintenance for children. *The Western Journal of Medicine, 141*(6), 816–823.

Ryberg, J. W., & Merrifield, E. B. (1984). What parents want to know. *Nurse Practitioner, 9*(6), 24–32.

Santrock, J. W. (2006). *Life-span development* (10th ed.). Boston: McGraw-Hill.

Snowman, J., & Biehler, R. (2006). *Psychology applied to teaching.* Boston, MA: Houghton Mifflin Company.

Taylor, K., Marienau, C., & Fiddler, M. (2000). *Developing adult learners: Strategies for teachers and trainers.* San Francisco: Jossey-Bass.

Theis, S. L., & Merritt, S. L. (1994). A learning model to guide research and practice for teaching of elder clients. *Nursing and Health Care, 15*(9), 464–468.

U.S. Department of Health and Human Services. (2000). *Healthy People 2010.* McClean, VA: International Publishing.

Vander Zanden, J. W., Crandell, T. L., & Crandell, C. H. (2007). *Human Development* (8th ed.). Boston: McGraw-Hill.

Vulcan, B. (1984). Major coping behaviors of a hospitalized 3-year-old boy. *Maternal-Child Nursing Journal, 13*(2), 113–123.

Weinrich, S. P., & Boyd, M. (1992). Education in the elderly. *Journal of Gerontological Nursing, 18*(1), 15–20.

Whitener, L. M., Cox, K. R., & Maglich, S. A. (1998). Use of theory to guide nurses in the design of health messages for children. *Advances in Nursing Science, 20*(3), 21–35.

Woodring, B. C. (2000). If you have taught—have the child and family learned? *Pediatric Nursing, 26*(5), 505–509.

Chapter 6

Compliance, Motivation, and Health Behaviors of the Learner

Eleanor Richards

Kirsty Digger

CHAPTER HIGHLIGHTS

KEY TERMS

- compliance
- adherence
- locus of control
- noncompliance
- motivation
- hierarchy of needs

- motivational incentives
- motivational axioms
- concept mapping
- motivational interviewing
- health belief model
- health promotion model

❏ self-efficacy theory
❏ protection motivation theory
❏ stages of change model
❏ theory of reasoned action

❏ therapeutic alliance model
❏ concordance
❏ educational contracting

OBJECTIVES

After completing this chapter, the reader will be able to

1. Define the terms *compliance, adherence,* and *motivation* relevant to behaviors of the learner.
2. Discuss compliance and motivation concepts and theories.
3. Identify incentives and obstacles that affect motivation to learn.
4. State axioms of motivation relevant to learning.
5. Assess levels of learner motivation.
6. Outline strategies that facilitate motivation and improve compliance.
7. Compare and contrast selected health behavior frameworks and their influence on learning.
8. Recognize the role of the nurse as educator in health promotion.

The concepts of compliance and motivation are used implicitly or explicitly in many health behavior models. This chapter discusses these concepts as they relate to health behaviors of the learner and presents an overview of selected theories and models for consideration in the teaching–learning process. The nurse as educator needs to understand what factors promote or hinder the acquisition and application of knowledge, and what drives the learner to learn.

Factors that determine health behaviors and outcomes are complex. Knowledge alone does not guarantee that the learner will engage in health-promoting behaviors, nor that the desired outcomes will be achieved. The most well-thought-out educational program or plan of care will not achieve the prescribed goals if the learner is not understood in the context of complex factors associated with compliance and motivation.

Compliance

The literature reveals continuing controversy about the term compliance, which implies that independent decisions about health care are not made by the individual whose health is at stake. *Compliance* is a term used to describe submission or yielding to predetermined goals. Defined as such, it has a manipulative or authoritative undertone in which the healthcare provider or educator is viewed as the traditional authority, and the consumer or learner is viewed as submissive. This term has not been well received in nursing, most likely due to self-reflective thought and the belief in the ethical principle of autonomy. Clients have the right to make their own healthcare decisions and not necessarily follow predetermined courses of action set by healthcare professionals.

Healthcare literature suggests that compliance is the equivalent of the achieved goal in a predetermined regimen. Compliance, as an end result, is different from motivation, which is viewed as means to an end. Compliance to a health regimen is an observable behavior and as such can be directly measured. Motivation, by comparison, is a precursor to action that can be indirectly measured through behavioral consequences or results.

Commitment or attachment to a regimen is known as *adherence*, which may be long-lasting. Both compliance and adherence refer to health-promoting regimens, which are determined largely by the healthcare provider. A subtle difference separates compliance and adherence. It is possible for an individual to comply with a regimen and not necessarily be committed to it. For example, a patient who is experiencing sleep disturbances may comply with medication as directed for a period of 1 week. The same patient may not continue to adhere to the regimen for an extended period of time, even though the sleep disturbances continue. In this situation, there is no commitment to follow through. Nonadherence can be intentional or unintentional and can be impacted by such variables as cognitive function, social support, or financial constraints. Erlen (2006) and colleagues continue to investigate "maintenance strategies, booster programs, and specific factors that can impede or enhance adherence" (p. 17). Both compliance and adherence are terms used in the measurement of health outcomes. For the purpose of this chapter, these terms are used interchangeably.

Multidisciplinary healthcare literature has traditionally focused on compliance or adherence to a predetermined regimen. This phenomenon may be the result of an emphasis on cost-effective health care, as seen, for example, in shorter lengths of hospital stays. The successes of educational programs in a fiscally responsible system will ultimately be linked to measurement of patient compliance relative to outcomes.

Perspectives on Compliance

The theories of compliance as described by Eraker, Kirscht, and Becker (1984) and Levanthal and Cameron (1987) can be viewed from various perspectives and are useful in explaining or describing compliance from a multidisciplinary approach including psychology and education. These theories are:

1. Biomedical theory, including patient demographics, severity of disease, and complexity of treatment regimen
2. Behavioral/social learning theory, using the behaviorist approach of rewards, cues, contracts, and social supports
3. Communication feedback loop of sending, receiving, comprehending, retaining, and acceptance
4. Rational belief theory, weighing the benefits of treatment and the risks of disease through the use of cost-benefit logic
5. Self-regulatory systems, in which patients are seen as problem solvers whose regulation of behavior is based on perception of illness, cognitive skills, and past experiences that affect their ability to plan and cope with illness

Locus of Control

The authoritative aspect of compliance infers that the educator makes an attempt to control, in part, decision making on the part of the learner. Some models of compliance have attempted to balance the issue of control by using terms such as *mutual contracting* (Steckel, 1982) or *consensual regimen* (Fink, 1976).

One way to view the issue of control in the learning situation is through the concept of *locus of control* (Rotter, 1954), or health locus of control (Wallston, Wallston, & DeVellis, 1978). Through objective measurement, individuals can be categorized as internals, whose health behavior is self-directed, or externals, whereby others are viewed as more powerful in influencing health outcomes. Externals believe that fate is a powerful external force that determines life's course, whereas internals believe that they control their own destiny. For instance, an external might say, "Osteoporosis runs in my family, and it will catch up with me." An internal might say, "Although there is a history of osteoporosis in my family, I will have necessary screenings, eat an appropriate diet, and do weight-bearing exercise to prevent or control this problem."

Locus of control has been linked to compliance with therapeutic regimens. Shillinger (1983) suggests that different teaching strategies are indicated for internals and externals. The literature, however, remains inconclusive as to the nature of the relationship between compliance and internals versus externals.

Noncompliance

Noncompliance describes resistance of the individual to follow a predetermined regimen. Ward-Collins (1998) notes that noncompliance can be a highly subjective judgmental term sometimes used synonymously with the term noncooperative, or disobedient. She suggests the elimination of the term from professional vocabulary. The literature is replete with studies that indicate patient noncompliance. Nevertheless, the question of why clients are noncompliant remains largely unanswered. The educator's self-awareness relative to the learner's personality characteristics and previous history of compli-

ance to health regimens could play an important role in the educational process.

In an overview of the nursing literature reported by Russell, Daly, Hughes, and op't Hoog (2003, p. 282), noncompliance was categorized as follows:

1. A patient problem to be solved by nursing interventions
2. Rationalization—critical of the term noncompliance but acknowledges its importance in healthcare issues
3. Evaluative—expresses concern about the term but offers various perspectives

Russell et al. note that the "labeling of noncompliance is predominantly based on nurses' opinions of patients' behavior" (2003, p. 283). The results of this intervention, rationalization, and evaluative review support a patient-centered approach that challenges nurses not to reeducate, or coerce, but rather to embrace a paradigm shift that changes patients' lives rather than health outcomes. They conclude that nurses need to act as advocates and acknowledge the importance of patients' self-knowledge and decision making. In light of this discussion, nursing research targeted at positively influencing lifestyles rather than specific health behaviors is an area that warrants investigation.

The expectation of total compliance in all spheres of behavior and at all times is unrealistic. At times, noncompliant behavior may be desirable and could be viewed as a necessary defensive response to stressful situations. The learner may use time-outs as the intensity of the learning situation is maintained or escalates. This mechanism of temporary withdrawal from the learning situation may actually prove beneficial. Following withdrawal, the learner could reengage, feeling renewed and ready to continue with an educational program or regimen. Viewed in this way, noncompliance is not an obstacle to learning and does not carry a negative connotation.

Motivation

Motivation, from the Latin word *movere,* means to set into motion. *Motivation* has been defined as a psychological force that moves a person toward some kind of action (Haggard, 1989). It has also been described as a willingness of the learner to embrace learning, with readiness as evidence of motivation (Redman, 2007). According to Kort (1987), motivation is the result of both internal and external factors and not the result of external manipulation alone. Implicit in motivation is movement in the direction of meeting a need or toward reaching a goal.

Lewin (1935), an early field theorist, conceptualized motivation in terms of positive or negative movement toward goals. Once an individual's equilibrium is disturbed, such as in the case of illness, forces of approach and avoidance may come into play. He noted that if avoidance endured in an approach–avoidance conflict, there would be negative movement away from a goal. His theory implies the existence of a critical time factor relative to motivation. This time factor, however, is generally not a serious consideration in motivational models of health behavior or motivational research.

Ideally, the nurse educator's role is to facilitate the learner's approach toward a desired goal and to prevent untimely delays. For example, nursing staff may request an in-service program about evidence-based practice. The in-service nurse educator may delay this request to the extent that the staff loses interest in the topic. Although untimely delays may be beyond the control of the educator, every effort should be made to capitalize on the staff's desire and readiness to learn.

Maslow (1943), another well-known early theorist, developed a theory of human motivation that is still widely used in the social sciences. The major premises of Maslow's motivation theory are integrated wholeness of the individual and a hierarchy of goals. Acknowledging the complexity of the concept of motivation, he noted that not all behavior is motivated and that behavior theories are not synonymous with motivation. Many determinants of behavior other than motives exist, and many motives can be involved in one behavior. Using the principles of *hierarchy of needs*— physiological, safety, love/belonging, self-esteem, and self-actualization—Maslow noted the relatedness of needs, which are organized by their level of potency. Some individuals are highly motivated, whereas others are weakly motivated. When a need is fairly well satisfied, then the next potent need emerges. An example of the hierarchy of basic needs is the potent need to satisfy hunger. This need may be met by the nurse who assists the post-stroke patient with feeding. The nurse–patient interaction may also satisfy the next most potent needs, those of love/belonging and self-esteem.

Relationships exist between motivation and learning; between motivation and behavior; and among motivation, learning, and behavior. Motivation may be viewed in relation to learning in many ways. Redman (2007) categorizes theories of motivation that direct learning as behavioral reinforcers, need satisfaction, reduction of discomforting inconsistencies as a result of cognitive dissonance, allocating causal factors known as attributions, personality in which motivation is acknowledged to be a stable characteristic, expectancy theory encompassing value and perceived chance of success, and humanistic interpretations of motivation that emphasize personal choice. Each theory attempts to address the complex and somewhat elusive quality of motivation.

Motivational Factors

Factors that influence motivation can serve as incentives or obstacles to achieve desired behaviors. Both creating incentives and decreasing obstacles to motivation pose a challenge for the nurse as educator. The cognitive (thinking processes), affective (emotions and feelings), social, and psychomotor (behavioral) domains of the learner can be influenced by the educator, who can act as a motivational facilitator or blocker.

Motivational incentives need to be considered in the context of the individual. What may be a motivational incentive for one learner may be a motivational obstacle to another. For example, a student who is assigned to work with an elderly woman may be motivated when the student holds older persons in high regard. Another student may be motivationally blocked by the same emotional domain because previous experiences with older women, such as a grandmother, were unrewarding.

Facilitating or blocking factors that shape motivation to learn can be classified into the following three major categories, which are not mutually exclusive:

1. Personal attributes, which consist of physical, developmental, and psychological components of the individual learner
2. Environmental influences, which include the physical and attitudinal climate

3. Learner relationship systems, such as those of significant other, family, community, and teacher–learner interaction

Personal Attributes

Personal attributes of the learner, such as developmental stage, age, gender, emotional readiness, values and beliefs, sensory functioning, cognitive ability, educational level, actual or perceived state of health, and severity or chronicity of illness, can shape an individual's motivation to learn. Functional ability to achieve behavioral outcomes is determined by physical, emotional, and cognitive dimensions. One's perception of disparity between current and expected states of health can be a motivating factor in health behavior and can drive readiness to learn.

The learner's views about the complexity or extent of changes that are needed can shape motivation. Values, beliefs, and natural curiosity can be firmly entrenched and enduring factors that can also shape desire to learn new behaviors. Other factors, such as sensory input and processing of information and short-term and long-term memory, can affect motivation to learn as well. Emerging interest about male–female behavioral and learning differences indicates the need for in-depth research on gender-related characteristics affecting motivation to learn (see Chapter 8).

Environmental Influences

Physical characteristics of the learning environment, accessibility and availability of human and material resources, and different types of behavioral rewards influence the motivational level of the individual. The environment can create, promote, or detract from a state of learning receptivity. Pleasant, comfortable, and adaptable individualized surroundings can promote a state of readiness to learn. Conversely, noise, confusion, interruptions, and lack of privacy can interfere with the capacity to concentrate and to learn.

The factors of accessibility and availability of resources include physical and psychological aspects. Can the client physically access a health facility, and once there, will the healthcare personnel be psychologically available to the client? Psychological availability refers to whether the healthcare system is flexible and sensitive to patients' needs. It includes factors such as promptness of services, sociocultural competence, emotional support, and communication skills. Attitude influences the client's engagement with the healthcare system.

The manner in which the healthcare system is perceived by the client affects the client's willingness to participate in health-promoting behaviors. Behavioral rewards permeate the foundations of the learner's motivation. Rewards can be extrinsic, such as praise or acknowledgment from the educator or caretaker. Alternatively, they can be intrinsically based, such as feelings of a personal sense of fulfillment, gratification, or self-satisfaction.

RELATIONSHIP SYSTEMS

Family or significant others in the support system; cultural identity; work, school, and community roles; and teacher–learner interaction all influence an individual's motivation. The interactional aspects of motivation are perhaps the most salient because the learner exists in the context of interlocking relationship systems. Individuals are viewed in the context of family/community/cultural systems that have lifelong effects on the choices that individuals make, including healthcare seeking and healthcare

decision making. These significant other systems may have even more of an influence on health outcomes than commonly acknowledged, and the health-promoting use of these systems needs to be taken into account by the nurse as educator. All of these factors interact to address the motivation of the learner. They are not meant to be construed as comprehensive theory constructs, but rather as forces that act on motivation, serving to facilitate or block the desire to learn.

Motivational Axioms

Axioms are premises on which an understanding of a phenomenon is based. The nurse as educator needs to understand the premises involved in promoting motivation of the learner. *Motivational axioms* are rules that set the stage for motivation. They include (1) the state of optimum anxiety, (2) learner readiness, (3) realistic goal setting, (4) learner satisfaction/success, and (5) uncertainty-reducing or uncertainty-maintaining dialogue.

STATE OF OPTIMUM ANXIETY

Learning occurs best when a state of moderate anxiety exists. In this optimum state for learning, one's ability to observe, focus attention, learn, and adapt is operative (Peplau, 1979). Perception, concentration, abstract thinking, and information processing are enhanced. Behavior is directed at a learning or challenging situation. Above this optimum level, at high or severe levels of anxiety, the ability to perceive the environment, concentrate, and learn is reduced. A moderate state of anxiety can be comfortably managed and is known to promote learning (Kessels, 2003; Ley, 1979; Stephenson, 2006). As anxiety escalates, however, attention to external stimuli is reduced, the learner becomes increasingly self-absorbed, and behavior becomes defensively reactionary rather than being cognitively generated (Shapiro, Boggs, Melamed, & Graham-Pole, 1992).

For example, a patient who has been recently diagnosed with insulin-dependent diabetes and who has a high level of anxiety will not respond at an optimum level of retention of information when instructed about insulin injections. When the nurse as educator is able to aid the client in reducing anxiety, through techniques such as guided imagery, use of humor, or relaxation tapes, the patient will respond with a higher level of information retention.

LEARNER READINESS

Desire to move toward a goal and readiness to learn are factors that influence motivation. Desire cannot be imposed on the learner. It can, however, be critically influenced by external forces and be promoted by the nurse as educator. Incentives are specific to the individual learner. An incentive for one individual can be a deterrent to another. For example, suggesting a method of weight reduction that includes physical exercise may be an incentive for one client, while totally unappealing for another. Incentives in the form of reinforcers and rewards can be tangible or intangible, external or internal.

As a facilitator to the learner, the nurse as educator offers positive perspectives and encouragement, which shape the desired behavior toward goal attainment. By ensuring that learning is stimulating, making information relevant and accessible, and creating an environment conducive to learning, educators can facilitate motivation to learn (see Chapter 4 on readiness to learn).

REALISTIC GOALS

Goals that are within one's grasp and possible to achieve are goals toward which an individual will work. Goals that are beyond one's reach are frustrating and counterproductive. Unrealistic goals with loss of valuable time can set the stage for the learner to give up.

Setting realistic goals is a motivating factor. The belief that one can achieve the task set before him or her facilitates behavior geared toward achieving that goal. Goals should parallel the extent to which behavioral changes are needed. Learning what the learner wants to change is a critical factor in setting realistic goals. Mutual goal setting between learner and educator reduces the negative effects of hidden agendas or the sabotaging of educational plans.

LEARNER SATISFACTION/SUCCESS

The learner is motivated by success. Success is self-satisfying and feeds one's self-esteem. In a cyclical process, success and self-esteem escalate, moving the learner toward accomplishment of goals. When a learner feels good about step-by-step accomplishments, motivation is enhanced. For example, in the instructor–student relationship, evaluations can be a valuable method of promoting learner success. Clinical evaluations, when focused on demonstration of positive behaviors, can encourage movement toward performance goals. Focusing on successes as a means of positive reinforcement promotes learner satisfaction and instills a sense of accomplishment. On the other hand, focusing on weak clinical performance can reduce students' self-esteem.

UNCERTAINTY REDUCTION OR MAINTENANCE

Uncertainty (as well as certainty) can be a motivating factor in the learning situation. Individuals have ongoing internal dialogues that can either reduce or maintain uncertainty. Individuals carry on "self-talk"; they think things through. When one wants to change a state of health, behaviors will often follow a dialogue that examines uncertainty, such as, "If I stop smoking, then my chances of getting lung cancer will be reduced." On the other hand, when the probable outcome of health behaviors is more uncertain, then behaviors may maintain uncertainty. One might say, "I am not sure that I need this surgery because the survival rates are no different for those who had this surgery and those who did not." Some learners may maintain current behaviors, given probabilities of treatment outcomes, thus maintaining uncertainty.

Mishel (1990) reconceptualized the concept of uncertainty in illness. She views uncertainty as a necessary and natural rhythm of life, rather than an adverse experience. Uncertainty in sufficient concentration influences choices and decision making, and it can capitalize on receptivity or readiness for change. Premature uncertainty reduction can be counterproductive to the learner who has not sufficiently explored alternatives. For example, when a staff nurse is uncertain about positions for catheterizing a debilitated female client and is presented with alternatives, then a thinking dialogue is carried out. If the decision to use a particular position is not premature, then uncertainty will promote exploration of alternative positions.

Assessment of Motivation

How does the nurse know when the learner is motivated? As a generic concept, assessment of motivation to learn has not been adequately addressed in the literature. The lack of adequate, conceptually based measurement tools could be a factor in this neglect.

Redman (2001) views motivational assessment as a part of general health assessment and states that it includes such areas as level of knowledge, client skills, decision-making capacity of the individual, and screening of target populations for educational programs. The educator can pose several questions in terms of the learner, such as those focusing on previous attempts, curiosity, goal setting, self-care ability, stress factors, survival issues, and life situations. Motivational assessment of the learner needs to be comprehensive, systematic, and conceptually based. Cognitive, affective, physiological, experiential, environmental, and learning relationship variables need to be considered. **Table 6–1** shows parameters for a comprehensive motivational assessment of the learner.

These multi-theory-based parameters incorporate several perspectives, including Bandura's (1986) construction of incentive motivators; Ajzen and Fishbein's (1980) intent and attitude; Becker, Drachman, and Kirscht's (1974) notion of likelihood of engaging in action; Pender's (1996) commitment to a plan of action; and Barofsky's (1978) focus on alliance in the learning situation. Additionally, the presence of cognitions in the form of facilitative beliefs proposed by Wright, Watson, and Bell (1996) provides a comprehensive and multidimensional assessment. This multidimensional guide allows for assessment of the level of learner motivation. If responses to dimensions are positive, then the learner is likely to be motivated.

Assessment of learner motivation involves the judgment of the educator, because teaching–learning is a two-way process. In particular, motivation can be assessed through both subjective and objective means. A subjective means of assessing level of motivation is through dialogue. Through the sense of nurse presence and use of communication skills, the nurse can

Table 6–1 Comprehensive Parameters for Motivational Assessment of the Learner

Cognitive Variables

- Capacity to learn
- Readiness to learn
  - Expressed self-determination
  - Constructive attitude
  - Expressed desire and curiosity
  - Willingness to contract for behavioral outcomes
- Facilitating beliefs

Affective Variables

- Expressions of constructive emotional state
- Moderate level of anxiety

Physiological Variables

- Capacity to perform required behavior

Experiential Variables

- Previous successful experiences

Environmental Variables

- Appropriateness of physical environment
- Social support systems
  - Family
  - Group
  - Work
  - Community resources

Educator–Learner Relationship System

- Prediction of positive relationship

obtain verbal information from the client, such as, "I really want to maintain my weight" or "I want to have a healthy baby." Both of these statements indicate an energized desire with direction of movement toward an expected health outcome. Nonverbal cues can also indicate motivation, such as browsing through lay literature about healthy pregnancy. Likewise, a staff member or student nurse may express a verbal desire to know more about a specific advanced procedure. A nonverbal motivational cue might be expressed by the staff member or student nurse carefully observing a senior nurse or clinical specialist performing an advanced technique, for example.

Measurement of motivation is another aspect to be considered. Subjective self-reports indicate the level of motivation from the learner's perspective. If desired, self-report measurements could be developed for educational programs. Objective measurement of motivation—an indirect measurement—can be quantified through observation of expected behaviors, the consequence of motivation. These behaviors can be observed in increments as the learner moves toward preset realistic health or practice goals.

Motivational Strategies

Finding the spark that motivates the learner to learn is challenging to the educator. The question remains, how does an educator motivate a seemingly unmotivated individual? As noted earlier, incentives viewed as appeals or inducements to motivation can be either intrinsically or extrinsically generated. Incentives and motivation are both stimuli to action. Bandura (1986) associates motivation with incentives. He noted, however, that intrinsic motivation, although highly appealing, is elusive. Only rarely does motivation occur without extrinsic influence. Green and Kreuter (1999) note that "strictly speaking we can appeal to people's motives, but we cannot motivate them" (p. 30). Extrinsic incentives are used for motivational strategizing in the educational situation.

Cognitive evaluation theory (Ryan & Deci, 2000) posits that knowing how to foster motivation becomes essential since educators cannot rely on intrinsic motivation to promote learning. They note, however, that autonomy and competence are intrinsic motivators that can be fostered by selected teaching strategies. One contemporary nursing educational strategy that can be used to promote motivation is *concept mapping*, which enables the learner to integrate previous learning with newly acquired knowledge through diagrammatic "mapping." As a motivational technique, concept mapping facilitates the acquisition of complex new knowledge through visual links that acknowledge previous learning. Learner interest is sustained by perceived competence and autonomy. Concept mapping as a less instructor-regulated learning activity promotes interest and value. Wilkes, Cooper, Lewin, and Batts (1999) reported that bachelor's degree nursing students produced high-level concept maps, indicating that the maps were valued as a learning experience.

Motivational strategies for the nurse as educator are extrinsically generated through the use of specific incentives. The critical question for the nurse as educator to ask is, "What specific behavior, under what circumstances, in what time frame, is desired by this learner?" Strategizing begins with a systematic assessment of learner motivation, like that outlined in Table 6–1. When an applicable dimension is absent or reduced, then incentive strategizing is likely to move the individual away from the desired outcome. When considering strategies to improve learner motivation, Maslow's (1943) hierarchy of needs can also be taken into consideration. An appeal can be made to the innate need for the learner to succeed, known as achievement motivation (Atkinson, 1964).

In the educational situation, clear communication, including clarification of directions and expectations, is critical. Organization of material in a way that makes information meaningful to the learner, environmental manipulation, positive verbal feedback, and providing opportunities for success are motivational strategies proposed by Haggard (1989). Reducing or eliminating barriers to achieve goals is an important aspect of maintaining motivation.

One particular model developed by Keller (1987), the attention, relevance, confidence, and satisfaction (ARCS) model, focuses on creating and maintaining motivational strategies used for instructional design. This model emphasizes strategies that the educator can use to effect changes in the learner by creating a motivating learning environment.

- Attention introduces opposing positions, case studies, and variable instructional presentations.
- Relevance capitalizes on the learners' experiences, usefulness, needs, and personal choices.
- Confidence deals with learning requirements, level of difficulty, expectations, attributions, and sense of accomplishment.
- Satisfaction pertains to timely use of a new skill, use of rewards, praise, and self-evaluation.

In motivational strategizing, it would also be beneficial to consider Damrosch's (1991) proposal that client health beliefs, personal vulnerability, efficacy of proposed change, and ability to effect the change are important in patient education efforts.

Beliefs are a major construct proposed by Wright, Watson, and Bell (1996) as the heart of healing in families. Facilitating beliefs can promote a desired change, whereas constraining beliefs can restrict options. Challenging constraining beliefs and promoting facilitating beliefs are, therefore, offered as motivational strategies.

An understanding of the individual's mental representations or beliefs is also foundational to the common sense model in the representational approach to patient education (Levanthal & Diefenbach, 1991). Beliefs constitute an underacknowledged and understudied phenomenon that needs to be further developed in the education literature in terms of motivational strategizing.

Motivational interviewing is a method of staging readiness to change for the purpose of promoting desired health behaviors. It is an individualized, flexible, patient-centered approach that is supportive, empathetic and goal directed. It takes into consideration problem solving, confidence in change and resistance to change. The interviewer seeks to gain knowledge about health beliefs (Rollnick, Mason, & Butler, 1999). This method has been used as a strategy to explore client motivation for adherence to health regimens (Gance-Cleveland, 2005). Zimmerman, Olsen, and Bosworth (2000) developed a readiness to change ruler for motivational interviewing in which the client self-reports preparedness to change. This could be a useful tool for the nurse as educator in motivational strategizing.

Selected Models and Theories

Compliance and motivation are concepts germane to health behaviors of the learner. The nurse as educator focuses on health education as well as the expected health behaviors. Health behavior frameworks are blueprints and, as such, serve as tools for the nurse as educator that can be used to maintain desired patient behaviors or promote changes. As a consequence, a familiarity with models and theories that describe, explain, or predict health behaviors will increase the range of health-promoting strategies for the nurse as educator. When these frameworks are understood, the principles inherent in each can be used either to promote compliance to a health regimen or facilitate motivation. This chapter presents an overview of the following selected models and theories: health belief model, health promotion model, self-efficacy theory, protection motivation theory, stages of change model, theory of reasoned action, and the therapeutic alliance model.

Health Belief Model

The original *health belief model* was developed in the 1950s from a social psychology perspective to examine why people did not participate in health-screening programs (Rosenstock, 1974). This model was modified by Becker et al. (1974) to address compliance to therapeutic regimens.

The two major premises on which the model is built are the eventual success of disease prevention and curing regimens that involve the clients' willingness to participate and the belief that health is highly valued (Becker, 1990). Both of these premises need to be present for the model to be relevant in explaining health behavior. The model is grounded on the supposition that it is possible to predict health behavior given these three major interacting components: individual perceptions, modifying factors, and likelihood of action (**Figure 6–1**).

Figure 6–1 The health belief model used as a predictor of preventive health behavior.

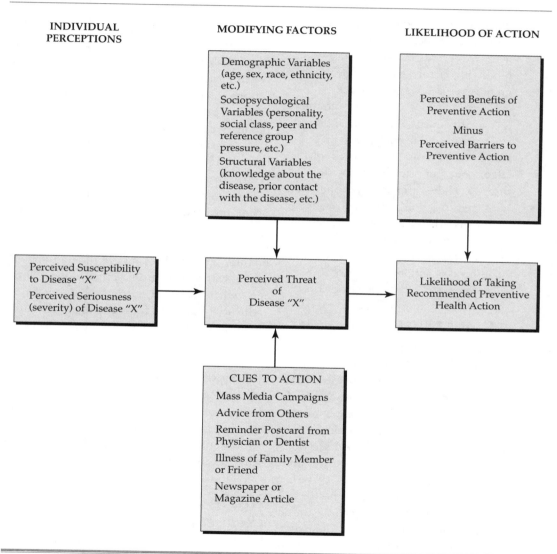

Source: From Becker, M., Drachman, R., & Kirscht, J. (1974). A new approach to explaining sick-role behavior in low-income populations. *American Journal of Public Health, 64*(3), 206. Copyright by American Public Health Association. Reprinted with permission.

Figure 6–1 shows the direction and flow of these interacting components, each of which is further divided into subcomponents:

1. Individual perceptions: comprised of subcomponents of perceived susceptibility or perceived severity of a specific disease.

2. Modifying factors: consist of demographic variables (age, sex, race, ethnicity), sociopsychological variables (personality, locus of control, social class, peer and reference group pressure), and structural variables (knowledge about and prior contact with disease). These variables, in conjunction with cues to action (mass media, advice, reminders, illness, reading material), influence the subcomponent of perceived threat of the specific disease.

3. Likelihood of action: consists of the subcomponents of perceived benefits of preventive action minus perceived barriers to preventive action.

All of the components are directed toward the likelihood of taking recommended preventive health action as the final phase of the model. In sum, individual perceptions and modifying factors interact. An individual appraisal of the preventive action occurs, which is followed by a prediction of the likelihood of action.

The health belief model has been the predominant explanatory model since the 1970s for uncovering differences in preventive health behaviors as well as differences in preventive use of health services (Langlie, 1977). Used to predict preventive health behavior and to explain sick-role behavior, it has been used widely in health behavior research across disciplines such as medicine, psychology, social behavior, and gerontology. The model has also been broadly used to study patient behaviors in relation to preventive behaviors and acute and chronic illnesses.

Over time, studies have supported the validity of this model. For instance, Jachna and Forbes-Thompson (2005) studied health belief constructs in an assisted living facility and found healthcare providers can influence health beliefs relative to osteoporosis, which has implications for gerontological nursing education. Charron-Prachnowik et al. (2001) studied reproductive health behaviors in adolescents with Type 1 diabetes and found that preconception counseling is a motivational cue that triggers positive health actions.

Findings from studies such as these can be operationalized through educational programs specific to high-risk populations. In an historical 10-year review of the health belief model literature, Janz and Becker (1984) found that the model was robust in predicting health behaviors, with perceived barriers being the most influential factor. As it applies today, the nurse as educator needs to take into consideration the availability of barrier-free educational resources.

Dutta-Bergman (2004) suggests a relationship between health beliefs, information seeking, and active versus passive learners with implications for type of health education delivery. They indicate that health educators need to be concerned with consumer health-seeking behaviors in the technology age.

Health Promotion Model (Revised)

The *health promotion model*, originally developed by Pender in 1987, has been primarily used in the discipline of nursing. This model, which describes major components and variables that factor into health-promoting behaviors, was revised by Pender in 1996 to increase the utility of its predictions and interventions (**Figure 6–2**). Its emphasis on actualizing health potential and increasing the level of well-being using approach behaviors rather than avoidance of disease behaviors distinguish this model as a health promotion rather than a disease-prevention model.

Figure 6–2 Revised health promotion model.

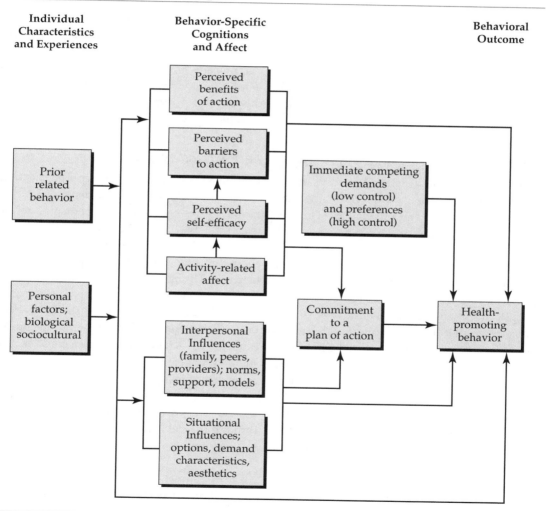

Source: From Pender, N. (1996). *Health promotion in nursing practice* (3rd ed., p. 67). Upper Saddle River, NJ: Pearson Education. Reprinted by permission of Pearson Education, Inc.

The sequence of major components and variables is clearly outlined as follows:

1. Individual characteristics and experiences: prior related behavior, and personal factors.
2. Behavior-specific cognitions and affect: perceived benefits of action, perceived barriers to action, perceived self-efficacy, activity-related affect, interpersonal influences, and situational influences.
3. Behavioral outcome: health-promoting behavior partially mediated by commitment to a plan of action and influenced by immediate competing demands and preferences.

The revised model was expanded to include these three variables: activity-related affect, commitment to a plan of action, and immediate competing demands and preferences. There is continuing discussion of this popular model (Pender, Murdaugh, & Parsons, 2002).

The health belief model and the health promotion model share several schematic similarities, seen in a comparison of Figures 6–1 and 6–2. Both models describe the use of factors or components that impact perceptions. Sequencing of factors in each of the models, however, shows some schematic dissimilarities. While the health belief model targets the likelihood of engaging in preventive health behaviors, the revised health promotion model targets positive health outcomes.

Research support for the health promotion model has been shown in a variety of settings. Buijs, Ross-Kerr, Cousins, and Wilson (2003) addressed community-based health promotion and used the health promotion model to interpret data and explain health behaviors of low-income senior citizens in a 10-month community-based health promotion program. The results of this qualitative study (N = 34) show Pender's model as a useful method of encouraging senior citizen participation in health-promoting activities. Rothman, Lourie, Brian, and Foley (2005) used the model in an underserved community to develop programs such as lead poisoning in children prevention, tobacco awareness, and prenatal education. These programs decreased barriers to healthcare access. Hjelm, Mufunda, Nambozi, and Kemp (2003) call for a curricular change that prepares nurses for new roles in health promotion in order to expand public awareness of the pandemic nature of Type 2 diabetes, and the need for lifestyle change.

Self-Efficacy Theory

Developed from a social-cognitive perspective, the *self-efficacy theory* is based on a person's expectations relative to a specific course of action (Bandura, 1977a, 1977b, 1986, 1997). It is a predictive theory in the sense that it deals with the belief that one can accomplish a specific behavior. The belief of competency and capability relative to certain behaviors is a precursor to expected outcomes. **Figure 6–3** shows an adaptation of Bandura's efficacy expectations model extended to include expected outcomes. In this adapted model, self-efficacy is used as an outcome determinant.

According to Bandura (1986, 1997), self-efficacy is cognitively appraised and processed through the following four principal sources of information:

1. Performance accomplishments evidenced in self-mastery of similarly expected behaviors
2. Vicarious experiences, such as observing successful expected behavior through the modeling of others

Figure 6–3 Determinants of expected outcomes using self-efficacy perceptions.

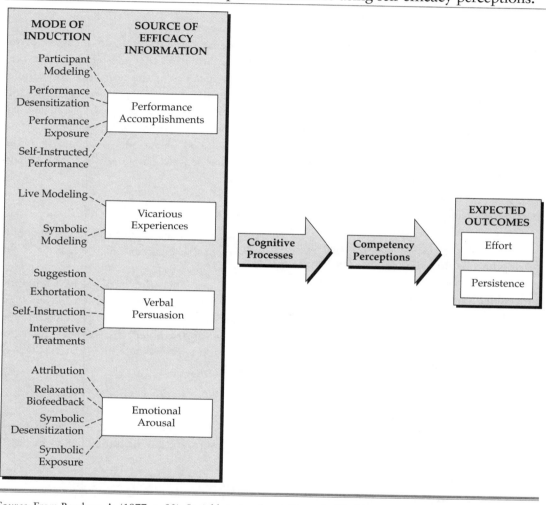

3. Verbal persuasion by others who present realistic beliefs that the individual is capable of the expected behavior
4. Emotional arousal through self-judgment of physiological states of distress

Bandura (1986, 1997) notes that the most influential source of efficacy information is that of previous performance accomplishments. Efficacy expectations (expectations relative to a specific course of action) are induced through certain modes. Modes of induction include, but are not limited to, desensitization, self-instruction, exposure, suggestion, and relaxation.

Self-efficacy has proved useful in predicting the course of health behavior. Kaewthummanukul and Brown (2006) reviewed the literature from 11 studies and concluded that self-efficacy was the best predictor in an employee physical activity program and could be used in occupational health nursing. Callaghan (2005) studied relationships between self-care behaviors and self-efficacy in the older adult population (N = 235). She found a significant relationship between self-care behaviors in older women and self-efficacy, noting that nurses are in a key position to promote self-care and healthy aging.

The use of the self-efficacy theory for the nurse as educator is particularly relevant in developing educational programs. The behavior-specific predictions of the theory can be used for understanding the likelihood of individuals to participate in existing or projected educational programs. Educational strategies such as modeling, demonstration, and verbal reinforcement parallel modes of self-efficacy induction.

Protection Motivation Theory

Protection motivation theory (Prentice-Dunn & Rogers, 1986) explains behavioral change in terms of threat and coping appraisal. A threat to health is considered a stimulus to protection motivation. This linear theory includes sources of information (environmental and intrapersonal) that are cognitively processed by appraisal of threat and coping to form protective motivation, which leads to intent and ultimately to action.

Influenced by crisis and self-efficacy theories, protection motivation theory has tested antecedents to health behaviors such as drug abuse, AIDS, smoking, and drinking behaviors. Wu, Stanton, Li, Galbraith, and Cole (2005) found that adolescent drug trafficking can be predicted by an overall level of health protection motivation. They suggested that the theory be considered in the design of drug-trafficking prevention programs.

Evidence-based research can uncover motivational information that can be used to inform health educators in the design of educational programs that specifically target high-risk individuals or groups for selected risk behaviors. The protection motivation theory goes beyond the likelihood of action in the health belief model and self-efficacy intent to health behavior action.

Stages of Change Model

Another model that informs us of the phenomenon of health behaviors of the learner is the *stages of change model,* also known as the transtheoretical model (Prochaska & Di Clemente, 1982). Originating from the field of psychology, this model (see **Table 6–2**) was developed around addictive and problem behaviors. Prochaska (1996) notes six distinct time-related stages of change:

1. Precontemplation—individuals have no current intention of changing. Strategies involve simple observations, confrontation, or consciousness raising.

Table 6–2 Six Stages of Change

- Precontemplation
- Contemplation
- Preparation
- Action
- Maintenance
- Termination

2. Contemplation—individuals accept or realize that they have a problem and begin to think seriously about changing it. Strategies involve increased consciousness raising.

3. Preparation—individuals are planning to take action within the time frame of 1 month. Strategies include a firm and detailed plan for action.

4. Action—there is overt/visible modification of behavior. This is the busiest stage, and strategies include commitment to the change, self-reward, countering (substitute behaviors), creating a friendly environment, and supportive relationships.

5. Maintenance—is a difficult stage to achieve and may last 6 months to a lifetime. There are common challenges to this stage, including overconfidence, daily temptation, and relapse self-blame. The strategies in this stage are the same for the action stage.

6. Termination—occurs when the problem no longer presents any temptation. However, some experts note that termination does not occur, only that maintenance becomes less vigilant.

The extent to which people are motivated and ready to change is seen as an important construct. It is useful in nursing to stage the client's intentions and behaviors for change as well as strategies that will enable completion of the specific stage. More recent use of the model in nursing research has focused on its value in health promotion and the processes by which people decide to change (or not to change) behaviors.

The stages of change model has been used to investigate health behaviors such as smoking cessation (Narsavage, 2003) and dietary habits (Frenn & Malin, 2003). Paul and Sneed (2004) examined readiness for behavior change in patients with heart failure and noted that it is "not realistic to expect patients to make changes that they are not prepared to make" (p. 313). This popular model can be used with children and adults, which has implications for a variety of educational settings. Recently, Kelly (2005) developed the commitment to health scale that shows potential as a research instrument for measuring the final stage of change. This stage could be viewed as an educational outcome in terms of health behaviors of the learner.

Theory of Reasoned Action

The *theory of reasoned action* emerged from a research program that began in the 1950s and is concerned with prediction and understanding of any form of human behavior within a social context (Ajzen & Fishbein, 1980). It is based on the premise that humans are rational decision makers who make use of whatever information is available to them. Attitudes toward persons are not an integral part of this theory; rather, the focus is on the predicted behavior. This theory is shown as a sequential model in **Figure 6–4**.

In a two-pronged linear approach, specific behavior is determined by (1) beliefs, attitude toward the behavior, and intention; and (2) motivation to comply with influential persons known as referents, subjective norms, and intention. The person's intention to perform can be measured by relative weights of attitude and subjective norms.

Kleier (2004), in a large scale (N = 1,490) study, tested the theory of reasoned action to determine nurse practitioner attitudes toward teaching testicular self-examination. The results showed that nurse practitioners were engaged in this teaching behavior and suggest the importance of including strategies to promote positive

Figure 6–4 Factors determining a person's behavior.

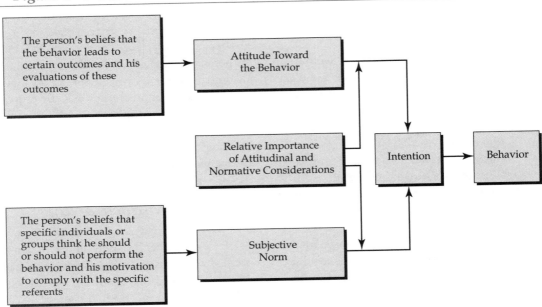

Note: Arrows indicate the direction of influence.

Source: From Ajzen, I., & Fishbein, M. (1980). *Understanding attitudes and predicting social behavior* (p. 8). Upper Saddle River, NJ: Prentice-Hall. Reprinted by permission of Prentice-Hall.

values as components of nurse [educational] preparation. McGahee, Kemp, and Tingen (2000) suggest the use of the theory as a framework for conducting empirical studies for smoking prevention in preteens, which has implications for educational program development. Hanson (2005) investigated ethnic differences in cigarette smoking intention among female teenagers and found attitude to be the greatest predictor of intention to smoke in Hispanic as well as non-Hispanic White teenagers.

The theory of reasoned action is useful in predicting health behaviors, particularly for educators who want to understand the attitudinal context within which behaviors are likely to change. Nurses as educators need to take beliefs, attitudinal factors, and subjective norms into consideration when designing educational programs relating to intent to change a specific health behavior.

Therapeutic Alliance Model

Barofsky's (1978) therapeutic alliance model addresses a shift in power from the provider to a learning partnership in which collaboration and negotiation with the consumer are key. A therapeutic alliance is formed between the caregiver and receiver in which each participant in this affiliation is viewed as having equal power. The client is viewed as active and responsible, with an outcome expectation of self-care. The shift toward self-determination and control over one's own life is fundamental to this model (**Figure 6–5**).

The therapeutic alliance model compares the components of compliance, adherence, and alliance. According to Barofsky (1978), change is needed in treatment determinants—change from coercion in compliance and from conforming in adherence to collaboration in alliance. The power in the relationship between the participants is equalized by alliance. The role of the patient is neither passive nor rebellious, but rather active and responsible. The expected outcomes are not compliant dependence or counterdependence, but responsible self-care.

Although not originally developed as an educational model, and not well known in nursing, the usefulness of this model to the nurse as educator is nevertheless acknowledged in the partnership of learning. This interpersonal model is appropriate in the educational process when shifting the focus from the patient as a passive-dependent learner to one of an active learner. It serves as a guide to refocus education efforts on collaboration rather than on compliance. The nurse as educator and the patient as learner form an alliance with the goal of self-care.

Hobden (2006), in a recent exploration of the concepts of compliance and adherence, notes that these terms have a negative connotation and a shift in the balance of power towards the patient lies in the consultative process known as *concordance*, which is "consultation that allows mutual respect for the patient's and professional's beliefs, and allows negotiation to take place about the best course of action for the patient" (p. 258). She notes there is a shift in the balance of power from the professional to the patient. Although concordance should lead to improved health outcomes, the focus is on the process.

Motivational interviewing also interfaces with the therapeutic alliance model. Duran (2003) notes that successful motivational interviewing takes place in an atmosphere of the client being understood and respected, and is collaborative in nature with the highest priority placed on the client's autonomy and freedom of choice.

Models for Health Education

Selection of models for educational use can be made with respect to (1) similarities and dissimilarities, (2) nurse as educator agreement with model conceptualizations, and (3) functional utility.

Similarities and Dissimilarities of Models

Models may be seen as so similar that there would be a negligible difference in choosing one over the other, or they may be seen as so

Figure 6–5 Continuum of the therapeutic alliance model.

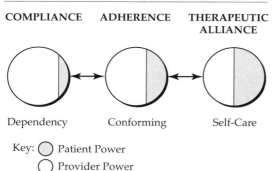

COMPLIANCE   ADHERENCE   THERAPEUTIC ALLIANCE

Dependency   Conforming   Self-Care

Key: ◐ Patient Power
      ○ Provider Power

dissimilar that one would be inappropriate for a specific educational purpose. A cursory comparative analysis of the different frameworks reveals that the health belief model and the health promotion model are similar. Each uses comparable salient factors of individual perceptions and competing variables. The differences appear in the models' basic premises and outcomes. The health belief model emphasizes susceptibility to disease and the likelihood of preventive action, whereas the health promotion model emphasizes health potential and health-promoting behaviors.

The self-efficacy theory and the theory of reasoned action are similar in that they focus on the predictions or expectations of specific behaviors. The theories lend themselves more easily to less complex model testing than either the health belief model or the health promotion model because the former are more linear in conceptualization. Specificity of behaviors may aid in targeting outcomes of educational programs. The stages of change model is similar to the self-efficacy theory and the theory of reasoned action in the sense that these models focus on intent. The stages of change model appears to be less complicated and does not take into account personal characteristics or experiences. It differs from the self-efficacy theory, the protection motivation theory, and the theory of reasoned action in that change is time relevant with implications for educational interventions.

Protection motivation theory is similar to the health promotion model and the theory of reasoned action in the sense that information is cognitively processed, followed by intent or commitment to action and the health behavior.

The health belief model, health promotion model, self-efficacy theory, protection motivation theory, and theory of reasoned action are similar in that they acknowledge factors such as experiences, perceptions, or beliefs relative to the individual and factors external to the individual that can modify health behaviors. These frameworks also recognize the multidimensional nature, complexity, and probability of health behaviors. One major difference between the health belief model and the protection motivation theory is that the latter has a component of fear appraisal and focuses on a specific vulnerability rather than general susceptibility to illness (Prentice-Dunn & Rogers, 1986).

All of the models acknowledge the importance of the patient in decision making with respect to health behaviors. The differences relate to patient focus, the relative importance of modifying factors, specificity of behavior, and outcomes.

The most dissimilar model is the therapeutic alliance model. Although it is relatively narrow in scope, its simplicity and parsimony are strengths. When applied to the educational arena, the educator–learner relationship is the critical factor. Addressing potentially frustrating patient education situations such as noncompliance, Hochbaum (1980) noted that patient educators, when frustrated, "are unable to understand the apparently irrational and self-destructive action of their patients, and sometimes throw their hands up in despair, bedeviled by the seeming irrationality of the patient's behavior . . . But this behavior may be altogether rational from the patient's perspective" (p. 7). Understanding of the client as learner can be uncovered in the therapeutic alliance model.

Educator Agreement With Model Conceptualizations

Nurses as educators have belief systems, which may or may not agree with some of the tenets of each of the models presented. The choice of a model, therefore, can be based on the educator's level of agreement with salient factors in each framework.

Likelihood of action is best addressed by the health belief model, while attaining positive health outcomes is the focus of the health promotion model and the protection motivation theory. Attitude and intention are best viewed through the theory of reasoned action. Belief in one's capabilities is best addressed by self-efficacy theory, and the therapeutic alliance model is best used for reduction of noncompliance through an educator–learner collaboration. Staging the individual's readiness for change and developing strategies for interventions are helpful in designing educational programs with the stages of change model.

Through in-depth analysis of each model, the attention of the educator may be drawn to other factors as well. Ultimately, the model or models that fit best with the educator's own beliefs are more likely to be chosen.

Functional Utility of Models

Model selection for educational purposes can also be based on functional utility. Questions to be asked to determine functional utility are as follows:

- Who is the target learner?
- What is the focus of the learning?
- When is the optimal time?
- Where is the process to be carried out?

The question of *who* the learner is deals with whether the target learner is the individual, family, or group. The health belief model, health promotion model, self-efficacy theory, protection motivation theory, stages of change model, and theory of reasoned action can be used across the range of these target learners. The important notion for the nurse as educator to remember is the probability of individual vari-

ation. Another consideration in terms of the target learner is categorical groups, such as those considered at high risk and those diagnosed with acute or chronic illnesses.

The functional use of the models can also be determined by the content needed, the timing of the educational experience, and the setting in which the learning is to take place. *What* is needed relates to the focus of the learning and addresses the content to be taught, such as disease processes, specific disease, promotion of wellness, expectations of specific health practices, or focus on self-care.

The question of *when* is one of optimal timing and refers to the readiness of the learner, a mutually convenient time, and prevention of untimely delays in moving toward a desired goal. Although considered important in the context of health education, this critical factor has received little specific reference in terms of health promotion models. Except for the stages of change model, timing is an often neglected factor in the models discussed. It is apparent that determining optimal time can be a motivational incentive in terms of meeting the health needs of the learner.

Addressing the question of *where* the educational process is to be carried out is another aspect of functional utility. The settings of home, workplace, school, institution, or specific community locations are all options. All of the models discussed in this chapter lend themselves to these diverse settings.

Integration of Models for Use in Education

Theories provide blueprints for interventions. From the previous discussion, it is clear that the integration of various components of health behavior models is advantageous in the educational process. When salient factors are taken into consideration in light of developmental stages of the learner, an integrated motivational model of learning in health promotion could emerge.

Recent literature proposes model integration. For example, Gebhardt and Maes (2001) advocate for a multitheory approach to promote health behaviors. Cautioning against the use of unidirectional and nondynamic views of behavioral change, they propose an integrative approach using goal theories and stages of change. Poss (2001) developed a new model synthesizing the health belief model and the theory of reasoned action, noting that a synthesized model is appropriate for the study of persons from varying cultural backgrounds. Chiu (2005) investigated the previously untested Bruhn and Parcel (1982) model of children's health promotion in adolescents with Type 1 diabetes using structural equation modeling analysis. She found only partial support for the model, suggesting a new model that would incorporate self-efficacy as well as locus of control.

The development of new models and/or the revision of older models are necessary steps in the evolution and delivery of health care, and it necessarily affects the educator concerned with motivational behaviors of the learner.

Salient health promotion factors that can be used in a multitheory approach to health education include, but are not limited to, level of knowledge, attitudes, values, beliefs, perceptions, level of anxiety, self-confidence, skills mastery, past experiences, intention, physiological capacity, sociocultural enablers, environment, educator–learner alliance, resources and reinforcements, mutual and realistic goal setting, hierarchy of needs, quality of life, and voluntary participation in learning.

Developmental stages of the learner incorporate principles of pedagogy (teaching children), andragogy (teaching adults), and gerogogy (teaching older adults) to meet the needs of the learner. A more comprehensive and holistic model for the nurse as educator could emerge when learning is viewed along a unidirectional developmental continuum, in combination with salient health promotion factors. (For a discussion on educational approaches with learners at different stages of development, see Chapter 5.)

The Role of Nurse as Educator in Health Promotion

Nurses as educators are in a position to promote healthy lifestyles. Combining content specific to the discipline of nursing, knowledge from educational theories, and health behavior models allows for an integrated approach to shaping health behaviors of the learner. The roles of the nurse as educator include facilitator of change, contractor, organizer, and evaluator.

Facilitator of Change

The goal of the nurse as educator is, of course, to promote health. Health education and health promotion are integral to this effort. At the same time, the nurse as educator is an important facilitator of change. When learning is viewed as an intervention, it needs to be considered in the context of other nursing interventions that will effect change. In 1987, deTornay and Thompson proposed that explaining, analyzing, dividing complex skills, demonstrating, practicing, asking questions, and providing closure are effective in facilitating change in the learning situation.

Contractor

Contracting has been a popular means of facilitating learning. Informal or formal contracts can delineate and promote learning objectives. Similar to the nursing process, *educational contracting* involves stating mutual goals to be accomplished, devising an agreed-upon plan of action, evaluating the plan, and deriving alternatives. (See discussion of learning contracts in Chapter 10.) The plan of action needs to be as specific as possible and include the who, what, when, where, and how of the learning process. Responsibilities that are clearly stated aid in evaluating the plan and directing plan revisions.

In light of our changing healthcare system, there needs to be an emphasis on patient–nurse partnerships, because patients are expected to take increasingly more responsibility and control in the decisions that affect their own health. Educational contracting is the key to informed decision making.

When education is viewed in the context of the client, rather than the client in the context of education, learning is individualized. The fit between the client as learner and the nurse as educator has the capacity to facilitate learning. Indeed, the goodness of fit between these two educational participants can be a motivating factor. Do the client and educator share an understanding of backgrounds or language? Is there a mutual understanding of goal setting? Are health beliefs respected?

A contract involves a trusting relationship. In a mutually satisfying teacher–learner relationship system, trust is a key ingredient. The learner trusts that the nurse as educator possesses a respectable, current body of theoretically based and clinically applicable knowledge. The nurse needs to be approachable, trustworthy,

and culturally sensitive, because the learner's own health status is often valued as a private matter. In turn, the nurse trusts that when the client enters into an agreement, the learner will demonstrate behaviors that will be health promoting. Newman and Brown (1986) list the following elements as part of the ideal relationship: both parties have trust and respect; the teacher assumes the student can learn and is sensitive to individual needs; and both feel free to learn and make mistakes.

Organizer

Organization of the learning situation, including manipulation of materials and space, sequential organization of content from simple to complex, and determining priority of subject matter, is a task taken on by the nurse as educator. Organization of learning material decreases obstacles to learning. Attendance at educational programs or individual sessions can be organized around the target learner as well as significant others to facilitate the learning process and promote motivation to learn.

Evaluator

Educational programs, like other healthcare projects, need to be accountable to the learner or consumer of the health service. This accountability is ensured by evaluation in the form of outcomes. Self-evaluation, learner evaluation, organization evaluation, and peer evaluation are not new concepts. Evaluative processes are an integral part of all learning.

As early as 1989, Luker and Caress challenged the nurse as educator role. They made a distinction between patient education and patient teaching, noting that the former is in the advanced practice province and that not all nurses are prepared to be patient educators. The difference between the specialist role and the generalist role in education remains largely unsubstantiated by evidence.

In the final analysis, application of knowledge that improves the health of individuals, families, and groups is the evaluative measure of learning.

State of the Evidence

The evidence is less than adequate for implementing nursing interventions that specifically address the variables of compliance and motivation as related to health behaviors of the learner. With the explosion of interest in evidence-based nursing practice, further conceptually based research that identifies, describes, explains, and predicts health behaviors of the learner needs to be conducted.

Healthy People 2010 (United States Department of Health and Human Services, 2000) has established two major goals: (1) to increase the quality and years of healthy life, and (2) to eliminate health disparities among different segments of the population. This document sets the stage for the nurse as educator to use theoretically based strategies to promote desirable health behaviors of the learner.

Carter and Kulbok (2002), in an integrative review of motivational research (conducted using the Cumulative Index of Nursing and Allied Health Literature database) concluded that no clear definition of motivation exists, certain populations have been underrepresented in motivational research, and that motivation may not be able to be effectively measured. They challenge researchers and practitioners to carefully examine the role of motivation in influencing health behaviors. Zinn (2005) argues that there is insufficient data to explain why people take health risks and that more research concerning how an individual's knowledge is shaped and how it impacts health behaviors is needed. A clarion call is needed for both qualitative and quantitative conceptually grounded research to be infused into the teaching–learning process. Forums for evidence-based learning ought to be widely established and should include discussion relative to compliance, motivation, and health behaviors of the learner. In light of the critical nursing workforce shortage and nursing faculty shortage, motivational factors should be a paramount focus of research in nursing education as well as client education.

Summary

Critical components of this chapter have included a discussion of concepts of compliance and motivation, assessment of level of learner motivation, identification of incentives and obstacles that affect motivation and compliance, and discussion of axioms of motivation relevant to learning. An overview of selected health behavior frameworks and their influence on learning have been compared and contrasted. In light of the role of nurse as educator, strategies that facilitate health behaviors of the learner have been outlined, and the need for continued evidence-based practice has been proposed.

When information is imparted, accepted, and applied, the foundation is set for change in health behaviors. When people are motivated and know that they can make a difference in their own lives, then a barrier to health has been lifted.

REVIEW QUESTIONS

1. How are the terms *compliance, adherence,* and *motivation* defined?
2. How do the terms defined in Question 1 relate to one another?
3. What are the three major motivational factors?
4. Which axioms (premises) are involved in promoting motivation of the learner?
5. What are the six parameters for a comprehensive motivational assessment of the learner?
6. What are seven major models or theories used to describe, explain, or predict health behaviors?
7. Which models/theories are used to facilitate motivation, and which ones are used to promote compliance to a therapeutic healthcare regimen?
8. What are the basic concepts particular to each model or theory?
9. What are the similarities and differences among the models with respect to who is the target audience, what is the focus of the learning, and what are the implications for education?
10. What is the role of the nurse in shaping health behaviors of the learner?

References

Ajzen, I., & Fishbein, M. (1980). *Understanding attitudes and predicting social behavior.* Englewood Cliffs, NJ: Prentice-Hall.

Atkinson, J. W. (1964). *An introduction to motivation.* Princeton, NJ: Van Nostrand.

Bandura, A. (1977a). Self-efficacy: Toward a unifying theory of behavioral change. *Psychological Review, 84*(2), 191–215.

Bandura, A. (1977b). *Social learning theory.* Englewood Cliffs, NJ: Prentice-Hall.

Bandura, A. (1986). *Social foundations of thought and action: A social cognitive theory.* Englewood Cliffs, NJ: Prentice-Hall.

Bandura, A. (1997). *Self-efficacy: The exercise of control.* New York: Freeman.

Barofsky, I. (1978). Compliance, adherence and the therapeutic alliance: Steps in the development of self-care. *Social Science and Medicine, 12,* 369–376.

Becker, M. (1990). Theoretical models of adherence and strategies for improving adherence. In S. A. Shumaker, E. B. Schron, & J. K. Ockene (Eds.), *The handbook of human health behavior* (pp. 5–43). New York: Springer.

Becker, M. W., Drachman, R. H., & Kirscht, J. P. (1974). A new approach to explaining sick-role behavior in low-income populations. *American Journal of Public Health, 64*(3), 205–216.

Bruhn, J. G., & Parcel, G. S. (1982). Current knowledge about the health behavior of young children: A conference summary. *Health Education Quarterly, 9,* 142–165.

Buijs, R., Ross-Kerr, J., Cousins, S., & Wilson, D. (2003). Promoting participation: Evaluation of a health promotion program for low income seniors. *Journal of Community Health Nursing, 20*(2), 93–107.

Callaghan, D. (2005). Health behaviors, self-efficacy, self-care and basic conditioning factors in older adults. *Journal of Community Health Nursing, 22*(3), 169–178.

Carter, K. F., & Kulbok, P. A. (2002). Motivation for health behaviours: A systematic review of the nursing literature. *Journal of Advanced Nursing, 40*(3), 316–330.

Charron-Prachnowik, D., Sereika, S., Becker, D., Jacober, S., Mansfield, J., White, N., et al. (2001). Reproductive health beliefs and behaviors in teens with diabetes: Application of the expanded health belief model. *Pediatric Diabetes, 2,* 30–39.

Chiu, H. J. (2005). A test of the Bruhn and Parcel model of health promotion. *The Journal of Nursing Research, 13*(3), 184–196.

Damrosch, S. (1991). General strategies for motivating people to change their behavior. *Nursing Clinics of North America, 26*(4), 833–843.

deTornay, R., & Thompson, M. A. (1987). *Strategies for teaching nursing* (3rd ed.). New York: Wiley.

Duran, L. S. (2003). Motivating health: Strategies for the nurse practitioner. *Journal of the American Academy of Nurse Practitioners, 15*(5), 200–203.

Dutta-Bergman, M. J. (2004). Primary sources of health information: Comparisons in the domain of health attitudes, health cognitions, and health behaviors. *Health Communication, 16*(3), 273–288.

Erlen, J. (2006, Winter). Adherence is a concept. *Pitt Nurse,* 15–17.

Eraker, S. A., Kirscht, J. P., & Becker, M. H. (1984). Understanding and improving patient compliance. *Annals of Internal Medicine, 100,* 258–268.

Fink, D. L. (1976). Tailoring in the consensual regimen. In D. L. Sackett & R. B. Haynes (Eds.), *Compliance with therapeutic regimens.* Baltimore: Johns Hopkins University Press.

Frenn, M., & Malin, S. (2003). Diet and exercise in low income diverse middle school students. *Public Health Nursing, 20*(5), 361–368.

Gance-Cleveland, B. (2005). Motivational interviewing as a strategy to increase families' adherence to treatment regimens. *Journal of Specialists in Pediatric Nursing, 10*(3), 151–155.

Gebhardt, W. A., & Maes, S. (2001). Integrating social-psychological frameworks for health behavior research. *American Journal of Health Behavior, 25*(6), 528–536.

Green, L. W., & Kreuter, M. W. (1999). *Health promotion planning: An educational and ecological approach* (3rd ed.). Mountain View, CA: Mayfield.

Haggard, A. (1989). *Handbook of patient education.* Rockville, MD: Aspen.

Hanson, M. S. (2005). An examination of ethnic differences in cigarette smoking intention among female teenagers. *Journal of the American Academy of Nurse Practitioners, 17*(4), 149–155.

Hjelm, K., Mufunda, E., Nambozi, G., & Kemp, J. (2003). Preparing nurses to face the pandemic of diabetes mellitus: A literature review. *Journal of Advanced Nursing, 41*(5), 424–434.

Hobden, A. (2006). Concordance: A widely used term, but what does it mean? *British Journal of Community Nursing, 11*(6), 257–260.

Hochbaum, G. M. (1980). *Patient counseling vs. patient teaching: Education for self-care.* Rockville, MD: Aspen.

Jachna, C. M., & Forbes-Thompson, S. (2005). Osteoporosis: Health beliefs and barriers to treatment in an assisted living facility. *Journal of Gerontological Nursing, 31*(1), 24–30.

Janz, N. K., & Becker, M. H. (1984). The health belief model: A decade later. *Health Education Quarterly, 11*(1), 1–47.

Kaewthummanukul, T., & Brown, K. C. (2006). Determinants of employee participation in physical activity: A review of the literature. *American Association of Occupational Health Nurses Journal, 54*(6), 249–261.

Keller, J. M. (1987). Development and use of the ARCS model of instructional design. *Journal of Instructional Development, 10*(3), 2–10.

Kelly, C. W. (2005). Commitment to health scale. *Journal of Nursing Measurement, 13*(3), 219–229.

Kessels, R. P. C. (2003). Patients' memory for medical information. *Journal of the Royal Society of Medicine, 96,* 219–222.

Kleier, J. A. (2004). Nurse practitioners' behavior regarding teaching testicular self-examination. *Journal of the American Academy of Nurse Practitioners, 16*(5), 206–208, 210, 212.

Kort, M. (1987). Motivation: The challenge for today's health promoter. *Canadian Nurse, 83*(9), 16–18.

Langlie, J. K. (1977). Social networks, health beliefs, and preventive health behavior. *Journal of Health and Social Behavior, 18,* 244–260.

Levanthal, H. C., & Cameron, L. (1987). Behavior theories and the problem of compliance. *Patient Education Counseling, 10,* 117–138.

Levanthal, H. C., & Diefenbach, M. (1991). The active side of illness cognition. In J. A. Skelton & R. T. Croyle (Eds.), *Mental representation in health and illness.* New York: Springer-Verlag, 245–271.

Lewin, K. (1935). *A dynamic theory of personality.* New York: McGraw-Hill.

Ley, P. (1979). Memory for medical information. *British Journal of Social and Clinical Psychology, 18,* 245–255.

Luker, K., & Caress, A. L. (1989). Rethinking patient education. *Journal of Advanced Nursing, 14,* 711–718.

Maslow, A. H. (1943). A theory of human motivation. *Psychological Review, 50*(4), 371–396.

McGahee, T. W., Kemp, V., & Tingen, M. (2000). A theoretical model for smoking prevention studies in preteen children. *Pediatric Nursing, 26*(2), 135–138, 141.

Mishel, M. H. (1990). Reconceptualization of the uncertainty in illness theory. *Image: Journal of Nursing Scholarship, 22*(4), 256–262.

Narsavage, G. (2003). Smoking cessation interventions for hospitalized patients with cardiopulmonary disorders. *Online Journal of Issues in Nursing, 8*(2), 16. http://www.nursingworld.org./ojin.

Newman, F., & Brown, R. (1986). Creating optimal conditions for learning. *Educational Horizons, 64*(4), 188–189.

Paul, S., & Sneed, N. V. (2004). Strategies for behavior change in patients with heart failure. *American Journal of Critical Care, 13*(4), 305–313.

Pender, N. (1987). *Health promotion in nursing practice* (2nd ed.). Norwalk, CT: Appleton-Lange.

Pender, N. (1996). *Health promotion in nursing practice* (3rd ed.). Upper Saddle River, NJ: Pearson Education.

Pender, N. J., Murdaugh, C. L., & Parsons, M. A. (2002). *Health promotion in nursing practice* (4th ed.). Upper Saddle River, NJ: Prentice Hall.

Peplau, H. E. (1979). *The psychotherapy of Hildegard E. Peplau.* Madison, WI: Atwood.

Poss, J. E. (2001). Developing a new model for cross-cultural research: Synthesizing the health belief model and the theory of reasoned action. *Advances in Nursing Science, 23*(4), 1–15.

Prentice-Dunn, S., & Rogers, W. R. (1986). Protection motivation theory and preventive health: Beyond the health belief model. *Health Education Research, 3,* 153–161.

Prochaska, J. O. (1996, September). Just do it isn't enough: Change comes in stages. *Tufts University Special Report Diet and Nutrition Letter.*

Prochaska, J. O., & Di Clemente, C. C. (1982). Transtheoretical therapy: Towards a more integrative model of change. *Psychotherapy, Theory, and Practice, 19*(3), 276–288.

Redman, B. K. (2001). *The practice of patient education* (9th ed.). St. Louis, MO: Mosby.

Redman, B. K. (2007). *The practice of patient education: A case study approach* (10th ed.). St. Louis, MO: Mosby.

Rollnick, S., Mason, P., & Butler, C. (1999). *Health behavior change: A guide for practitioners.* London: Churchill Livingstone.

Rosenstock, I. M. (1974). Historical origins of the health belief model. In M. H. Becker (Ed.), *The health belief model and personal health behavior.* Thorofare, NJ: Slack.

Rothman, N. L., Lourie, R. J., Brian, D., & Foley, M. (2005). Temple health connection: A successful collaborative model of community-based primary health care. *Journal of Cultural Diversity, 12*(4), 145–151.

Rotter, J. B. (1954). *Social learning theory and clinical psychology.* Englewood Cliffs, NJ: Prentice-Hall.

Russell, S., Daly, J., Hughes, E., & op't Hoog, C. (2003). Nurses and "difficult" patients: Negotiating noncompliance. *Journal of Advanced Nursing, 43*(3), 281–287.

Ryan, R. M., & Deci, E. L. (2000). Intrinsic and extrinsic motivations: Classic definitions and new directions. *Contemporary Educational Psychology, 25,* 54–67.

Shapiro, D. E., Boggs, S. R., Melamed, B. G., & Graham-Pole, J. (1992). The effect of varied physician affect on recall, anxiety, and perceptions in women at risk for breast cancer: An analogue study. *Health Psychology, 11*(1), 61–66.

Shillinger, F. (1983). Locus of control: Implications for nursing practice. *Image: Journal of Nursing Scholarship, 15*(2), 58–63.

Steckel, S. B. (1982). Predicting, measuring, implementing and following up on patient compliance. *Nursing Clinics of North America, 17*(3), 491–497.

Stephenson, P. L. (2006). Before the teaching begins: Managing patient anxiety prior to providing education. *Clinical Journal of Oncology Nursing, 10*(2), 241–245.

United States Department of Health and Human Services. (2000). *Healthy People 2010* (Conference edition). Washington, DC: U.S. Government Printing Office.

Wallston, K. A., Wallston, B. S., & DeVellis, R. (1978, Spring). Development of the multidimensional health locus of control (MHLC) scales. *Health Education Monographs,* 160–170.

Ward-Collins, D. (1998). Noncompliant: Isn't there a better way to say it? *American Journal of Nursing, 98*(5), 17–31.

Wilkes, L., Cooper, K., Lewin, J., & Batts, J. (1999).
Concept mapping: Promoting science learning in
BN learners in Australia. *Journal of Continuing
Education in Nursing, 30*(1), 37–44.

Wright, L. M., Watson, W. L., & Bell, J. M. (1996).
Beliefs: The heart of healing in families and illness.
New York: Basic Books.

Wu, Y., Stanton, B. F., Li, X., Galbraith, J., & Cole,
M. L. (2005). Protection motivation theory and
adolescent drug trafficking: Relationship between
health motivation and longitudinal risk involvement. *Journal of Pediatric Psychology, 30*(2),
127–137.

Zimmerman, G. L., Olsen, C. G., & Bosworth, M. F.
(2000). A stages of change approach to helping
patients change behavior. *American Family
Physician, 61*(5), 1409–1416.

Zinn, J. O. (2005). The biographical approach: A better
way to understand behaviour in health and illness.
Health, Risk, and Society, 7(1), 1–9.

Chapter 7

Literacy in the Adult Client Population

Susan B. Bastable

CHAPTER HIGHLIGHTS

KEY TERMS

- ❑ literacy
- ❑ literate
- ❑ illiterate
- ❑ low literacy
- ❑ functional illiteracy

- ❑ health literacy
- ❑ reading
- ❑ readability
- ❑ comprehension
- ❑ numeracy

OBJECTIVES

After completing this chapter, the reader will be able to

1. Define the terms *literacy, illiteracy, health literacy, low literacy, functional illiteracy, reading, readability, comprehension,* and *numeracy.*
2. Identify the magnitude of the literacy problem in the United States.
3. Describe the characteristics of those individuals at risk for having difficulty with reading and comprehension of written and oral language.
4. Discuss common myths and assumptions about people with illiteracy.
5. Identify clues that are indicators of reading and writing deficiencies.
6. Assess the impact of illiteracy and low literacy on client motivation and compliance with healthcare regimens.
7. Recognize the role of the nurse as educator in the assessment of clients' literacy skills.
8. Critically analyze the readability and comprehension levels of printed materials and the reading skills of clients using specific formulas and tests.
9. Describe specific guidelines for writing effective education materials.
10. Outline various teaching strategies useful in educating clients with low literacy skills.
11. Recognize the research and policy-making issues that must be addressed to solve the health literacy problem.

Over the past 2 decades, literacy in the U.S. population has been the subject of increasing interest and concern by educators as well as by government officials, employers, and media experts. Adult illiteracy continues to be a major problem in this country despite public and private efforts at all levels to address the issue through testing of literacy skills and development of literacy training programs.

Today, the fact remains that many individuals do not possess the basic literacy abilities to function effectively in our technologically complex society. Many adult citizens have difficulty reading and comprehending information well enough to be able to perform such common tasks as filling out job and insurance applications, interpreting bus schedules and road signs, completing tax forms, applying for a driver's license, registering to vote, or ordering from a restaurant menu (Weiss, 2003).

In the early 1980s, President Reagan launched the National Adult Literacy Initiative, which was followed by the United Nations' declaration of 1990 as the International Literacy Year (Belton, 1991; Wallerstein, 1992). In 1992, the National Adult Literacy Survey (NALS) was conducted by the U.S. Department of Education. The results of this survey revealed a shockingly high prevalence of illiteracy in this country (Weiss, 2003; Weiss et al., 2005; Zarcadoolas, Pleasant, & Greer, 2006). Since then, awareness about illiteracy, thought previously to be a problem mainly confined to developing countries, has taken on new meaning (Lasater & Mehler, 1998; Schwartzberg, VanGeest, & Wang, 2004).

However, in light of the relatively recent attention given to this problem in the last twenty years, it must be acknowledged that Literacy Volunteers of America, Inc. and Lauback Literacy International have for many decades served as advocates for the most marginalized adult population in this country and around the globe. Today, ProLiteracy Worldwide, recently formed from the merger of these two entities, is the world's largest organization for adult literacy. It operates 1,200 literacy programs across the United States and partners with 120 other organizations in 62 countries worldwide. Syracuse, New York, has been the birthplace of all three of these organizations and central New York is now recognized as the capital of the literacy movement. America's literacy problem has become a national crisis because for too long this country has ignored those who are unseen and unheard (Wedgeworth, 2007).

Particularly in the past 10 years as a result of the NALS report, nursing and medical literature has focused significant attention on the effects of patient illiteracy on healthcare delivery and health outcomes. Today, the emphasis is on health literacy—that is, the extent to which Americans can read and comprehend health information well enough to function successfully in a healthcare environment and make appropriate decisions for themselves. Although a great deal more research needs to be done on the causes and effects associated with poor health literacy as well as the methods available to screen and teach patients, much has been learned about the magnitude and consequences of the health literacy problem (Gazmararian, Curran, Parker, Bernhardt, & DeBuono, 2005; Pignone, DeWalt, Sheridan, Berkman, & Lohr, 2005).

With respect to the subject of literacy, the nurse educator's attention specifically focuses on adult client populations. Literacy levels are not an issue in teaching staff nurses or nursing students because of their level of formal education. However, literacy levels remain a concern if the audience for in-service programs includes less educated, more culturally and socioeconomically diverse support staff (Hess, 1998), or if a member of the audience has been diagnosed with a learning disability, such as dyslexia.

What must be of particular concern to the healthcare industry are the numbers of consumers who are illiterate, functionally illiterate, or marginally literate. Researchers have discovered that people with poor reading and comprehension skills have disproportionately higher medical costs, increased number of hospitalizations and readmissions, and more perceived physical and psychosocial problems than do literate persons (Baker, Parker, Williams, & Clark, 1998; Baker, Williams, Parker, Gazmararian, & Nurss, 1999; Weiss, 2003; Weiss et al., 2005).

In today's world of managed care, the literacy problem is perceived to have grave consequences.

Clients are expected to assume greater responsibility for self-care and health promotion, yet this expanded role depends on increased knowledge and skills. If people with low literacy abilities cannot fully benefit from the type and amount of information they are typically given, then they cannot be expected to maintain health and manage independently. The result is a significant negative impact on the cost of health care and the quality of life (Kogut, 2004; Pignone et al., 2005; Williams, Davis, Parker, & Weiss, 2002; Wood, Kettinger, & Lessick, 2007).

Traditionally, healthcare professionals have relied heavily on printed education materials as a cost-effective and time-efficient means to communicate health messages. For years, nurses and physicians have assumed that the written materials commonly distributed to clients were sufficient to ensure informed consent for tests and procedures, to promote compliance with treatment regimens, and to guarantee adherence to discharge instructions.

Only recently have healthcare providers begun to recognize that the scientific and technical terminology inherent in the ubiquitous printed teaching aids is a bewildering set of written instructions little understood by the majority of people. Kessels (2003) pointed out that 40–80% of medical information provided by health professionals is forgotten immediately, not only because medical terminology is too difficult to understand, but too much information leads to poor recall. He also noted that half of the information remembered is incorrect. Unless education materials are written at a level and style appropriate for their intended audiences, clients cannot be expected to be able or willing to accept responsibility for self-care.

An essential prerequisite for implementing health education programs is to know the literacy skills of audiences for whom these programs are intended (Quirk, 2000). Yet calls for assessment of literacy and recommendations for appropriate interventions for clients with poor literacy skills have largely been ignored. Even though illiteracy and low literacy are quite prevalent in the U.S. population, problems with literacy frequently continue to go undiagnosed (Doak, Doak, & Root, 1996; Zarcadoolas et al., 2006).

This chapter examines the magnitude of the literacy problem, the myths associated with it, the factors that influence literacy levels, the important role nurses play in assessing clients' literacy skills, and the effects of illiteracy on the health and well-being of the public. In addition, the formulas and tests used to evaluate readability of printed tools and to assess clients' comprehension and reading skills are reviewed, specific guidelines are put forth for writing effective health education materials, and teaching strategies are recommended as a means for breaking down the barriers of illiteracy.

Definition of Terms

For many years, there was no clear agreement of what it has meant to be literate in our society. A literate person was loosely described as someone who possessed socially required and expected reading and writing abilities, such as being able to sign his or her name and read and write a simple sentence. Over time, performance on reading tests in school became the conventional method to measure grade-level achievement.

However, because it is difficult, if not impossible, to measure reading abilities on a population-wide basis, the U.S. Bureau of the Census still continues to this day to use the number of years of schooling attended to define literacy levels (Giorgianni, 1998). This remains, though, an imprecise estimation of someone's true reading skills. Many researchers have found that the reported grade level achieved in school is an inadequate predictor of reading ability (Chew, Bradley, & Boyko, 2004; Doak et al., 1996; Weiss, 2003; Winslow, 2001).

In the United States, the term literacy is generally defined as the ability to read and speak English (Andrus & Roth, 2002). In the 1992 National Adult Literacy Survey (NALS), the U.S. Department of Education (1993) defined *literacy* as "the ability to use printed and written information to function in society, to achieve one's goals, and to develop one's knowledge and potential" (p. 6).

NALS categorized literacy into three general kinds of tasks (U.S. Department of Education, 1993):

- Prose tasks, which measure reading comprehension and the ability to extract themes from newspapers, magazines, poems, and books
- Document tasks, which assess the ability of readers to interpret documents such as insurance reports, consent forms, and transportation schedules
- Quantitative tasks, which assess the ability to work with numerical information embedded in written material such as computing restaurant menu bills, figuring out taxes, interpreting paycheck stubs, or calculating calories on a nutrition checklist

Although no precise cut-off point defines the difference between literacy and illiteracy, the commonly accepted working definition of what is meant to be *literate* is the ability to write and to read, understand, and interpret information written at the eighth-grade level or above. On the other end of the continuum, *illiterate* is defined as someone who is unable to read or write at all or whose reading and writing skills are at the fourth-grade level or below.

Low literacy, also termed marginally literate or marginally illiterate, refers to the ability of adults to read, write, and comprehend information between the fifth- and eighth-grade level of difficulty. Persons with low literacy have trouble using commonly printed and written information to meet their everyday needs such as reading a TV schedule, taking a telephone message, or filling out a relatively simple application form (Doak et al., 1996).

Functional illiteracy means that adults lack the fundamental reading, writing, and comprehension skills that are needed to operate effectively in today's society. Functional illiteracy is a relatively new term. People who are functionally illiterate have very limited competency to perform the tasks of everyday life (Giorgianni, 1998). They do not read well enough to understand and interpret what they have read or use the information as it was intended (Doak et al., 1996). For example, someone who is functionally illiterate may be able to read the simple words on a label of a can of soup that directs them to "Pour soup into pan. Add one can water. Heat until hot." However, they cannot comprehend the meaning and sequence of the words to carry through with these directions.

These operational definitions are, at best, approximations. Conventional grade-level definitions of literacy are considered conservative because even an adult with the ability to read at the eighth-grade level will encounter difficulties in functioning in our advanced society. However, although an individual may have poor reading skills, this does not necessarily imply a lack of intelligence. Low literacy or illiteracy cannot be equated with IQ level. A person can be illiterate or low literate, yet intellectually be within at least normal IQ range (Doak et al., 1996).

Health literacy refers to how well an individual can read, interpret, and comprehend health information for maintaining an optimal level of wellness. The Ad Hoc Committee on Health Literacy for the Council on Scientific Affairs of the American Medical Association (1999) defined health literacy as "a constellation of skills, including the ability to perform basic reading and numerical tasks required to function in the health care environment" (p. 553). This committee identified the scope and consequences of poor health literacy in the United States. They concluded that an individual's functional health literacy is likely to be significantly worse than his or her general literacy skills because of the complicated language (medicalese) used in the healthcare field.

The U.S. Department of Health and Human Services (2000) more explicitly defined health literacy as "the degree to which individuals have the capacity to obtain, process, and understand basic health information and services needed to make appropriate health decisions." Health literacy potentially enables individuals to make informed choices, reduce their health risks, and increase their quality of life (Wood et al., 2007). The 2003 National Assessment of Adult Literacy (NAAL), which was a 10-year follow-up to the original NALS study, was the first national assessment designed specifically to measure the literacy skills of adults in understanding health-related information (National Center for Education Statistics, 2006).

With managed care requiring individuals to take more responsibility for self-care and symptom management, health literacy is becoming an important determinant of health status. Poor health literacy may lead to serious negative consequences, such as increased morbidity and mortality, when a person is unable to read and comprehend instructions for medications, follow-up appointments, diet, procedures, and other regimens. Patients cannot be expected to be compliant, autonomous, and self-directed in navigating the healthcare system if they do not have the ability to follow basic instructions (Fetter, 1999; Williams, Baker, Honig, Lee, & Nowlan, 1998). Health knowledge, health status, and the use of health services are all related to health literacy levels.

Reading, readability, and comprehension also are terms frequently used when determining levels of literacy. Fisher (1999) defines *reading* or word recognition as "the process of transforming letters into words and being able to pronounce them correctly" (p. 57). Word recognition test scores, which can be misleading because they only indicate a person's ability to identify words, not understand them, are usually three grade levels higher than comprehension scores (Fisher, 1999). Hirsch (2001) addressed the public's confusion between reading in the sense of being able to decode words fluently and reading in the sense of being able to comprehend the meaning of words.

Readability is defined as the ease with which written or printed information can be read. It is based on a measure of a number of different elements within a given text of printed material that influence with what degree of success a group of readers will be able to read the style of writing of a selected printed passage (Fisher, 1999).

Comprehension, on the other hand, is the degree to which individuals understand what they have read (Fisher, 1999; Koo, Krass, & Aslani, 2005). It is the ability to grasp the meaning of a message—to get the gist of it. A healthcare professional can determine whether comprehension of health instruction has occurred by noting whether clients are able to correctly demonstrate or recall in their own words the message that was received.

The ability to read does not alone guarantee reading comprehension. Comprehension is affected by the amount, clarity, and complexity of the information presented. If the elements of logic, language, and experience in health instruction are compatible with and culturally appropriate to the clients' background, the message likely will be clear and relevant to them (Doak et al., 1996). A mismatch will likely make the message confusing, incomprehensible, and useless to the individual.

Also, illness or other disruptive life situations, which cause stress and anxiety, have been found to significantly interfere with comprehension. The ability to take in medical information, store it in memory, and recall it when necessary is affected by many other factors as well, such as the length of time between information disclosure and the need to remember the information, the nature of the information (how threatening), and the method of presentation (Doak et al., 1996; Doak, Doak, Friedell, & Meade, 1998; Kessels, 2003; Ley, 1979).

Readability and comprehension, therefore, are particularly complex activities involving many variables with respect to both the reader and the actual written material (Doak et al., 1996; Fisher, 1999). Both are commonly determined by using one or more measurement formulas (see the later discussions of measurement tools in this chapter). **Table 7–1** shows examples of elements that affect readability and comprehension.

Another term used when discussing literacy is *numeracy*, which is the ability to read and interpret numbers. Overwhelmingly, those with limited literacy also have limited skills in numeracy (Andrus & Roth, 2002; Doak et al., 1996; Fisher, 1999; Williams et al., 1995).

Literacy Relative to Oral Instruction

To date, very little attention has been paid to the role of oral communication in the assessment of illiteracy. Certainly, inability to comprehend the spoken word or oral instruction above the level

Table 7–1 Examples of Elements that Affect Readability and Comprehension

Material Variables	Reader Variables
Legibility (e.g., print size, spacing)	Health status
Organization and flow of content	Perceived threat of illness
Concept level	Effects of illness/stress
Length of text	Physical and mental energy
Sentence structure	Level of motivation
Level of vocabulary	Visual and auditory acuity
Relevance to the reader	Educational attainment
Jargon (medical terminology)	Background knowledge
Number of polysyllabic words	Ability to decipher language of message

of understanding simple words, phrases, and slang words should be considered an important element in the definition or assessment of literacy. Kessels (2003) pointed out that although most health information is spoken, oral instruction alone is not a very successful method of teaching. "Written information is better remembered and leads to better treatment adherence" (p. 221).

Doak, Doak, and Root (1985) addressed the fact that there is no universally accepted way to test the degree of difficulty with oral language. However, as these authors observed, "it is believed that some of the same characteristics that are critical for written materials will also affect the comprehensibility of spoken language" (p. 40). Much more research needs to be done on "iloralacy," or the inability to understand simple oral language, as a generic concept of illiteracy (Hirsch, 2001; Zarcadoolas et al., 2006).

Literacy Relative to Computer Instruction

The literacy issue has always been examined from the standpoint of readability and comprehension of printed materials. However, computer literacy is an increasingly popular concern as an important dimension of the literacy issue. More and more, educators and consumers are relying on computers as educational tools and the potential of this technology is transforming the way healthcare information is accessed and shared. Those clients who are well educated and career oriented are already likely to own a computer and be computer literate, but those with limited resources, literacy skills, and technological know-how are being left behind (Zarcadoolas et al., 2006).

As healthcare organizations and agencies continue to invest more resources in computer tech-

nology and software programs for educational purposes, computer literacy in the overall client population must be addressed. Computers not only are used to convey instructional messages, but also serve as a valuable tool for access to a wide array of additional sources of information (see Chapters 12 and 13).

The opportunity to expand clients' knowledge base through telecommunications requires nurse educators to attend to computer literacy levels of their audiences. In the same way that they now recognize the negative effects that illiteracy and low literacy have had in restricting the information base of consumers of health care when printed materials are relied upon, nurses must begin to advocate for computer literacy in the public they serve (Doak et al., 1996). Computer software programs can be made suitable for use by low-literate learners as long as these individuals have the basic capacity to access and operate computers, and if the information is simplified for readability and comprehension.

Scope and Incidence of the Problem

Literacy has been termed the "silent epidemic," the "silent barrier," the "silent disability," and "the dirty little secret" (Conlin & Schumann, 2002; Doak & Doak, 1987; Kefalides, 1999; Wedgeworth, 2007). Based on available statistics over the past 20 years, it is evident that the United States has significant literacy problems. In fact, this country only ranked among the middle of industrialized nations on most measures of adult literacy, and yet many of our educators, elected representatives, and social advocates have remained blind to this significant problem (Kogut, 2004).

The first national assessment of adult literacy, known as the Young Adult Literacy Survey, was undertaken in 1985 by the U.S. Department of Education. Since then, two subsequent large-scale assessments have been conducted by the federal government (U.S. Department of Health and Human Services, 2003).

The 1992 National Adult Literacy Survey (NALS), considered to be a highly accurate and detailed profile on the condition of English language literacy in the United States, revealed surprising statistics. NALS interviewed and collected data from a representative sample of 26,000 individuals, aged 16 years and older. Based on the findings from an assessment of literacy skills in three areas (prose, document, and quantitative), literacy abilities were categorized into five levels, with Level 1 being the lowest and Level 5 being the highest.

About 21–23%, or approximately 40–44 million of the 191 million adults in the country at that time, scored in the lowest level of the three skill areas. They were considered to be functionally illiterate. Another 25–28%, or approximately 50 million adults, scored in the Level 2 category. That is, they were considered to have low literacy skills. Thus, the number of illiterate and low-literate adults in the United States conservatively was estimated to be approximately 90–94 million in total (**Figure 7–1**).

This figure represented about one half of the adult population in this country who had deficiencies in reading, writing, and math skills (Fisher, 1999; Weiss, 2003). The researchers

Figure 7–1 Literacy levels in U.S. adults.

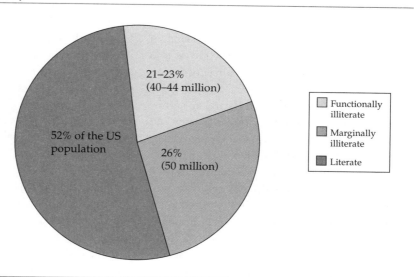

21–23%
(40–44 million)

52% of the US population

26%
(50 million)

Functionally illiterate

Marginally illiterate

Literate

Source: Bastable, L. C., Chojnowski, D., Goldberg, L., McGurl, P., & Riegel, B. (2005). Comparing heart failure patient literacy levels with available educational materials. Poster presented at the Heart Failure Society of America, 9th Annual Scientific Conference, September 18–21, 2005, Boca Raton, FL.

found that those individuals with poor literacy skills (Levels 1 and 2) were disproportionately more often from minority populations, from lower socioeconomic groups, and had poorer health status (Fisher, 1999; Andrus & Roth, 2002; Weiss, 2003).

In 2003, building on the NALS of 10 years earlier, the NAAL (National Assessment of Adult Literacy) was the first study to identify the literacy of America's adults in the 21st century. New, more sensitive instruments were designed to enhance measurement of the literacy abilities of the least-literate adults. Most importantly, it included a health literacy component to assess adults' understanding of health-related materials and forms (National Center for Education Statistics, 2006).

The NAAL categorized literacy skills into four levels, and the findings revealed the following percentages and total numbers: below basic (14% or 30 million), basic (29% or 63 million), intermediate (44% or 95 million), and proficient (13% or 28 million). Of the overall 216 million adults in the U.S. population in 2003, 43% (93 million) fell into the lowest two categories (National Center for Education Statistics, 2006).

The average score results indicated no significant change in prose and document literacy and only a slight increase in quantitative literacy between 1992 and 2003. However, a higher proportionate percentage of several population groups, such as those who did not graduate from high school, Hispanics, and those over 65 years of age, fell into the below basic level of prose literacy (Kutner, Greenberg, Jin, & Paulsen, 2006). The NAAL's *Health Literacy Report* specifically found that 36% (47 million) of adults had basic or below basic health literacy and older adults (65 years and older) had the lowest health literacy levels (National Center for Education Statistics, 2006). For more detailed information on the NAAL survey, visit the National Center for Education Statistics at http://www.nces.ed .gov/NAAL.

In addition to the NAAL survey, in 2004, the Institute of Medicine (IOM), the Agency for Healthcare Research and Quality (AHRQ), and the American Medical Association (AMA) issued their own reports on the status of health literacy in this country. All three reports revealed that as many as 50% of all American adults lack the basic reading and numerical skills essential to function adequately in the healthcare environment (Aldridge, 2004; Institute of Medicine, 2004; Schwartzberg et al., 2004; Weiss et al., 2005). For more information on health literacy, see **Table 7–2** for Web sites.

Limited literacy leads to poor health outcomes. In fact, literacy skills are "a stronger predictor of an individual's health status than age, income, employment status, education level, and racial or ethnic group" (Weiss, 2003, p. 11). Individuals with limited literacy skills are less knowledgeable about their health problems, have higher hospitalization rates, higher healthcare costs, and poorer health status (Weiss et al., 2005). To obtain a CD with video entitled *Health Literacy: A Prescription to End Confusion,* go to The National Academies Press at http://www.nap.edu. Also see **Table 7–3** for a list of additional audiovisuals on health literacy.

Thus, according to the findings of NALS and NAAL reports, about 4 to 5 out of every 10 Americans lack the basic reading and comprehension skills to perform simple, everyday literacy tasks (U.S. Department of Education, 1993; National Center for Education Statistics, 2006). Because the mean reading level of the U.S. population is at or below the eighth grade

---

Table 7–2 HEALTH LITERACY WEB SITES

The National Center for the Study of Adult Learning and Literacy (NCSALL): http://www.ncsall.net

Harvard School of Public Health, Health Literacy Studies: http://www.hsph.harvard.edu/healthliteracy

The National Library of Medicine, Current Bibliographies in Medicine 2000–2001, Health Literacy:
 http://www.nlm.nih.gov/archive//20061214/pubs/cbm/hliteracy.html

American Medical Association, Health Literacy: http://www.ama-assn.org

National Health Council, Health Literacy Initiatives:
 http://www.nhcouncil.org/initiatives/health_literacy.htm

National Institute for Literacy: http://www.nifl.gov

Maine AHEC Health Literacy Center: http://www.une/com/ahec

World Education: http://www.worlded.org

Health Literacy Consulting: http://www.healthliteracy.com

Healthy People 2010: http://www.health.gov/healthypeople

System for Adult Basic Education Support (SABES): http://www.sabes.org

Pfizer Health Literacy: http://www.pfizerhealthliteracy.com

Center for Health Care Strategies, Inc.: http://www.chcs.org

Health Literacy Resources: http://www.mlanet.org

HHS/Office of Minority Health Resource Center: http://www.omhrc.gov

National Center for Education: http://nces.ed.gov/naal

ProLiteracy Worldwide: http://www.proliteracy.org/downloads/proliteracystateofliteracy.pdf

America's Literacy Directory: http://www.literacydirectory.org

National Center for Family Literacy: http://www.famlit.org

---

and many people read two to four grades below their reported level of formal education achieved, millions are challenged by the demands of common, day-to-day activities (Winslow, 2001). For example, one needs to be able to read at the sixth-grade level to understand a driver's license manual, at the eighth-grade level to follow directions on a frozen dinner package, and at the tenth-grade level to read instructions on a bottle of aspirin (Doak et al., 1985). The literacy problem is so widespread that the government, in an effort to reduce traffic accidents, has replaced some conventional printed road signs with road signs using symbols (Loughrey, 1983).

Because of the difficulty inherent in defining and testing literacy, the lack of inclusion of unidentified illegal immigrants in the sample populations studied, and the fact that few people with limited reading skills admit to having any difficulty, the scope of the literacy problem is thought to be much greater than the estimates found in formal studies (Brownson, 1998; Doak et al., 1996; Weiss, 2003).

Table 7–3 HEALTH LITERACY AUDIOVISUALS

Health Literacy: A Prescription to End Confusion. (2004). CD-ROM. Institute of Medicine (IOM) of The National Academies. Includes an executive summary of the report *Health Literacy* and video clips of patients discussing their health literacy experiences. Requires a Windows Media Player, Adobe Acrobat Reader, and a Web browser. For more information contact ORAC@NAS.edu.

Providing Patient Education to Meet JCAHO Standards. (2003). DVD. MedCom, Cypress, California (23 minutes in length).

Patient Education Takes Center Stage. (1999). VHS tape. *Creative Health Care Management.* Underscores the value of helping patients and families learn. Expands perspectives on patient education as the central aspect of health care by providing a real-life example of a person with a kidney transplant (28 minutes in length).

Low Health Literacy: You Can't Tell by Looking. (2000). VHS tape. American Medical Association, Chicago. Case studies of four patients with low health literacy (20 minutes in length).

Teaching Patients With Low Literacy Skills. (2001). VHS tape. Concept Media, Inc. Irvine, California ISBN 1564376524 (26 minutes in length).

Reading Between the Lines. (2003). VHS tape. Medical Library Association. Chicago. Concepts of health information literacy to enhance knowledge of information professionals in the provision of quality consumer health with patient education information services.

Overcoming Patient Language Barriers: Caring for Patients With Limited English Proficiency. (2001). VHS tape. Concept Media. ISBN 156437653-2 (25 minutes in length).

Health Literacy: Help Your Patients Understand. (2003). VHS tape. American Medical Association. Chicago (20 minutes in length).

The rates of illiteracy and low literacy in general and health literacy in particular continue to pose a major threat to many segments of our society. The problem is expected to grow worse in light of the many forces operating in our country and worldwide unless specific measures are taken to curb the tide. To be literate 100 years ago meant that people could read and write their own name. Today, being literate means that one is able to learn new skills, think critically, problem solve, and apply general knowledge to various situations (Weiss, 2003).

Trends Associated with Literacy Problems

The trend toward an increased proportion of Americans with literacy levels that are inadequate for active participation in our advanced society is due to such factors as the following (Gazmararian et al., 1999; Giorgianni, 1998; Hayes, 2000; Hirsch, 2001; Kogut, 2004; Weiss, 2003):

- A rise in the number of immigrants
- The aging of the population

- The increasing amount and complexity of information
- The increasing sophistication of technology
- More people living in poverty
- Changes in policies and funding for public education
- Disparities between minority versus nonminority populations

All of these factors correlate significantly with the level of formal schooling attained and the level of literacy ability. Although research indicates the number of years of schooling is not a good predictor of literacy level, there remains a correlation between someone's educational background and the ability to read. As our society becomes more and more high tech, with new products and more complicated functions to perform, the basic language requirements needed for survival will continue to rise. Many more people are beginning to fall behind, unable to keep up with our increasingly sophisticated world.

In cases of both illiteracy and low literacy, the level of readability is measured in terms of performance, not years of school attendance. The mean literacy level of the U.S. population is at or below eighth grade. Medicaid enrollees, on average, read at the fifth-grade level (Andrus & Roth, 2002; Giorgianni, 1998; Winslow, 2001). Many people read at least two to four grade levels below their reported level of formal education. For those in poverty, the gap between grade level completed and actual reading level was even greater (Andrus & Roth, 2002). This deficiency persists because schools have a tendency to promote students for social and age-related reasons rather than for academic achievement alone (Feldman, 1997), because clients may report inaccurate histories of years

of school attended, and because reading skills may be lost over time through lack of practice (Davidhizar & Brownson, 1999; Miller & Bodie, 1994; Weiss, 2003; Williams et al., 2002).

Levels of literacy are often seen as indicators of the well-being of individuals, and the literacy problem has greater implications for the social and economic status of the country as a whole (Kogut, 2004). Low levels of literacy have been associated with marginal productivity, high unemployment, minimum earnings, high costs of health care, and high rates of welfare dependency (Andrus & Roth, 2002; Giorgianni, 1998; Winslow, 2001; Ziegler, 1998).

Also, illiteracy is considered to be an element that is contributing to many of the grave social issues confronting the United States today, such as homelessness, teen pregnancy, unemployment, delinquency, crime, and drug abuse (Fleener & Scholl, 1992; Kogut, 2004). Deficiencies in basic literacy skills compound to create devastating cumulative effects on individuals, which creates a social burden that is extremely costly for the American people. Illiteracy and low literacy are not necessarily the reasons for these ills, but the high correlation between literacy levels and social problems is a marker for disconnectedness from society in general (Kogut, 2004; U.S. Department of Health and Human Services, 2003).

Those at Risk

Illiteracy has been portrayed "as an invisible handicap that affects all classes, ethnic groups, and ages" (Fleener & Scholl, 1992, p. 740). It is a silent disability. Illiteracy knows no boundaries and exists among persons of every race and ethnic background, socioeconomic class, and age category (Duffy & Snyder, 1999; Weiss, 2003).

It is true, however, that illiteracy is rare in the higher socioeconomic classes, for example, and that certain segments of the U.S. population are more likely to be affected than others by lack of literacy skills.

According to Cole (2000); Winslow (2001); Hayes (2000); Wood (2005); Kogut (2004); Schultz (2002); Nath, Sylvester, Yasek, and Gunel (2001); Schillinger et al. (2002); Montalto and Spiegler (2001); Williams, Baker, Parker, and Nurss (1998); and Rothman et al. (2004), populations that have been identified as having poorer reading and comprehension skills than the average American include the following:

- The economically disadvantaged
- Older adults
- Immigrants (particularly illegal ones)
- Racial minorities
- High school dropouts
- The unemployed
- Prisoners
- Inner-city and rural residents
- Those with poor health status due to chronic mental and physical problems

With respect to demographics, statistics indicate that 34 million Americans are presently living in poverty and that nearly half (43%) of all adults with low literacy live in poverty (Darling, 2004). Although the disadvantaged represent many diverse cultural and ethnic groups, including millions of poor White people, one third of the disadvantaged in this country are minorities, and a larger percentage of minorities fall into the disadvantaged category (Giorgianni, 1998; Weiss et al., 2005).

In this 21st century, the major growth in the population will come from the ranks of minority groups. By 2010, one out of every three people in the United States is projected to belong to a racial or ethnic minority (Robinson, 2000); in 53 of the 100 largest cities, minorities will be in the majority. In 2000, the U.S. Bureau of the Census reported that approximately 31 million immigrants reside in this country, more than triple the number in 1970. One third of the foreign-born population has arrived since 1990, one in five children is from an immigrant family, and 30% of immigrants do not have a high school diploma (3.5 times the rate for native Americans). Of the 1,200 community-based adult literacy programs run by ProLiteracy of America, 90% are teaching English as a second language (ESL) (Kogut, 2004). Nurse educators must recognize how these demographic changes will affect the way in which services need to be rendered, educational materials need to be developed, and information needs to be marketed (Andrus & Roth, 2002; Borrayo, 2004; Nurss et al., 1997; Robinson, 2000).

Many minority and economically disadvantaged people, as well as the prison population—which has the highest concentration of adult illiteracy (Duffy & Snyder, 1999)—are not benefactors of mainstream health education activities, which often fail to reach them. Overall, they are not active seekers of health information because they tend to have weaker communication skills and inadequate foundational knowledge on which to better understand their needs. Many lack enough fluency to make good use of written health education materials. Also, not only are the majority of printed education materials written in English, but fluency in verbal skills in another language does not guarantee functional literacy in that native language (Horner, Surratt, & Juliusson, 2000). Areas with the highest percentage of minorities and high rates of poverty and immigration also have the highest percentage of functionally illiterate people. When these people need medical care, they tend to require more resources, have longer hospital stays, and have a greater number of readmissions (Weiss, 2003). The challenge now and in the future will be to find improved ways of communicating with these population groups and to develop innovative strategies in the delivery of medical and nursing care.

Of the Americans older than 65 years of age, two out of five adults (approximately 40%) are considered functionally illiterate (Davidhizar & Brownson, 1999; Gazmararian et al., 1999; Williams et al., 2002). In 2003, the population of older adults was approximately 36 million (more than 12% of the total population) and the individuals older than 85 years of age make up the fastest-growing age group in the country. At the turn of the century, they numbered 4.2 million people, but it is projected that by 2050 that number could reach 21 million. Children born today can expect to live to an average age of at least 80. Statistics indicate that the U.S. population is growing older as people live longer. By 2030, it is expected that the 65-and-older population will double from what it was at the beginning of the 21st century (Santrock, 2006; Vander Zanden, Crandell, & Crandell, 2007).

As time goes on, the older population will be more educated and demand more services. In 1960, only 20% of older people were high school graduates, whereas by the beginning of the 21st century, 64% were educated at the high school level. Although these statistical trends indicate there will be a more highly educated group of older adults in the future, the information explosion and rapid technological advances may cause them to fall behind relative to future standards of education. Today, the illiteracy problem in the aged is due to the facts that not only did these individuals have less education in the past, but also that their reading skills have declined over time because of disuse. If a person does not use a skill, he or she loses the skill. Reading ability can deteriorate over time if not exercised regularly (Brownson, 1998).

In addition, cognition and some types of intellectual functioning are affected by aging (Kessels, 2003; Santrock, 2006; Vander Zanden et al., 2007). The vast majority of older people have some degree of cognitive changes and sensory impairments, such as vision and hearing loss. About one fourth of people aged 65 and one half over 75 years of age have serious hearing impairment (Vander Zanden et al., 2007). Along with these normal physiological changes, many suffer from chronic diseases, and large numbers are taking prescribed medications. All of these conditions can interfere with the ability to learn or negatively affect thought processes, which contributes to the high incidence of illiteracy in this population group.

Beyond the issue of prevalence, illiteracy also presents unique psychosocial problems for the older adult. Because older persons tend to process information more slowly than do young adults, they may become more easily frustrated in a learning situation (Kessels, 2003; Vander Zanden et al., 2007). Furthermore, many older individuals have developed ways to compensate for missing skills through their support network. Lifetime patterns of behavior have been set such that they may lack the motivation to improve their literacy skills. Today and in the years to come, those involved with providing health education will be challenged to overcome these obstacles to learning in the older adult.

Cultural diversity, although not considered to be directly related to illiteracy, may also serve as a barrier to effective client education. According to Davidhizar and Brownson (1999) and backed up by the NAAL's 2003 statistics, most adults with illiteracy problems in this country are White, native-born, English-speaking Americans. However, when examining the proportion of the population that has poor literacy skills, minority ethnic groups are at a disproportionately higher risk (Andrus & Roth, 2002).

When healthcare providers are communicating with clients from cultures different than those of their own, it is important to be aware that their clients may not be fluent in English. Furthermore, even if people speak the English language, the meanings of words and the understanding of facts may vary significantly based on life experiences, family background, and culture of origin, especially if English is the client's second language (Purnell & Paulanka, 2003). In conversation, an individual must be able to understand undertones, voice intonations, and in what context (slang, terminology, or customs) the message is being delivered.

Purnell and Paulanka (2003) stress the importance of assessing other elements of verbal and nonverbal communication, such as emotional tone of speech, gestures, eye contact, touch, voice volume, and stance, between persons of different cultures that may affect the interpretation of behavior and the validating of information received or sent (see Chapter 8). Educators must be aware of these potential barriers to communication when interacting with clients from other cultures whose literacy skills may be limited. Given the increasing diversity of the U.S. population, most currently available written materials are inadequate based on the literacy level of minority groups and the fact that the majority of printed education materials are available only in English.

Thus, individuals with less education, which often includes the groups of low-income per-sons, older adults, racial minorities, and people with ethnic origins for whom English is a second language, are likely to have more difficulty with reading and comprehending written materials as well as understanding oral instruction (Winslow, 2001). This profile is not intended to stereotype illiterate people but rather to give a broad picture of who most likely lacks literacy skills. It is essential that nurses and other healthcare providers be aware of those susceptible to having literacy problems when carrying out assessments on their patient populations.

Myths, Stereotypes, and Assumptions

Rarely do people voluntarily admit that they are illiterate. Illiteracy is a stigma that creates feelings of shame, inadequacy, fear, and low self-esteem (Weiss, 2003; Williams et al., 2002). Most individuals with poor literacy skills have learned that it is dangerous to reveal their illiteracy because of fear that others such as family, strangers, friends, or employers would consider them dumb or incapable of functioning responsibly. In fact, the majority of people with literacy problems have never told their spouse or children of their disability (Quirk, 2000; Williams et al., 2002).

People also tend to underreport their limited reading abilities because of embarrassment or lack of insight about the extent of their limitation. The NALS report revealed that the majority of adults performing at the two lowest levels of literacy skill describe themselves as proficient in being able to read and/or write English (Ad Hoc Committee on Health Literacy, 1999). Because self-reporting is so unreliable and because illiteracy and low literacy are so common, many experts suggest that screening of all patients should be done to identify clients who have reading difficulty to determine the extent of their impairment (Andrus & Roth, 2002; Weiss, 2003; Weiss et al., 2005).

Most people with limited literacy abilities are masters at concealment. Typically, they are ashamed by their limitation and attempt to hide the problem in clever ways. Often, they are resourceful and intelligent about trying to conceal their illiteracy and have developed remarkable memories to help them cope with family and career situations (Doak et al., 1996; Kanonowicz, 1993). Many have discovered ways to function quite well in society without being able to read by memorizing signs and instructions, by making intelligent guesses, or by finding employment opportunities that are not heavily dependent on reading and writing skills.

An important thing to remember is that there are many myths about illiteracy. It is very easy for healthcare providers to fall into the trap of wrongly labeling someone as illiterate or, for that matter, assuming that they are literate based on stereotypical images. Some of the most common myths about people who struggle with literacy skills are outlined next (Andrus & Roth, 2002; Doak et al., 1996; Weiss, 2003; Williams et al., 2002; Winslow, 2001).

Myth No. 1: They are intellectually slow learners or incapable of learning at all. (In fact, many have average or above-average IQs.)

Myth No. 2: They can be recognized by their appearance. (In fact, appearance alone is an unreliable basis for judgment; some very articulate, well-dressed people have no visible signs of a literacy disability.)

Myth No. 3: The number of years of schooling completed correlates with literacy skills. (In fact, grade-level achievement does not correspond well to reading ability. The number of years of schooling completed overestimates reading levels by four to five grade levels.)

Myth No. 4: Most are foreign-born, poor, and of ethnic or racial minority. (In fact, they come from very diverse backgrounds and the majority are White, native-born Americans.)

Myth No. 5: Most will freely admit that they do not know how to read or do not understand. (In fact, most try to hide their reading deficiencies and will go to great lengths to avoid discovery, even when directly asked about their possible limitations.)

Assessment: Clues to Look For

So the question remains: How does one recognize an illiterate person? Identifying illiteracy is not easy because there is no stereotypical pattern. It is an impairment easily overlooked because illiteracy has no particular face, age, socioeconomic status, or nationality (Cole, 2000; Hayes, 2000).

Nurses, because of their highly developed assessment skills and frequent contact with clients, are in an ideal position to determine the literacy levels of individuals (Cutilli, 2005; Monsivais & Reynolds, 2003). Because of the prevalence of illiteracy, nurses should never assume that their clients are literate. Knowing a person's ability to read and comprehend is critical in providing teaching–learning encounters that are beneficial, efficient, and cost effective.

There are a number of informal clues or red flags to watch out for that indicate reading and writing deficiencies. The caveat is: do not rely on the obvious but look for the unexpected. In so many instances when someone does not fit the stereotypical image, nurses and physicians have never even considered the possibility that an illiteracy problem exists.

Overlooking the problem has the potential for grave consequences in treatment outcomes and has resulted in frustration for both the client and the caregiver (Cole, 2000; Weiss, 2003). Unfortunately, healthcare providers are often hesitant to infer that a patient may have low literacy skills because there is an implication of personal inadequacy associated with the failure to have learned to read (Quirk, 2000).

Because people with illiteracy or marginal literacy skills often have had many years of practice at disguising the problem, they will go to elaborate lengths to hide the fact that they do not possess a skill already acquired by most elementary schoolchildren. The observant practitioner should always be on the lookout for possible signs of poor reading abilities. If healthcare providers become aware of a client's literacy problem, they must convey sensitivity and maintain confidentiality to prevent increased feelings of shame (Quirk, 2000).

During assessment, the nurse educator should take note of the following clues that clients with illiteracy or low literacy may demonstrate (Andrus & Roth, 2002; Davis, Michielutte, Askov, Williams, & Weiss, 1998; Weiss, 2003):

- Reacting to complex learning situations by withdrawal, complete avoidance, or being repeatedly noncompliant
- Using the excuse that they were too busy, too tired, too sick, or too sedated with medication to maintain their attention span when given a booklet or instruction sheet to read
- Claiming that they just did not feel like reading, that they gave the information to their spouse to take home, or that they lost, forgot, or broke their glasses

- Camouflaging their problem by surrounding themselves with books, magazines, and newspapers to give the impression they are able to read
- Circumventing their inability by insisting on taking the information home to read or having a family member or friend with them when written information is presented
- Asking you to read the information for them under the guise that their eyes are bothersome, they lack interest, or they do not have the energy to devote to the task of learning
- Showing nervousness as a result of feeling stressed by the threat of the possibility of getting caught or having to confess to illiteracy
- Acting confused, talking out of context, holding reading materials upside down, or expressing thoughts that may seem totally irrelevant to the topic of conversation
- Showing a great deal of frustration and restlessness when attempting to read, often mouthing words aloud (vocalization) or silently (subvocalization), substituting words they cannot decipher (decode) with meaningless words, pointing to words or phrases on a page, or exhibiting facial signs of bewilderment or defeat
- Standing in a location clearly designated for authorized personnel only
- Listening and watching very attentively to observe and memorize how things work
- Demonstrating difficulty with following instructions about relatively simple activities such as breathing exercises or with operating the TV, electric bed, call

light, and other simple equipment, even when the operating instructions are clearly printed on them

- Failing to ask any questions about the information they received
- Revealing a discrepancy between what is understood by listening and what is understood by reading

In summary, although it has been clearly pointed out that the level of completed formal education is an inaccurate presumption by which to predict reading level, it is certainly one estimate that nurses should incorporate into their methods of assessment. Also, negative feedback and clues from the client in the form of puzzled looks, inappropriate behaviors, excuses, or irrelevant statements may give the nurse the intuitive feeling that the message being communicated has neither been received nor understood. Not only do illiterate people become confused and frustrated in their attempts to deal with the complex system of health care, which is so dependent on written and verbal information, but they also become stressed in their efforts to cover up their disability.

Nurses, in turn, can feel frustrated when those who have undiagnosed literacy problems seem at face value to be unmotivated and noncompliant in following self-care instructions. Many times nurses wonder why clients make caregiving so difficult for themselves as well as for the provider. It is not unusual for nurses to conclude, "He's too proud to bend," "She's in denial," or "He's just being stubborn—it's a control issue."

Nurses in their role as educators must go beyond their own assumptions, look beyond a client's appearance and behavior, and seek out the less than obvious by conducting a thorough initial assessment of variables to uncover the possibility that a literacy problem exists. An

awareness of this possibility and good skills at observation are key to diagnosing illiteracy or low literacy in learners. Early diagnosis will enable nurses to intervene appropriately to avoid disservice to those who do not need condemnation but nurses' support and encouragement.

Impact of Illiteracy on Motivation and Compliance

In addition to the fact that poor literacy skills affect the ability to read as well as to understand and interpret the meaning of written and verbal instructions, a person with illiteracy or semiliteracy struggles with other significant interrelated limitations with communication that negatively influence healthcare teaching (Doak et al., 1998; Kalichman, Ramachandran, & Catz, 1999). The person's organization of thought, perception, vocabulary and language/fluency development, and problem-solving skills are adversely affected, too (Giorgianni, 1998).

Fleener and Scholl (1992) investigated characteristics of those who had self-identified themselves as literacy disabled. For the functionally illiterate, the most common deficiencies found were in phonics, comprehension, and perception. Difficulties in perception were evident in the reversal of letters and words, miscalling letters, and adding and omitting letters. Also, a major problem was comprehension, identification of words without knowing their meaning. Some individuals needed to read aloud to understand, and others read so slowly that they lost the meaning of a paragraph before they had finished it. Still other subjects perceived difficulty in remembering as a factor in their lack of reading skill.

People with poor reading skills have difficulty analyzing instructions, assimilating and correlating new information, and formulating questions (Giorgianni, 1998). They may be reluctant to ask questions because of concerns that their inquiries will be regarded as incomprehensible or irrelevant. Often they do not even know what to ask, but they also fear if they try others will think of them as ignorant or lacking in intelligence.

Hussey and Guilliland (1989) provided a poignant example, which remains as relevant today as it was then, of a young pregnant girl prescribed antiemetic suppositories to control her nausea. When she had no relief of symptoms, questioning by the nurse revealed that she was swallowing the medication. Obviously, not only did she not understand how to take the medicine, but she also likely had never seen a suppository and was not even able to read or understand the word. She did not ask what it was, probably because she did not know what to ask in the first place, and she may have been reluctant to question the treatment out of fear that she would be regarded as ignorant.

If past experiences with learning have been less than positive, some people may prefer not knowing the answers to questions and may withdraw altogether to avoid awkward or embarrassing learning situations. Also, they may react to complicated, fast-paced instruction with discouragement, low self-esteem, and refusal to participate because their process of interpretation is so slow. Even when questioned about their understanding, persons with low literacy skills will most likely claim that the information was understood even when it was not (Doak et al., 1996).

Another characteristic of illiterate individuals is that they have difficulty synthesizing information in a way that fits into their behavior patterns. If they are unable to comprehend a required

behavior change or cannot understand why it is needed, then any health teaching will be disregarded (Weiss, 2003). For example, cardiac patients who are told via verbal and written instructions to lose weight, increase exercise, decrease dietary fat, and begin taking medications may fail to comply with this regimen because of lack of understanding of the information and how to go about incorporating these changes into their lifestyle (Schultz, 2002).

Persons with poor literacy skills may also think in only concrete, specific, and literal terms. An example of this limitation is the diabetic patient whose glucose levels were out of control even when the patient insisted he was taking his insulin as instructed—injecting the orange and then eating the fruit (Hussey & Guilliland, 1989).

The person with limited literacy also may experience difficulty handling large amounts of information and classifying it into categories. Older adults, in particular, who need to take several different medications at various times and in different dosages may either become confused with the schedule or ignore the instruction. If asked to change their daily medication routine, a great deal of retraining may be needed to convince them of the benefits of the new regimen (Kessels, 2003).

Another major factor in noncompliance is the lack of adequate and specific instructions about prescribed treatment regimens. Unfortunately, poor literacy skills are seldom assessed by healthcare personnel when, for example, teaching a patient about medications. Literacy problems tend to limit the patient's ability to understand the array of instructions regarding medication labels, dosage scheduling, adverse reactions, drug interactions, and complications (Williams et al., 2002). No wonder those who lack the required vocabulary, organized thinking skills, and the ability to formulate questions, coupled with inadequate instruction, become confused and easily frustrated to the point of taking medications incorrectly or refusing to take them at all.

Thus, illiteracy, functional illiteracy, and low literacy significantly affect both motivation and compliance levels (see Chapter 6). What is often mistaken for noncompliance is, instead, the simple inability to comply. Although almost one half of the adult population is functionally illiterate, this statistic is overlooked by many healthcare professionals as a major factor in noncompliance with prescribed regimens, follow-up appointments, and measures to prevent medical complications (Andrus & Roth, 2002; Doak et al., 1996; Weiss, 2003; Williams et al., 2002).

A number of studies have correlated literacy levels with noncompliance (Doak et al., 1998; Kalichman et al., 1999; Mayeaux et al., 1996; Weiss, 2003). Individuals with poor literacy skills that coincide with inadequate language skills have difficulty following instructions and providing accurate and complete health histories, which are vital to the delivery of good health care. The burden of illiteracy leads patients into noncompliance not because they do not want to comply, but rather because they are unable to do so (Hayes, 2000; Williams, Counselman, & Caggiano, 1996).

Numerous research studies indicate that the impact of illiteracy is broader than just the inability to read; it alters the way a person organizes, interprets, analyzes, and summarizes information (Giorgianni, 1998). Caregivers often overestimate an individual's ability to understand instructions and are quick to label someone as uncooperative. In reality, the underlying problem may be limited cognitive processing that impedes comprehending and following written and oral communication.

Ethical, Financial, and Legal Concerns

Sources of printed education materials (PEMs) include healthcare facilities, commercial vendors, government services, voluntary health agencies, nonprofit charitable organizations, pharmaceutical firms, and medical equipment supply companies. These materials are distributed primarily by nurses and physicians and are the major sources of information for clients participating in health programs in many settings.

Written health information materials are intended to reinforce learning about health promotion, disease prevention, illness management, diagnostic procedures, drug and treatment modalities, rehabilitative course, and self-care regimens. Unfortunately, many of these sources fail to take into account the educational level, preexisting knowledge base, cultural influences, language barriers, or socioeconomic backgrounds of persons with limited literacy skills.

As compared with people who have adequate health literacy, it is estimated that expenditures for health care for those with limited literacy cost our country between $32 billion and $58 billion in 2001 (Center for Health Care Strategies, 2003; Wood, 2005). Unless patients are competent in reading and comprehending the literature given to them, these tools are useless as adjuncts for health education. They are neither a cost-effective nor a time-efficient means for teaching and learning. Materials that are widely distributed, but little or not at all understood, pose not only a health hazard for clients but also an ethical, financial, and legal liability for healthcare providers (Ad

Hoc Committee, 1999; French & Larrabee, 1999; Gazmararian et al., 2005; Giorgianni, 1998; Schultz, 2002).

Materials that are too difficult to read or comprehend serve little purpose. Health education cannot be considered to have taken place if the written information that has been distributed to clients does not enhance their knowledge and requisite skills necessary for self-care. Ultimately, indiscriminate or nonselective use of PEMs can result in complete or partial lack of communication between healthcare providers and consumers (Andrus & Roth, 2002; Fisher, 1999; Weiss, 2003; Winslow, 2001).

Initial standards for health education put forth in 1993 by the Joint Commission for Accreditation of Healthcare Organizations (JCAHO)—now known as the Joint Commission (JC)—still remain as a current standard requiring "the patient and/or, when appropriate, his/her significant other(s) are provided with education that can enhance their knowledge, skills, and those behaviors necessary to fully benefit from the health care interventions provided by the organization" (JCAHO, 1993, p. 1030).

In 1996, JCAHO identified additional standards necessary for client care to meet accreditation mandates. Not only is patient and family (or significant other) instruction required, but education must be provided by all relevant members of the interdisciplinary healthcare team, with special consideration being given to the client's literacy level, educational level, and language. All clients must have an assessment of their readiness to learn and an identification of any obstacles to learning.

Emphasis on such standards has prompted healthcare agencies and providers to reexamine their teaching practices, educational materials, and systems of documenting evidence of teaching interventions to better match the reading levels and cultural diversity of the clients being served. These JC standards further specify that education relevant to a person's healthcare needs must be understandable and culturally appropriate to the patient and/or significant others. Therefore, PEMs must be written in ways that assist clients in comprehending their health needs and problems to undertake self-care regimens such as medications, diet, exercise therapies, and use of medical equipment (Fisher, 1999; Weiss, 2003).

Furthermore, the federally mandated Patient's Bill of Rights has established the rights of patients to receive complete and current information regarding their diagnoses, treatments, and prognoses in terms they can understand (Duffy & Snyder, 1999). It is imperative that the reading levels of PEMs match the patients' reading abilities and vice versa. Compounding the need for appropriately written materials is the fact that research reveals that people forget almost immediately about one half of any instruction they receive orally (Kessels, 2003). Failure to retain information combined with inappropriate reading levels of materials used to reinforce or supplement verbal teaching methods decreases compliance, increases morbidity, and results in misuse of healthcare facilities (Weiss et al., 2005).

Encouraging self-care through client education for purposes of health promotion, disease prevention, health maintenance, and rehabilitation is not a new concept to either consumers or providers of health care. However, the trends in the current healthcare system in the United States have impinged on the professional ability of nurses to provide needed information to ensure self-care that is both safe and effective. Patient education has assumed an even more vital role in assisting clients to independently manage their own healthcare needs given such factors as:

- Early discharge
- Decreased reimbursement for direct care
- Increased emphasis on delivery of care in the community and home setting
- Greater demands on nursing personnel time
- Increased technological complexity of treatment
- Assumption by caregivers that printed information is an adequate substitute for direct instruction of patients

These constraints do not allow for sufficient opportunities for clients in various healthcare settings to receive the necessary education they need for self-management after discharge. Most outpatient care, such as that given in clinics, doctors' offices, and same-day surgery centers, requires patients and their families to understand both written and oral instruction (Wood, 2005). Consequently, professional nurses are relying to a greater extent than ever before on PEMs to supplement their teaching (Horner et al., 2000).

Thus, the burden of becoming adequately educated falls on the shoulders of patients, their families, and significant others. Often unprepared because of shortened hospital stays or limited contact with healthcare providers, consumers have to assume a greater role in their own recovery and the maximization of their health potential (Weiss, 2003; Wood, 2005).

The burden also falls on nurses to safeguard the lives of their clients by becoming better, more effective communicators of written health information. Since 1990, the Maine Area Health Education Center (AHEC) Literacy Center at the University of New England has been holding summer institutes for healthcare professionals to learn about literacy issues, to share resources with colleagues from around the world, and to acquire skills in writing and critiquing health information documents (Andrus & Roth, 2002; Osborne, 1999).

It is only recently that research in the area of written health education materials in relation to clients' literacy skills has examined and attempted to answer even the most basic questions, such as the following:

- Do consumers read the health education literature provided them?
- Are they capable of reading it?
- Can they comprehend what they read?
- Are written materials appropriate and sufficient for the intended target audience?

In our increasingly litigious and ethically conscious society, growing attention is being paid by health professionals to informed consent and teaching for self-care via both verbal and written healthcare instruction (Gazmararian et al., 2005). The potential for misinterpretation of instructions not only can adversely affect treatment but also raises serious concerns about the ethical and legal implications with respect to professional responsibility and liability when information is written at a level incomprehensible to many patients (French & Larrabee, 1999; Weiss, 2003). A properly informed consumer is not only a legal concern in health care today but an ethical one as well (see Chapter 2).

Readability of Printed Education Materials

Many studies on literacy have attempted to document the disparity between the reading levels of consumers and the estimated readability demand of printed health information. Given that the health of people depends in part on their ability to understand information contained in food labeling, over-the-counter and prescription medication instructions, environmental safety warnings, discharge instructions, health promotion and disease prevention flyers, and the like, the focus of attention on identifying this discrepancy is more than warranted.

A substantial body of evidence in the literature indicates that there is a significant gap between patients' reading and comprehension levels and the level of reading difficulty of printed education materials (PEMs) (Andrus & Roth, 2002; Weiss, 2003; Winslow, 2001). A variety of education materials available from sources such as the government, health agencies, professional associations, health insurance companies, and industries are written beyond the reading ability of the majority of clients.

Healthcare providers are beginning to recognize that the reams of written materials relied on by so many of them to convey health information to consumers are essentially closed to those with illiteracy and low-literacy problems. For example, look at the text below on information about colonoscopy:

Your naicisyhp has dednemmocer that you have a ypocsonoloc. A ypocsonoloc is a test for noloc recnac. It sevlovni gnitresni a elbixelf gniweiv epocs into your mutcer. You must drink a laiceps diuqil the thgin erofeb the noitanimaxe to naelc out your noloc.

Does it make sense, or are you confused? If the words appear unreadable, that is exactly what written teaching instructions look like to someone who cannot read (Weiss, 2003).

Many researchers have assessed specific population groups in a variety of healthcare settings based on the ability of clients to meet the literacy demands of written materials related to their care. All of these investigators used commonly accepted readability formulas to test consumers' understanding of printed health information. Their findings revealed:

- Emergency department instructional materials (average 10th-grade readability) are written at a level of difficulty out of the readable range for most patients (Duffy & Snyder, 1999; Lerner, Jehle, Janicke, & Moscati, 2000; Williams et al., 1996).

- A significant mismatch exists between the reading ability of older adults and the readability levels of documents essential to their gaining access to health-related services offered through local, state, and federal government programs (Winslow, 2001).

- A large discrepancy exists between clients' average reading comprehension levels and the readability demand of PEMs used in ambulatory care settings (Lerner et al., 2000; Schillinger et al., 2002; Wood, 2005).

- Standard consent forms used in hospitals, private physician offices, and clinics, as well as by institutional review boards (IRBs) to protect potential research subjects require high school- to college-level reading comprehension (Doak et al., 1998; Paasche-Orlow, Taylor, & Brancati, 2003).

- Physicians' letters to their patients required an average of 16th–17th-grade reading ability, and, likewise, health articles in newspapers ranged from 12th- to 14th-grade level (Conlin & Schumann, 2002)

- The reading grade levels of 15 psychotropic medication handouts for patient education ranged from 12th to 14th grade, well above the 5th-grade level recommended by the National Cancer Institute guidelines (Myers & Shephard-White, 2004)

Thus, numerous investigators have demonstrated that PEMs for the purpose of disseminating health information are written at grade levels that far exceed the reading ability of the majority of consumers. Results from these studies reveal that most health education literature is written above the 8th-grade level, with the average level falling between the 10th and 12th grade. Many PEMs exceed this upper range, even though the average reading level of adults falls at the 8th-grade level. Millions of people in our population read at considerably lower levels and need materials written at the 5th-grade level or lower (Bastable, Chojnowski, Goldberg, McGurl, & Riegel, 2005; Brownson, 1998; Doak et al., 1998; Davis, Williams, Marin, Parker, & Glass, 2002).

Furthermore, the health education literature indicates that people typically read at least two grade levels below their highest level of schooling and prefer materials that are written below their literacy abilities. In fact, contrary to popular belief, sophisticated readers also prefer simplified PEMs when ill due to low energy and concentration levels, and even when they are well due to the demands of their busy schedules and the fact that even highly educated people do not know the vocabulary of medicine, known as medicalese (Giorgianni, 1998; Lasater & Mehler, 1998; Winslow, 2001).

The conclusion to be drawn is that complex and lengthy PEMs serve no useful teaching purpose if healthcare consumers are unable to understand them or unwilling to read them. Literacy levels of clients compared with literacy demands of PEMs, whether in hospital or community-based settings, are an important factor in the rehabilitation and recidivism of those who are recipients of healthcare services.

The Internet is an excellent resource for nurse educators to locate easy-to-read PEMs. See **Table 7–4** for sources of low-literacy education materials.

Measurement Tools to Test Literacy Levels

Healthcare professionals continually struggle with the task of effectively communicating highly complex and technical information to their consumers, who often lack sufficient background knowledge to understand the sophisticated content of instruction relevant to their care. Whether they author or merely distribute printed education information, nursing and other healthcare practitioners are responsible for ensuring the appropriate literacy level of the materials given to their clients.

If the literacy of education materials matches the readers' literacy skills, consumers may be better able to understand and comply with healthcare regimens, thereby reducing the costs of care and improving their quality of life (Ad Hoc Committee, 1999). Because nurses rely heavily on PEMs to convey necessary information to their clients, the usefulness and efficacy of these materials must be determined in relation to the readers' abilities to decipher information.

To objectively evaluate the difficulty of written materials, two basic measurement methods exist: formulas and tests. Various formulas measure

---

Table 7-4 SOURCES OF LOW-LITERACY EDUCATION MATERIALS

Agency for Healthcare Research and Quality (AHRQ). Web site: www.ahcpr.gov; phone: (315) 594-1364

National Institutes of Health (NIH). Web site: www.nih.gov

National Heart, Lung, and Blood Institute (NHLBI). Web site: www.nhlbi.nih.gov; phone: (301) 251-1222

United States Pharmacopeia (Library of Pictograms). Web site: www.usp.org; phone: (800) 227-8772

The Indian Health Service. Web site: www.ihs.gov

National Cancer Institute, Cancer Information Services. Web site: www.nci.nih.gov; phone: (800) 4-CANCER

American Cancer Society. Web site: www.cancer.org; phone: (800) ACS-2345

American Heart Association. Web site: www.americanheart.org; phone: (800) 242-1793

National Institute for Literacy. Web site: www.nifl.gov; phone: (202) 632-1500

American Dietetic Association. Web site: www.eatright.org; phone: (312) 899-0400

Office of Minority Health. Web site: www.omhrc.gov; phone: (800) 444-6472

Channing L. Bete Company, Inc. Web site: www.channing-bete.com; phone: (800) 477-4776

Krames Communication. Web site: www.krames.com; phone: (800) 333-3032

Mosby Consumer Health. Web site: www.mosby.com; phone: (800) 325-4177

Ask me 3. Web site: www.askme3.org

Executive Secretariat: The Plain Language Initiative. Web site: execsec.od.nih.gov/plainlang/guidelines/index.html

National Cancer Institute. Web site: cancer.gov/cancerinformation/clearandsimple

---

readability of PEMs and are based on ascertaining the average length of sentences and words (vocabulary difficulty) to determine the grade level at which they are written. Standardized tests, which measure actual comprehension and reading skills, involve readers' responses to instructional materials or the ability to decode and pronounce words to determine their grade level (see Appendix A).

Both methods, although not ideal, are considered to have a sufficient relationship to literacy ability to justify their use. The most widely used readability formulas and standardized tests for comprehension and reading skill rate high on reliability and predictive validity. They also do not require elaborate training to use, but they do vary in the amount of time required to administer. In addition, the advent of computerized readability analysis (nearly all word-processing programs, such as Microsoft Word, will produce readability statistics with just a click of the mouse) has made evaluating the reading grade level of written materials much easier and quicker. All of these methods are most useful to nurse educators for designing and evaluating PEMs.

Formulas to Measure Readability of PEMs

Readability is not a new concept and has been a concern of primary and secondary school educators and educational psychologists for years. In the 1940s, there was a great upswing in attempts by educators and reading specialists to develop systematic procedures by which to objectively evaluate reading materials. Readability is defined as "characteristics of reading materials that make material 'easy' or 'difficult' to read" (Aldridge, 2004). Today, more than 40 formulas are available to measure the readability levels of PEMs.

Readability indices have been devised to determine the grade level demand of specific written information. Although they can predict a level of reading difficulty of material based on an analysis of sentence structure and word length, they do not take into account the within or inherent individual variables that affect the reader, such as interest in or familiarity with the subject itself or the actual content of the materials (Doak et al., 1996).

Even though materials may have similar readability levels as measured by some formula, not all readers will have equal competence in reading them. For example, a patient with a long-standing chronic illness may already be familiar with vocabulary related to the disease and, therefore, may be able to read similar grade-level materials much more easily than a newly diagnosed patient, even though both individuals may have equal literacy skill with other types of material (Doak et al., 1985).

As assessment tools, readability formulas are useful but must be employed with caution, because the match between reader and material does not necessarily guarantee comprehension (Aldridge, 2004; Davis et al., 1998). Readability formulas originally were designed as predictive averages to rank the difficulty of books used in specific grades of school—not to determine exactly which factors contribute to the difficulty of a text. Educators should be careful in assuming that people can or cannot read instructional material simply because a formula-based readability score does or does not match their educational level.

Even though these simple instruments are practical for assessment of literacy, they are limited in that they cannot determine the cause or type of reading and learning problems (Davis et al., 1998). Therefore, while readability formulas are easily applied and have proved useful in determining the reading grade level of a text, when used alone they are not an adequate index of readability (Davis et al., 1998; Doak et al., 1996).

Readability formulas are merely one useful step in determining reading ease of a document. Many researchers suggest using a multi-method approach to ascertain readability—that is, they suggest applying a number of readability formulas to any given piece of written material as well as taking into consideration the reader and other material variables (Doak et al., 1996; Ley & Florio, 1996). Formula scores are simply rough approximations of text difficulty. Human judgment is always needed in conjunction with formula-based estimates to determine the quality of PEMs.

Readability formulas are mathematical equations derived from multiple regression analysis that describe the correlation between an author's style of writing and a reader's ability at identifying words as printed symbols within a context (Doak et al., 1996). Most of them provide fairly accurate grade-level estimates, give or take one grade level with 68% confidence. In many respects, a readability formula is like a reading test, except that it does not test people but rather written material (Fry, 1977).

The first guideline to remember is that readability formulas should not be the only tool used for assessing PEMs. The second rule is to select readability formulas that have been validated on the reader population for whom the PEM is intended. Several formulas are geared to specific types of materials or population groups.

Ley and Florio (1996) and Meade and Smith (1991) conducted extensive studies of the most commonly used formulas and reported on their reliability and validity when used to measure health-related information. In particular, the Flesch, Fog, and Fry formulas showed strong correlations with health-based literature (Horner et al., 2000). Since so many readability formulas are available for assessment of reading levels of PEMs, only those that are relatively simple to work with, are accepted as reliable and valid, and are in widespread use have been chosen for review here.

Spache Grade-Level Score

What is unique about the Spache grade-level formula (Spache, 1953) is that, unlike the other leading formulas that focus largely on the evaluation of materials written for adults, this score is specifically designed to judge materials written for children at grade levels below fourth grade (elementary grades one through three). The Spache grade-level score should not be used to assess adult reading materials (Spache, 1953). The elements used to estimate reading difficulty using the Spache formula are sentence length and the number of words outside the Dale easy word list of 769 words required for formula calculation. See Appendix A for the method of formula analysis.

Flesch-Kincaid Scale

The Flesch-Kincaid formula was developed as an objective measurement of readability of materials between grade five and college level. Its use has been validated repeatedly over more than 50 years for assessing news reports, adult education materials, and government publications. The Flesch formula is based on a count of two basic language elements: average sentence length (in words) of selected samples and average word length measured as syllables per 100 words of sample. The reading ease (RE) score is calculated by combining these two variables (Flesch, 1948; Spadero, 1983; Spadero, Robinson, & Smith, 1980). See Appendix A for the method of formula analysis.

Fog Index

The Fog formula developed by Gunning (1968) is appropriate for use in determining readability of materials from fourth grade to college level. It is calculated based on average sentence length and the percentage of multisyllabic words in a 100-word passage. The Fog index is considered one of the simpler methods because it is based on a short sample of words (100), it does not require counting syllables of all words, and the rules are easy to follow (Spadero, 1983; Spadero et al., 1980). See Appendix A for the method of formula analysis.

Fry Readability Graph—Extended

The contribution of the Fry formula comes from the simplicity of its use without sacrificing accuracy, as well as its wide and continuous range of testing readability of materials (especially books, pamphlets, and brochures) at the level of grade one through college (grade 17). It is well accepted by literature and reading specialists and is not copyrighted (Doak et al., 1996). A series of simple rules can be applied to plot two language elements—the number of syllables and the number of sentences in three 100-word selections (Fry, 1968; Fry, 1977; Spadero et al., 1980). If a very long text is being analyzed, such as a 50-page or more book, one should use six 100-word samples rather than three (Doak et al., 1996). With some practice, this formula takes only about 10 minutes to determine the readability level of a document. See Appendix A for directions on how to use the Fry readability graph.

SMOG Formula

The SMOG (simplified measure of gobbledygook) formula by McLaughlin (1969) is recommended not only because it offers relatively easy computation (simple and fast) but also because it is one of the most valid tests of readability. The SMOG formula measures readability of PEMs from grade four to college level based on the number of polysyllabic words within a set number of sentences (Doak et al., 1996). It evaluates the readability grade level of PEMs to within 1.5 grades of accuracy (Myers & Shepard-White, 2004). Thus, when using the SMOG formula to calculate the grade level of material, the SMOG results are usually about two grades higher than the grade levels calculated by the other methods (Spadero, 1983).

The SMOG formula has been used extensively to judge grade-level readability of patient education materials. It is one of the most popular measurement tools because of its reputation for reading-level accuracy, its simple directions, and its speed of use, which is a particularly

important factor if computerized resources for analysis of test samples are not available (Meade & Smith, 1991). See Appendix A for the method of formula analysis and for an example of how to apply the SMOG formula to a short passage.

In summary, Doak et al. (1996) state that it is critically important to determine the readability of all written materials at the time they are drafted or adopted by using one or more of the many available formulas. They contend that you cannot afford to fly blind by using health materials that are untested for readability difficulty. Pretesting PEMs before distribution is the way to be sure they fit the literacy level of the audience for which they are intended. It is imperative that the formulas used to measure grade-level readability of PEMs are appropriate for the type of material being tested (see **Table 7–5**).

Computerized Readability Software Programs

Computerized programs have helped tremendously in facilitating the use of readability formulas. Some software programs are capable of applying a number of formulas to analyze one text selection. In addition, some packages are able to identify difficult words in written passages that may not be understood by patients. Dozens of user-friendly, menu-driven commercial software packages can automatically calculate reading levels as well as provide advice on how to simplify text (Aldridge, 2004; Doak et al., 1996).

Computerized assessment of readability is fast and easy, and it provides a high degree of reliability, especially when several formulas are used. Determining readability by computer programs rather than doing so manually is also

Table 7–5 Appropriate Readability Formula Choice

Formula	Selection Shorter Than 300 Words	Selection Longer Than 300 Words	Entire Piece	Grade Level
Spache score	Yes	Yes	Yes	1–3
Flesch formula	Yes	Yes	Yes	5 to college
Fog formula	Yes (minimum of 100 words)	Yes	Yes	4 to college
Fry graph	Not recommended	Yes	Yes	1 to college
SMOG formula	Yes	Yes	Yes	4 to college

Source: Adapted from Spadero, Robinson, & Smith (1980), p. 216.

more accurate in calculating reading levels because it eliminates human error in scoring and because entire articles, pamphlets, or books can be scanned (Duffy & Snyder, 1999). It is advisable to take an average across several pieces of literature, using several different formulas and software programs, when calculating estimates of readability.

Tests to Measure Comprehension of PEMs

A number of standardized tests have proved reliable and valid to measure comprehension of readers, a relatively new concept in health education (Doak et al., 1996). Usually pretests and posttests used in institutional settings measure recall of knowledge rather than comprehension. However, the determination of readers' abilities to comprehend information is essential. Health education materials must serve a useful purpose, both from the standpoint of assisting patients to assume self-care and for protecting the health professional from legal liability.

Comprehension implies that the reader has internalized the information found in PEMs (Aldridge, 2004). The two most popular standardized methods to measure comprehension of written materials are the cloze test and the listening test. These tests can be used to assess how much someone understands from reading or listening to a passage of text.

Cloze Procedure

The cloze test (derived from the term *closure*) has been specifically recommended for assessing understanding of health education literature. Although it takes more time and resources to compute than do readability formulas, the cloze procedure has been validated for its adequacy in ranking reading difficulty of medical literature, which typically has a high concept load. This procedure is not a formula that provides a school grade-type level of readability like the formulas already described, but rather takes into consideration the context of a written passage (Doak et al., 1996).

The cloze test can be administered to individual clients who demonstrate difficulty comprehending health materials used for instruction. Nevertheless, it is suggested that this test not be administered to every client in a particular health setting but rather to a representative sample of consumers. The cloze test should be used only with those individuals whose reading skills are at sixth grade or higher (approximately Level 1 on the NALS scale); otherwise, it is likely that the test will prove too difficult (Doak et al., 1996).

The cloze test is best used when reviewing the appropriateness of several texts of the same content for a particular audience. The reader may or may not be familiar with the material being tested. This procedure is designed so that every fifth word is systematically deleted from a portion of a text. The reader is asked to fill in the blanks with the *exact* word replacements. One point is scored for every missing word guessed correctly by the reader. The final cloze score is the total number of blanks filled in correctly by the reader.

To be successful, the reader must demonstrate sensitivity to clues related to grammar, syntax, and semantics. If the reader is able to fill in the blanks with appropriate words, this process is an indication of how well the material has been comprehended—that is, how much knowledge was obtained from the set surrounding the blank spaces and how well the information was used to supply the additional information (Dale & Chall, 1978; Doak et al., 1996). The underlying theory is that the more readable a passage is, the better it will be understood even when words are omitted. The resulting score can be converted to a percentage for ease in interpreting and analyzing the data (Pichert & Elam, 1985).

A score for the cloze test is obtained by dividing the number of exact word replacements by the total number of blanks. A score of 60% or better indicates that the passage was sufficiently understood by the patient. A score of 40–59% indicates a moderate level of difficulty, where supplemental teaching is required for the patient to understand the message. A score of less than 40% indicates the material is too difficult to be understood and is not suitable to be used for teaching (Doak et al., 1996).

Instead of using packaged cloze tests available from commercial sources, it is suggested that educators devise their own tests so that the resultant scores will indicate a client's comprehension of their own instructions. Then problem words or sentences within these PEMs can be revised accordingly to make them more understandable. See Appendix A for an outline of the steps for constructing a cloze test, test scoring methodology, and a sample test.

Because the cloze procedure is a test of learners' ability to understand what they have read, be sure to be honest about the purpose of the test. For example, you might state that it is important for them to understand what they are to do when on their own after discharge, so you want to be sure they understand the written instructions they will need to follow. Doak et al. (1985) found that most people are willing to participate in the testing activity. They suggest that the following guidelines should be used before taking the cloze test:

1. Encourage participants to read through the entire test passage before attempting to fill in the blanks.
2. Tell them that only one word should be written in each blank.
3. Let them know that it is all right to guess, but that they should try to fill in every blank as accurately as possible.

4. Reassure them that spelling errors are all right just as long as the word they have put in the blank can be recognized.

5. Explain to them that this exercise is not a timed test. (If readers struggle to complete the test, tell them not to worry, that it is not necessary for them to fill in all the blanks, and set the test aside to go on to something else less frustrating or less threatening.)

Listening Test

Unlike the cloze test, which may be too difficult for clients who read below the sixth-grade level—that is, those who likely lack fluency and read with hesitancy—the listening test is a good approach to determining what a low-literate person understands and remembers when listening to oral instruction (Doak et al., 1996). Although it may take a couple of hours to develop this test, it takes only about 10–20 minutes to administer.

The procedure for administering the listening test is to select a passage from instructional materials that takes about 3 minutes to read aloud and is written at approximately the fifth-grade level. Formulate 5–10 short questions relevant to the content of the passage by selecting key points of the text. Read the passage to the person at a normal rate. Ask the listener the questions orally and record the answers (Doak et al., 1996).

To determine the percentage score, divide the number of questions answered correctly by the total number of questions. The instructional material will be appropriate for the client's comprehension level if the score is approximately 75–89% (some additional assistance when teaching the material may be necessary for full comprehension). A score of 90% or higher indicates that the material is easy for the client and can be

fully comprehended independently. A score of less than 75% means that the material is too difficult and simpler instructional material will need to be used when teaching the individual. Doak et al. (1996) provide an example of a sample passage and questions for a listening comprehension test.

Tests to Measure Reading Skills of Clients

The three most popular standardized methods to measure reading skill are the wide range achievement test (WRAT), the rapid estimate of adult literacy in medicine (REALM), and the test of functional health literacy in adults (TOFHLA). The literacy assessment for diabetes (LAD) is a relatively new instrument specific to clients with diabetes.

WRAT (Wide Range Achievement Test)

The WRAT is a word recognition screening test. It is used to assess a learner's ability to recognize and pronounce a list of words out of context as a criterion for measuring reading skills. There are a number of word recognition tests available, but the WRAT requires the least time to administer (approximately 5 minutes as compared with 30 minutes or more for the other tests).

Although it is limited to measuring only word recognition and does not test other aspects of reading such as vocabulary and comprehension of text material, this test is nevertheless useful for determining an appropriate level of instruction and for establishing a client's level of literacy. It is based on the belief that reading skill is associated with the ability to look at written words and put them into oral language, a necessary first step in comprehension (Doak et al., 1996).

As designed, it should be used only to test people whose native language is English. The WRAT tests on two levels: Level I is designed for children 5 to 12 years of age, and Level II is intended for testing persons older than age 12. The WRAT scores are normed on age but can be converted to grade levels.

The WRAT consists of a graduated list of 42 words. Starting with the most easy and ending with the most difficult, the person taking the test is asked to pronounce the words from the list, starting from the top, where the easiest words are located. The individual administering the test listens carefully to the patient's responses and scores those responses on a master score sheet. Next to those words that are mispronounced, a checkmark should be placed. When five words are mispronounced, indicating that the patient has reached his or her limit, the test is stopped.

To score the test, the number of words missed or not tried is subtracted from the list of words on the master score sheet to get a raw score. Then a table of raw scores is used to find the equivalent grade rating (GR). For more information on this test, see Doak et al. (1996), Davis et al. (1998), and Quirk (2000).

REALM (Rapid Estimate of Adult Literacy in Medicine)

The REALM test has advantages over the WRAT and other word tests because it measures a patient's ability to read medical and health-related vocabulary, it takes less time to administer, the scoring is simpler, and is well received by most clients (Davis et al., 1998; Duffy & Snyder, 1999; Foltz & Sullivan, 1998). This instrument has been field tested on large populations in public health and primary care settings (Davis et al., 1993). Although it has established validity, this test offers less precision than other word tests (Hayes, 2000). The raw score is converted to a range of grade levels rather than an exact grade level, but this result correlates well with the WRAT reading scores.

The procedure for administering the test is to ask patients to read aloud words from three word lists. Sixty-six medical and health-related words are arranged in three columns of 22 words each, beginning with short, easy words such as fat, flu, pill, and dose, and ending with more difficult words such as anemia, obesity, osteoporosis, and impetigo. Clients are asked to begin at the top of the first column and read down, pronouncing all the words that they can from the three lists. If they come upon a word they cannot pronounce, they are told to skip it and proceed to the next word. There is no time limit. The examiner keeps score on a separate copy of the list and places a plus sign next to words correctly pronounced and a minus next to those mispronounced or skipped (Davis et al., 1993). The total number of words pronounced correctly is the client's raw score, which is converted to a grade ranging from third grade and below (score of 0–18) to ninth grade and above (score of 61–66). Those whose scores fall at sixth grade or below have literacy skills equivalent to NALS levels 1 and 2 (Weiss, 2003; Schultz, 2002).

TOFHLA (Test of Functional Health Literacy in Adults)

The TOFHLA is a relatively new instrument developed in the mid-1990s for measuring patients' literacy skills using actual hospital materials, such as prescription labels, appointment slips, and informed consent documents. The test consists of two parts: reading comprehension and numeracy. It has demonstrated reliability and validity, requires approximately 20 minutes to administer, and is available in a Spanish version (TOFHLA-S) as well as an English version (Parker, Baker, Williams, & Nurss, 1995; Quirk, 2000; Williams et al., 1995). A more recent abbreviated version, known as the S-TOFHLA, was developed in 1999; it takes only 12 minutes to administer. Not only has it been tested for reliability and validity, but it is a more practical measure of functional health literacy to determine who needs assistance with achieving learning goals (Baker et al., 1999). A copy of the TOFHLA instrument and directions can be accessed at http://www.peppercornbooks.com/catalog/information.php?info_id=5

Readability formulas and standardized tests for comprehension and reading skills were never designed for the purpose of serving as writing guides. Patient educators may be tempted to write PEMs to fit the formulas and tests, but they should be aware that doing so places emphasis on structure, not content, and that comprehensibility of a written message may be greatly compromised. Pichert and Elam (1985) recommend that readability formulas should be used solely to judge material written without formulas in mind. Formulas are merely methods to check readability, and standardized tests are merely methods to check comprehension and word recognition. Neither method guarantees good style in the form of direct, conversational writing.

LAD (Literacy Assessment for Diabetes)

The LAD was specifically developed in 2001 to measure word recognition in adult patients with diabetes. This reading skills test, compared with WRAT3 (3rd version) and the REALM, was assessed to have strong reliability and validity. It consists of three word lists presented in ascending order of difficulty. The majority of terms are at the fourth-grade reading level, but the remaining words range from sixth- through sixteenth-grade levels. The LAD can be administered in 3 minutes or less. It was tested on a group of 200 people at a primary care clinic, a senior center, and three prisons. The subjects ranged in age from 20 to 85 years (mean age = 43.5). This standardized test was modeled after the REALM but emphasizes common words used when teaching self-care management of diabetes. The LAD instrument is copyrighted but is available with permission from Robert C. Byrd Health Sciences Center, Department of Family Medicine, PO Box 9152, Morgantown, WV 26505-9152, attn. Charlotte Nath, EdD, (Nath et al., 2001) or via the Internet at http://tde.sagepub.com

SAM (Instrument for Suitability Assessment of Materials)

In addition to using formulas and tests to measure readability, comprehension, and reading skills, Doak et al. (1996) designed a tool to rapidly and systematically assess the suitability of instructional materials for a given population of learners. Ideally, instructional tools should be evaluated with a sample of the intended audience, but limited time and resources may preclude such an approach. In response to this dilemma, these literacy experts developed the (suitability assessment of materials) SAM instrument. Not only can the SAM be used with print material and illustrations, but it has also been designed to be applied to video- and audiotaped instructions.

The SAM yields a numerical (percent) score, with materials tested falling into one of three categories: superior (70–100%), adequate (40–69%), or not suitable (0–39%). The application of the SAM can identify specific deficiencies in instructional materials that reduce their suitability. The SAM includes 22 factors to assess the content, literacy demand, graphics, layout and typography, learning stimulation and motivation, and cultural appropriateness of instructional materials being developed or already in use. The maximum score possible is 44 points (equals 100%). If one or more SAM factors do not apply to the material being tested, the test administrator should subtract two points each for every not applicable factor. For example, if the material tests at 36 but two factors did not apply, the maximum possible score would be 40. Thus, 36/40 = 90% (Doak et al., 1996). See Appendix A for the SAM instrument and directions for scoring.

Simplifying the Readability of PEMs

The suitability of written materials for different audiences depends not only on actual grade-level demand, which can be measured by readability formulas, but also on those elements within a text such as technical format, concept density, and accuracy and clarity of the message. It must never be forgotten that knowing the target audience in terms of the members' level of motivation, reading abilities, experiential factors, and cultural background is also of crucial importance in determining the appropriateness of printed health information as effective communication tools (Meade & Smith, 1991; Weiss, 2003). Even good readers may fail to respond to important health education literature if they lack the motivation to do so or if the material is not appealing to them.

Despite the well-documented potential of written materials to increase knowledge, compliance, and satisfaction with care, PEMs are often too difficult for even motivated clients to read. Clearly, the technical nature of health education literature lends itself to high readability levels, often requiring college-level reading skills to fully comprehend (Winslow, 2001).

Even though printed materials are the most commonly used form of media, as currently written, they remain the least effective means for reaching a large proportion of the adult population who have marginal literacy skills (Monsivais & Reynolds, 2003). What the nurse in the role of educator must strive to achieve when designing or selecting health-based literature is a good and proper fit between the material and the reader. Choosing and designing PEMs is a difficult, time-consuming, and challenging task that often becomes the responsibility of the nurse (Winslow, 2001).

Certainly the best solution for improving the overall comprehension and reading skills of clients would be to strengthen their basic general education, but this process will require decades to accomplish. What is needed now are ways in which to write or rewrite educational materials commensurate with the current comprehension and reading skills of learners. Nathaniel Hawthorne was once reported to have said, "Easy reading is damned hard writing" (Pichert & Elam, 1985, p. 181). He was correct in his perception that clear and concise writing is a task that takes effort and practice.

It is possible, though, to reduce the disparity between the literacy demand of written instructional materials and the actual reading level of clients by attending to some basic linguistic, motivational, organizational, and content principles. *Linguistics* refers to the type of language and grammatical style used. *Motivation principles* focus on those elements that stimulate the reader, such as relevance and appeal of the material. *Organizational factors* deal with layout and clarity. *Content principles* relate to load and concept density of information (Bernier, 1993). Wood et al. (2007) describe the language, information, and design (LID) method to create easy-to-read materials. These elements will be examined as they relate to designing or revising instructional materials for the marginally literate reader.

Prior to writing or rewriting a text for easier reading, however, some preliminary planning steps need to be taken to ensure that the final written material will be geared to the target audience (Davis et al., 1998; Doak et al., 1996; Kessels, 2003). The steps are:

1. Decide what the client should do or know. In other words, what is the purpose of the instruction? What outcomes do you hope learners will achieve?

2. Choose information that is relevant and needed by the client to achieve the behavioral objectives. Limit or cut out altogether extraneous and nice to know information such as the history or detailed physiological processes of a disease. Include only survival skills and essential main ideas of who, what, where, and when, with new information related to what the reader already knows. **Remember: a person does not have to know how an engine works to drive a car.**

3. Select other media to supplement the written information, such as pictures, demonstrations, models, audiotapes, and videotapes. Even poor readers will benefit from written material if it is combined with other forms of delivering a message. Consider the field of advertising, for example. Advertisers get their message across with words but often in combination with strong, action-packed visuals.

4. Organize topics into chunks that follow a logical sequence. Prioritize to present the most important information first. If topics are of equal importance, proceed from the more general as a basis on which to build to the more specific. Begin with a statement of purpose. In a list of items, place key facts at the top and bottom, because readers best remember information presented first and last in a series.

5. Determine the preferred reading level of the material. If the readers have been tested, preferably write two to four grades below the reading grade-level score. If the audience has not been tested, the group is likely to display a wide range of reading skills. When in doubt, write instructional materials at the fifth-grade level, which is the lowest common denominator, keeping in mind that the average reading level of the population is approximately eighth grade, that more than 20% read below the fifth-grade level, and that fewer than 50% read above the tenth-grade level.

To cover a wide range of reading skills, it is also possible to develop two sets of instructions— one at a higher grade level and one at a lower grade level—and allow patients to select the one they prefer (**Table 7–6**). Once the reading grade level of a piece of written material is determined, it should be printed on the back of the document in coded form as, for example, RL = 7 (reading level = seventh grade), for easy reference.

The literature contains numerous references related to techniques for writing effective educational materials (Aldridge, 2004; Andrus & Roth, 2002; Buxton, 1999; Doak et al., 1996; Doak et al., 1998; Duffy & Snyder, 1999; Horner et al., 2000; Mayer & Rushton, 2002; Monsivais & Reynolds, 2003; Pignone et al., 2005; Weiss, 2003). Recommendations have been put forth for developing written instructions that can be more easily understood by a wide audience.

The strategies described in this section are specific with regard to simplifying written health information for clients with low literacy skills. The key factor in accommodating low-literate readers is to write in plain, familiar language using an easy visual format. The following general guidelines are some basic linguistic,

---

Table 7–6 EXAMPLE OF LOWERED READABILITY LEVEL

NINTH-GRADE LEVEL

Smoking contributes to heart disease in the following ways:

1. When you smoke, you inhale carbon monoxide and nicotine, which causes your blood vessels to narrow, your heart rate to increase, and your blood pressure to go up. All of these factors increase the workload for your heart.

2. Carbon monoxide stimulates your body to produce more red blood cells. The presence of more red cells means that your blood will clot more readily, leading to increased risk of coronary artery disease and stroke.

3. Carbon monoxide and nicotine may also increase your risk of atherosclerotic buildup by causing damage to your artery walls.

4. Smoking raises blood cholesterol level and has been known to cause irregular heartbeats.

FOURTH-GRADE LEVEL

Smoking hurts your heart in many ways:

1. Smoking makes your heart beat faster, raises your blood pressure, and makes your blood vessels smaller. All these things cause your heart to work harder.

2. Smoking makes your blood clot easier. This increases your chance of having a heart attack or a stroke.

3. Smoking makes your cholesterol level go up. It may also damage your blood vessels.

4. Smoking may make your heartbeat less regular.

Source: From Wong, M. (1992, Feb.). Self-care instructions: Do patients understand educational materials? *Focus on Critical Care, 19*(1), 47–49. Reprinted with permission of American Association of Critical-Care Nurses.

motivational, organizational, and content principles to adhere to when writing effective PEMs:

1. Write in a conversational style using the personal pronoun *you* and the possessive pronoun *your*. Use an active voice in the present tense rather than a passive voice in the past or future tense. The message is more personalized, more imperative, more interesting, and easier to understand if instruction is written as "Take your medicine . . ." instead of "Medicine should be taken . . ." This rule is considered to be the most important technique to reduce the level of reading difficulty and to improve comprehension of what is read. Directly addressing the reader through personal words and sentences engages the reader. For example:

LESS EFFECTIVE
People who sunburn easily and have fair skin with red or blond hair are most prone to develop skin cancer. The amount of time spent in the sun affects a person's risk of skin cancer.[1]

MORE EFFECTIVE
If you sunburn easily and have fair skin with red or blond hair, you are more likely to get skin cancer. How much time you spend in the sun affects your risk of skin cancer.

2. Use short words and common vocabulary with only one or two syllables as much as possible. Rely on sight words, known as high-frequency words, which are recognized by almost everyone. The key is to choose words that sound familiar and natural and are easy to read and understand, such as *shot* rather than *injection* and *use* instead of *utilize*. Avoid compound words, such as *lifesaver*, and words with prefixes or suffixes, such as *reoccur* or *emptying*, that create multisyllable words.

Also, try to avoid technical words and medical terms (medicalese), and substitute common, nontechnical, lay terms such as *stroke* instead of *cardiovascular accident*. Be sure to select substitutions carefully, because they may have a different meaning for some people than for others or in one context versus another. For example, if the word *medicine* is replaced with the word *drug*, the latter may be interpreted as the illegal variety. Using modest words is not considered talking down to readers; it is considered talking to them at a more comfortable level.

3. Spell words out rather than using abbreviations or acronyms. *That is* should be used instead of *i.e.* and *for example* instead of *e.g.* Abbreviations for the months of the year (such as Sept.) or the days of the week (Wed., for example) are a real problem for clients with limited vocabulary. Also do not use acronyms, such as CVA or NPO, unless these medical abbreviations are clearly defined beforehand in the text.

4. Organize information into chunks, which improves recall. Also, use numbers sparingly and only when absolutely necessary. Statistics are usually mean-

---

[1] Fry Now, Pay Later, American Cancer Society pamphlet, No. 2611, 1985.

ingless and are another source of confusion for the low-literate reader. Limit the number of items in any list to no more than seven. People have a difficult time remembering more than seven consecutive items (Baddeley, 1994).

5. Keep sentences short, preferably not longer than 20 words and fewer if possible, because they are easier to read and understand for clients with short-term memories or who struggle decoding words of a sentence. Avoid subordinate (dependent) clauses that make the reading more difficult. The use of commas, colons, or dashes result in long, complex sentences that turn off the reader. Titles also should be short and convey the purpose and meaning of the material that follows.

6. Clearly define any technical or unfamiliar words by using parentheses that include simple terms after difficult words—for example, "bacteria (germ)." A glossary that provides definitions of each difficult term is a helpful tool, but it is highly recommended to phonetically spell out terms immediately following the unfamiliar word within the text; for example, "Alzheimer's (pronounced Alts-hi-merz)." If a new technical vocabulary word needs to be introduced, such as diabetes or hypertension, it should be used and repeated frequently (Byrne & Edeani, 1984; Spees, 1991). Standal's (1981) method suggests identifying words whose meanings should be taught to the reader prior to introducing the instructional material to increase reader comprehension and to avoid having to make major revisions to a printed piece.

7. Use words consistently throughout the text and avoid interchanging words. For example, if discussing diet, adhere to the word *diet* rather than substituting other terms for it, such as *meal plan, menu, food schedule,* and *dietary prescription,* which merely confuse readers and can lead to misunderstanding of instruction.

8. Avoid value judgment words with many interpretations, such as *excessive, regularly,* and *frequently.* How much pain or bleeding is excessive? How often is regularly or frequently? Use exact terms to describe what you mean by using, for example, a scale of 1–5 or explaining frequency in terms of minutes, hours, or days. Instead of saying, "drink milk frequently," you should be more specific by stating, "drink three full glasses of milk every day."

9. Put the most important information first by prioritizing the need to know. Place essential messages up front and get rid of extraneous details.

10. Use advance organizers (topic headings or headers) and subheadings. They clue the reader in to what is going to be presented and help focus the reader's attention on the message.

11. Limit the use of connectives such as *however, consequently, even though,* and *in spite of* that lengthen sentences and make them more complex. Also, avoid *and* if it connects two different ideas; instead break the ideas into two sentences.

12. Make the first sentence of a paragraph the topic sentence, and, if possible, make the first word the topic of the sentence. For example:

LESS EFFECTIVE

Even though overexposure to the sun is the leading cause, it isn't necessary to give up the outdoors in order to reduce your chances of developing skin cancer.[1]

MORE EFFECTIVE

Enjoying the outdoors is still possible if you take steps to reduce your risk of skin cancer when in the sun.

OR

Your chance of skin cancer can be reduced even when enjoying the outdoors.

13. Reduce concept density by limiting each paragraph to a simple message or action and include only one idea per sentence. In the following example, the original paragraph contains at least six concepts. As rewritten, the revised paragraph has been reduced to four concepts (and is written using the second person pronoun, which is a much more personalized approach):

ORIGINAL PARAGRAPH

A person who has had a stroke may or may not be able to return to his or her former level of functioning, depending on the extent and location of brain damage. Mental attitude, efforts of the rehabilitation team and the understanding of family and friends also affect the patient's progress. Recovery must be gradual, but it should begin the moment the patient is hospitalized. After the patient is tested to determine the extent of brain damage, rehabilitation such as physical, speech,

and occupational therapy should begin. Family and friends should be told how to handle special problems the stroke victim may have, such as irrational behavior or difficulty communicating.[2]

REVISED PARAGRAPH

Getting back to your normal life after a stroke is an important part of your recovery. Each stroke patient is different. Your progress depends on where and how much your brain is damaged. Getting better will take time. The care you get will begin while you are in the hospital. How you think and feel about what happened to you will help you handle special problems. Also helpful to you is the care given by the nurses, doctors, and others. The support you get from your family and friends is important, too.

14. Keep density of words low by not exceeding 30–40 characters (letters) per line. The number of words in each line is influenced by the size of the font.

15. Allow for plenty of white space in margins, and use generous spacing between paragraphs and double spacing within paragraphs to reduce density. Pages that are not crowded seem less overwhelming to the reader with low-literacy skills.

16. Keep right margins unjustified because the jagged right margins help the reader distinguish one line from another. In this way, the eye does not have to adjust

---

[1] Fry Now, Pay Later, American Cancer Society pamphlet, No. 2611, 1985.

[2] Adapted from American Heart Association (1983). *An Older Person's Guide to Cardiovascular Health,* National Center, 7320 Greenville Avenue, Dallas, TX 75321. The information from this book is not current and is used for illustration purposes only.

to different spacing between letters and words as it does with justified type.

17. Design layouts that encourage eye movement from left to right, as in normal reading. In simple drawings and diagrams, using arrows or circles that give direction is helpful, but do not add too many elements to a schematic.

18. Select a simple type style (serif, Times New Roman, or Courier) and a large font (14 or 16 point size) in the body of the text for ease of reading and to increase motivation to read. A sans serif font (without little hooks at the top and bottom of letters) or other type of clean style should be used only for titles to give style to the page. Avoid *italics,* *fancy lettering,* and ALL CAPITAL letters. Low-literate readers are not fluent with the alphabet and need to look at each letter to recognize a word. To facilitate their decoding of words in titles, headings, and subheadings, use uppercase and lowercase letters, which provide reading cues given by tall and short letters on the type line. Avoid using a large stylized letter to begin a new paragraph, such as:

This looks attractive, but it is confusing to a poor reader who cannot decode the word minus the first letter.

19. Highlight important ideas or key terms with bold type or underlining, but never use all capital letters or italics.

20. If using color, employ it consistently throughout the text to emphasize key points or to organize topics. Color, if applied appropriately, attracts the reader. Red, yellow, and orange are warm colors that are more eye-catching and easier to read than cold colors such as violet, blue, and green. Use bold, solid colors and avoid pastel colors that all look gray to older adults with vision problems, such as cataracts.

21. Create a simple cover page with a title (in uppercase and lowercase lettering) that clearly and succinctly states the topic to be addressed. The title should ideally be one to four words in length.

22. Limit the entire length of a document—the shorter, the better. It should be long enough just to cover the essential, need-to-know information. Too many pages with nice-to-know information will turn off even the most eager and capable reader.

23. Select paper that is attractive and on which the typeface is easy to read. Black print on white paper is most easily read and most economical. Dull finishes reduce the glare of light. Avoid high-gloss paper, which reflects light into the eyes of the reader and is usually too formal and not in harmony with the purpose and informal tone of your message.

24. Use bold line drawings and simple, realistic pictures and diagrams. Basic visuals aid the reader to better understand the text information. Use cartoons judiciously, however, because they can trivialize the message and make it less credible.

Graphic designs that are strictly decorative should never be used because they are distracting and confusing. Also, never superimpose words on a background design because it makes reading the letters of the words very difficult.

Only illustrations that enhance understanding of the text and that relate specifically to the message should be used.

Be careful to use pictures that portray the messages intended. For example, avoid using a picture of a pregnant woman smoking or drinking alcohol because this negative message is dependent on careful reading of the text to correct a faulty impression. The visuals should clearly show only those actions that you want the reader to do and remember. Be sure that visuals do not communicate cultural bias.

Use simple subtitles and captions for each picture. Also, be sure drawings are recognizable to the audience. For instance, if you draw a picture of the lungs, be certain they are within the outline of the person's body to accurately depict the location of the organs. The person with low literacy may not know what they are looking at if the lungs are not put in context with the body's torso. However, pictures do not necessarily make the text easier to read if the readability level remains high.

25. Include a summary section using bullet points or a numbered list to review what has already been presented. A question-and-answer format using the client's point of view is an effective way to summarize information in single units using a conversational style. The following example is adapted from an American Cancer Society pamphlet.[1]

Q: Am I likely to get skin cancer?

A: If you have spent a lot of time in the sun, you have a greater chance of getting skin cancer than people who have stayed out of the strong sunlight. If you sunburn easily, you are at more risk for skin cancer. If you have fair skin with red or blond hair, you are more likely to get skin cancer than people with dark skin.

Q: How can I tell if I have skin cancer?

A: The only way to know for certain is to see your doctor. Your doctor may want to take a sample of skin to test for cancer. If you have a red, scaly patch, a mole that has changed, or an area of the skin that does not heal, see your doctor right away.

Q: How can I prevent skin cancer?

A: Stay out of direct sunlight between 11:00 a.m. and 2:00 p.m. When outside in the sun, cover up with clothing, wear a wide-brimmed hat, and use sunscreens that block out the sun's harmful rays.

Ask for feedback after clients have read your instructions. Either have readers explain the information in their own words or have them demonstrate the desired behavior. If learners can do so correctly, it is a good indication that the information is understood. Do not ask questions such as "Do you understand?" because you are likely to get a "yes" or "no" answer, not a substantive response.

26. Put the reading level (RL) on the back of a PEM for future reference—for example, if the PEM is readable at the sixth-grade level, the designation would be RL6.

27. Determine readability by applying at least two formulas (SMOG, Fog, and

[1] Fry Now, Pay Later, American Cancer Society pamphlet, No. 2611, 1985.

Fry are suggested). Also, you can measure comprehension by applying the cloze or listening test and check reading skills by applying the WRAT, REALM, or TOFHLA.

It does not take a great deal of effort, just know-how and common sense, to improve the readability and comprehensibility of instructional materials (see **Table 7–7** for a summary of tips). The benefits are significant in terms of

---

Table 7–7 SUMMARY OF TIPS FOR DESIGNING EFFECTIVE LOW-LITERACY PRINTED MATERIALS

CONTENT

Clearly define the purpose of the material.
Decide when and how the information will be used.
Use behavioral objectives that cover the main points.
Verify the accuracy of content with experts.
Give "how to" information for the learner to achieve objectives.
Present only the most essential information (three to four main ideas: who, what, where, and when).
Relate new information to what the audience already knows.
Present content relevant to the audience and avoid cultural bias in writing and graphics.

ORGANIZATION

Keep titles short, yet use words that clearly convey the meaning of the content.
Provide a table of contents for lengthy material and a summary to review content presented.
Present the most important information first.
Use topic headings (advance organizers).
Make the first sentence of each paragraph the topic sentence.
Include only a few concepts per paragraph.
Use short, simple sentences that convey only one idea at a time; limit the length of the entire text.
Limit lists to no more than seven items.
Present each idea in logical sequence.

LAYOUT/GRAPHICS

Select large, easily read print (minimum 12-point type) and use nonglossy paper.
Write headings and subheadings in both lowercase and uppercase letters; avoid fancy lettering.
Use bold type or underlining to emphasize important information.
Use lots of white space between segments of information.
Use generous margins and keep right-hand margins unjustified.
Provide a question-and-answer format for patient–nurse interaction.
Select double spacing (between lines of type), type style (serif), and font (print size) for ease of reading.
Design a colorful, eye-catching cover that suggests the message contained in the text.

continues

Table 7-7 SUMMARY OF TIPS FOR DESIGNING EFFECTIVE LOW-LITERACY PRINTED MATERIALS (CONTINUED)

LINGUISTICS

Keep sentences short (ideally 8–10 words, but no more than 20 words).

Write in the active voice, using the present tense and the pronouns *you* and *your* to engage the reader.

Use one- to two-syllable words as much as possible; avoid multisyllabic (polysyllabic) words.

Use words familiar and understandable to the target audience.

Avoid complex grammatical structures (i.e., multiple clauses).

Limit the number of concepts.

Focus content on what the audience should do as well as know.

Use positive statements; avoid negative messages.

Use questions throughout the text to encourage active learning.

Provide examples the audience can use to relate to personal experiences/circumstances.

Avoid using double negatives and value judgment words.

Clearly define terms likely to be unclear to audience.

VISUALS

Include simple, culturally sensitive illustrations and pictures.

Use simple drawings, but only if they improve the understanding of essential information.

Choose illustrations and photographs free of clutter and distractions.

Convey a single message or point of information in each visual.

Use visuals that are relevant to the text and meaningful to the audience.

Use drawings recognizable to the audience that reflect familiar images.

Use adult rather than childlike images (use cartoons sparingly).

Use captions to describe illustrations.

Use cues such as arrows, underlines, circles, and color to give direction to ideas and to highlight the most important information.

Use appealing and appropriate colors for the audience (for older adults, use black and white, and avoid pastel shades, especially blue, green, and violet hues).

READABILITY AND COMPREHENSION

Perform analysis with readability formulas and comprehension tests to determine reading level of material.

Write materials two to four grade levels below the determined literacy level of the audience.

Pilot test the material to determine readability, comprehensibility, and appeal before its widespread use.

Source: Adapted from Bernier, M.J. (1993). Developing and evaluating printed education materials: A prescriptive model for quality. *Orthopedic Nursing, 12*(6), 42, and from papers from the 16th Annual Conference on Patient Education, Nov. 17–20, 1994, Orlando, FL—sponsored by American Academy of Family Physicians and Society of Teachers of Family Medicine.

compliance and quality of care when marginally literate patients are given PEMs that effectively communicate messages they can read and understand.

Always remember to test any new materials before printing and distributing them. Not only will this effort save the cost of printing handouts that might not be useful, but patients will have the opportunity to participate in the evaluative process. Readily understandable materials also reduce time and frustration on the part of the nurse educator and avoid the possibility of litigation when better-quality and more appropriate healthcare instructions are used. The important role of printed media to communicate health information should compel all writers of PEMs to use the techniques recommended in this chapter. As Doak and Doak (1987) so aptly summarize, "With so much to be gained, the investments of a little time and thoughtful attention to the materials provided to patients can pay back dividends too important to ignore" (p. 8).

Teaching Strategies for Clients with Low Literacy

Working with clients who are illiterate and marginally literate requires more than designing simple-to-read instructional literature. It also calls for using alternative and innovative teaching strategies to break down the barriers of illiteracy. Using techniques to improve communication with clients has the potential to greatly enhance their understanding (Mayeaux et al., 1996; Weiss, 2003).

Teaching clients with poor reading skills does not have to be viewed as a problem, but rather can be seen as a challenge (Dunn, Buckwalter, Weinstein, & Palti, 1985). Existing teaching methods

and tools can be adapted to meet the logic, language, and experience of the patient who has difficulty with reading and comprehension (Doak et al., 1998). Incidentally, many literate and highly motivated clients also can benefit from some of these same teaching strategies.

Many authors (Austin, Matlock, Dunn, Kesler, & Brown, 1995; Davis et al., 2002; Doak et al., 1998; Houts et al., 1998; Kessels, 2003; Lerner et al., 2000; Mayeaux et al., 1996; Pignone et al., 2005; Rothman et al., 2004; Schultz, 2002; Webber, Higgins, & Baker, 2001; Weiss, 2003; Winslow, 2001) suggest the following tips as useful strategies for the nurse educator to employ:

1. *Establish a trusting relationship before beginning the teaching–learning process.* Start by getting to know the clients to reduce their anxiety. Because many poor readers have a history of being defensive, the nurse educator must attempt to overcome their defense mechanisms by casting aside communication barriers such as any preconceived notions, including myths and stereotypes. Also, focus on clients' strengths. Demonstrate your belief in them as responsible individuals. Be open and honest about what specifically needs to be learned to build up their confidence in their ability to perform self-care activities. Encourage family and friends to help reinforce the clients' self-confidence. Remember, your role as educator is to facilitate learning by providing guidance and support.

2. *Use the smallest amount of information possible to accomplish the predetermined behavioral objectives.* Stick to the essentials, paring down the information you teach to what the client must learn. Prioritize

behavioral objectives, and select only one or two concepts to present and discuss in any one session. Present the context of the message first before giving any new information. Remember, clients with poor comprehension and reading skills are easily overwhelmed. Information about the history of treatment, general principles, statistics, detailed physiology, and extraneous facts about a topic are not necessary for them to know. Keep teaching sessions short, limiting them to no more than 20–30 minutes, but 15–20 minutes is the ideal time limit.

3. *Make points of information as vivid and explicit as possible.* Explain information in simple, concrete terms using everyday, living-room language. Provide personal examples relevant to the client's background. Visual aids, such as signs and pictographs, should be large with readable print and contain only one or two messages. For example, a sign reading "NOTHING BY MOUTH" or, worse yet, "NPO" should be changed to "Do not eat or drink anything" (remember to avoid using all-capital letters and abbreviations).

   Underlining, highlighting, color coding, arrows, and common international symbols can be used effectively to give directions and draw attention to important information. For example, different-colored signs, pictorial cues, and other visual stimuli, such as strips on the floor tiles that lead to specific areas of the hospital, are valuable for increasing independence and safety.

4. *Teach one step at a time.* Teaching in increments and organizing information into segments of information (chunks) help to reduce anxiety and confusion and give enough time for clients to understand each item before proceeding to the next unit of information. Also, these techniques give clients a sense of order and a chance to ask questions after each block of information has been presented. In addition, you have the opportunity to assess their progress and reward them with words of encouragement, praise, and reinforcement every step of the way. Most importantly, the pacing of instruction allows for more adequate time between sessions for learners to assimilate information.

5. *Use multiple teaching methods and tools requiring fewer literacy skills.* Oral instruction contains cues such as tone, gestures, and expressions that are not found in written materials. However, the spoken word lacks other signals, such as punctuation and capital letters. Therefore, a person with poor reading skills may likely have some trouble with understanding spoken language as well. The listening test, as previously described, can be used to measure comprehension of oral instruction. Another way to test the difficulty level of information presented verbally is to begin by taping a spoken message, then converting it into a written form, and finally applying a readability formula to it.

   Exposing clients to repetition and multiple forms of the same message is highly recommended. Audiotaped instruction, used in combination with other visual resources such as simple lists, pictorials, and videotapes, can help to improve comprehension and reduce learning time. These media forms, as more permanent sources of information, can also be sent home with the client for added reinforcement of health messages. Also, interactive computer programs, which allow clients to proceed at their own pace, can be programmed developmentally to match a user's literacy skill level.

6. *Allow patients the chance to restate information in their own words and to demonstrate any procedures being taught.* Use the teach back or show me method to verify that information shared with the learner was, in fact, understood. Encouraging them to explain something in their own words may take longer and requires patience on the part of the educator, but feedback in this manner can reveal gaps in knowledge or misconceptions of information. Return demonstration, hands-on practice, role-playing real-life situations, and sharing personal stories in dialogue form are communication modes that provide you with feedback as to the client's level of functioning.

Trying to elicit feedback by asking questions does not always work, because people with low literacy skills often do not have the right vocabulary or fluency to explain what they do and do not understand. Remember, do not ask questions that will elicit only a yes or no response. This is because learners will likely respond in the affirmative, even when they have no clue as to what you are talking about, just so they do not have to admit their ignorance.

Furthermore, they are unlikely to ask questions of you for fear of embarrassment at not understanding instructions.

Use open-ended statements, such as "Tell me what you understand about . . . ," to obtain feedback from them to verify their comprehension. Encouraging clients to repeat instructions in their own words or physically demonstrate an activity is an effective approach to verifying what they really understand.

Chew et al. (2004), based on their research, developed the following three questions as a practical and quick method for identifying literacy skills in patients: (1) "How often do you have someone help you read hospital materials?" (2) "How confident are you filling our medical forms by yourself?" and (3) "How often do you have problems learning about your medical condition because of difficulty understanding written information?" They found these three questions to be effective screening tests for inadequate health literacy in patients at the VA preop clinic, but not as effective for detecting patients with marginal health literacy.

7. *Keep motivation high.* It is important to recognize that people with limited literacy may feel like failures when they cannot work through a problem. Reassure them that it is normal to have trouble with new information and that they are doing well. Encouraging them to keep trying and recognizing any progress they make, even if in small increments, is motivating to the slow learner. Rewards—not punishments—are excellent motivators. Sticking to the basics and keeping the information relevant and succinct will maintain a learner's interest and willingness to learn.

8. *Build in coordination of procedures.* A way to facilitate learning is to simplify information by using the principles of tailoring and cuing. *Tailoring* refers to coordinating recommended regimens into the daily schedules of clients rather than forcing them to adjust their lifestyles to these regimens. Otherwise, they may feel that changes are being imposed on them. Tailoring allows new tasks to be associated with old behaviors. It personalizes the message so that instruction is individualized to meet the client's learning needs. For example, coordinating a medication schedule to a patient's mealtimes does not drastically alter everyday lifestyle and tends to increase motivation and compliance. *Cuing* focuses on the appropriate combination of time and situation using prompts and reminders to get a person to perform a routine task. For example, placing medications where they best can be seen on a frequent basis or keeping a simple chart to check off each time a pill is taken serves as a reminder to comply with taking medications as prescribed.

Both of these principles are related to the behavior modification theory and are especially useful techniques to encourage compliance with medications. Because poor readers often cannot decipher schedules, tailoring and cuing can assist them to adhere to time frames.

9. *Use repetition to reinforce information.* Repetition, at appropriate intervals, is a key strategy to use with clients who have low literacy. Each major point made along the way should be reviewed. Therefore, time must be set aside to remind learners of what has come before and to prepare them for what is to follow. But this is time well spent. Repetition, in the form of saying the same thing in different ways, is one of the most powerful tools to help clients understand their situations and learn important self-care measures.

All of these teaching strategies are especially well suited to the individual needs of people with low-literacy skills. As noted earlier, nurses must empower consumers by providing health information that is culturally and linguistically appropriate. Creating an open, trusting, and accepting environment that makes it acceptable for the client to say "I don't understand" is the cornerstone of effective communication (Cole, 2000).

It is always a challenge to teach clients who, because of illness or a threat to their well-being, may be anxious, frightened, depressed, in denial, or in pain. Teaching patients, in particular, is even more of a special challenge in today's healthcare environment, when varying degrees of literacy compound the ability of a significant portion of the adult population to understand information vital to their health and welfare.

State of the Evidence

In 1999, the Ad Hoc Committee on Health Literacy for the Council on Scientific Affairs of the American Medical Association acknowledged that, although a great deal had been learned to that date about the magnitude and consequences of the problem of illiteracy and low literacy, further research efforts had to focus on four areas:

1. Literacy screening
2. Methods of health education
3. Medical outcomes and economic costs
4. Understanding the causal pathway of how health literacy influences health status

The committee also called for healthcare policies to address the issue of health literacy for the following reasons:

1. Low-literate patients cannot be empowered consumers in a market-driven healthcare system.
2. Patients who cannot understand healthcare instructions will not receive quality health care.
3. Healthcare professionals are subject to liability for adverse outcomes by patients who do not understand important health information.
4. Clinical management problems likely result in substantial but avoidable costs for the U.S. healthcare system.
5. Health literacy problems are more prevalent in certain populations (Medicare beneficiaries, Medicaid recipients, and uninsured individuals).

Indeed, as a result of the findings of the NALS and NAAL reports, a broad policy agenda on health literacy has been put forth in the 10-year goals and objectives of *Healthy People 2010* (U.S. Department of Health and Human Services, 2003). Specifically, objective 11-2 (Improvement of Health Literacy) addresses three major health literacy initiatives: prevention measures, interaction activities between healthcare providers and clients, and navigation of the healthcare system. Although the literacy and verbal skills of individuals is a concern of critical importance, so too are the demands made by PEMs, the need to improve communication skills of health professionals, and the need to make the healthcare system less complex.

The specific reports by the Institute of Medicine (IOM), the Agency for Healthcare Research and Quality (AHRQ), and the American Medical Association (AMA), all released in 2004, recognized that health literacy is a key priority in transforming the U.S. healthcare system (Aldridge, 2004; Weiss et al., 2005). In particular, AHRQ examined the relationship between literacy and adverse outcomes as well as interventions to improve outcomes for people who are low literate (Pignone et al., 2005).

The interest in the literacy problem has escalated tremendously in the past 5–10 years and numerous research studies have been conducted to examine many aspects of the problem. Pignone et al. (2005) conducted a systematic review of intervention studies designed to improve health outcomes of clients with low health literacy. These authors called for further research to understand the types of interventions that would be most effective and efficient. Also, Williams et al. (2002) examined patient–physician communication as a critical factor affecting health outcomes. These researchers, noted experts in the field of health literacy, have called for additional research on the optimal methods for interacting with people who have limited literacy skills. Nursing research must specifically focus on nurse–client interaction techniques that improve understanding of health information, which would lead to a higher level of motivation and compliance.

Baker et al. (1998) studied health literacy and the risk of increased hospital admissions. They called for further research that would lead to a more accurate assessment of the impact of low literacy on healthcare costs. If the consequences of inadequate literacy result in poorer health outcomes and higher costs for health care, then this would be an incentive for all types of payers to develop education programs to better reach patients with different levels of reading ability.

However, it is not yet well understood if health education materials for clients with low literacy do, in fact, improve health outcomes. In addition, more evidence is needed on the benefits of nonprint media, such as videos, audiotapes, and computers, in helping clients to overcome barriers of health illiteracy to improve their quality of life. In addition, much more attention must be paid to the ethical and legal implications of providing education materials to clients with limited literacy skills that are suitable to meet their health information needs. Nurses, in the role of educators, must empirically explore teaching and learning approaches to find those most effective in working with clients who suffer the burden of illiteracy and low literacy.

Summary

The ability to learn from health instruction varies for clients, depending on such factors as educational background, motivational levels, reading and comprehension skills, and readability level of the materials used for instruction. The prevalence of functional illiteracy and low literacy is a major problem in the adult population of this country. Nurses in the role of educators serve as communicators and interpreters of health information. They must always be alert to the potentially limited capacity of their clients to grasp the meaning of written and oral instruction. Nurse educators need to know how to identify clients with literacy problems, assess their needs, and choose appropriate interventions that create a supportive environment directed toward helping those with poor reading and comprehension skills to better and more safely

care for themselves. An awareness of the incidence of illiteracy, the populations most at risk, and the effects that literacy levels have on motivation and compliance with self-management regimens are key to understanding the barriers to communication between nurses and clients.

The first half of this chapter focused on the magnitude of the illiteracy problem, the myths and stereotypes associated with poor literacy skills, the assessment of variables affecting reading and comprehension of information, and the readability levels of patient education materials. The remainder of the chapter examined in detail the measurement tools available to test for readability, comprehension, and reading skills, guidelines for writing and evaluating education materials, and specific teaching strategies to be used to match the logic, language, and experience of clients with literacy problems.

Data suggest that written materials are an important source of health information to reinforce and complement other methods and tools of instruction. PEMs are the most cost-effective and time-efficient means to communicate health messages, but research suggests that there is a large discrepancy between the average comprehension and reading skills of clients and the readability level of current written instructional aids. Unless this gap is narrowed, printed sources of information will serve no useful purpose for adults who suffer with illiteracy and low literacy.

Removing the barriers to communication between clients and healthcare providers offers an ideal opportunity for nurse educators to function as facilitators and work collaboratively with other health professionals to improve the quality of care delivered to consumers. It is our mandated responsibility to teach in understandable terms so that clients we serve can fully benefit from our nursing interventions.

REVIEW QUESTIONS

1. What are the definitions of the terms *literacy, illiteracy, low literacy, functional illiteracy,* and *health literacy*?
2. Approximately how many millions of Americans are considered to be illiterate or functionally illiterate? This represents what percentage of the U.S. population?
3. Why are the rates of low literacy and illiteracy potentially on the rise in the United States?
4. Why is the number of years of schooling a poor indicator of someone's literacy level?
5. What segments of the U.S. population are more likely to be at risk for having poor reading and comprehension skills?
6. Why are problems with low literacy and functional illiteracy greater in older adults than in younger age groups?
7. What are three common myths about people who are illiterate?
8. What are seven clues that clients who are illiterate may demonstrate?
9. What impact does illiteracy or low literacy have on a person's level of motivation and compliance?
10. How does reliance on printed education materials to supplement teaching pose an ethical or legal liability for nurse educators?
11. Which measurement tools (formulas and standardized tests) are used specifically to test readability, comprehension, and reading skills?
12. What are 10 general guidelines to simplify written educational materials for clients with low literacy skills?
13. What 5 teaching strategies can be used by the nurse educator to make health information more understandable for clients with poor reading and comprehension skills?

References

Ad Hoc Committee on Health Literacy for the Council on Scientific Affairs, American Medical Association. (1999). Health literacy: Report of the Council on Scientific Affairs. *Journal of the American Medical Association, 281*(6), 552–557.

Aldridge, M. D. (2004). Writing and designing readable patient education materials. *Nephrology Nursing Journal, 31*(4), 373–377.

Andrus, M. R., & Roth, M. T. (2002). Health literacy: A review. *Pharmacotherapy, 22*(3), 282–302.

Austin, P. E., Matlock, R., Dunn, K. A., Kesler, C., & Brown, C. K. (1995). Discharge instructions: Do illustrations help our patients understand them? *Annals of Emergency Medicine, 25*(3), 317–320.

Baddeley, A. (1994). The magical number seven: Still magic after all these years? *Psychological Review, 101*(2), 353–356.

Baker, D. W., Parker, R. M., Williams, M. V., & Clark, W. S. (1998). Health literacy and the risk of hospital admission. *Journal of General Internal Medicine, 13,* 791–798.

Baker, D. W., Williams, M. V., Parker, R. M., Gazmararian, J. A., & Nurss, J. (1999). Development of a brief test to measure functional health literacy. *Patient Education and Counseling, 38*, 33–42.

Bastable, L. C., Chojnowski, D., Goldberg, L., McGurl, P., & Riegel, B. (2005). Comparing heart failure patient literacy levels with available educational materials. Poster presentation at the Heart Failure Society of America, 9th Annual Scientific Conference, September 18–21, 2005, Boca Raton, FL.

Belton, A. B. (1991). Reading levels of patients in a general hospital. *Beta Release, 15*(1), 21–24.

Bernier, M. J. (1993). Developing and evaluating printed education materials: A prescriptive model for quality. *Orthopedic Nursing, 12*(6), 39–46.

Borrayo, E. A. (2004). Where's Maria? A video to increase awareness about breast cancer and mammography screening among low-literacy Latinas. *Preventive Medicine, 39*, 99–110.

Brownson, K. (1998). Education handouts: Are we wasting our time? *Journal for Nurses in Staff Development, 14*(4), 176–182.

Buxton, T. (1999). Effective ways to improve health education materials. *Journal of Health Education, 30*(1), 47–50, 61.

Byrne, T., & Edeani, D. (1984). Knowledge of medical terminology among hospital patients. *Nursing Research, 33*(3), 178–181.

Center for Health Care Strategies. (2003). *Impact of low health literacy skills on annual health care expenditures.* Retrieved July 16, 2003, from www.chcs.org

Chew, L. D., Bradley, K. A., & Boyko, E. J. (2004). Brief questions to identify patients with inadequate health literacy. *Family Medicine, 36*(8), 588–594.

Cole, M. R. (2000). The high risk of low literacy. *Nursing Spectrum, 13*(10), 16–17.

Conlin, K. K., & Schumann, L. (2002). Literacy in the health care system: A study on open heart surgery patients. *Journal of the American Academy of Nurse Practitioners, 14*(1), 38–42.

Cutilli, C. C. (2005). Do your patients understand? Determining your patient's health literacy skills. *Orthopaedic Nursing, 24*(5), 372–377.

Dale, E., & Chall, J. S. (1978). The cloze procedure: Measuring the readability of selected patient education materials. *Health Education, 9*, 8–10.

Darling, S. (2004, Spring). Family literacy: Meeting the needs of at-risk families. *Phi Kappa Phi Forum,* 18–21.

Davidhizar, R. E., & Brownson, K. (1999). Literacy, cultural diversity, and client education. *Health Care Manager, 18*(1), 39–47.

Davis, T. C., Long, S. W., Jackson, R. H., Mayeaux, E. J., George, R. B., Murphy, P. W. et al. (1993). Rapid estimate of adult literacy in medicine: A shortened screening instrument. *Family Medicine, 25*(6), 391–395.

Davis, T. C., Michielutte, R., Askov, E. N., Williams, M. V., Weiss, B. D. (1998). Practical assessment of adult literacy in health care. *Health Education & Behavior, 25*(5), 613–624.

Davis, T. C., Williams, M. V., Marin, E., Parker, R. M., & Glass, J. (2002). Health literacy and cancer communication. *CA: A Cancer Journal for Clinicians, 52*(3), 134–151.

Doak, C. C., Doak, L. G., Friedell, G. H., & Meade, C. D. (1998). Improving comprehension for cancer patients with low literacy skills: Strategies for clinicians. *CA: A Cancer Journal for Clinicians, 48*(3), 151–162.

Doak, C. C., Doak, L. G., & Root, J. H. (1985). *Teaching patients with low literacy skills.* Philadelphia: Lippincott.

Doak, C. C., Doak, L. G., & Root, J. H. (1996). *Teaching patients with low literacy skills* (2nd ed.). Philadelphia: Lippincott.

Doak, L. G., & Doak, C. C. (1987, July/August). Lowering the silent barriers to compliance for patients with low literacy skills. *Promoting Health,* 6–8.

Duffy, M. M., & Snyder, K. (1999). Can ED patients read your patient education materials? *Journal of Emergency Nursing, 25*(4), 294–297.

Dunn, M. M., Buckwalter, K. C., Weinstein, L. B., & Palti, H. (1985). Teaching the illiterate client does not have to be a problem. *Family & Community Health, 8*(3), 76–80.

Feldman, S. (1997). Passing on failure: Social promotion is not the way to help children who have fallen behind. *American Educator, 21*(3), 4–10.

Fetter, M. S. (1999). Recognizing and improving health literacy. *MEDSURG Nursing, 8*(4), 226.

Fisher, E. (1999). Low literacy levels in adults: Implications for patient education. *Journal of Continuing Education in Nursing, 30*(2), 56–61.

Fleener, F. T., & Scholl, J. F. (1992). Academic characteristics of self-identified illiterates. *Perceptual and Motor Skills, 74*(3), 739–744.

Flesch, R. (1948). A new readability yardstick. *Journal of Applied Psychology, 32*(3), 221–233.

Foltz, A., & Sullivan, J. (1998). Get real: Clinical testing of patients' reading abilities. *Cancer Nursing, 21*(3), 162–166.

French, K. S., & Larrabee, J. H. (1999). Relationships among educational material readability, client literacy, perceived beneficence, and perceived quality. *Journal of Nursing Care Quality, 13*(6), 68–82.

Fry, E. (1968). A readability formula that saves time. *Journal of Reading, 11*, 513–516, 575–579.

Fry, E. (1977). Fry's readability graph: Clarifications, validity, and extension to level 17. *Journal of Reading, 21*, 242–252.

Gazmararian, J. A., Baker, D. W., Williams, M. V., Parker, R. M., Scott, T. L., Green, D. C., et al. (1999). Health literacy among Medicare enrollees in a managed care organization. *JAMA, 281*(6), 545–551.

Gazmararian, J. A., Curran, J. W., Parker, R. M., Bernhardt, J. M., & DeBuono, B. A. (2005). Public health literacy in America: An ethical perspective. *American Journal of Preventive Medicine, 28*(3), 317–322.

Giorgianni, S. J. (Ed.). (1998). Perspectives on health care and biomedical research: Responding to the challenge of health literacy. *The Pfizer Journal, 2*(1), 1–37.

Gunning, R. (1968). The Fog index after 20 years. *Journal of Business Communications, 6*, 3–13.

Hayes, K. S. (2000). Literacy for health information of adult patients and caregivers in a rural emergency department. *Clinical Excellence for Nurse Practitioners, 4*(1), 35–40.

Hess, V. T. (1998). Literacy and learning for hospital employees. *Journal for Nurses in Staff Development, 14*(3), 143–146.

Hirsch, E. D. (2001). Overcoming the language gap. *American Educator, 4*, 6–7.

Horner, S. D., Surratt, D., & Juliusson, S. (2000). Improving readability of patient education materials. *Journal of Community Health Nursing, 17*(1), 15–23.

Houts, P. S., Bachrach, R., Witmer, J. T., Tringali, C. A., Bucher, J. A., & Localio, R. A. (1998). Using pictographs to enhance recall of spoken medical instructions. *Patient Education and Counseling, 35*, 83–88.

Hussey, L. C., & Guilliland, K. (1989). Compliance, low literacy, and locus of control. *Nursing Clinics of North America, 24*(3), 605–611.

Institute of Medicine. (2004). *IOM report calls for national effort to improve health literacy.* Retrieved July 1, 2007, from http://www4.nationalacademies.org/news

Joint Commission on Accreditation of Healthcare Organizations. (1993). *Accreditation manuals for hospitals—1993.* Chicago: JCAHO.

Kalichman, S. C., Ramachandran, B., & Catz, S. (1999). Adherence to combination antiretroviral therapies in HIV patients of low health literacy. *Journal of General Internal Medicine, 14*, 267–273.

Kanonowicz, L. (1993). National project to publicize link between literacy, health. *Canadian Medical Association Journal, 148*(7), 1201–1202.

Kefalides, P. T. (1999). Illiteracy: The silent barrier to health care. *Annals of Internal Medicine, 130*(4), 333–336.

Kessels, R. P. C. (2003). Patients' memory for medical information. *Journal of the Royal Society of Medicine, 96*, 219–222.

Kogut, B. H. (2004, Spring). Why adult literacy matters. *Phi Kappa Phi Forum*, 26–28.

Koo, M. M., Krass, I., & Aslani, P. (2005). Patient characteristics influencing evaluation of written medicine information: Lessons for patient education. *Annals of Pharmacotherapy, 39*(9), 1434–1440.

Kutner, M., Greenberg, E., Jin, Y., & Paulsen, C. (2006, September). *The Health Literacy of America's Adults: Results from the 2003 National Assessment of Adult Literacy*, from http://nces.ed.gov, retrieved July 1, 2007.

Lasater, L., & Mehler, P. S. (1998). The illiterate patient: Screening and management. *Hospital Practice, 33*(4), 163–165, 169–170.

Lerner, E. B., Jehle, D. V. K., Janicke, D. M., & Moscati, R. M. (2000). Medical communication: Do our patients understand? *American Journal of Emergency Medicine, 18*(7), 764–766.

Ley, P. (1979). Memory for medical information. *British Journal of Social and Clinical Psychology, 18*(2), 245–255.

Ley, P., & Florio, T. (1996). The use of readability formulas in health care. *Psychology, Health & Medicine, 1*(1), 7–28.

Loughrey, L. (1983). Dealing with the illiterate patient . . . You can't read him like a book. *Nursing, 13*(1), 65–67.

Mayeaux, E. J., Murphy, P. W., Arnold, C., Davis, T. C., Jackson, R. H., & Sentell, T. (1996). Improving patient education for patients with low literacy skills. *American Family Physician, 53*(1), 205–211.

Mayer, G. G., & Rushton, N. (2002). Writing easy-to-read teaching aids. *Nursing 2002, 32*(3), 48–49.

McLaughlin, G. H. (1969). SMOG—grading: A new readability formula. *Journal of Reading, 12,* 639–646.

Meade, C. D., & Smith, C. F. (1991). Readability formulas: Cautions and criteria. *Patient Education and Counseling, 17,* 153–158.

Miller, B., & Bodie, M. (1994). Determination of reading comprehension level for effective patient health-education materials. *Nursing Research, 43*(2), 118–119.

Monsivais, D., & Reynolds, A. (2003). Developing and evaluating patient education materials. *The Journal of Continuing Education in Nursing, 34*(4), 172–176.

Montalto, N. J., & Spiegler, G. E. (2001). Functional health literacy in adults in a rural community health center. *The West Virginia Medical Journal, 97*(2), 111–114.

Myers, R. E., & Shepard-White, F. (2004). Evaluation of adequacy of reading level and readability of psychotropic medication handouts. *Journal of the American Psychiatric Nurses Association, 10,* 55–59.

Nath, C. R., Sylvester, S. T., Yasek, V., & Gunel, E. (2001). Development and validation of a literacy assessment tool for persons with diabetes. *The Diabetes Educator, 27*(6), 857–864.

National Center for Education Statistics. (1993). *Adult Literacy in America: National Adult Literacy Survey.* Washington, DC: U.S. Department of Education.

National Center for Education Statistics. (2006). *National Assessment of Adult Literacy (NAAL): Health Literacy Component.* Retrieved April 29, 2006, from http://nces.ed.gov/NAAL/index.asp?file=highlights/healthliteracyfactsheet.asp

Nurss, J. R., El-Kebbi, I. M., Gallina, D. L., Ziemer, D. C., Musey, V. C., Lewis, S., et al. (1997). Diabetes in urban African Americans: Functional health literacy of municipal hospital outpatients with diabetes. *The Diabetes Educator, 23*(5), 563–568.

Osborne, H. (1999). In other words . . . Getting through . . . Lives can depend on simplifying the written word. *On-Call, 2*(9), 42–43.

Paasche-Orlow, M. K., Taylor, H. A., & Brancati, F. L. (2003). Readability standards for informed-consent forms as compared with actual readability. *New England Journal of Medicine, 348*(8), 721–726.

Parker, R., Baker, D., Williams, M., & Nurss, J. (1995). The test of functional health literacy in adults (TOFHLA): A new instrument for measuring patients' literacy skills. *Journal of General Internal Medicine, 10,* 537–545.

Pichert, J. W., & Elam, P. (1985). Readability formulas may mislead you. *Patient Education and Counseling, 7,* 181–191.

Pignone, B. D., DeWalt, D. A., Sheridan, S., Berkman, N., & Lohr, K. W. (2005). Interventions to improve health outcomes for patients with low literacy. *Journal of Internal Medicine, 20,* 185–192.

Purnell, L. D., & Paulanka, B. J. (2003). *Transcultural health care: A culturally competent approach* (2nd ed.). Philadelphia: F.A. Davis.

Quirk, P. A. (2000). Screening for literacy and readability: Implications for the advanced practice nurse. *Clinical Nurse Specialist, 14*(1), 26–32.

Robinson, J. H. (2000). Increasing students' cultural sensitivity: A step towards greater diversity in nursing. *Nurse Educator, 25*(3), 131–135, 144.

Rothman, R. L., DeWalt, D. A., Malone, R., Bryant, B., Shantani, A., Crigler, B., et al. (2004). Influence of patient literacy on the effectiveness of a primary care-based diabetes disease management program. *JAMA, 292*(14), 1711–1716.

Santrock, J. W. (2006). *Life-span development* (10th ed.). Boston: McGraw-Hill.

Schillinger, D., Grumbach, K., Piette, J., Wang, F., Osmond, D., Daher, C., et al. (2002). Association of health literacy with diabetes outcomes. *JAMA, 288*(4), 475–482.

Schultz, M. (2002). Low literacy skills needn't hinder care. *RN, 65*(4), 45–48.

Schwartzberg, J., VanGeest, J., & Wang, C. (Eds.). (2004). *Understanding health literacy: Inspirations for medicine and public health.* Chicago: American Medical Association Press.

Spache, G. (1953). A new readability formula for primary-grade reading materials. *Elementary School Journal, 53*(7), 410–413.

Spadero, D. C. (1983). Assessing readability of patient information materials. *Pediatric Nursing, 9*(4), 274–278.

Spadero, D. C., Robinson, L. A., & Smith, L. T. (1980). Assessing readability of patient information materials. *American Journal of Hospital Pharmacy, 37,* 215–221.

Spees, C. M. (1991). Knowledge of medical terminology among clients and families. *Image: Journal of Nursing Scholarship, 23*(4), 225–229.

Standal, T. C. (1981). How to use readability formulas more effectively. *Social Education, 45,* 183–186.

U.S. Department of Health and Human Services. (2000). *Healthy People 2010* (Vol. II). Washington, DC: U.S. Government Printing Office.

U.S. Department of Health and Human Services. (2003). *Community Health: Priorities and Strategies for Success.* Washington, DC: Office of Disease Prevention and Health Promotion. Retrieved April 6, 2004, from http://odphp.osophs.dhhs .gov/projects/healthcomm/

Vander Zanden, J. W., Crandell, T. L., & Crandell, C. H. (2007). *Human Development* (8th ed.). Boston: McGraw-Hill.

Wallerstein, N. (1992). Health and safety education for workers with low-literacy or limited-English skills. *American Journal of Industrial Medicine, 22*(5), 751–765.

Webber, D., Higgins, L., & Baker, V. (2001). Enhancing recall of information from a patient education booklet: A trial using cardiomyopathy patients. *Patient Education and Counseling, 44,* 263–270.

Wedgeworth, R. (2007). Fundraising letter. Syracuse, NY: ProLiteracy Worldwide,

Weiss, B. D. (2003). *Health literacy: A manual for clinicians.* Chicago: American Medical Association and American Medical Association Foundation.

Weiss, B. D., Mays, M. Z., Martz, W., Castro, K. M., DeWalt, D. A., Pignone, M. A., et al. (2005). Quick assessment of literacy in primary care. *Annals of Family Medicine, 3*(8), 514–522.

Williams, D. M., Counselman, F. L., & Caggiano, C. D. (1996). Emergency department discharge instructions and patient literacy: A problem of disparity.

American Journal of Emergency Medicine, 14(1), 19–22.

Williams, M. V., Baker, D. W., Honig, E. C., Lee, T. M., & Nowlan, A. (1998). Inadequate literacy is a barrier to asthma knowledge and self-care. *Chest, 114*(4), 1008–1015.

Williams, M. V., Baker, D. W., Parker, R. M., & Nurss, J. R. (1998, January 26). Relationship of functional health literacy to patients' knowledge of their chronic disease. *Archives of Internal Medicine, 158,* 166–172.

Williams, M. V., Davis, T., Parker, R. M., & Weiss, B. D. (2002). The role of health literacy in patient-physician communication. *Family Medicine, 34*(5), 383–389.

Williams, M. V., Parker, R. M., Baker, D. W., Parikh, W. S., Pitkin, K., Coates, W. C., et al. (1995). Inadequate functional health literacy among patients at two public hospitals. *Journal of the American Medical Association, 274*(21), 1677–1682.

Winslow, E. H. (2001). Patient education materials: Can patients read them, or are they ending up in the trash? *American Journal of Nursing, 101*(10), 33–38.

Wood, F. G. (2005). Health literacy in a rural clinic. *Journal of Rural Nursing and Health Care, 5*(1). Retrieved July 27, 2006, from http://www.rno .org/journal/issues/Vol-5/issue-1/wood_article .htm

Wood, M. R., Kettinger, C. A., & Lessick, M. (2007). Knowledge is power: How nurses can promote health literacy. *Nursing for Women's Health, 11*(2), 180–188.

Zarcadoolas, C., Pleasant, A. F., & Greer, D. J. (2006). *Advancing health literacy: A framework for understanding and action.* San Francisco: Jossey-Bass.

Ziegler, J. (1998). How literacy drives up health care costs. *Business & Health, 16*(4), 53–54.

Chapter 8

Gender, Socioeconomic, and Cultural Attributes of the Learner

Susan B. Bastable

CHAPTER HIGHLIGHTS

Gender Characteristics
    Cognitive Abilities
    Personality Traits
Socioeconomic Characteristics
    Teaching Strategies
Cultural Characteristics
    Definition of Terms
    Assessment Models for the Delivery of Culturally
      Sensitive Care
    General Assessment and Teaching Interventions
    Use of Translators

The Four Major Ethnic Groups
    Hispanic/Latino Culture
    Black/African American Culture
    Asian/Pacific Islander Culture
    American Indian/Alaskan Native
      Culture
Preparing Nurses for Diversity Care
Stereotyping: Identifying the Meaning,
    the Risks, and the Solutions
State of the Evidence

KEY TERMS

- ❑ gender-related cognitive abilities
- ❑ gender-related personality behaviors
- ❑ gender gap
- ❑ gender bias
- ❑ socioeconomic status (SES)
- ❑ poverty circle (cycle of poverty)
- ❑ acculturation
- ❑ assimilation
- ❑ cultural awareness
- ❑ cultural competence

- ❑ cultural diversity
- ❑ cultural relativism
- ❑ culture
- ❑ ethnic group
- ❑ ethnocentrism
- ❑ ideology
- ❑ subculture
- ❑ transcultural
- ❑ primary characteristics of culture
- ❑ secondary characteristics of culture

❑ cultural encounter
❑ spirituality
❑ religiosity
❑ stereotyping

❑ cultural assessment
❑ worldview
❑ cultural knowledge
❑ cultural skill

OBJECTIVES

After completing this chapter, the reader will be able to

1. Identify gender-related characteristics in the learner based on social and hereditary influences on brain functioning, cognitive abilities, and personality traits.
2. Recognize the influence of socioeconomics in determining health status and health behaviors.
3. Define the various terms associated with diversity.
4. Examine cultural assessment from the perspective of different models of care.
5. Distinguish between the beliefs and customs of the four predominant ethnic groups in the United States.
6. Suggest teaching strategies specific to the needs of learners belonging to each of the four ethnic groups.
7. Examine ways in which transcultural nursing can serve as a framework for meeting the learning needs of various ethnic populations.
8. Identify the meaning of stereotyping, the risks involved, and ways to avoid stereotypical behavior.

Gender, socioeconomic level, and cultural background have a significant influence on a learner's willingness and ability to respond to and make use of the teaching–learning situation. Two of these factors—gender and socioeconomic status—have been given very little attention to date by nurse educators. The third factor, cultural and ethnic diversity, has been the focus of considerable study in recent years with respect to its effects on learning. Understanding diversity, particularly those variations among learners related to gender, socioeconomics, and culture, is of major importance when designing and implementing education programs to meet the needs of an increasingly unique population of learners.

This chapter explores how individuals respond differently to healthcare interventions through examination of gender-related variations resulting from heredity or social conditioning that affects how the brain functions for learning. Secondly, the influence of environment on the learner from a socioeconomic viewpoint is examined. Thirdly, consideration is given to the significant effects cultural norms have on the behaviors of learners from the perspective of the four major ethnic groups in the United States. In addition, models for cultural assessment and the planning of care are highlighted. This chapter also includes ways to prepare nurses for diversity care and to deal with the issue of stereotyping.

Gender Characteristics

Most of the information on gender variations with respect to learning can be found in the educational psychology and neuroscience literature. Nursing literature contains scant information about this subject from a teaching–learning perspective. There are, however, characteristics of male and female orientations that affect learning, which need to be addressed more closely. Two well-established facts exist. First, individual differences within a group of males or females are usually greater than differences between groups of males versus groups of females. Second, studies that compare the sexes seldom are able to separate genetic differences from environmental influences on behavior (Santrock, 2006; Vander Zanden, Crandell, & Crandell, 2007).

There remains a gap in knowledge of what the sexes would be like if humans were not subject to behavioral conditioning. No person can survive outside a social matrix, and, therefore, individuals begin to be shaped by their environment right from birth. For example, our U.S. culture exposes girls and boys, respectively, to pink and blue blankets in the nursery, dolls and trucks in preschool, ballet and basketball in the elementary grades, and cheerleading and football in high school. These social influences continue to affect the sexes throughout the life span.

Of course, men and women are different. But the question is: are they different or the same when it comes to learning, and to what can the differences and similarities be attributed? Biological and behavioral scientists have, to date, been unable to quantify the exact impact that genetics and environment have on the brain. Opinions are rampant, and research findings are inconclusive.

To date, there has been a great divide between neuroscience and education. What is needed is multidisciplinary research to bridge the gap in the discoveries being made in cognitive science laboratories and the application of this information to teaching in the real world. To address this need, the National Science Foundation in 2005 pledged $90 million in grants over 5 years to support four teams of cognitive neuroscientists, psychologists, computer scientists, and educationalists to "give the craft of teaching a solid scientific underpinning" (Gura, 2005, p. 1156). By discovering how the brain works in learning, teaching methods and tools can be designed "to complement the brain's natural development" (Gura, 2005, p. 1156). This is "a massive effort to put the way children are taught on a sounder scientific footing" (Gura, 2005, p. 1156).

The fact remains that there are gender differences as to how males and females act, react, and perform in situations affecting every aspect of life (Cahill, 2006). As Cahill contends, the issue of gender influences is much too important to be ignored or marginalized. The national Academy of Sciences reports "sex does matter in ways that we did not expect. Undoubtedly, it matters in ways that we have not yet begun to imagine" (Cahill, 2006, p. 7).

For example, when it comes to human relationships, intuitively women tend to pick up subtle tones of voice and facial expressions, whereas men tend to be less sensitive to these communication cues. In navigation, women tend to have difficulty finding their way, while men seem to have a better sense of direction. In cognition, females tend to excel in languages and verbalization, and men are likely to demonstrate stronger spatial abilities and interest in mathematical problem solving. Scientists are beginning to believe that gender differences have as much to do with the biology of the brain as with the way people are raised (Baron-Cohen,

2005; Gorman, 1992). Kimura (1999) reported on the many different patterns of behavior and cognition between men and women that are thought to be due to varying hormonal influences on brain development.

Some would argue that these examples are representative of stereotyping. But as generalizations, these statements seem to hold some truth. Neuroscientists have begun to detect structural as well as functional differences in the brains of males and females. These early findings have led to an upsurge in neuroscience research into the mental lives of men and women (Baron-Cohen, 2005).

Neurobiologists are just at the dawn of understanding how the human brain works and exactly the types of sensory input that wire the brain and how that input affects it. Scientists suspect that cognitive abilities work much like sensory ones in that they are promoted by those activities and experiences to which a person is exposed right from birth. Circuits in different regions of the brain are thought to mature at different stages of development. These circuits are critical windows of opportunity at different ages for the learning of math, music, language, and emotion.

Brain development is much more sensitive to life experiences than once believed (Begley, 1996; Hancock, 1996). A baby's brain is like "a work in progress, trillions of neurons waiting to be wired . . . to be woven into the intricate tapestry of the mind" (Begley, 1996, pp. 55–56). Some of the neurons of the brain have been hard wired by genes, but trillions more have almost infinite potential and are waiting to be connected by the influence of environment. The first 3 years of life, it is being discovered, are crucial in the development of the mind. The wiring of the brain, a process both of nature and

nurture, dubbed the "dual sculptors," forms the connections that determine the ability to learn and the interest for learning different types of skills (Harrigan, 2007; Nash, 1997).

Thanks to modern technology, imaging machines are revolutionizing the field of neuroscience. Functional magnetic resonance imaging (fMRI) and positron emission tomography (PET) are being used to observe human brains in the very act of thinking, feeling, or remembering (Kawamura, Midorikawa, & Kezuka, 2000; Monastersky, 2001; Speck et al., 2000; Yee et al., 2000). Amazing discoveries through brain scanning have been made, such as where the emotion of love resides in the brain. Although machines can measure the brain's blood flow that supports nerve activity, no machines have been developed to date that can read or interpret a person's thoughts. The field of brain scanning still has far to go, but experts consider its potential to be incredible.

The trend in current studies is to focus on how separate parts of the brain interact while performing different tasks rather than focusing on only isolated regions of the brain associated with certain tasks (Monastersky, 2001). Researchers have already reported that men and women use different clusters of neurons when they read than when their brains are idling. For example, Kawamura and colleagues (2000) focused on the cerebral localization of the center for reading and writing music of a male patient. They concluded that the left side of the brain is involved in this type of task, just as it is in an individual's ability to read and write language.

Also, gender differences in brain activity during working memory—an important component for performing many higher functions—have been examined with fMRI. For example, in a study of verbal working memory by Speck et al.

(2000), the amount of brain activity increased with task difficulty. Interestingly, male subjects demonstrated more right-sided hemispheric dominance, whereas females showed more left-sided hemispheric dominance, with higher accuracy and slightly slower reaction times than their male counterparts. The results revealed significant gender differences in the functional brain organization for working memory.

In general, the brains of men and women seem to operate differently. Provocative new studies are revealing that women engage more of their brains when thinking sad thoughts. When men and women subjects were asked to conjure up sad memories, the front of the limbic system in the brain of women glowed with activity eight times more than in men. Although men and women were able to perform equally well in math problems, tests indicated that they seemed to use the temporal lobes of the brain differently to figure out problems. Also, it has been found that men and women employ different parts of their brains to figure out rhymes. These results are just a few examples of some of the tentative, yet tantalizing, findings from research that are beginning to show that male and female identity is a creation of both nature and nurture. Along with genetics, life experiences and the choices men and women make in the course of a lifetime help to mold personal characteristics and determine gender differences in the very way the sexes think, sense, and respond (Begley, Murr, & Rogers, 1995).

In comparing how men and women feel, act, process information, and perform on cognitive tests, scientists have been able to identify only a few gender differences in the actual brain structure of humans (**Table 8–1**). Most differences that have been uncovered are quite small, as measured statistically. Even the largest differences in *gender-related cognitive abilities* are not as significant as, for example, the disparity found between male and female height. There seems to be, in fact, a great deal of overlap in how the brains of the two sexes work. Otherwise, "women could never read maps and men would always be left-handed. That flexibility within the sexes reveals just how complex a puzzle gender actually is, requiring pieces from biology, sociology, and culture" (Gorman, 1992, p. 44).

With respect to brain functioning, there is likely a mix between the factors of heredity and environment that accounts for gender characteristics. The following is a comparison of cognitive abilities between the genders based on developmental and educational psychology findings in Vander Zanden et al. (2007), Santrock (2006), Snowman and Biehler (2006), and Baron-Cohen (2005).

Cognitive Abilities

General intelligence: Various studies have not yielded consistent findings on whether males and females differ in general intelligence. But if any gender differences exist, they seem to be attributed to patterns of ability rather than IQ (Kimura, 1999). When mean differences have occurred, they are small. However, what is well documented is the strong correlation between IQ and heredity (Santrock, 2006). On IQ tests during preschool years, girls score higher; in high school, boys score higher on these tests. Differences may be due to greater dropout rates in high school for low-ability boys and gender identity formation in adolescence. Thus, overall no dramatic differences between the sexes have been found on measures of general intelligence (Vander Zanden et al., 2007).

However, a very interesting trend in IQ scores has been noted. IQs (as measured by the Stanford-Binet intelligence test) are increasing

Table 8–1 Gender Differences in Brain Structure

	Men	Women
Temporal Lobe		
Regions of the cerebral cortex help to control hearing, memory, and a person's sense of self and time.	In cognitively normal men, a small region of the temporal lobe has about 10% fewer neurons than it does in women.	More neurons are located in the temporal region where language, melodies, and speech tones are understood.
Corpus Callosum		
The main bridge between the left and right brain contains a bundle of neurons that carry messages between the two brain hemispheres.	This part of the brain in men takes up less volume than a woman's does, which suggests less communication between the two brain hemispheres.	The back portion of the callosum in women is bigger than in men, which may explain why women use both sides of their brains for language.
Anterior Commissure		
This collection of nerve cells, smaller than the corpus callosum, also connects the brain's two hemispheres.	The commissure in men is smaller than in women, even though men's brains are, on average, larger in size than women's brains.	The commissure in women is larger than in men, which may be a reason why their cerebral hemispheres seem to work together on tasks from language to emotional responses.
Brain Hemispheres		
The left side of the brain controls language, and the right side of the brain is the seat of emotion.	The right hemisphere of men's brains tends to be dominant.	Women tend to use their brains more holistically, calling on both hemispheres simultaneously.
Brain Size		
Total brain size is approximately 3 pounds.	Men's brains, on average, are larger than women's.	Women have smaller brains, on average, than men because the anatomical structure of their entire bodies is smaller. However, they have more neurons than men (an overall 11%) crammed into the cerebral cortex.

Source: Adapted from Begley, S., Murr, A., & Rogers, A. (1995, March 27). Gray matters. *Newsweek,* 51.

rapidly worldwide. In America, children seem to be getting smarter. As compared with IQs tested in 1932, if people took the same test today, a large percentage would score much higher. Since the increase has occurred over such a relatively short time, heredity is not the cause. It is thought that increasing levels of education and the information-age explosion are the reasons. This increase in IQ scores is known as the *Flynn effect* after the researcher who discovered it (Santrock, 2006).

Verbal ability: Girls learn to talk, form sentences, and use a variety of words earlier than boys. In addition, girls speak more clearly, read earlier, and do consistently better on tests of spelling and grammar. Originally, researchers believed females performed better than males on measures of verbal fluency, but recent research has questioned this early superiority of females in the verbal domain. On tests of verbal reasoning, verbal comprehension, and vocabulary, the findings are not consistent. The conclusion is that no significant gender differences in verbal ability exist.

Mathematical ability: During the preschool years, there appear to be no gender-related differences in ability to do mathematics. By the end of elementary school, however, boys show signs of excelling in mathematical reasoning, and the differences in math abilities of boys over girls become even greater in high school. Recent studies reveal that any male superiority likely is related to the way math is traditionally taught—as a competitive individual activity rather than as a cooperative group learning endeavor.

When the approach to teaching math is taken into consideration, only about a 1% variation in quantitative skills is seen in the general population. In our culture, math achievement differences may result from different role ex-

pectations. The findings on math ability and achievement can also be extended to science ability and achievement, as these two subjects are related.

Spatial ability: The ability to recognize a figure when it is rotated, to detect a shape embedded in another figure, or to accurately replicate a three-dimensional object is consistently better for males than for females. Of all possible gender-related differences in cognitive activity, the spatial ability of males is consistently higher than that of females and probably has a genetic origin. Rubin Gur, a noted researcher on gender differences in the brain, concurs with other research findings that men do perform better on spatial tasks than women (Gur et al., 2000). However, the magnitude of this sex difference accounts for only about 5% of the variation in spatial ability.

Interestingly, women surpass men in the ability to discern and later recall the location of objects in a complex, random pattern (Kimura, 1999). Scientists have reasoned that historically men may have developed strong spatial skills so as to be successful hunters, while women may have needed other types of visual skills so as to excel as gatherers and foragers of food (Gorman, 1992).

Problem solving: The complex concepts of problem solving, creativity, analytical skill, and cognitive styles, when examined, have led to mixed findings regarding gender differences. Men tend to try new approaches in problem solving and are more likely to be field independent. That is, they are less influenced by irrelevant cues and more focused on common features in certain learning tasks (see Chapter 4 on learning styles). Males also show more curiosity and significantly less conservatism than women in risk-taking situations. In the area of human relations, however, women perform better at problem solving than do men.

School achievement: Without exception, girls get better grades on average than boys, particularly at the elementary school level. Scholastic performance of girls is more stable and less fluctuating than that of boys.

Although no compelling evidence proves significant gender-linked differences in the areas of cognitive functioning, except in spatial ability as mentioned above, some findings do reveal sex differences when it comes to personality characteristics. Evidence reported by Vander Zanden and others (2007), Santrock (2006), and Snowman and Biehler (2006) was used to substantiate the following summary findings unless otherwise noted.

Personality Traits

Most of the observed *gender-related personality behaviors* are thought to be largely determined by culture but are, to some extent, a result of mutual interaction between environment and heredity.

Aggression: Males of all ages and in most cultures are generally more aggressive than females (Baron-Cohen, 2005). The role of the gender-specific hormone testosterone is linked as a possible cause of the more aggressive behavior demonstrated by males (Kimura, 1999). However, anthropologists, psychologists, sociologists, and scientists in other fields continue to disagree about whether aggression is biologically based or environmentally influenced. Nevertheless, male and female roles differ widely in most cultures, with males usually being more dominant, assertive, energetic, active, hostile, and destructive.

Conformity and dependence: Females have been found generally to be more conforming and more influenced by suggestion. The gender biases of some studies have made these findings open to suspicion, however.

Emotional adjustment: The emotional stability of the sexes is approximately the same in childhood, but differences do arise in how emotional problems are manifested. Some evidence indicates that adolescent girls and adult females have more neurotic symptoms than males. However, this tendency may reflect how society defines mental health in ways that coincide with male roles. Also it has been pointed out that tests to measure mental health usually have been designed by men and, therefore, may be biased against females.

Values and life goals: In the past, men have tended to show greater interest in scientific, mathematical, mechanical, and physically active occupations as well as to express stronger economic and political values. Women have tended to choose literary, social service, and clerical occupations and to express stronger aesthetic, social sense, and religious values. These differences have become smaller over time as women have begun to think differently about themselves, have more freely pursued career and interest pathways, and society has begun to take a more equal opportunity viewpoint for both sexes.

Achievement orientation: Females are more likely to express achievement motivation in social skills and social relations, whereas men are more likely to try to succeed in intellectual or competitive activities. This difference is thought to be due to sex-role expectations that are strongly communicated at very early ages.

How do the preceding observations on gender characteristics in intellectual functioning and personality relate to the process of teaching clients whom the nurse as educator encounters? It is very difficult to differentiate between biological and environmental influences simply because these two factors are intertwined and influence each other. The cause, meaning, and outcome of these differences remain speculative at this time, and further research needs to be conducted.

The behavioral and biological differences between males and females, known as the *gender gap*, are well documented. Also well documented is *gender bias*, "a preconceived notion about the abilities of women and men that prevented individuals from pursuing their own interests and achieving their potentials" (Santrock, 2006, p. 66). Females have an accelerated biological timetable and, in general, are more prone to have early verbal ability. Conversely, males lag behind females in biological development and attention span but tend to excel in visual-spatial ability and mathematical pursuits (Vander Zanden et al., 2007). During adolescence, they also are likely to surpass females in physical strength.

With respect to gender differences and aging, as suggested by current life-span mortality rates, White females have a life expectancy of approximately 80 years compared to approximately 73 years for White males. Also, men have higher mortality rates for each of the 10 leading causes of death (U.S. Department of Health and Human Services, 2000). However, more needs to be understood about women's health because for years their health issues have been underrepresented in research studies. Fortunately, this trend has changed within the last 2 to 3 decades and significant evidence is beginning to surface about the physical and mental health status of females (Dignam, 2000; Kato & Mann, 1996; U.S. DHHS, 2000).

However, what has been known is that women are likely to seek health care more often than men do (U.S. Census Bureau, 2006). It is suspected that one of the reasons women have more contact with the healthcare system is that they traditionally have tended to be the primary caretakers of their children, who need pediatric services. In addition, during childbearing years, women seek health services for care surrounding pregnancy and childbirth (Kato & Mann, 1996).

Perhaps the reason that men tend not to rely as much as women on care from health providers is because of the sex-role expectation by our society that men should be stronger. They also have a tendency to be risk takers and to think of themselves as more independent. Although men are less likely to pursue routine health care for purposes of health and safety promotion and disease and accident prevention, they typically face a greater number of health hazards, such as a higher incidence of automobile accidents, use of drugs and alcohol, suicide, heart disease, and engaging in dangerous occupations. Furthermore, men are less likely to notice symptoms or report them to physicians (Kato & Mann, 1996).

TEACHING STRATEGIES

As health educators, nurses must become aware of the extent to which social and heredity-related characteristics of the genders affect health-seeking behaviors and influence individual health needs. As stated previously, in some areas males and females display different orientations and learning styles (Severiens & Ten Dam, 1994). The differences seem to depend on their interests and past experiences in the biological and social roles of men and women in our society.

Women and men are part of different social cultures, too. They use different symbols, belief systems, and ways to express themselves, much in the same manner that different ethnic groups have distinct cultures (Tear, 1995). In the future, these gender differences may become less pronounced as the sex roles become more blended.

In addition, one of the two major goals of *Healthy People 2010* (goal No. 2) is to eliminate health disparities among segments of the population. This includes differences that occur by gender, such as men are two times more likely to die from injuries than women, and women are at greater risk for Alzheimer's disease and two times as likely to be affected by depression as men (U.S. DHHS, 2000).

Nurse educators are encouraged to include information on general health disparities when educating clients and staff. They also are encouraged to use versatile teaching style strategies so as not to perpetuate stereotypical approaches to teaching and learning with the two genders. In addition, the nursing profession has a responsibility to incorporate gender issues into nursing education curricula.

Socioeconomic Characteristics

Socioeconomic status (SES), in addition to gender characteristics, influences the teaching–learning process. SES is considered to be the single most important determinant of health in our society (Crimmins & Saito, 2001; Singh-Manoux, Ferrie, Lynch, & Marmot, 2005). Socioeconomic class is an aspect of diversity that must be addressed in the context of education and in the process of teaching and learning.

Class is the "unmentionable five-letter word" (Rhem, 1998, p. 1). Many people are hesitant to categorize themselves according to class. They also are reluctant to discuss the issue of class differences because of the widespread idea that the United States should be a classless society (Felski, 2002; Rhem, 1998). It is a myth, though, that America is a country without classes (McGoldrick, 1995). Class, as universal as race or gender, hides in the shadows. However, class consciousness seems to be a commonality shared by everyone. Those who are privileged often feel guilty about their advantages. Those who are poor feel ashamed or embarrassed about their disadvantages (Rhem, 1998).

Social and economic levels of individuals have been found to be significant variables affecting health status, literacy levels, and in determining health behaviors (Crimmins & Saito, 2001; Monden, van Lenthe, & Mackenbach, 2006). Approximately 34 million Americans are living in poverty. The poverty threshold for a family of four is defined as an income of $18,400 and severe poverty is an annual income of at most half ($9,200) of this amount (Darling, 2004).

Disadvantaged people—those with low incomes, low educational levels, and/or social deprivation—come from many different ethnic groups, including millions of poor White people (U.S. DHHS, 2000). SES takes into account the variables of educational level, family income, and family structure (Vander Zanden et al., 2007). See **Figure 8–1** for the relationship between educational level and household income. All of these variables influence health beliefs, health practices, and readiness to learn (Darling, 2004; Mackenbach et al., 2003).

The relationships among socioeconomic position, cognitive ability, and health status have been explored, but the mechanics and processes involved are highly complex and remain poorly understood (Batty, Der, Macintyre, & Deary, 2006; Singh-Manoux et al., 2005). Heredity and environment usually vary together; that is, people who are genetically related (parents and

Figure 8–1 Relationship between education and median household income among adults aged 25 years and older, by gender, United States, 1996.

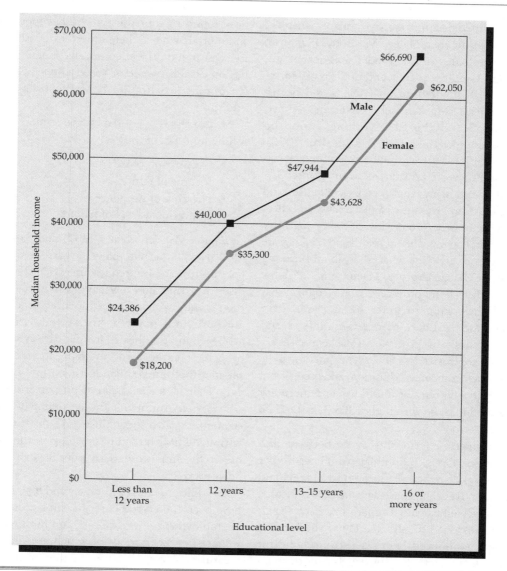

Source: U.S. Department of Commerce, Bureau of the Census. (1997, March). Current population survey. In *Healthy People 2010: Understanding and improving health* (p. 101). Rockville, MD: U.S. Department of Health and Human Services.

their children) tend to have similar environments. Evidence suggests that variations in heredity are equally as powerful as variations in environmental conditions in producing individual differences in cognitive ability (Santrock, 2006; Turkheimer, Haley, Waldron, D'Onofrio, & Gottesman, 2003; Vander Zanden et al., 2007). Also, low socioeconomic class is correlated with low educational levels and health inequalities (Mackenbach, Cavelaars, Kunst, Groenhof, and the EU Working Group on Socioeconomic Inequalities in Health, 2000). The significant correlation between literacy levels and SES is well documented in Chapter 7.

Although many educators, psychologists, and sociologists have recognized that a cause and effect relationship exists among low SES, low cognitive ability, and poor quality of health and life, they are hard pressed to know what to do about breaking the cycle (Batty, Deary, & Macintyre, 2006). So, too, are healthcare providers, who recognize that clients belonging to lower social classes have higher rates of illness, more severe illnesses, and reduced rates of life expectancy (Mackenbach et al., 2003). People with low SES, as measured by indicators such as income, education, and occupation, have increased rates of morbidity and mortality compared to those with higher SES (U.S. DHHS, 2000).

An inverse relationship exists between SES and health status. Individuals who have higher incomes and are better educated live longer and healthier lives than those who are of low income and poorly educated (Rognerud & Zahl, 2005; Crimmins & Saito, 2001). Thus, the level of socioeconomic well-being is a strong indicator of health outcomes. See **Figure 8–2** for the relationship between SES and health status.

These findings raise serious questions about health differences among our nation's people as a result of unequal access to health care due to SES. These unfortunate health trends are costly to society in general and to the healthcare system in particular. Although adverse health-related behavior and less access to medical care have been found to contribute to higher morbidity and mortality rates, there is newer but still limited research on the effect socioeconomic status has on disability-free or active life expectancy (Crimmins & Saito, 2001; Mackenbach et al., 2003).

Social class is measured by one or more of the following types of indices:

- Occupation of parents
- Income of family
- Location of residence
- Educational level of parents

Vander Zanden et al. (2007) and Santrock (2006) explain that many factors, including poor health care, limited resources, family stress, discrimination, and low-paying jobs, maintain the cycle by which generation after generation are born into poverty. Elstad and Krokstad (2003) found that health inequalities as a result of socioeconomic factors are reproduced as people mature from young adulthood into middle age. That is, a social causation pattern exists whereby environments are the source of socioeconomic health inequalities. As such, people with good health tend to move up in the social hierarchy and those with poor health move downward.

In addition, rates of illiteracy and low literacy have been linked to poorer health status, high unemployment, low earnings, and high rates of welfare dependency, all of which are common measures of a society's economic well-being (Giorgianni, 1998; Weiss, 2003). Whatever the factors that keep particular groups from achieving at higher levels, these groups are likely to remain on the lower end of the occupational

Figure 8–2 Percentage of persons with perceived fair or poor health status by household income, United States, 1995.

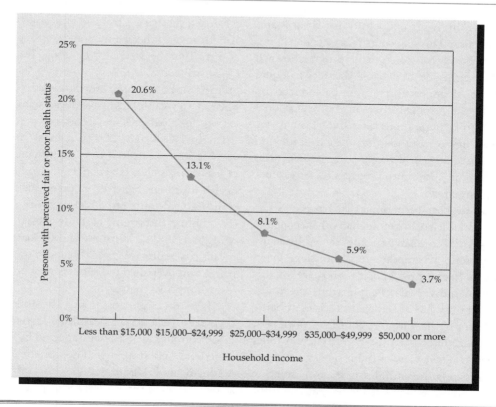

Source: Centers for Disease Control and Prevention, National Center for Health Statistics. (1995). National health interview survey. In *Healthy People 2010: Understanding and improving health* (p. 101). Rockville, MD: U.S. Department of Health and Human Services.

structure. This cycle has been coined the *poverty circle* (Gage & Berliner, 1998) or the *cycle of poverty*. The poverty circle is described as follows:

> *Parents low in scholastic ability and consequently in educational level create an environment in their homes and neighborhoods that produce children who are also low in scholastic ability and academic attainment. These children grow up and become parents, repeating the*

> *cycle. Like them, their children are fit only for occupations at lower levels of pay, prestige, and intellectual demand. (Gage & Berliner, 1998, p. 61)*

Family structure and the home environment are not the only factors affecting proficiency in learning. Hirsch (2001) contends that the alarming verbal and reading gap between rich and poor students "represents the single greatest failure in American public schooling" (p. 5). Many low-income children entering kindergarten have heard only half the words and understand only half the meanings of language than the high-income child has heard and understands. This gap continues to widen along the same trajectory as students progress in each succeeding grade in school. Barriers to equal educational opportunity must be reduced by putting the responsibility on the educational system to become more intensive. That is, we need to develop standards for each grade and make sure each child meets these expectations before being allowed to progress to subsequent grades in school.

The lower socioeconomic class has been studied by social scientists more than other economic classes. This is probably because the health views of this group deviate the most from those viewpoints of health professionals who care for this group of individuals. People from the lower social stratum have been characterized as being indifferent to the symptoms of illness until poor health interferes with their lifestyle and independence. Their view of life is one of a sense of powerlessness, meaninglessness, and isolation from middle-class knowledge of health and the need for preventive measures, such as vaccination for their children (U.S. DHHS, 2000; Lipman, Offord, & Boyle, 1994; Winkleby, Jatulis, Frank, & Fortmann, 1992).

The high cost of health care may well be a major factor affecting health practices of people in the lower socioeconomic classes. Individuals with adequate financial and emotional resources are able to purchase services and usually have support systems on which to rely to sustain them during recovery or augment their remaining functions after the course of an acute illness. Conversely, individuals deprived of monetary and psychosocial resources are at a much greater risk for failing to reach an optimal level of health and well-being. Unfortunately, the number of Americans at or below the national poverty level is at 12.6% and almost 47 million Americans lack health insurance, an increase of 1.3 million between 2004 and 2005 (U.S. Census Bureau, 2006).

Just as SES can have a negative effect on illness, so, too, can illness have devastating implications for a person's socioeconomic well-being (Elstad & Krokstad, 2003). A catastrophic or chronic illness can lead to unemployment, loss of health insurance coverage or ineligibility for health insurance benefits, enforced social isolation, and a strain on social support systems (Lindholm, Burstrom, & Diderichsen, 2001; Mulligan, 2004). Without the socioeconomic means to counteract these threats to their well-being, impoverished individuals may be powerless to improve their situation.

These multiple losses tax the individual, their families, and the healthcare system. Low-income groups are especially affected by changes in federal and state assistance in the form of Medicare and Medicaid. The spiraling costs associated with illness and consequent overuse of the healthcare system have resulted in increased interest on the part of the public and healthcare providers to control costs (Baker, Parker, Williams, & Clark, 1998). Today, more emphasis is being given to health promotion, health maintenance, and disease prevention.

Teaching Strategies

The current trends in health care, as a result of these economic concerns, are directed toward teaching individuals how to attain and maintain health. The nurse plays a key role in educating the consumer about avoiding health risks, reducing illness episodes, establishing healthful environmental conditions, and accessing healthcare services. Educational interventions by nurses for those who are socially and economically deprived have the potential for yielding short-term benefits in meeting these individuals' immediate healthcare needs. However, more research must be done to determine whether teaching can ensure the long-term benefits of helping deprived people develop the skills needed to reach and sustain independence in self-care management.

Nurse educators must be aware of the probable effects of low SES on an individual's ability to learn as a result of suboptimal cognitive functioning, poor academic achievement, low literacy, high susceptibility to illness, and disintegration of social support systems. Low-income people are at greater risk for these factors that can interfere with learning, but one cannot assume that everyone at the poverty or near-poverty level is equally influenced by these threats to their well-being. To avoid stereotyping, it is essential that each individual or family be assessed to determine their particular strengths and weaknesses for learning. In this way, teaching strategies unique to particular circumstances can be designed to assist socioeconomically deprived individuals in meeting their needs for health care.

Nevertheless, it is well documented that individuals with literacy problems, poor educational backgrounds, and low academic achievement are likely to have low self-esteem, feelings of helplessness and hopelessness, and low expectations. They also tend to think in concrete terms, are more focused on satisfying immediate needs, have a more external locus of control, and have decreased attention spans. They have difficulty in problem solving and in analyzing and synthesizing large amounts of information.

With these individuals, the nurse educator will most likely have to rely on specific teaching methods and tools similar to those identified as appropriate for intervening with clients who have low literacy abilities (see Chapter 7).

Cultural Characteristics

At the beginning of the 21st century, the composition of the U.S. population was approximately 71.3% White, 12.2% Black/African American, 11.2% Hispanic/Latino, 3.8% Asian/Pacific Islander, 0.7% American Indian/Alaskan Native, and 0.8% other. Thus, more than one quarter (28.7%) of the U.S. population consists of people from culturally diverse ethnic groups (U.S. Census Bureau, 2006). By 2010, one out of every three people in the United States is projected to belong to a racial or ethnic minority (Robinson, 2000). In addition, 7 million people indicated in their responses to the U.S. census survey taken in 2000 that they belonged to more than one race (Tashiro, 2002). By 2050, it is projected that people belonging to cultural subgroups will account for close to half of the U.S. total population (U.S. Census Bureau, 2006). If predictions prove true, by the middle of this century, it will be the first time in U.S. history that people from ethnic groups (subcultures) will constitute the majority of the total population.

To keep pace with a society that is increasingly more culturally diverse, nurses will need to have sound knowledge of the cultural values and beliefs of specific ethnic groups as well as be aware of individual practices and preferences (Price & Cortis, 2000; Purnell & Paulanka, 2003). In the past, healthcare providers have experienced difficulties in caring for clients whose cultural beliefs differ from their own because beliefs about health and illness vary considerably among ethnic groups. Lack of cultural sensitivity by healthcare professionals has resulted in millions of dollars wasted annually through misuse of healthcare services, the alienation of large numbers of people, and the misdiagnosis of health problems with often tragic and dangerous consequences.

In addition, underrepresented ethnic groups are beginning to demand culturally relevant health care that respects their cultural rights and incorporates their specific beliefs and practices into the care they receive. This expectation is in direct conflict with the unicultural, Western, biomedical paradigm taught in many nursing and other healthcare provider programs across the country (Purnell & Paulanka, 2003). A serious conceptual problem exists within the nursing profession because nurses are presumed to understand and be able to meet the healthcare needs of a culturally diverse population, even though they do not have the formal educational preparation to do so (Boss, 2007; Carthron, 2007).

Definition of Terms

Before examining the major ethnic (subcultural) groups within the United States, it is imperative to define the following terms, as identified by Purnell and Paulanka (2003), that are commonly used in addressing the subject of culture:

Acculturation: A willingness to adapt or "to modify one's own culture as a result of contact with another culture" (p. 351).

Assimilation: The willingness of an individual or group "to gradually adopt and incorporate characteristics of the prevailing culture" (p. 351).

Cultural awareness: Recognizing and appreciating "the external signs of diversity" in

other ethnic groups, such as their art, music, dress, and physical features (p. 352).

Cultural competence: A conscious process of recognizing one's own culture so as to avoid "undue influence on those from other cultural backgrounds" (p. 352).

Cultural diversity: A term meaning "representing a variety of different cultures" (p. 352).

Cultural relativism: "The belief that the behaviors and practices of people should be judged only from the context of their cultural system" (p. 352).

Culture: "The totality of socially transmitted behavioral patterns, arts, beliefs, values, customs, lifeways, and all other products of human work and thought characteristic of a population of people that guide their worldview and decision making. These patterns may be explicit or implicit, are primarily learned and transmitted within the family, and are shared by the majority of the cultures" (p. 352–353).

Ethnic group: Also referred to as a subculture are populations of "people who have experiences different from those of the dominant culture" (p. 4).

Ethnocentrism: "The tendency of human beings to think that [their] own ways of thinking, acting, and believing are the only right, proper, and natural ones and to believe that those who differ greatly are strange, bizarre, or unenlightened" (p. 353).

Ideology: "Consists of the thoughts, attitudes, and beliefs that reflect the social needs and desires of an individual or ethnocultural group" (p. 3).

Subculture: A group of people "who have had different experiences from the dominant culture by status, ethnic background, residence, religion, education, or other factors that functionally unify the group and act collectively on each other" (p. 357).

Transcultural: "Making comparisons for similarities and differences between cultures" (p. 358).

Worldview: Refers to "the way individuals or groups of people look at the universe to form values about their lives and the world around them" (p. 4).

Assessment Models for the Delivery of Culturally Sensitive Care

Given increases in immigration and birth rates in the United States as well as the significant increased geographical mobility of people around the globe, our system of health care and our educational institutions must respond by shifting from a dominant monocultural, ethnocentric focus to a more multicultural, transcultural focus (Narayan, 2003).

Tripp-Reimer and Afifi (1989) describe the interpretation of American cultural ideal from a historical perspective:

In the United States, the myth of the melting pot emerged largely from a combination of a cultural ideal of equality and a European ethnocentric perspective. This myth promoted the notion that all Americans are alike—that is, like white, middle-class persons. For many years, the notion that ethnicity should be discounted or ignored was prominent in the delivery of health care, including health teaching programs . . . (p. 613)

The question posed by Leininger (1994) still remains relevant today: How can nurses competently respond to and effectively care for people from diverse cultures who act, speak, and behave in ways different than their own? Studies indicate that health professionals are often unaware of the complex factors influencing clients' responses to health care.

From a sociological perspective, the symbolic interaction theory provides a theoretical framework for interacting with ethnic groups. It emphasizes social and group identities rather than just individual identity. Tashiro (2002) points out that this framework is useful to understand the situational nature of identity and the negotiation and renegotiation necessary when working with groups.

Purnell and Paulanka (2003) propose that there are a number of factors that influence an individual's identification with an ethnic group and that cause the individual to share his or her worldview. They have labeled these factors as primary and secondary characteristics of culture. *Primary characteristics of culture* include nationality, race, color, gender, age, and religious affiliation. *Secondary characteristics of culture* include many of a person's attributes that are addressed in this chapter and this text, such as SES, physical characteristics, educational status, occupational status, and place of residence (urban versus rural). These two major characteristics affect one's worldview and belief system.

The *Purnell model for cultural competence* is presented as a popular organizing framework for understanding the complex phenomenon of culture and ethnicity. This framework "provides a comprehensive, systematic, and concise" approach that can assist healthcare providers in teaching students in educational settings and clients and staff in practice settings for the delivery of "holistic, culturally competent, therapeutic interventions" (Purnell & Paulanka, 2003, p. 8).

The Purnell model, depicted in a circle format, includes the macro layers of the metaparadigm concepts of:

1. Global society (outermost sphere)
2. Community (second sphere)
3. Family (third sphere)
4. Individual (innermost sphere)

The interior of the circle is cut into 12 equally sized, pie-shaped wedges that represent the following 12 cultural domains that should be assessed when planning for educational interventions for clients in any setting:

1. Communication (e.g., dominant language and nonverbal expressions and cues)
2. Family roles and organization (e.g., head of household, gender roles, developmental tasks, social status, alternative lifestyles, roles of older adults)
3. Workforce issues (e.g., language barriers, autonomy, acculturation)
4. Biocultural ecology (e.g., heredity, biological variations, genetics)
5. High-risk behaviors (e.g., smoking, alcoholism, physical activity, safety practices)
6. Nutrition (e.g., common foods, rituals, deficiencies, limitations)
7. Pregnancy (e.g., fertility, practices, views toward childbearing, beliefs about pregnancy, birthing practices)
8. Death rituals (e.g., views of death, bereavement, burial practices)
9. Spirituality (e.g., religious beliefs and practices, meaning of life, use of prayer)
10. Healthcare practices (e.g., traditions, responsibility for health, pain control, sick role, medication use)
11. Healthcare practitioners (e.g., folk practitioners, gender issues, perceptions of providers)
12. Overview/heritage (e.g., origins, economics, education, occupation, economics)

These two authors also put forth 19 explicit assumptions upon which the model is based, some of which are most pertinent to this chapter, such as:

- One culture is not better than another—they are just different.
- The primary and secondary characteristics of culture determine the degree to which one varies from the dominant culture.
- Culture has a powerful influence on one's interpretation of and responses to health care.
- Each individual has the right to be respected for his or her uniqueness and cultural heritage.
- Prejudices and biases can be minimized with cultural understanding.
- Caregivers who intervene in a culturally competent manner improve the care of clients and their health outcomes.
- Cultural differences often require adaptations to standard professional practices.

Four other models for conducting a nursing assessment include Giger and Davidhizar's (2004) model of six cultural phenomena that need to be taken into account: (1) communication, (2) personal space, (3) social organization, (4) time, (5) environmental control, and (6) biological variations (**Figure 8–3**) and Price and Cordell's (1994) model outlining a four-step approach to help nurses provide culturally sensitive patient teaching (**Figure 8–4**).

The third model, *the nurse–client negotiations model,* was developed in the mid-1980s for the purpose of *cultural assessment* and planning for care of culturally diverse people. The negotiations model, although 20 years old, is still relevant. It recognizes discrepancies that exist between notions of the nurse and client about health, illness, and treatments. This model attempts to bridge the gap between the scientific perspectives of the nurse and the popular perspectives of the client. (Anderson, 1990).

The nurse–client negotiations model serves as a framework to attend to the culture of the nurse as well as the culture of the client. In addition to the professional culture, each nurse has his or her own personal beliefs and values, which

Figure 8–3 Six cultural phenomena.

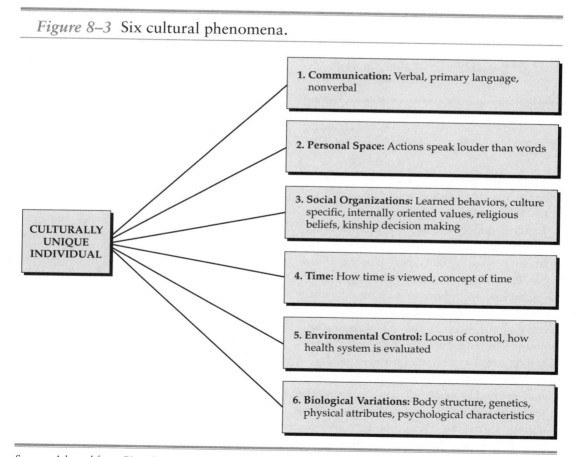

CULTURALLY UNIQUE INDIVIDUAL

1. **Communication:** Verbal, primary language, nonverbal

2. **Personal Space:** Actions speak louder than words

3. **Social Organizations:** Learned behaviors, culture specific, internally oriented values, religious beliefs, kinship decision making

4. **Time:** How time is viewed, concept of time

5. **Environmental Control:** Locus of control, how health system is evaluated

6. **Biological Variations:** Body structure, genetics, physical attributes, psychological characteristics

Source: Adapted from Giger, J. N., & Davidhizar, R. E. (1995). *Transcultural nursing: Assessment and intervention* (2nd ed., p. 9). St. Louis: Mosby–Year Book.

Figure 8–4 Four-step approach to providing culturally sensitive care.

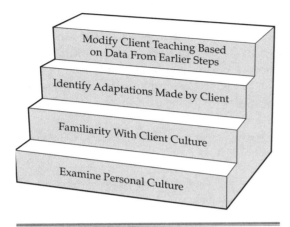

Source: Reprinted with permission from Price, J. L., & Cordell, B. (1994). Cultural diversity and patient teaching. *Journal of Continuing Education in Nursing, 25*(4), 164.

may operate without the nurse being fully aware of them. These beliefs and values may influence nurses' interactions with patients and families.

Explanations of the same phenomena may yield different interpretations based on the cultural perspective of the layperson or the professional. For example, putting lightweight covers on a patient may be interpreted by family members as placing their loved one at risk for getting a chill, whereas the nurse will use this technique to reduce a fever. As another example, a Jehovah's Witness family considers a blood transfusion for their child as contamination of the child's body, whereas the nurse and other healthcare team members believe a transfusion is a lifesaving treatment (Anderson, 1987). The important aspect of this model is that it can open lines of communication between the nurse and the patient/family. It helps each understand how the other interprets or

values a problem or practice such that they respect one another's goals.

Negotiation implies a mutual exchange of information between the nurse and client. The nurse should begin negotiation by learning from the clients about their understanding of their situation, their interpretations of illness and symptoms, the symbolic meanings they attach to an event, and their notions about treatment. The goal is to actively involve clients in the learning process so as to acquire healthy coping mechanisms and styles of living. Together, the nurse and client then need to engage in a transaction to work out how the popular and scientific perspectives can be meshed to achieve goals related to the individual client's interests (Anderson, 1990).

General areas to assess when first meeting the client include the following:

1. The client's perceptions of health and illness
2. His or her use of traditional remedies and folk practitioners
3. The client's perceptions of nurses, hospitals, and the care delivery system
4. His or her beliefs about the role of family and family member relationships
5. His or her perceptions of and need for emotional support (Anderson, 1987; Jezewski, 1993)

According to Anderson (1990) and Narayan (2003), the following are some questions that can be used as a means for understanding the client's perspectives or viewpoints. The answers then serve as the basis for negotiation:

- What do you think caused your problem?
- Why do you think the problem started when it did?
- What major problems does your illness cause you?

- How has being sick affected you?
- How severe do you think your illness is? Do you see it as having a short- or long-term course?
- What kinds of treatments do you think you should receive?
- What are the most important results you hope to obtain from your treatments?
- What do you fear most about your illness?

The fourth model, *the culturally competent model of care* proposed by Campinha-Bacote (1995), serves as a resource for conducting a thorough and sensitive cultural assessment. Cultural competence, as defined by this author, is as a set of congruent behaviors, attitudes, and policies that enable a system, agency, or professional to work effectively in a cross-cultural situation. Through this model, cultural competence is seen as a continuous process involving four components: (1) cultural awareness, (2) cultural knowledge, (3) cultural skill, and (4) cultural encounter.

Cultural awareness is the process of becoming sensitive to interactions with other cultural groups. It requires nurses to examine their biases and prejudices toward others of another culture or ethnic background. *Cultural knowledge* is the process in which nurses acquire an educational foundation with respect to various cultural worldviews. *Cultural skill* involves the process of learning how to conduct an accurate cultural assessment. *Cultural encounter* encourages nurses to expose themselves in practice to cross-cultural interactions with clients of diverse cultural backgrounds. All four components are essential if one is to deliver culturally competent nursing care (**Figure 8–5**).

Figure 8–5 Culturally competent model of care.

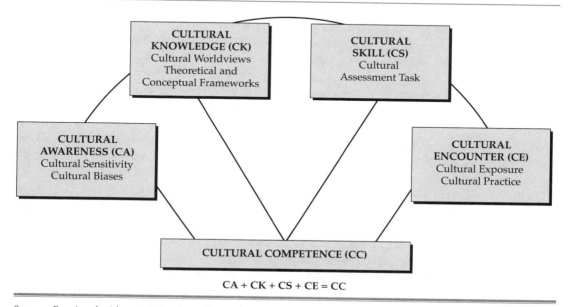

Source: Reprinted with permission from Campinha-Bacote, J. (1995). The quest for cultural competence in nursing care. *Nursing Forum, 30*(4), 20.

Nurse educators who are competent in cultural assessment and negotiation likely will be the most successful at designing and implementing culturally effective teaching programs. They also will be able to assist their colleagues in working with clients who may be considered uncooperative, noncompliant, or difficult. In addition, they can help with identifying potential areas of cultural conflict and select teaching interventions that minimize conflict. Nurses must understand how the reactions of practitioners influence labeling of clients' behaviors and, therefore, eventually influence nurse–client interactions (Anderson, 1987, 1990; Gutierrez & Rogoff, 2003).

There is one very important caveat for the educator to remember when conducting a cultural assessment of any client:

> *Nurses must be especially careful not to overgeneralize or stereotype clients on the basis of their ethnic heritage. Just because someone belongs to a particular subculture does not necessarily mean they adhere to all the beliefs, values, customs, and practices of that ethnic group. Nurses should never assume a client's learning needs or preferences for treatment will be alike simply based on the individual's ethnicity.*

As Andrews and Boyle (1995) so aptly explained, "Sometimes cultural stereotyping may be perpetuated when a recipe-like approach to clients from specific cultural groups is used: i.e., there is a tendency by the nurse to view all members of a group homogenously and to expect certain beliefs or practices because of presumptions that may or may not apply to the client" (p. 50). Knowledge of cultural variations should serve only as background cues for obtaining additional information through assessment.

General Assessment and Teaching Interventions

As a first step in the teaching process, assessment should determine health beliefs, values, and practices. The nurse in the role of educator must implement successful teaching interventions using the universal skills of establishing rapport, assessing readiness to learn, and using active listening to understand problems. Nurses need to be aware of the established customs that influence the behavior one is attempting to change (Tripp-Reimer & Afifi, 1989). The nurse should, however, keep in mind that belonging to an ethnic group does not always mean a person follows or buys into all of the traditions or customs of the group to which they belong. Given that culture affects the way someone perceives a health problem and understands its course and possible treatment options, it is essential to carry out a thorough assessment prior to establishing a plan of action for long-term behavioral change.

Different cultural backgrounds not only create different attitudes and reactions to illness, but also can influence how people express themselves, both verbally and nonverbally, which may prove difficult to interpret. For example, asking a patient to explain what they believe to be the cause of a problem will help to reveal whether the patient thinks it is due to a spiritual intervention, a hex, an imbalance in nature, or other culturally based beliefs. The nurse should accept the client's explanation (most likely reflecting the beliefs of the support system as well) in a nonjudgmental manner.

Culture also guides the way an ill person is defined and treated. For example, some cultures believe that once the symptoms disappear, illness is no longer present. This belief can be problematic for individuals suffering from an acute illness, such as a streptococcal infection, when a 1- or 2-day course of antibiotic therapy relieves the soreness in the throat. This belief also can be a problem for the individual afflicted with a chronic disease that is manifested by periods of remission or exacerbation.

In addition, readiness to learn must be assessed from the standpoint of a person's culture. Patients and their families, for instance, may believe that behavior change is context specific, such that they will adhere to a recommended medical regimen while in the hospital setting but fail to follow through with the guidelines once they return to the home setting. Also, the nurse and other health-care providers must be cautious not to assume that the values adhered to by professionals are equally important or cherished by the patient and significant others. Consideration, too, must be given to barriers that might exist, such as time, financial, and environmental variables, which may hinder readiness to learn (see Chapter 4). Finally, the client needs to believe that new behaviors are not only possible, but also beneficial if the new information is to be remembered and interpreted correctly for behavioral change to be maintained over the long term (Kessels, 2003).

The following specific guidelines for assessment should be used regardless of the particular cultural orientation of the client (Anderson, 1987; Uzundede, 2006):

1. **Observe the interactions between client and his/her family members as well as among family members.** Determine who makes the decisions, how decisions are made, who is the primary caregiver, what type of care is given, and what foods and other objects are important to them.

2. **Listen to the client.** Find out what the person wants, how his/her wants differ from what the family wants, and how they differ from what you think is appropriate.

3. **Consider communication abilities and patterns.** Identify the client's primary language (which may be different from your own). Also, note manners of speaking (rate of speech, expressions used) and nonverbal cues that can enhance or hinder understanding. In addition, be aware of your own nonverbal behaviors and etiquettes of interaction that may be acceptable or unacceptable to the client and family members.

4. **Explore customs or taboos.** Observe behaviors and clarify beliefs and practices that may interfere with care or treatment.

5. **Determine the notion of time.** Become oriented to the individual's and family members' sense of time and importance of time frames.

6. **Be aware of cues for interaction.** Determine which communication approaches are appropriate with respect to what is the most comfortable way to address the person(s) with whom you are interacting. Also, find out the symbolic objects or the activities that provide comfort and security.

These guidelines will assist in the exchange of information between the educator and client. The nurse/client role is a mutual one in which the nurse is both learner and teacher and the client is also both learner and teacher. The goal of negotiation is to arrive at ways of working together to solve a problem or to determine a course of action (Anderson, 1987, 1990). The objective is not to take a totally fact-centered approach or pretend you are completely color blind, but to recognize each person as an individual and that differences exist within ethnic and racial groups as well as between these groups.

Use of Translators

If the client speaks a foreign language, the nurse should use the client's primary language whenever possible. When the nurse does not fluently speak the same language, it is necessary to secure the assistance of a translator. Translators may be family members, neighbors and friends, other healthcare staff, or professional interpreters.

For many reasons, the use of family or friends for translation of communication is not as desirable as using professionally trained interpreters. First, family members and friends may not be sufficiently fluent to assume the role. Second, they may choose to omit portions of the content they believe to be unnecessary or unacceptable. Third, their presence may inhibit peer communication and violate the patient's right to privacy and confidentiality (Baker et al., 1996; Poss & Rangel, 1995), especially in light of the recent HIPAA (Health Information Portability and Accountability Act) regulations.

Thus it is optimal if professionally trained interpreters can be used. They can translate instructional messages verbatim, and they work under an established code of ethics and confidentiality. If there is no bilingual person available to facilitate communication, the AT&T Language Line provides 24-hour access to translators who are fluent in 144 languages (Duffy & Snyder, 1999).

In teaching clients who are only partially fluent in English, the following strategies are rec-

ommended (Poss & Rangel, 1995; Stanislav, 2006; Tripp-Reimer & Afifi, 1989) to help the nurse alter the style of interaction when no translator is used:

- Speak slowly and distinctly, allowing for twice as much time as a typical teaching session would take.
- Use simple sentences, relying on an active rather than a passive voice.
- Avoid technical terms (e.g., use *heart* rather than *cardiac*, or *stomach* rather than *gastric*). Also avoid medical jargon (e.g., use *blood pressure* rather than *BP*) and American idioms (e.g., *it's just red tape you have to go through* or *I heard it straight from the horse's mouth*).
- Organize instructional material in the sequence in which the plan of action should be carried out.
- Make no assumptions that the information given has been understood. Ask for clients to explain in their own words what they heard, and, if appropriate, request a return demonstration of a skill that has been taught.

The Four Major Ethnic Groups

The U.S. Census Bureau (2000) defines the major ethnic groups in this country as follows: Black/African American (of African, Haitian, and Dominican Republic descents), Hispanic/Latino (of Mexican, Cuban, Puerto Rican, and other Latin descents), Asian/Pacific Islander (of Japanese, Chinese, Filipino, Korean, Vietnamese, Hawaiian, Guamian, Samoan, and Asian Indian descents), and American Indian/Alaskan Native (descendents of hundreds of tribes of Native Americans and of Eskimo descent).

Given the fact that there are many ethnic groups (subcultures) in the United States, and hundreds worldwide, it is impossible to address the cultural characteristics of each one of them. The following is a review of the beliefs and health practices of the four major ethnic groups in this country as identified by the U.S. Census Bureau. These groups, who have been historically underrepresented, account for almost one third (28.7%) of the total U.S. population. These groups are recognized by the U.S. government as disadvantaged due to low income, low education, and/or sociocultural deprivation. The Hispanic/Latino and Asian/Pacific Islander groups are the fastest growing ethnic subcultures in this country (U.S. Census Bureau, 2006).

It must be remembered that one of the most important roles of the nurse as educator is to serve as an advocate for clients—as a representative of their interests. If nurses are to assume this role, then their efforts should be directed at making the healthcare setting as similar to the client's natural environment as possible. To do so, they must be aware of clients' customs, beliefs, and lifestyles.

In addition to information provided below on the four major ethnic groups, the following references are recommended as sources of additional information on particular tribes or subcultures specifically not addressed: Purnell and Paulanka (2003), Kelley and Fitzsimons (2000), Vivian and Dundes (2004), Chideya (1999), Chachkes and Christ (1996), Cantore (2001), Lowe and Struthers (2001), Parker and Kiatoukaysy (1999), Young, McCormick, and Vitaliano (2002), Cohen (1991), Kniep-Hardy and Burkhardt (1977), Pang (2007), Horton and Freire (1990), and Smolan, Moffitt, and Naythons (1990).

Hispanic/Latino Culture

According to the U.S. Census Bureau (2006), the Hispanic/Latino group is the largest and the fastest-growing subculture in the United States. As of the last full census survey of 2000, they represent 11.9% of the total population of the United States. The number of Hispanic Americans has increased significantly since 1970 as a result of a higher birth rate in this group than the rest of the population, an increase in immigration, as well as improved census procedures.

Hispanic or Latino Americans derive from diverse origins. This heterogeneous group of Americans with varied backgrounds in culture and heritage are of Latin American or Spanish origin who use Spanish (or a related dialect) as their dominant language. Those of Mexican heritage comprise the largest number of people (approximately 60%) of this subculture, followed by Puerto Rican, Central and South American, and Cuban Americans. They are found in every state but are concentrated in just nine states. California and Texas together have one half of the Hispanic population, but other large concentrations are found in New York, New Jersey, Florida, Illinois, Arizona, New Mexico, and Colorado (U.S. Census Bureau, 2006). Nurse educators who practice in the Southwestern states are most likely to encounter clients of Mexican heritage, those practicing in the Northeast states will most likely be caregivers of clients of Puerto Rican heritage, and nurses in Florida will be delivering care to a large number of Cuban Americans. Also, Hispanic people are more likely to live in metropolitan or rural areas than are non-Hispanic Americans (Purnell & Paulanka, 2003). While Hispanic

Americans have many common characteristics, each subgroup has unique characteristics.

The people of Hispanic heritage have particular healthcare needs that must be addressed. They are disproportionately affected by certain cancers, alcoholism, drug abuse, obesity, hypertension, diabetes, adolescent pregnancy, dental disease, and HIV/AIDS. Unlike in non-Hispanic Whites, homicide, AIDS, and perinatal conditions rank in the top 10 as causes of mortality. Hispanics are more prone to certain diseases, are less likely to receive preventive care, often lack health insurance, and have less access to health care than Whites living in the United States (Fernandez & Hebert, 2000; Hebert & Fernandez, 2000; Pacquiao, Archeval, & Shelley, 2000; Purnell & Paulanka, 2003; U.S. DHHS, 2000).

Unfortunately, both the curricula in nursing schools nationwide and the literature in nursing with respect to patient education efforts geared toward Hispanic Americans have paid little attention to the healthcare needs of this minority group. Although Hispanics are a culturally diverse group of people with varying health needs, avenues for including Hispanic healthcare issues in nursing curricula have been minimal and especially need to be developed in schools located in areas with high population concentrations of this ethnic group (Kelley & Fitzsimons, 2000; Sullivan & Bristow, 2007).

Fluency in Spanish as a foreign language is a necessity, or at least highly recommended, when practitioners are responsible for delivering care to this growing, underserved, culturally diverse ethnic group. Spanish-speaking people represent 54% of all non–English-speaking persons in the United States (U.S. Census Bureau, 2006). In proportion to the U.S. population, those of Hispanic heritage are underrepresented

in nursing education. Only 1.7 % of all graduates of basic nursing programs are of Hispanic descent (see Figure 8–6). Far too few graduates are available to satisfy the increasing need for Hispanic healthcare professionals. The lack of representation of people from this subculture in the health professions is not thought to result from low aspirations on their part. Indeed, many Hispanic high school students rank health/medical services among their top 10 career choices. Unfortunately, the often poor academic achievement of Hispanic students in high schools and colleges is associated with a number of factors related to socioeconomic and educational disadvantages (Educating the Largest Minority Group, 2003).

Access to health care by Hispanics is limited both by choice and by unavailability of health services. Only one fifth of Puerto Rican, one fourth of Cuban, and one third of Mexican/Americans see a physician during the course of a year. Even when Hispanic people have access to the healthcare system, they may not receive the care they need. Difficulty in obtaining services, dissatisfaction with the care provided, and inability to afford the rising costs of medical care are major factors that discourage them from using the healthcare system (Fernandez & Hebert, 2000; Purnell & Paulanka, 2003).

Approximately 23% of Hispanic families live below the poverty line; members of this ethnic group are 2.5 times more likely to be below the poverty level than members of other subcultural groups in the United States. Economic disadvantage leaves little disposable income for paying out-of-pocket expenses for health care. When they do seek a regular source of care, many people of this minority group rely on public health facilities, hospital outpatient clinics, and emergency rooms (Fernandez & Hebert,

2000; Purnell & Paulanka, 2003). Also, they are very accepting of health care being delivered in their homes, where they feel a sense of control, stability, and security (Pacquiao et al., 2000).

The health beliefs of Hispanic people also affect their decisions to seek traditional care. Many studies dating back to the 1940s on Hispanic health beliefs and practices stressed exotic folklore practices, such as their use of herbs, teas, home remedies, and over-the-counter drugs for treating symptoms of acute and chronic illnesses. In addition, they place a high degree of reliance on health healers, known as *curenderos* or *esperitistas*, for health advice and treatment (Fernandez & Hebert, 2000; Purnell & Paulanka, 2003). For example, illnesses of Mexican Americans as an Hispanic subgroup could be organized into the following categories (Caudle, 1993; Markides & Coreil, 1986; Purnell & Paulanka, 2003):

1. Diseases of hot and cold, believed to be due to an imbalanced intake of foods or ingestion of foods at extreme opposites in temperature. In addition, cold air was thought to lead to joint pain, and a cold womb resulted in barrenness in women. Heating or chilling was the cure for parts of the body afflicted by disease.
2. Diseases of dislocation of internal organs, cured by massage or physical manipulation of body parts.
3. Diseases of magical origin, caused by *mal ojo*, or evil eye, a disorder of infants and children as a result of a woman's looking admiringly at someone else's child without touching the child, resulting in crying, fitful sleep, diarrhea, vomiting, and fever.

4. Diseases of emotional origin, attributed to sudden or prolonged terror called *susto*.
5. Folk-defined diseases, such as *latido*.
6. Standard scientific diseases.

Recent research reveals that overall health status of Hispanic Americans is determined by key health indicators on infant mortality, life expectancy, and mortality from cardiovascular disease, cancer, and measures of functional health. This research concludes that the health of people of Hispanic heritage is much closer to that of White Americans than to African Americans, even though the Hispanic and Black populations share similar socioeconomic conditions. Concerning the incidence of diabetes and infectious and parasitic diseases, however, Hispanic people are clearly at a disadvantage in relation to White people.

Possible explanations for the relative advantages and disadvantages in health status of Hispanic Americans involve such factors as the following, which were outlined by Purnell and Paulanka (2003):

- Cultural practices favoring reproductive success
- Early and high fertility contributing to low breast cancer but high cervical cancer rates
- Dietary habits linked to low cancer rates but high prevalence of obesity and diabetes
- Genetic heritage
- Extended family support reducing the need for psychiatric services
- Low socioeconomic status that contributes to increased infectious and parasitic diseases

Alcoholism also represents a serious health problem for many Hispanic Americans. Furthermore, as the Hispanic population becomes more acculturated, certain risk factors conducive to cardiovascular disease and certain cancers are expected to play larger roles in this group (Markides & Coreil, 1986; Purnell & Paulanka, 2003).

Today, the literature disagrees about the extent and frequency to which Hispanic people use home remedies and folk practices. In the southwestern United States, the Hispanic population has been found to use herbs and other home remedies to treat illness episodes—twice the proportion reported in the total U.S. population. Other studies claim that the use of folk practitioners has declined and practically disappeared in some Hispanic subgroups (Purnell & Paulanka, 2003).

Knowing where people get their health information can provide clues to practitioners as to how to reach particular population groups. For example, Mexican Americans receive almost as much information from mass media sources (TV, magazines, and newspapers) as they do from physicians and nurses. As a consequence, mass media could play an important role in disseminating information to a large portion of the Mexican American population (Purnell & Paulanka, 2003).

Because of the centrality of the family in Hispanic peoples' lives, the extended family serves as the single most important source of social support to its members. This culture is characterized by a pattern of respect and obedience to elders as well as a pattern of male dominance. Caregivers' focus, therefore, needs to be on the family rather than on the individual. It is likely, for example, that a woman would be reluctant to make a decision about her or her child's health care without consulting her husband first (Purnell & Paulanka, 2003).

Gender and family member roles are changing, however, as Hispanic women are taking jobs outside the home. Also, children are picking up the English language more quickly than their parents and are ending up in the powerful position of acting as interpreters for their adult relatives. The heavy reliance on family has been linked to this minority group's low utilization of healthcare services. In addition, levels of education correlate highly with access to health care. That is, as clearly depicted in Figure 8–1, the less education members within a household have, the poorer the family's health status and access to health care (Purnell & Paulanka, 2003; U.S. DHHS, 2000). Hispanic Americans are more likely than the general U.S. population to read English below the basic health literacy level (National Center for Education Statistics, 2006) and to have lower educational attainment than non-Hispanic Whites (Massett, 1996).

Teaching Strategies

Only about 40% of the Hispanic population has completed 4 years of high school or more, and only 10% have completed college, as compared with approximately 80% and 20%, respectively, of the rest of the non-Hispanic population (Purnell & Paulanka, 2003; Educating the Largest Minority Group, 2003). Both the educational level and the primary language of Hispanic clients need to be taken into consideration when selecting instructional materials (Massett, 1996; National Center for Education Statistics, 2006). Sophisticated teaching methods and tools would be inappropriate for those who have minimal levels of education.

The age of the population also can affect health and client education efforts. According to the

U.S. Census Bureau (2006), the Hispanic population is young as a total group (30% are younger than 20 years of age). Thus, the school system is an important setting for educating members of the Hispanic community. Education programs in the school system for Hispanic students on alcohol and drug abuse and on cardiovascular disease risk reduction proved successful if:

- Cultural beliefs were observed.
- The educator was first introduced by an individual accepted and respected by the learners.
- Family members were included.
- The community was encouraged to take responsibility for resolving the health problems discussed.

Morbidity, mortality, and risk factor data also provide clues to the areas in which patient education efforts should be directed. As mentioned earlier, Hispanic people have higher rates of diabetes, AIDS, obesity, alcohol-related illnesses, and mortality from homicide than the general population. All of these topics should be targeted for educational efforts at disease prevention and health promotion (Caudle, 1993).

Until recently, little data existed regarding patient education for Hispanic Americans. Purnell and Paulanka (2003), Fernandez and Hebert (2000), Hebert and Fernandez (2000), Pacquiao and others (2000), and Caudle (1993) have contributed significantly to our understanding of the traditions and practices surrounding health and illness in the various Hispanic subgroups. The following general suggestions are useful when designing and implementing education programs for Hispanic Americans:

1. Identify the Hispanic American subgroups (e.g., Mexican, Cuban, and Puerto Rican) in the community whose needs differ in terms of health beliefs, language, and general health status. Design education programs that can be targeted to meet their distinct ethnic needs.

2. Be aware of individual differences within subgroups as to age, years of education, income levels, job status, and degree of acculturation.

3. Take into account the special health needs of Hispanic Americans with respect to incidences of diseases and risk factors to which they are vulnerable—breast cancer in women (Borrayo, 2004), diabetes, AIDS, obesity, alcohol-related illnesses, homicide, and accidental injuries.

4. Be aware of the importance of the family so as to direct education efforts to include all interested members. Remember that Hispanic families on the whole are very supportive of each other, and decision making rests with the male and elder authority figures in the traditional families.

5. Provide adequate space for teaching to accommodate family members who typically accompany patients seeking health care.

6. Be cognizant of the importance of the Roman Catholic religion in the lives of the Hispanic people when dealing with such issues as contraception, abortion, and family planning.

7. Demonstrate cultural sensitivity to health beliefs by respecting ethnic values and taking time to learn about Hispanic beliefs.

8. Consider other sources of care that this ethnic group might be using, such as home remedies, before they enter or while they are within the healthcare system.

9. Be aware of the modesty felt by some Hispanic women and girls, who may be particularly uncomfortable in talking about sexual issues in mixed company.

10. Display warmth, friendliness, and tactfulness when developing a relationship with people of Hispanic heritage because they expect healthcare providers to be informal and interested in their lives.

11. Determine whether Spanish is the language by which the client best communicates. Many Hispanic Americans prefer to speak Spanish, but they are not always literate in reading their native language.

12. Speak slowly and distinctly, avoiding the use of technical words and slang if the client has limited proficiency in the English language.

13. Do not assume that a nod of the head or a smile indicates understanding of what has been said. Even if Hispanic clients are not familiar with English, they respect authority and, therefore, it is not uncommon for them to display nonverbal cues that may be misleading or misinterpreted by the nurse. Ask clients to repeat in their own words what they have been told or use the teach back method to determine their level of understanding (Weiss, 2003).

14. If interpreters are used, be sure they speak the dialect of the learner. Be certain that the interpreter interprets instructions, rather than just translates them so that the real meaning gets conveyed. Also, be sure to talk to and with the client, not to the interpreter. If an interpreter is not available, use the AT&T hotline telephone number for a direct link to Spanish-speaking interpreters.

15. Provide written and audiovisual materials in Spanish that reflect linguistic appropriateness and cultural sensitivity. An increasing number of health education materials are available in Spanish (Borrayo, 2004).

Much more must be learned by nurse educators about the Hispanic American population with respect to their cultural beliefs and their health and education needs. It is evident that many members of this cultural group are not receiving the kind and amount of health services they desire and deserve. Nurses need to extend themselves to Hispanics in a culturally sensitive manner to effectively and efficiently address the needs of this rapidly growing segment of the U.S. population (Borrayo, 2004).

Black/African American Culture

According to the 2000 U.S. Census, members of the Black/African American culture make up the largest ethnic group in the United States. Currently, Black Americans constitute 12.2% of the U.S. population as compared with 11.9% for Hispanics. However, the most recent 2004 statistics indicate that the Hispanic population has surpassed this group in population growth (U.S. Census Bureau, 2006).

The cultural origins and heritage of Black Americans are quite diverse. Their roots are mainly from Africa and the Caribbean Islands.

They speak a variety of languages, including French, Spanish, African dialects, and various forms of English. Depending on the age cohort group to which they belong, African Americans may prefer to identify themselves differently as a racial group. For example, the youngest generation often refers to themselves (and likes to be referred by others) by the term *African American*. By contrast, middle-aged members of this ethnic group may prefer the term Black or Black American. Either designation is politically correct according to the U.S. Census Bureau's identification of this ethnic group as Black/African American. However, because the diversity of cultural heritage varies within the many Black subgroups, healthcare providers need to be aware of intraethnic differences in cultural beliefs, customs, and traditions (Purnell & Paulanka, 2003).

The one distinguishing factor of this ethnic group, in comparison to other subcultures, is that quite a few Black families have ancestry dating back to the early colonization of America in the 1600s when millions of Africans were brought forcibly to this country as slaves. The rich history of African heritage and American slavery has been passed on from generation to generation (Purnell & Paulanka, 2003).

The majority of this ethnic population resides in the South (54%). Approximately 19% live in the Midwest, 18% in the Northeast, and 9% in the West. The greatest concentration resides in large metropolitan areas, such as New York City; Chicago; Atlanta, Georgia; Washington, D.C.; Baltimore; Detroit, Michigan; and New Orleans, Louisiana (U.S. Census Bureau, 2006).

Unfortunately, African Americans have suffered a long history of inequality in educational opportunity. They were victims of school segregation and inferior facilities until the 1954 Supreme Court decision, *Brown v. Board of Education of Topeka*, outlawed the separation of Blacks and Whites in the public school systems. However, this educational deprivation has had long-term consequences, such as unequal access to higher paying and higher status job opportunities, which has led to low wages and a disproportionate number (approximately one third) of African Americans living at or below the poverty level (U.S. Census Bureau, 2006). In turn, poverty has resulted in low educational attainment, high rates of school dropout, drug and alcohol abuse, decreased health status, and a lower quality of life altogether (Forrester, 2000; Purnell & Paulanka, 2003). Nevertheless, many African Americans value education, which they see as the means to raise their standard of living by being able to secure better jobs and a higher social status.

Black Americans constitute a large segment of blue-collar workers and are not well represented in managerial and professional positions of employment. Discrimination in employment and job advancement is thought to be a major variable contributing to problems with career mobility. The government has taken major steps in the past 30 years to reverse discrimination in social and employment settings so as to give Black Americans more equal opportunities, but the majority of working-class Black people still do not typically advance to higher-level occupations.

Also, poverty and low educational attainment have had major consequences for the Black American community in terms of social and medical issues. Although Black families value education highly, there continues to be a greater than average high school dropout rate among Blacks, and many individuals remain poorly educated with concomitant literacy problems. Low educational levels and socioeconomic deprivation are strongly correlated with higher incidences of disease, poor nutrition, lower survival rates, and a decreased quality of life in general. Increased exposure to hazardous working conditions in low paying, manual labor jobs has also resulted in a greater incidence of occupation-related diseases and illnesses among this population (Dignam, 2000; Mackenbach et al., 2000; Monden et al., 2006; Rognerud & Zahl, 2005). In addition, the majority of Blacks reside in inner-city areas where exposure to violence and pollution puts them at greater risk for disease, disability, and death. The average life span of Black Americans is shorter than that of White Americans due to high death rates from cancer, cardiovascular disease, cirrhosis, diabetes, accidents, homicides, and infant mortality (Anderson et al., 2000; Dignam, 2000; Forrester, 2000; Holt, Kyles, Wiehagen, & Casey, 2003; Keyserling et al., 2000; Samuel-Hodge, Keyserling, France, Ingram, Johnston, Davis et al., 2006; Yanek, Becker, Moy, Gettelsohn, & Koffman, 2001). Also, Blacks are at higher risk for drug addiction, teenaged pregnancy, and sexually transmitted diseases (Purnell & Paulanka, 2003).

Purnell and Paulanka (2003) reported findings that African Americans are pessimistic about human relationships and their belief system emphasizes three major themes:

1. The world is a hostile and dangerous place to live.
2. The individual is vulnerable to attack from external forces.
3. The individual is considered helpless with few internal resources to combat adversity.

Because many African Americans tend to be suspicious of Western ethnomedical practitioners, they often seek the assistance of physicians and nurses only when absolutely necessary (Purnell & Paulanka, 2003). Instead, folk practitioners are held in higher esteem than the Western biomedical healthcare team.

Common to the Black culture is the concept of extended family, consisting of several households, with the older adults often taking the leadership role within the family constellation. Respect for elders and ancestors is valued. They are held in high esteem because living a long life indicates that the individual had more opportunities to acquire much experience and knowledge. Decision making regarding healthcare issues is, therefore, often left to the elders. Family ties are especially strong between grandchildren and grandparents. It is not unusual for grandmothers to want to stay at the hospital bedside when their grandchildren are ill. This extended family network provides emotional, physical, and financial support to members during times of illness and other crises (Forrester, 2000; Purnell & Paulanka, 2003).

Single parenting within the African American culture is an accepted position without stigma attached to it. Becoming a mother at a young age, although not highly desirable or condoned by Black women, does have a fairly high level of tolerance in this cultural group (Purnell & Paulanka, 2003). In fact, Black women do not perceive negative sanctions within their culture if they do not meet the ideal norm of getting an education or job prior to marriage and children. Relatives are supportive of each other if help is needed with childbearing.

Spirituality and religiosity are very much a prominent cultural component of this ethnic group's community. They are at the center of and are a defining feature of African American life and serve as a source of hope, renewal, liberation, and unity among its members. *Spirituality* is defined as a belief in a higher power, a sacred force that exists in all things. *Religiosity* is defined as an individual's level of adherence to beliefs and ritualistic practices associated with religious institutions (Holt, Clark, & Kreuter, 2003; Mattis, 2000; Mattis & Jagers, 2001; Puchalski & Romer, 2000).

Both spirituality and religion play a role in the development and maintenance of social relationships throughout the developmental life span. Blacks, moreso than Whites, turn to religion to cope with health challenges. Religious practices also have been found to influence health beliefs and positively influence health status and outcomes in the African American community (Newlin, Knafl, & Melkus, 2002). These strong religious values and beliefs may extend to their feelings about illness and health. A majority of Black Americans find inner strength from their trust in God. Some believe that whatever happens is God's will. This belief has led to the perception that Black Americans have a fatalistic view of life (Purnell & Paulanka, 2003) and are governed by a relatively strong external locus of control (Holt, Clark et al., 2003).

A traditional folk practice, known as voodoo, consists of beliefs about good or evil spirits inhabiting the world. A religious leader or voodoo doctors have the power to appease or release hostile spirits. Illness, or disharmony, is thought to be caused by evil spirits because a person failed to follow religious rules or the dictates of ancestors. Curative measures involve finding the cause of an illness—a hex or a spell placed on a person by another or the breaking of a taboo—and then finding someone with magical healing powers or witchcraft to rid the afflicted individual of the evil spirit(s). Some Black American families also continue to practice home remedies such as the use of mustard plasters, taking of herbal medicines and teas, and wearing of amulets to cure or ward off a variety of illnesses and afflictions (Purnell & Paulanka, 2003).

TEACHING STRATEGIES

In teaching Black Americans preventive and promotion measures, as well as caring for them during acute and chronic illnesses, the nurse must explore the client's value systems. Generally, any folk practices or traditional beliefs should be respected and allowed (if they are not harmful) and incorporated into the recommended treatment or healthcare interventions used by western medicine. The following discussion offers more specific recommendations for rendering culturally appropriate care for Black Americans.

Black Americans tend to be very verbal, dynamic, animated, and interpersonal, whereby they express feelings openly to family and friends. However, they are much more private about family matters when in the company of strangers. Even though Black Americans are very informal when they interact among themselves, they prefer to be greeted in a more formal manner with the use of their surnames, which demonstrates the respect and pride they have in their family heritage.

Also, Black Americans tend to feel comfortable with less personal space than do some other ethnic groups. Humor, joking, and teasing one another are ways to reduce stress and tension, but these types of communication can be misinterpreted as aggressive behavior if not understood within the context of their culture (Purnell & Paulanka, 2003).

Generally, African Americans are also more present than past or future oriented. Thus, they tend to be more relaxed about specific time frames, evincing a more circular rather than linear sense of time, which is more characteristic of the dominant White culture. Health providers must be careful not to misinterpret nonverbal and verbal behaviors when delivering care and must be flexible in the timing of appointments, as Blacks will usually keep their appointments but may not always be on schedule.

Traditionally, the family structure has been matriarchal; this pattern persists to the present day due to a high percentage of households run by a female single parent. It is imperative that healthcare providers acknowledge the dominant role that Black women play in decision making and the importance of sharing health information directly with them. Grandmothers continue to play a central role in the Black American family and are often involved in providing economic support and child care for their grandchildren (Forrester, 2000).

With respect to prevalent diseases and health issues within this population group, diabetes and hypertension continue to be the most serious health problems. The group as a whole suffers higher morbidity and mortality rates from these diseases than do other Americans (Samuel-Hodge et al., 2006; Yanek et al., 2001). Also, Blacks are at higher risk for being victims of violence, accidents, disabilities, and cancer (Forrester, 2000; Purnell & Paulanka, 2003). Obesity is another major problem among Black Americans. Food to them is a symbol of health and wealth, and a higher than ideal body weight is viewed as positive by this ethnic group.

Nurse educators must concentrate on disease prevention measures, institute early screening for high blood pressure, cancer, and diabetes, as well as screening for signs and symptoms of other diseases common in this population, and provide culturally congruent health education to improve the overall health status of Black Americans (Bailey, Erwin, & Belin, 2000; Powe, Daniels, Finnie, & Thompson, 2005). Strong family ties encourage individuals to be treated by the family before seeking care from health professionals. This cultural practice may be a factor contributing to the delay or failure of Blacks to seek treatment of diseases at the early stages of illness. An effective approach to providing care can be to conduct health screening programs in conjunction with community and church activities (Samuel-Hodge et al., 2006). "The church is a viable health education venue for this population" (Holt, Kyles et al., 2003).

Due to economic factors, Black Americans are likely to have less ready access to healthcare services. Identified barriers to Black Americans seeking the health care they need include lack of culturally relevant care, perceptions of racial discrimination, and a general distrust of both healthcare professionals and the healthcare system. Establishing a trusting relationship, therefore, is an essential first step to be taken by healthcare professionals if Blacks are to receive and accept the health services they require and deserve. Recognizing their unique responses to health and illness based on their spiritual and religious foundations, their strong family ties, and other traditional beliefs is essential if therapeutic interventions developed by the healthcare team are to be successful. Efforts to recruit more Blacks into the nursing profession would help most assuredly to reduce some of the barriers to caring for this population of Americans.

Asian/Pacific Islander Culture

People from Asian countries and the Pacific Islands constitute the third major ethnic group. Many Southeast Asian refugees have come to the U.S. mainly as a result of World War II, the Korean War in the 1950s, the fall of the South

Vietnam government in 1975, and the successive disintegrations of the governments of Laos and Cambodia. Primarily, they have settled on the West Coast, particularly in the San Francisco Bay area of California and in Washington state (Villanueva & Lipat, 2000; Young et al., 2002). Also, the states of New York, New Jersey, and Texas have experienced a large influx of Asian peoples, particularly from China, the Philippines, and Japan. In the decades following political and social upheavals in Southeast Asia, almost three quarters of a million people of Asian/Pacific Islander origin immigrated into the United States. As of 2004, more than 12 million Asian/Pacific Islanders (3.8% of the total U.S. population) live in the country (U.S. Census Bureau, 2006).

Although Asian/Pacific Islander people have been classified as a single ethnic group by many researchers and census takers, the culture of all these people is not the same. In fact, a wide variety of cultural, religious, and language backgrounds are represented. Some similarities exist among members of the Asian/Pacific Islander group, but there are also many differences (Purnell & Paulanka, 2003). By understanding the basic beliefs of the Asian/Pacific Islander people, nurses and other healthcare practitioners can be better prepared to understand and accept their cultural differences and varied behavior patterns (Villanueva & Lipat, 2000; Young et al., 2002).

The major philosophical orientation of the Asian/Pacific Islander people is a blend of four philosophies—Buddhism, Confucianism, Taoism, and Phi. Four common values are strongly reflected in all of these philosophies:

1. Male authority and dominance
2. Saving face (behavior as a result of a sense of pride)
3. Strong family ties
4. Respect for parents, elders, teachers, and other authority figures

The following is a brief review of the beliefs and healthcare practices of the Asian/Pacific Islander people (Pang, 2007; Purnell & Paulanka, 2003).

BUDDHISM

The fundamental belief is that all existence is suffering. The continuation of life, and therefore suffering, arises from desires and passions. According to the Buddhist philosophy, no humans are limited to a single existence terminating in death. Instead, everyone is reincarnated. Cambodians, who are in particular strongly influenced by the Buddhist philosophy, strive to accumulate religious merits or good deeds to ensure a better life to come. They adhere to a deep belief in karma, whereby things done in this existence will help or hinder their ascension on the ladder to nirvana. Good deeds, sharing, donating, and being generous and kind are all ways to accumulate merits.

CONFUCIANISM

Moral values and beliefs are heavily influenced by this philosophy, which focuses on the moral aspects of one's personality. Two predominant moral qualities, developed through cultivation of the personality, include humaneness (the attitude shown toward others) and a sense of moral duty and obligation (attitudes persons display toward themselves). The principles that guide the social behavior of people who adhere to Confucianism are described as follows.

Patterns of Authority The following five relationships run from inferior to superior to form a pattern of obligation and authority in the family as well as in social and political realms:

1. Son (child) to father
2. Wife to husband
3. Younger brother to older brother
4. Friend to friend
5. Subject to ruler

These patterns of authority and obligation influence decision making and social interactions. For example, a friend is to regard a friend as a younger or older brother. Women's subservience to men is reflected in a woman's behavior to always seek the advice of her husband when making decisions. This authority needs to be respected by nursing staff when, for instance, a woman refuses to choose a contraceptive method until she asks for her husband's advice and permission.

Man in Harmony with the Universe   In the Confucian system, people are seen as being between heaven and earth, and life has to be in harmony with the universe. An example of this principle in action is when an Asian responds passively to new information, quietly accepting it rather than actively seeking to clarify it. Given this perspective, it is important for the nurse when instructing the client to ask for an explanation of the information to ascertain if it was understood.

Ancestor Worship   Concern for the moral order of relationships is reflected in a deep reverence for tradition and prescribed rites. Great emphasis is placed on funerals, etiquette for mourning, and the sharing of a communal meal with the dead.

The Asian/Pacific Islander culture values harmony in life and a balance of nature. Shame is something to be avoided, families are the center of life, elders are respected, and ancestors are worshiped and remembered. Children are highly valued because they carry on the family name and are expected to care for aging parents. The woman's role is one of subservience throughout her entire life—she will follow the advice of parents while unmarried, the husband's advice while married, and the children's advice when widowed. This subservient role is in direct conflict with U.S. social and family values, which expect women to take a more independent, assertive, and self-determined role.

TAOISM

The Tao philosophy has its roots in the belief of two opposing magical forces in nature, the negative (yin) and the positive (yang), which affect the course of all material and spiritual life. The basic concepts of Chinese philosophy, the beliefs in tao (the way of nature) and yin and yang (the principle of balance), stress that human achievement in harmony with nature should be accomplished through nonaction.

Common also is the idea that good health depends on the balance between hot and cold. Equilibrium of hot and cold elements produces good health. Drugs, natural elements, and foods are classified as either hot or cold. It is believed that sickness can be caused by eating too much hot or cold food. Hot foods include meats, sweets, and spices. Cold foods include rice and vegetables.

The Chinese people believe in strong family ties, respect for elders, and the authority of men as the head of the household. As a consequence, sons are highly valued. Illness is believed to result from an imbalance in the forces of nature. Ill health is believed to be a curse from heaven, with mental illness being the worst possible curse, because the individual was irresponsible in not obtaining the right amount of rest, food, and work.

Phi

Phi worship is a belief in the spirits of dead relatives or the spirits of animals and nature. Phi ranges from bad to good. If a place has a strong phi, the individual must make an offering before doing anything in that place, such as building a house or tilling the land. If someone violates a rule of order, an atmosphere of bad phi can result in illness or death. Redemption can be sought from a phi priest as a hope of getting relief from suffering. Offerings are made and special rites are performed to rid the person of a bad phi.

Worshipers of this philosophy respect elders and avoid conflict by doing things in a pleasant manner. Those who adhere to the phi philosophy are hospitable and generous. They show respect to others by the way a person is addressed, and tend to prize hard work and ambition.

For people of the Asian/Pacific Islander ethnic group, marked cultural differences confront them when they live in the United States with respect to ways of life, ways of thinking, values orientation, social structure, and family interactions (Chao, 1994; Young et al., 2002). Children may adapt quickly, but the older generations tend to have difficulty acculturating.

Their medical practices, like their other unique cultural practices, differ significantly from Western ways. The health-seeking behaviors of immigrants tend to be crisis oriented, following the pattern in their homelands where medical care was not readily available. They are likely to seek health care only when seriously ill. Reinforcement is needed to encourage them to come for follow-up visits after an initial encounter with the health-care system. Sometimes they are viewed by practitioners as noncompliant when they do not do exactly what is expected of them, when they withdraw from follow-up treatments, or when they do not keep prearranged appointments.

Asian people make great use of herbal remedies to treat various ills, such as fevers, diarrhea, and coughs. Dermabrasion, often misunderstood by U.S. practitioners, is a home remedy to cure a wide variety of problems such as headaches, cold symptoms, fever, and chills. In their traditional healthcare system, Asian individuals rely on folk medicines from healers, sorcerers, and monks.

Western medicine is thought to be "shots that cure," and Asian patients expect to get some form of medicine (injections or pills) whenever they seek medical help in the United States. If no medication is prescribed, the person, if not given an explanation, may feel that care is inadequate and fail to return for future care.

Common to many Southeast Asians is the idea that illnesses, just like foods, are classified as hot and cold. This belief coincides with the yin and yang philosophy of the principles of balance. If a disease is considered hot in origin, then giving cold foods is believed to be the proper treatment.

Conflict and fear are the most likely responses to laboratory tests and having blood drawn. It is the belief of this ethnic group that removing blood makes the body weak and that blood is not replenished. Fear of surgery may result from the conviction that souls inhabit the body and may be released. Another major fear is the loss of privacy leading to extreme embarrassment and humiliation.

Teaching Strategies

Respect is automatically endowed on most healthcare providers and teachers because they are seen as knowledgeable. Asians are sensitive and formal people, so making a friendly and nonthreatening approach to them is necessary before giving care. They must be given permission to ask a question but are not offended by questions from others.

One salient characteristic to be noted of the Japanese subculture is a childlike dependency known as *amae,* which continues through adulthood but is especially evident when people are ill or going through hardships. This behavior conflicts with the Western nursing philosophy of helping those they care for to become independent in self-care. Awareness of this characteristic dependent behavior will allow American nurses to approach clients of Japanese heritage in a culturally relevant and tolerant manner (Hisama, 2000).

Language barriers are usually the first and biggest obstacle to overcome in working with people of Asian/Pacific Islander descent. The learning style of Asians is essentially passive—no personal opinions, no confrontations, no challenges, and no outward disagreements. Nurses and other healthcare practitioners should be aware that in the Asians' wish to save face for themselves and others, they avoid being disruptive and will agree to what is said so as not to be offensive.

The approach to learning is done primarily by repetition and rote memorization of information. It must be remembered that decision making is a family affair. Consequently, family members need to be included, especially the male authority figure, in the process of deciding the best solution for a situation. They are easily shamed, so clients must be reassured and told what is considered acceptable behavior by Western moral and legal standards. Nods of the head do not necessarily mean agreement or

understanding. Questions directed to them need to be asked in several ways to confirm that they understand any instructional messages given.

American Indian/Alaskan Native Culture

The U.S. Census Bureau (2006) has identified more than 2.8 million people (almost 1% of the U.S. population) who are of this ethnic group living in the United States. There are more than 500 distinct tribes of American Indians and Native Alaskans, including Eskimo and Aleut tribes (Lowe & Struthers, 2001). The largest of these tribes is the Cherokee. Other tribes of significant size are the Navaho, Sioux, Chippewa, Choctaw, Pueblo, and the Latin American Indian. These tribes reside primarily in the Northwestern, Central, and Southwestern regions of the United States (U.S. Census Bureau, 2006). The term Native American will be used throughout this section of the chapter to include both the American Indian and Native Alaskan people.

Of these people, approximately one half are eligible for health services provided by the federal government. Medical care to American Indian people has a long history. As far back as 1832, the War Department undertook a smallpox vaccination campaign for tribes of American Indian people, largely to protect military troops from infection. In 1849, healthcare responsibility was transferred to the newly created Bureau of Indian Affairs. In 1954, the Department of Health, Education, and Welfare of the U.S. Public Health Service (USPHS) took over jurisdiction. Today, the Indian Health Service (IHS) of the USPHS maintains responsibility for providing health care to members of this ethnic group (Mail, McKay, & Katz, 1989).

The current challenge to healthcare practitioners is to integrate Western medicine with traditional non-Western tribal folk medicine to provide cross-cultural health education to Native Americans in reservation-based communities across the nation. To do so, nurses must understand contemporary Native American cultural patterns, including theories of disease causality and associated therapies. It is also essential for nursing professionals to become focused on a more ethnomedical orientation. This means delineating the nature and consequences of illness problems and disease interventions from the ethnic group's perspective, rather than adhering to the biomedical orientation of defining diseases and illness interventions from only a Western perspective.

In the ethnomedical context, the concept of health and illness incorporates the relationship of humans with their universe—a concept that bridges culture with a sensitivity toward the daily practices inherent within specific ethnic groups. The challenge for the nurse educator is to understand the world perspective of contemporary American Indian and Native Alaskan people that sets them apart from non–Native Americans (Cantore, 2001; Lowe & Struthers, 2001; Mail et al., 1989).

As outlined by Purnell and Paulanka (2003), Lowe and Struthers (2001), Harding (1998), Scharnberg (2007), Joho and Ormsby (2000), and Cantore (2001), Native American culture has the following major characteristics:

1. A spiritual attachment to the land and harmony with nature
2. An intimacy of religion and medicine
3. Emphasis on strong ties to an extended family network, including immediate family, other relatives, and the entire tribe
4. The view that children are an asset, not a liability
5. A belief that supernatural powers exist in animate as well as in inanimate objects
6. A desire to remain Native American and avoid acculturation, thereby retaining one's own culture and language
7. A lack of materialism, lack of time consciousness, and a desire to share with others

Unless the awareness of non–Native American healthcare workers is raised, these common characteristics can easily be overlooked by them when care is being provided to clients of this ethnic group. Although Anglo-American culture and Western healthcare practices have been integrated to some extent into the Native American way of life, the preceding characteristics still predominate today to set this subculture apart as a unique entity.

Native Americans see a close connection between religion and health. When a family member becomes ill, witchcraft is still perceived by some tribes as the real cause of illness. In traditional societies, witchcraft functions to supply answers to perplexing or disturbing questions. It also explains personal insecurities, intragroup tensions, fears, and anxieties.

Witches, with their supernatural powers, have served as convenient scapegoats on which to blame the misfortunes in life and provided tribes with a mechanism for social control. It is hypothesized that as the cultural practices of witchcraft were increasingly denigrated by missionaries and bureaucrats, substitutions such as compulsive drinking and frequent use of narcotics (peyote) emerged as culturally sanctioned outlets for aggressive impulses and frustrations.

These behaviors were seen as less disruptive than demonstrating overt hostilities. This hypothesis has been proposed as an explanation of the high prevalence of substance abuse by Native Americans.

Some Native American tribes still practice witchcraft but tend to deny it as a reality because of the negative stereotype and stigma attached to it by outsiders. Nevertheless, the intimacy between religion and medicine persists and is exhibited in the form of "sing" prayers and ceremonial cure practices. However, few nurses would think of providing space and privacy for several relatives to be able to conduct a ceremony for a hospitalized family member.

Some Native American tribal beliefs also require incorporating the medicine man (shaman) into the system of care given to patients. The central and formal aspects of Native American medicine are ceremonial, embracing the notion of a supernatural power. Although the ceremonies vary from tribe to tribe, the ideas of causation and cure are common to all Native Americans. The ritual performed is determined by the signs and symptoms of an illness. Sometimes rituals are conducted by family members. Cornmeal, from the sacred food of corn, is one item that is frequently used in a variety of curative ceremonies. Herbal remedies have for generations served native healers as their pharmacopoeia. The nurse must demonstrate legitimate respect for such ritualistic symbols and ceremonial activities.

To be considered really poor in the Native American world is to be devoid of relatives. The family and tribe are of utmost importance, which is a belief that children learn from infancy. It is not unusual for many family members—sometimes large groups of 10 to 15 people—to arrive at the hospital and camp out on the hospital grounds to be with their sick relative. Talking

is unnecessary, but simply being there is highly important for everyone concerned. Hospital personnel have often labeled this behavior as useless and disruptive and deem the patient and family to be uncooperative.

Grandmothers, in particular, have great importance to a sick child, and they frequently must give permission for a child to be hospitalized and treated. The Native American kinship system, in fact, allows for a child to have several sets of grandparents, aunts, uncles, cousins, brothers, and sisters. Sometimes a number of women substitute as a mother figure for a child, which may cause role confusion for the non-Native American healthcare provider.

Children are given a great deal of freedom and independence to learn by their decisions and live by the consequences of their actions. Their entire childhood years consist of experiential learning to develop skills and self-confidence to function as adults. They may appear spoiled, but in fact they are taught self-care and respect for others at a very early age. Children are doted on by family members, and, in turn, they have high regard for their elders. In fact, the older adults in Native American communities are highly respected and looked to for advice and counsel. Outside of their private domain, such as in the public school system, Native American children tend not to be seen as very competitive or assertive. However, to call attention to oneself is interpreted by Native Americans as showy and inappropriate.

Another characteristic of Native Americans is that they generally are not very future oriented; they take one day at a time and do not feel they have control over their own destiny. Time is seen as being on a continuum with no beginning and no end. Native Americans tend not to live by clocks and schedules. In fact, many of their homes do not have clocks, and family members eat meals and do other activities when they please.

Members of this ethnic group tend to be more casual in their approach to life than many non-Native American people. This lack of time consciousness and pressure is a crucial factor to be remembered by healthcare providers when a prescribed regimen calls for the patient to follow a medication, exercise, or dietary schedule. This attitude or way of thinking also has proved to be a significant obstacle when health educators have attempted to provide preventive care. Inattention to time, in addition, can interfere with their keeping scheduled appointments, although lack of funds rather than time seems to be the main cause of missed appointments.

Another aspect of time is reflected in their belief that death is just a part of the life cycle—a much healthier and more accepting attitude toward dying than that held by most White Americans. Their grief process is culturally very different. Funerals are accompanied by large feasts and the sharing of gifts with relatives of the deceased. There is no belief in a life hereafter as a reward for a lifetime of good deeds while on earth. Life after death is, instead, viewed as an opportunity to join the world of long-ago ancestors. Their view of death is closely related to their opinion about the appropriate disposal of amputated limbs. Because diabetes is so prevalent in the Native American population, it is important to know that they usually want to reclaim an amputated body part for proper burial.

Sharing is another core value of Native Americans. The concept of *being* is fundamental, and there is little stress on achievement or the worth of material wealth. Individuals are valued much more highly than material goods. Overall, Native Americans are a proud, sensitive, cooperative, passive people, devoted to tribe and family, and willing to share possessions and self with others. They are very vulnerable when it comes to their pride and dignity. They can be easily offended by nonsensitive caregivers.

In terms of human relationships, it is important to note that Native Americans believe that to look someone in the eye is considered disrespectful. Some tribes feel that looking into the eyes of another person reveals and may even steal someone's soul. As a friendly handshake and eye contact are acceptable and even expected in the Anglo-American culture, it must be acknowledged that these gestures do not have the same meaning for the Native American. In fact, eye contact by White American definition is interpreted to mean that someone is paying attention, is interested, or understands. Non-Native American healthcare workers, therefore, may consider lack of eye contact to mean that these patients are shiftless, shifty, uninterested in learning, or inattentive, when in fact all along they were taking in the message of instruction being given. If asked, they can often repeat verbatim what someone just said to them.

The type and incidence of health problems faced by Native Americans have undergone significant change over the years. In the first half of the 20th century, acute and infectious diseases were prevalent and were the principal cause of death. Today, as a result of increased life expectancy, Native Americans are succumbing to many lifestyle diseases and chronic conditions. Chief among the causes of morbidity and mortality are heart disease, cancer, diabetes, and drug and alcohol abuse—all of which to some extent are amenable to educational intervention.

TEACHING STRATEGIES

Nurse educators need to focus on giving information about these diseases and risk factors, emphasize the teaching of skills related to changes in diet and exercise, and help clients to build positive coping mechanisms to deal with emotional problems. For the most part, acute and infectious diseases, with the exception of a recurrence in tuberculosis, are no longer a major cause of illness and death among Native Americans. This is due to modern drug therapy, early case findings, improved sanitary conditions, and better provision of health education.

Another positive influence has been the greater availability of community health representatives (CHRs). These indigenous community outreach workers have played a significant role in case finding, early diagnosis, and reinforcement of patient and other health education recommendations. As Mail and others (1989) stated: "Involving the CHR in patient education is an important cross-cultural consideration, because this is the individual who will reinforce behavior changes with the community and home" (p. 97).

Although all Native Americans share some of the core beliefs and practices of their culture, each tribe is unique in its customs and language. Finding the ways and means to integrate Western medicine with the traditional Native American folk medicine in caring for the varied needs of this population group presents a challenge to the nurse educator. It also presents a learning opportunity for the recipient of these health education services.

Preparing Nurses for Diversity Care

America is no longer the homogeneous melting pot society it once was. Today, myriad cultures are present in the United States, and we face an increasing trend toward global migration of people and globalization of nursing practice. The delivery of appropriate health care now and in the future will depend on use of a culturally informed approach that goes beyond simple language translation and an understanding of the characteristics of different cultures. As caregivers, we must learn how to relate to people, both clients, fellow healthcare practitioners, and nursing students, who come from a variety of cultural backgrounds, and discover the cultural meaning of various health events (Career Directory, 2005).

The nursing profession must be prepared to pursue this relatively new paradigm for creating and managing diversity within our workforce as well as within the healthcare marketplace consisting of consumers and staff from multicultural backgrounds. Diversity has the potential to positively affect our profession by increasing organizational effectiveness, creating greater access to care, lifting morale of clients and staff, and enhancing productivity in the workforce (Cooper, Grywalski, Lamp, Newhouse, & Studlien, 2007; Marquand, 2001; Thomas & Ely, 1996).

As a result of former President Clinton's national leadership to eliminate cultural disparities in health by the year 2010, the U.S. government introduced a series of initiatives put forth in the *Healthy People 2010* document. One goal of this 10-year plan was to eliminate racial and ethnic disparities in health (U.S. DHHS, 2000). This current initiative is lauded as "the first explicit commitment by the government to achieve equity in health outcomes" (Jones, 2000, p. 214). The nursing profession has embraced this goal and its objectives to eradicate discrepancies in health outcomes among minority populations. The profession has begun contributing to this expectation by focusing on change in both the academic and the practice settings as well as through clinical research (Carol, 2001).

One important step to assure culturally competent nursing care in this new century is to increase minority representation in nursing. The profession needs to recruit and retain more minority students and faculty to expand diversity within its ranks. Unfortunately, the nursing workforce comprises only 10% of people from minority groups (see **Figure 8–6**), whereas more than 28% of the total U.S. population belongs to a variety of cultural subgroups (Robinson, 2000).

Another initiative to break down cultural barriers to health care is to strengthen multicultural perspectives in the curriculum of nursing education programs (Bond, Kardong-Edgren, & Jones,

Figure 8–6 Distribution of registered nurses by racial/ethnic background, March 2004.

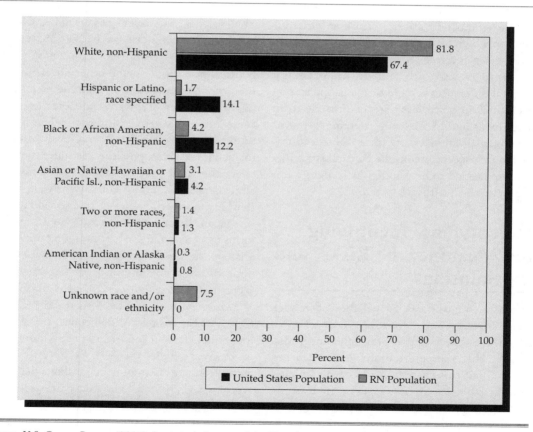

Source: U.S. Census Bureau (2006). Statistical abstract of the United States, resident population by sex, race, and Hispanic origin status: 2000 to 2004, Table 13. Retrieved from http://www.census.gov/prod/2005pubs/06statab/pop.pdf.

Note: Census reports that, of the 293,655,000 in the U.S. population for 2004, 197,841,000 are of White race and non-Hispanic. Thus, while 67.4% of the U.S. population are White, non-Hispanic, 32.6% are non-White or Hispanic.

2001; Kelley & Fitzsimons, 2000). Innovative nursing education means incorporating social values that recognize diverse lifestyles and acknowledge multicultural and multiracial perspectives (Rew, Becker, Cookston, Khosropour, & Martinez, 2003). As these authors pointed out, nurses must not only better understand the cultural characteristics and traits of patients and families from different ethnic backgrounds, but also improve the relationship between nurses and clients from different cultural backgrounds.

Nurses must be able to create an environment in which people are encouraged to express themselves and freely describe their needs. As Dreher (1996) so aptly stated, "Transcending cultural differences is more than an appreciation of cultural diversity. It is transcending one's own investment in the social and economic system as one knows it and lives it" (p. 4). Nurse educators must concentrate on the cultural strategies that are needed to help individuals and groups negotiate the healthcare system.

Stereotyping: Identifying the Meaning, the Risks, and the Solutions

In addressing the diversity issues of gender, socioeconomics, and culture, one must acknowledge the risks of stereotyping inherent in discussing these three attributes of the learner. Throughout this chapter, it has been explicitly recognized that differences exist in learning based on gender, socioeconomics, and culture and often require alternative approaches to teaching. It is important to realize that differences should not be equated with judgments as to what is good or bad, right or wrong; rather, one should not ignore the need to attend to

these differences in a sensitive, open, and fair manner.

Nurse educators must relate to each person as an individual. It is important to develop an awareness that although a person can be considered as a member—or may identify with members—of a certain ethnic group, the individual has his or her own abilities, experiences, preferences, and practices. Learning needs, learning styles, and readiness to learn are all factors that influence lifestyle behaviors.

Nevertheless, everyone has been socialized in subtle and not so subtle ways according to one's own diversity attributes, socioeconomic and political backgrounds, and other life exposures. It is imperative to acknowledge the prejudices, biases, and stereotypical tendencies that can come into play when dealing with others like or unlike ourselves. We must consciously attempt to recognize these possible attitudes and the effect they may have on others in our care. To address the dangers of stereotyping on more than just a superficial level, this section examines examples of what constitutes unacceptable forms of stereotyping, what common pitfalls can arise in dealing with diversity, and what can be done to avoid stereotypical behaviors in ourselves and others.

Stereotyping is defined by Purnell and Paulanka (2003) as "an oversimplified conception, opinion, or belief about some aspect of an individual or group of people" (p. 357). Exaggerated generalizations are commonly made about the characteristics, behaviors, and motives associated with any person or group of people. Actually, stereotyping can be positive or negative, depending on how, where, when, why, and about whom it is applied (Satel, 2002).

For example, stereotyping can be a useful and legitimate process to organize or classify people if based on logical reasoning and accumulated facts. A system of organization and classification helps people to identify and understand information—for example, "he's Jewish," "she's Italian," or "they're Democrats." Conversely, stereotyping can be negative if it is used to place people in a mold or an artificial, unfair position based on over-simplification without true substantiation by facts. Negative stereotyping leads to disrespect, dehumanization, and denigration of others and serves as a barrier to equality and fairness toward others.

Stereotyping deserves a bad name when associated with bias or clichés. There is a huge emotional component to stereotyping. The language that we use, the attitudes that we project, the conclusions that we draw, and the context in which we employ stereotyping all determine its positive or negative quality.

Unfortunately, classification by association is often perfunctory and, therefore, laden with bias. Stereotyping in this sense is used to label someone. For example, we, as Americans, think of ourselves as the freedom fighters and liberty lovers of the world; in the same breath, we may describe members of other groups or nationalities as violators of human rights or terrorists. This threat of stereotyping is even greater in light of the infamous September 11, 2001, attack on our country. Simple appearance, such as a beard, attire, or form of speech, can be the basis of broad and deep prejudices.

People particularly tend to use an excuse to classify individuals when they do not like or respect others whose backgrounds, attitudes, abilities, values, or beliefs are different from or opposed to their own or are misunderstood or misinterpreted. Stereotyping, conscious or subconscious, results in intolerance toward others and engenders the belief that our way is the only

way or the right way. Corley and Goren (1998) discuss the ways in which labeling, stereotyping, and stigmatizing responses by nurses tend to marginalize clients.

Attitudes toward sex-role competencies are considered a type of stereotyping. Gender bias has produced inequality in education, employment, and other social spheres. This is an especially relevant caveat for nurses in relating with colleagues as more and more men choose the nursing profession as a career (Coleman, 2002).

Research into gender stereotyping in the past 20 years has documented that elementary and secondary school teachers interact more actively with boys by asking them more questions, giving them more feedback (praise and positive encouragement), and providing them with more specific and valuable comments and guidance. In these subtle ways, these stereotypical expectations are reinforced (Snowman & Biehler, 2006).

Also, it used to be that an extensive list of personality differences between the sexes would be included in education and developmental psychology textbooks. However, recent psychology research has revealed that these sex-role lists are gender biased. Today, it is recognized that few personality characteristics associated with gender are consistent across cultures, except for aggression (Vander Zanden et al., 2007; Santrock, 2006; Snowman & Biehler, 2006).

As another example of gender bias, women have been labeled as attentive listeners and men as poor listeners when, in fact, listening behavior is not a measure of attentiveness but a matter of behavioral style. Men, when listening, move around and make sporadic eye contact, whereas women are likely to remain still and maintain steady eye contact with occasional nodding or smiling. As a result, the listening

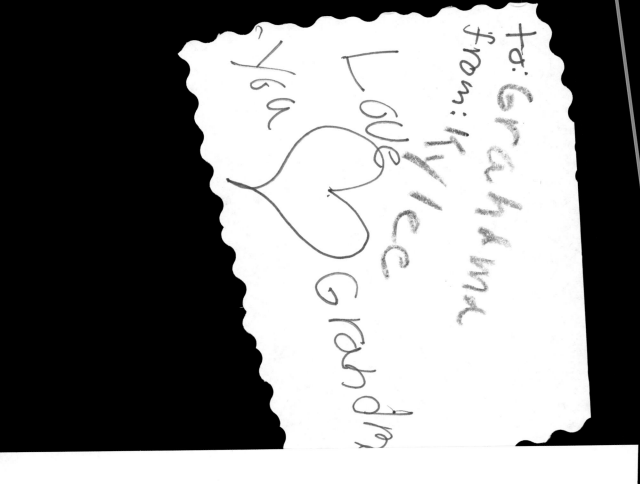

style of men is often misinterpreted as inattentive or rude, and the style of females is often mistaken for encouragement or agreement with what is being said (Tear, 1995).

Interruptions when engaging in dialogue also have been noted as a misinterpretation of communication differences between the sexes. Men frequently speak in a steady flow and interrupt each other to take turns, whereas women tend to speak with frequent pauses to allow others to have their say. Pause-free male speech is often misinterpreted as a device to discourage females from participating and as an attempt to be pushy. The tendency for females to pause in speaking is seen as being timid or courteous. These misinterpretations reinforce stereotypes of men as dominating, insensitive, and controlling and women as unassertive, passive, and oversensitive (Tear, 1995).

Nurses must concentrate on treating the sexes equally when providing access to health education, delivering health and illness care, and designing health education materials that contain bias-free language. For example, they must avoid gender-specific terms and choose words that minimize ambiguity in gender identity, unless critical to the content. They should avoid using the pronouns *he* or *she* and instead use the plural pronoun *they*. If at all possible, nurses should avoid beginning or ending words with man or men, such as *man-made*, *mankind*, or *chairmen*. Do not specify marital status unless necessary by using *Ms.* instead of *Mrs.* Guidelines for nonsexist language can be found in *McGraw-Hill Guidelines for Bias-Free Publishing* or *The Bias-Free Word Finder*.

With respect to age, socioeconomics, culture and race, religion, or disabilities, stereotyping most definitely exists. Throughout this chapter, there are many cautions against stereotyping of

individuals and groups. For example, just because someone belongs to a specific ethnic group does not necessarily mean that the individual adheres to all of the beliefs and practices of that particular culture.

A thorough and accurate assessment of the learner is the key to determining the particular abilities, preferences, and needs of each individual. The nurse educator should choose words that are accurate, clear, and free from bias whenever speaking or writing about various individuals or groups. Nurses should refer to someone's ethnicity, race, religion, age, and socioeconomic status only when it is essential to the content being addressed. For instance, it is more politically and socially correct to use the term *older adult* than the term *elderly* or *aged*. Do not label a member of a special population as a *disabled person* but rather as a *person with a disability*. Also, it is more appropriate and more acceptable to refer to a *person with diabetes* rather than a *diabetic* or to a *person with AIDS* rather than an *AIDS victim*.

To avoid stereotyping, nurses should ask themselves the following questions:

- Do I use neutral language when teaching clients and families?
- Do I confront bias when evidenced by other healthcare professionals?
- Do I request information equally from clients regardless of gender, socioeconomic status, age, or culture?
- Are my instructional materials free of stereotypical terminology and expressions?
- Am I an effective role model of equality for my colleagues?
- Do I treat all clients with fairness, respect, and dignity?
- Does someone's appearance influence (raise or lower) my expectations of that

person's abilities or affect the quality of care I deliver?

- Do I routinely assess the educational backgrounds, experiential backgrounds, personal attributes, and economic resources of clients to ensure appropriate health teaching?
- Am I knowledgeable enough of the cultural traditions of various groups to provide sensitive care in our multicultural, pluralistic society?

It is easy to stereotype someone, not out of malice, but out of ignorance. Nurse educators have a responsibility to keep informed of the most current beliefs and facts about various gender attributes, socioeconomic influences, and cultural traditions that could impact positively or negatively on teaching and learning. Every day, research in nursing, social science, psychology, and medicine is yielding information that will assist in planning and revising appropriate nursing interventions to meet the needs of our diverse client populations.

State of the Evidence

It is essential that nurses base their practice on evidence from empirical studies and expert opinion to deliver the highest, most scientifically sound care to clients. Such evidence also is important as a basis for the educational preparation of staff nurses and future members of the nursing profession to give them the most up-to-date knowledge and skills needed to function competently and confidently in today's healthcare environment.

With respect to gender attributes of the learner, it is evident that understanding how the human brain works and the differences between the sexes in how they think, feel, and respond is still in its infancy. Neuroscience is just beginning to unravel the mysteries and discover the differences and similarities in the way male and female brains are wired. In the last 5–10 years, there has been an upsurge of interest and fascination with the discoveries in the field of neurobiology. New brain imaging instruments are beginning to reveal which individual portions of the brain are responsible for cognition, emotions, and tasks, but even more importantly is how the different parts of the brain operate or interact in concert with one another.

Brain research is an exciting, largely uncharted field, and some of the research findings are conflicting or inconclusive. Therefore, the challenge is to incorporate what is currently known for the refinement of our approaches to teaching and learning, but not to be too quick in jumping to assumptions or generalizations in the application of preliminary research findings before the evidence is conclusive.

Research into the impact of socioeconomics on health outcomes also needs to be further conducted. For example, currently, scant information is available about IQ and socioeconomics in relation to health status and health inequalities. The research of Batty et al. (2006) has shown that although cognitive abilities are related to health, the association between socioeconomic environment, social position, educational attainment, and employment status on the health inequalities in morbidity and mortality is still not altogether clear (Elstad & Krokstad, 2003; Singh-Manoux et al., 2005). Much more research needs to be done to understand the impact of socioeconomic position in relation to the ability, preference, and motivation for learning.

Nursing research priorities on the influence of cultural diversity on the health of individuals and groups must be identified and defined. Knowledge gaps remain despite the increase in the number of new studies being conducted. For example, the growing multicultural nature of our American society requires that we understand the impact of ethnic beliefs on the epidemiology of various diseases, on the effectiveness of health promotion efforts, on illness prevention measures, and on health maintenance and rehabilitation interventions. Bolton and colleagues (2001) posed the question: Are there ethnic variations in response to chronic illness and the performance in functional abilities of daily living? A need exists for funding to support research investigation into so many issues related to health, such as nutrition, mental status, social isolation, and prenatal to postmenopausal phases of women's lives.

Also, research is just in its initial stages in developing instruments that give insight into cultural effects of clients' perspectives on health and responses to illness. Harris, Belyea, Mishel, and Germino (2003) call for exploration into creating as well as adopting reliable and valid instruments to measure health beliefs, attitudes, customs, and patterns of behavior in males and females of different ethnic backgrounds. It is clear that health providers lack substantial evidence on how the context of culture impacts health and illness.

Summary

This chapter explored the influence of gender characteristics, socioeconomic status, and cultural beliefs on both the ability and willingness of clients to learn healthcare measures. The in-depth examination of these three factors serves as an explanatory model for certain behaviors observed or potentially encountered in a teaching–learning situation. Even though the emphasis of this chapter was on clients of diverse backgrounds with whom nurse educators interact, an understanding of gender, socioeconomic, and cultural characteristics also can be a useful source of information when teaching nursing students or staff who may come with a variety of experiences and orientations.

The most important message to remember from this chapter is the care one must take not to stereotype or generalize common characteristics of a group to all members associated with that particular group. For example, if the nurse does not know much about an ethnic subculture, he or she should ask clients about their beliefs rather than just assuming they abide by the tenets of a certain cultural group. In that way, nurses can avoid offending learners.

In their role as teachers, nurses must be cautious to treat each learner as an individual. They must determine the extent to which clients ascribe to, exhibit beliefs in, or adhere to ways of doing things that might affect their learning. Humans live in a double environment—an outer layer of social and cultural experiences and an inner layer of innate strengths and weaknesses—which influences how they perceive and respond to their world (Griffith, 1982).

Nurses, as professionals, should constantly strive to improve the delivery of care to all people regardless of their gender orientation, ethnic origin, creed, nationality, or socioeconomic background. There is much more for nurses to know about how these three factors of gender, socioeconomics, and culture affect the teaching–learning process before we can competently, confidently, and sensitively deliver care to satisfy the needs of our socially, intellectually, and culturally diverse clientele.

REVIEW QUESTIONS

1. What are five gender-related characteristics in cognitive functioning and personality behavior that affect learning?
2. How does the environment versus heredity influence gender-specific approaches to learning?
3. In what ways does SES negatively affect a person's health, and, conversely, how does illness impact an individual's socioeconomic well-being?
4. How does the SES of individuals influence the teaching–learning process?
5. What is meant by the term *poverty circle*?
6. What is the definition of each of the following terms: *assimilation, acculturation, culture, ethnic group,* and *ethnocentrism*?
7. How can the concept of transcultural nursing be applied to the assessment and teaching of clients from culturally diverse backgrounds?
8. What are the 12 cultural domains identified in Purnell's model of cultural competence that should be taken into account when conducting a nursing assessment?
9. What are the four major ethnic groups in the United States?
10. What are the salient characteristics of each of the four major ethnic groups?
11. Which teaching strategies are most appropriate to meet the needs of individuals from each of the four major ethnic groups?
12. What can the nurse do to avoid cultural stereotyping?

References

Anderson, J. M. (1987, December). The cultural context of caring. *Canadian Critical Care Nursing Journal,* 7–13.

Anderson, J. M. (1990). Health care across cultures. *Nursing Outlook, 38*(3), 136–139.

Anderson, R. M., Funnell, M. M., Arnold, M. S., Barr, P. A., Edwards, G. J., & Fitzgerald, J. T. (2000). Assessing the cultural relevance of an education program for urban African Americans with diabetes. *The Diabetes Educator, 26*(2), 280–289.

Andrews, M. M., & Boyle, J. S. (1995). Transcultural nursing care. In M. M. Andrews & J. S. Boyle (Eds.), *Transcultural concepts in nursing care* (2nd ed., pp. 49–95). Philadelphia: Lippincott.

Bailey, E. J., Erwin, D. O., & Belin, P. (2000). Using cultural beliefs and patterns to improve mammography utilization among African-American women: The Witness project. *Journal of the National Medical Association, 92*(3), 136–142.

Baker, D. W., Parker, R. M., Williams, M. V., & Clark, W. S. (1998). Health literacy and the risk of hospital admission. *Journal of General Internal Medicine, 13*, 791–798.

Baker, D. W., Parker, R. M., Williams, M. V., Coates, W. C., & Pitkin, K. (1996). Use and effectiveness of interpreters in an emergency department. *Journal of the American Medical Association, 275*(10), 783–788.

Baron-Cohen, S. (2005). The essential difference: The male and female brain. *Phi Kappa Phi Forum, 85*(1), 23–26.

Batty, G. D., Deary, I. J., & Macintyre, S. (2006). Childhood IQ in relation to risk factors for premature mortality in middle-aged persons: The Aberdeen children of the 1950's study. *Journal of Epidemiology and Community Health, 61*, 241–247.

Batty, G. D., Der, G., Macintyre, S., & Deary, I. J. (2006). Does IQ explain socioeconomic inequalities in health? Evidence from a population based cohort study in the west of Scotland. *BMJ, 332*, 580–584. Retrieved July 5, 2007, from http://bmj.com/cgi/content/full/332/7541/580

Begley, S. (1996, February 19). Your child's brain. *Newsweek*, 55–62.

Begley, S., Murr, A., & Rogers, A. (1995, March 27). Gray matters. *Newsweek*, 48–54.

Bolton, L. B., Bennett, C., Richards, H., Gary, F., Harris, L., Millon-Underwood, S., et al. (2001). Nursing research priorities of the National Black Nurses Association. *Nursing Outlook, 49*(6), 258–262.

Bond, M. L., Kardong-Edgren, S., & Jones, M. E. (2001). Assessment of professional nursing students' knowledge and attitudes about patients of diverse cultures. *Journal of Professional Nursing, 17*(6), 305–312.

Borrayo, E. (2004). Where's Maria? A video to increase awareness about breast cancer and mammography screening among low-literacy Latinas. *Preventive Medicine, 39*, 99–110.

Boss, D. M. (2007). Teaching pluralism: Values to cross-cultural barriers. In M. L. Kelley & V. M. Fitzsimons (Eds.), *Understanding cultural diversity: Culture, curriculum, and community nursing* (54–56). Sudbury, MA: Jones and Bartlett.

Cahill, L. (2006). Why sex matters in neuroscience. *Nature Reviews/Neuroscience*. Retrieved July 3, 2007, from www.nature.com/nrn/index.html

Campinha-Bacote, J. (1995). The quest for cultural competence in nursing care. *Nursing Forum, 30*(4), 19–25.

Cantore, J. A. (2001, Winter). Earth, wind, fire and water. *Minority Nurse*, 24–29.

Carol, R. (2001, Fall). Taking the initiative. *Minority Nurse*, 24–27.

Career directory. (2005). Understanding transcultural nursing. *Nursing 2005*, 14–23.

Carthron, D. (2007). A splash of color: Increasing diversity among nursing students and faculty. *Journal of Best Practices in Health Professions Diversity: Research, Education and Policy, 1*(1), 13–23.

Caudle, P. (1993). Providing culturally sensitive health care to Hispanic clients. *Nurse Practitioner, 18*(12), 40, 43–44, 46, 50–51.

Chachkes, E., & Christ, G. (1996). Cross cultural issues in patient education. *Patient Education & Counseling, 27*, 13–21.

Chao, R. K. (1994). Beyond parental control and authoritarian parenting style: Understanding Chinese parenting through the cultural notion of training. *Child Development, 65*, 1111–1119.

Chideya, F. (1999). *The color of our future*. New York: William Morrow.

Cohen, D. (Ed.). (1991). *The circle of life: Rituals from the human family album*. New York: HarperCollins.

Coleman, S. (2002, January 21). You've got males! *Advance for Nurses*, 13.

Cooper, M., Grywalski, M., Lamp, J., Newhouse, L., & Studlien, R. (2007). Enhancing cultural competence: A model for nurses. *Nursing for Women's Health, 11*(2), 148–159.

Corley, M. C., & Goren, S. (1998). The dark side of nursing: Impact of stigmatizing responses on patients. *Scholarly Inquiry for Nursing Practice: An International Journal, 12*(2), 99–118.

Crimmins, E. M., & Saito, Y. (2001). Trends in healthy life expectancy in the United States, 1970–1990: Gender, race, and educational differences. *Social Science & Medicine, 52*, 1629–1641.

Darling, S. (2004). Family literacy: Meeting the needs of at-risk families. *Phi Kappa Phi Forum, 84*(2), 18–21.

Dignam, J. J. (2000). Differences in breast cancer prognosis among African-American and Caucasian women. *CA-A Cancer Journal for Clinicians, 50*(1), 50–64.

Dreher, M. C. (1996, 4th quarter). Nursing: A cultural phenomenon. *Reflections*, 4.

Duffy, M. M., & Snyder, K. (1999). Can ED patients read your education materials? *Journal of Emergency Nursing, 25*(4), 294–297.

Educating the largest minority group. (2003, November 28). *The Chronicle of Higher Education*, B6–B9.

Elstad, J. I., & Krokstad, S. (2003). Social causation, health-selective mobility, and the reproduction of socioeconomic health inequalities over time: Panel study of adult men. *Social Science & Medicine, 57*, 1475–1489.

Felski, R. (2002, January 25). Why academics don't study the lower middle class. *The Chronicle of Higher Education, 48*(2), B24.

Fernandez, R. D., & Hebert, G. J. (2000). Rituals, culture, and tradition: The Puerto Rican experience. In M. L. Kelley & V. M. Fitzsimons (Eds.), *Understanding cultural diversity: Culture, curriculum and community in nursing* (pp. 241–251). Sudbury, MA: Jones and Bartlett.

Forrester, D. A. (2000). Minority men's health: A review of the literature with special emphasis on African American men. In M. L. Kelley & V. M. Fitzsimons (Eds.), *Understanding cultural diversity: Culture, curriculum, and community in nursing* (pp. 283–305). Sudbury, MA: Jones and Bartlett.

Gage, N. L., & Berliner, D. C. (1998). *Educational psychology* (6th ed.). Boston: Houghton Mifflin.

Giger, J. N., & Davidhizar, R. E. (2004). *Transcultural nursing: Assessment and intervention* (2nd ed.). St. Louis: Mosby–Year Book.

Giorgianni, S. S. (1998). Responding to the challenge of health literacy. *The Pfizer Journal, 2*(1), 1–39.

Gorman, C. (1992, January 20). Sizing up the sexes. *Time*, 42–51.

Griffith, S. (1982). Childbearing and the concept of culture. *Journal of Obstetrics, Gynecological, and Neonatal Nursing, 11*(3), 181–184.

Gur, R. C., Alsop, D., Glahn, D., Petty, R., Swanson, C. L., Maldjian, J. A., et al., (2000). An fMRI study of sex differences in regional activation to a verbal and a spatial task. *Brain and Language, 74*, 157–170.

Gura, T. (2005). Big plans for little brains. *Nature, 435*, 1156–1158.

Gutierrez, K. D., & Rogoff, B. (2003). Cultural ways of learning individual traits or repertoires of practice. *Educational Research, 32*(5), 19–25.

Hancock, L. (1996, February 19). Why do schools flunk biology? *Newsweek*, 59.

Harding, S. (1998, June). Native healers: Part 2—The circle in practice. *Alternative & Complementary Therapies*, 173–179.

Harrigan, D. O. (Ed.). (2007). The young brain: Handle with care. *SUNY Upstate Medical University Outlook, 6*(3), 3–31.

Harris, L., Belyea, M., Mishel, M., & Germino, B. (2003). Issues in revising research instruments for use with Southern populations. *Journal of National Black Nurses Association, 14*(2), 44–50.

Hebert, G. J., & Fernandez, R. D. (2000). A challenge to the Puerto Rican community: An untold story of the AIDS epidemic. In M. L. Kelley & V. M. Fitzsimons (Eds.), *Understanding cultural diversity: Culture, curriculum, and community in nursing* (pp. 253–261). Sudbury, MA: Jones and Bartlett.

Hirsch, E. D. (2001, Summer). Overcoming the language gap. *American Educator*, 5–7.

Hisama, K. K. (2000, First Quarter). Japanese theory and practice: Carrying your own lamp. *Reflections on Nursing*, 30–32.

Holt, C. L., Clark, E. M., & Kreuter, M. W. (2003). Spiritual health locus of control and breast cancer beliefs among urban African American women. *Health Psychology, 22*(3), 294–299.

Holt, C. L., Kyles, A., Wiehagen, T., & Casey, C. (2003). Development of a spiritually based breast cancer educational booklet for African American women. *Cancer Control, 10*(5), 37–44.

Horton, M., & Freire, P. (1990). *We make the road by walking*. Philadelphia: Temple University Press.

Jezewski, M. A. (1993). Culture brokering as a model for advocacy. *Nursing & Health Care, 14*(2), 78–85.

Joho, K. A., & Ormsby, A. (2000). A walk in beauty: Strategies for providing culturally competent nursing care to Native Americans. In M. L. Kelley & V. M. Fitzsimons (Eds.), *Understanding cultural diversity: Culture, curriculum, and community in nursing* (pp. 209–218). Sudbury, MA: Jones and Bartlett.

Jones, C. P. (2000). Levels of racism: A theoretical framework and a gardener's tale. *American Journal of Public Health, 90*(8), 1212–1214.

Kato, P. M., & Mann, T. (1996). *Handbook of diversity issues in health psychology*. New York: Plenum Press.

Kawamura, M., Midorikawa, A., & Kezuka, M. (2000). Cerebral localization of the center for reading and writing music. *NeuroReport, 11*(14), 3299–3303.

Kelley, M. L., & Fitzsimons, V. M. (2000). *Understanding cultural diversity: Culture, curriculum, and community in nursing*. Sudbury, MA: Jones and Bartlett.

Kessels, R. P. C. (2003). Patients' memory for medical information. *Journal of the Royal Society of Medicine, 96*, 219–222.

Keyserling, T. C., Ammerman, A. S., Samuel-Hodge, C. D., Ingram, A. T., Skelly, A. H., Elasy, T. A., et al. (2000). A diabetes management program for African American women with Type 2 diabetes. *The Diabetes Educator, 26*(5), 796–805.

Kimura, D. (1999, Summer). The hidden mind: Sex differences in the brain. *Scientific American*, 32–37.

Kniep-Hardy, M., & Burkhardt, M. A. (1977). Nursing the Navajo. *American Journal of Nursing, 77*(1), 95–96.

Leininger, M. (1994). Transcultural nursing education: A worldwide imperative. *Nursing & Health Care, 15*(5), 254–257.

Lindholm, C., Burstrom, B., & Diderichsen, F. (2001). Does chronic illness cause adverse social and economic consequences among Swedes? *Scandinavian Journal of Public Health, 29*, 63–70.

Lipman, E. L., Offord, D. R., & Boyle, M. H. (1994). Relation between economic disadvantage and psychosocial morbidity in children. *Canadian Medical Association Journal, 151*(4), 431–437.

Lowe, J., & Struthers, R. (2001, Third Quarter). A conceptual framework of nursing in Native American culture. *Journal of Nursing Scholarship*, 279–283.

Mackenbach, J. P., Bos, V., Andersen, O., Cardano, M., Costa, G., Harding, S., et al. (2003). Widening socioeconomic inequalities in mortality in six Western European countries. *International Journal of Epidemiology, 32*, 830–837.

Mackenbach, J. P., Cavelaars, A. E. J. M., Kunst, A. E., Groenhof, F., & the EU Working Group on Socioeconomic Inequalities in Health. (2000). Socioeconomic inequalities in cardiovascular disease mortality: An international study. *European Heart Journal, 21*(14), 1141–1151.

Mail, P. D., McKay, R. B., & Katz, M. (1989). Expanding practice horizons: Learning from American Indian patients. *Patient Education & Counseling, 13*, 91–102.

Markides, K. S., & Coreil, J. (1986). The health of Hispanics in southwestern U.S.: An epidemiological paradox. *Public Health Reports, 101*(3), 253–265.

Marquand, B. (2001, Fall). On the front lines of diversity. *Minority Nurse*, 46–49.

Massett, H. A. (1996). Appropriateness of Hispanic print materials: A content analysis. *Health Education Research, 11*(2), 231–242.

Mattis, J. S. (2000). African American women's definitions of spirituality and religiosity. *Journal of Black Psychology, 26*(1), 101–122.

Mattis, J. S., & Jagers, R. J. (2001). A relational framework for the study of religiosity and spirituality in the lives of African Americans. *Journal of Community Psychology, 29*(5), 519–539.

McGoldrick, M. (1995). *You can go home again.* New York: W. W. Norton.

Monastersky, R. (2001, November 2). Land mines in the world of mental maps. *The Chronicle of Higher Education*, A20–A21.

Monden, C. W. S., van Lenthe, F. J., & Mackenbach, J. P. (2006). A simultaneous analysis of neighborhood and childhood socioeconomic environment with self-assessed health and health-related behaviors. *Health & Place, 12*, 394–403.

Mulligan, K. (2004). Chronic illness a prescription for financial distress. *Psychiatric News, 39*(23), 17. Retrieved July 3, 2007, from http://pn.psychiatryonline.org/cgi/content/full/39/23/17?eaf

Narayan, M. C. (2003). Cultural assessment. *Home Healthcare Nurse, 21*(9), 173–178.

Nash, J. M. (1997). Fertile minds. *Time, 149*(5), 48–56.

National Center for Education Statistics. (2006). *National Assessment of Adult Literacy (NAAL): Health literacy component.* Retrieved April 29, 2006, from http://nces.ed.gov/NAAL/index.asp?

Newlin, K., Knafl, K., & Melkus, G. D. (2002). African-American spirituality: A concept analysis. *Advances in Nursing Science, 25*(2), 57–70.

Pacquiao, D. F., Archeval, L., & Shelley, E. E. (2000). Hispanic client satisfaction with home health care: A study of cultural context of care. In M. L. Kelley & V. M. Fitzsimons (Eds.), *Understanding cultural diversity: Culture, curriculum, and community nursing* (pp. 229–240). Sudbury MA: Jones and Bartlett.

Pang, K. Y. C. (2007). The importance of cultural interpretation of religion/spirituality and depression in Korean elderly immigrant women Buddhists and Christians. *Journal of Best Practices in Health Professions Diversity: Research, Education and Policy, 1*(1), 57–89.

Parker, M., & Kiatoukaysy, L. N. (1999). Culturally responsive health care: The example of the Hmong in America. *Journal of the American Academy of Nurse Practitioners, 11*(12), 511–518.

Poss, J. E., & Rangel, R. (1995). Working effectively with interpreters in the primary care setting. *Nurse Practitioner, 20*(12), 43–44, 46–47.

Powe, B. D., Daniels, E. C., Finnie, R., & Thompson, A. (2005). Perceptions about breast cancer among African American women: Do selected educational materials challenge them? *Patient Education and Counseling, 56,* 197–204.

Price, J. L., & Cordell, B. (1994). Cultural diversity and patient teaching. *Journal of Continuing Education in Nursing, 25*(4), 163–166.

Price, K. M., & Cortis, J. D. (2000). The way forward for transcultural nursing. *Nurse Education Today, 20,* 233–243.

Puchalski, C., & Romer, A. L. (2000). Taking a spiritual history allows clinicians to understand patients more fully. *Journal of Palliative Medicine, 3*(1), 129–137.

Purnell, L. D., & Paulanka, B. J. (2003). *Transcultural health care: A culturally competent approach.* Philadelphia: F. A. Davis.

Rew, L., Becker, H., Cookston, J., Khosropour, S., & Martinez, S. (2003). Measuring cultural awareness in nursing students. *Journal of Nursing Education, 42*(6), 249–257.

Rhem, J. (1998). Social class and student learning. *National Teaching & Learning Forum, 7*(5), 1–4.

Robinson, J. H. (2000). Increasing students' cultural sensitivity. *Nurse Educator, 25*(3), 131–135.

Rognerud, M. A., & Zahl, P-H. (2005). Social inequalities in mortality: Changes in the relative importance of income, education, and household size over a 27-year period. *European Journal of Public Health, 16*(1), 62–68.

Samuel-Hodge, C. D., Keyserling, T. C., France, R., Ingram, A. F., Johnston, L. F., Davis, L. P., et al. (2006). A church-based diabetes self-management education program for African Americans with Type 2 diabetes. *Preventing Chronic Disease, 3*(3), 1–16.

Santrock, J. W. (2006). *Life-span development* (10th ed.). Boston: McGraw-Hill.

Satel, S. (2002, May 26). I am a racially profiling doctor. *The Post Standard,* D–6.

Scharnberg, K. (2007). Medicine men for the 21st century. *Chicago Tribune.* Retrieved June 25, 2007, from http://www.chicagotribune.com/news/nationworld/chi-ptsd_04_scharnbergjun04,1,1567532.story

Severiens, S. E., & Ten Dam, G. T. M. (1994). Gender differences in learning styles: A narrative review and quantitative meta-analysis. *Higher Education, 27,* 487–501.

Singh-Manoux, A., Ferrie, J. E., Lynch, J. W., & Marmot, M. (2005). The role of cognitive ability (intelligence) in explaining the association between socioeconomic position and health: Evidence from the Whitehall II prospective cohort study. *American Journal of Epidemiology, 161,* 831–839.

Smolan, R., Moffitt, P., & Naythons, M. (1990). *The Power to Heal: Ancient Arts and Modern Medicine.* New York: Prentice Hall Press.

Snowman, J., & Biehler, R. (2006). *Psychology Applied to Teaching.* Boston: Houghton Mifflin.

Speck, O., Ernst, T., Braun, J., Koch, C., Miller, E., & Chang, L. (2000). Gender differences in the functional organization of the brain for working memory. *NeuroReport, 11*(11), 2581–2585.

Stanislav, L. (2006, October). When language gets in the way. *Modern Nurse,* 32–35.

Sullivan, C. W., & Bristow, L. R. (2007). *Summary proceedings of the national leadership symposium on increasing diversity in the health professions.* The Sullivan Alliance, 1–12.

Tashiro, C. J. (2002). Considering the significance of ancestry through the prism of mixed-race identity. *Advances in Nursing Science, 25*(2), 1–21.

Tear, J. (1995, November 20). They just don't understand gender dynamics. *Wall Street Journal,* A14.

Thomas, D. A., & Ely, R. J. (1996). Making differences matter: A new paradigm for managing diversity. *Harvard Business Review, 74*(5), 79–90.

Tripp-Reimer, T., & Afifi, L. A. (1989). Cross-cultural perspectives on patient teaching. *Nursing Clinics of North America, 24*(3), 613–619.

Turkheimer, E., Haley, A., Waldron, M., D'Onofrio, B., & Gottesman, I. I. (2003). Socioeconomic status modifies heritability of IQ in young children. *Psychological Science, 14*(6), 623–628.

U.S. Census Bureau. (2000). *Population estimates program.* Washington, DC: Author.

U.S. Census Bureau. (2006). *Statistical abstract of the United States.* Retrieved July 9, 2007, from http://www.census.gov/prod/www/statistical-abstract.html

U.S. Department of Health and Human Services. (2003a). *Communicating health: Priorities and strategies for progress*. Retrieved April 26, 2004, from http://odphp.osophs.dhhs.gov/projects/healthcomm

U.S. Department of Health and Human Services. (2000). *Healthy People 2010: Understanding and improving health, Volume 1*. Rockville, MD: Author.

Uzundede, S. (2006, October). Respecting diversity: One patient at a time. *Modern Nurse*, 28–30.

Vander Zanden, J. W., Crandell, T. L., & Crandell, C. H. (2007). *Human development* (8th ed.). Boston: McGraw-Hill.

Villanueva, V., & Lipat, A. S. (2000). The Filipino American culture: The needs for transcultural knowledge. In M. L. Kelley & V. M. Fitzsimons (Eds.), *Understanding cultural diversity: Culture, curriculum, and community in nursing* (219–228). Boston: Jones and Bartlett.

Vivian, C., & Dundes, L. (2004, First Quarter). The crossroads of culture and health among the Roma (Gypsies). *Journal of Nursing Scholarship*, 86–91.

Weiss, B. D. (2003). *Health literacy: A manual for clinicians* (1–49). Chicago: American Medical Association and the American Medical Association Foundation.

Winkleby, M. A., Jatulis, D. E., Frank, E., & Fortmann, S. P. (1992). Socioeconomic status and health: How education, income, and occupation contribute to risk factors for cardiovascular disease. *American Journal of Public Health, 82*(6), 816–820.

Yanek, L. R., Becker, D. M., Moy, T. F., Gettelsohn, J., & Koffman, D. M. (2001). Project Joy: Faith based cardiovascular health promotion for African-American women. *Public Health Reports, 116*, 68–81.

Yee, S-H., Liu, H-L., Hou, J., Pu, Y., Fox, P. T., & Gao, J-H. (2000). Detection of the brain response during a cognitive task using perfusion-based event-related functional MRI. *NeuroReport, 11*(11), 2533–2536.

Young, H. M., McCormick, W. M., & Vitaliano, P. P. (2002). Evolving values in community-based long-term care services for Japanese Americans. *Advances in Nursing Science, 25*(2), 40–56.

Chapter 9

Special Populations

Kay Viggiani

CHAPTER HIGHLIGHTS

KEY TERMS

- habilitation
- rehabilitation
- disability
- sensory deficits
- hearing impairment
- visual impairment
- learning disability
- input disabilities
- output disabilities
- attention deficit hyperactivity disorder
- developmental disability
- expressive aphasia
- receptive aphasia
- dysarthria
- augmentative and alternative communication
- assistive technology

OBJECTIVES

After completing this chapter, the reader will be able to

1. Describe how visual and hearing deficits require adaptive intervention.
2. Identify the various teaching strategies that are effective with learning disabilities.
3. Describe the different physical and mental disabilities for appropriate adaptation of the teaching–learning plan.
4. Enhance the teaching–learning process for someone with a communication disability.
5. Discuss the effects of a chronic illness on people and their families in the teaching–learning process.
6. Describe assistive technology and its application for people with disabilities.

Teaching others to be independent in self-management of their lives is a critical and challenging role for the nurse in any setting and with any population of individuals. However, the teaching–learning process is especially challenging when dealing with patients who have altered functional status due to a disabling condition affecting their physical, cognitive, or sensory capacities. The educational component of the practice of nursing becomes paramount in importance as the nurse's efforts are directed toward assisting patients and their significant others to maintain already established patterns of living or to develop new ones to accommodate changes in functional ability.

This chapter on special populations is a unique aspect of this book on the role of the nurse as educator. Few other publications address the subject or suggest nursing interventions involving teaching self-care measures to individuals with a wide range of disabilities. Although the information presented here focuses specifically on patient populations, the same principles of teaching and learning can be extrapolated to apply to other categories of learners. For example, the nurse educator may be responsible in the position of in-service educator, faculty member, or staff development coordinator for teaching hospital personnel or nursing students who may have a physical or learning disability.

This chapter provides an overview of some of the more common disabilities. It addresses the learning problems inherent in population groups with various types of deficits and highlights the role of the nurse as educator in designing and implementing specific teaching strategies that can be used to overcome communication difficulties. It also suggests ways in which nurse educators can incorporate appropriate adaptations into their teaching plans to accommodate the needs of disabled patients and their families. A resource list is provided in Appendix B as a further reference to the reader who seeks additional information about a specific disability.

Definition of Terms

The terms *habilitation* and *rehabilitation* are frequently used to differentiate approaches for managing both developmental and acquired types of disabilities. Adsit and Hertzberg define the term habilitation as "needing new skills and abilities to meet maximum potential and the term rehabilitation to mean relearning skills and abilities or adjusting existing function to meet age-related developmental expectations" (Edwards, 2000, p. 319). Thus, habilitation and rehabilitation are futuristic processes that focus on helping individuals learn to live with their disability in their own environment through identification and use of tools that allow them to cope with the ramifications of their altered functional status.

Unfortunately, an increasing number of people are faced with having to deal with a disability caused by an injury, a disease, or a birth defect that is permanent and has long-term consequences on their mode of living. Nurses and other healthcare providers need to be prepared to provide those services that will meet the demands of a broad range of clients whose problems and situations are the result of a developmental or acquired disability.

With respect to patient populations, the teaching–learning process is an integral element in the habilitation and rehabilitation of disabled clients who need assistance in making the transition from being a recipient of care to assuming a self-care role. Certainly the disabled patient's family members and significant others are also major players in the habilitation and rehabilitation experience.

If we stopped for a moment to conjure up a mental picture of a person with a disability, what would we envision? People in this special population group may look like the average person, but then again, they may not. Some will have overt physical disabilities, whereas others may have a cognitive or mental impairment that on the surface may make them indistinguishable from anyone else. The one thing that they will have in common is a problem that makes learning more difficult for them. For the purpose of this chapter, the term *disability*, defined in 1980 by the World Health Organization (WHO) international classification is still relevant today, and is the "restriction or lack (resulting from an impairment) of ability to perform an activity in the manner or within the range considered normal for a human being" (DeLisa & Gand, 1998, p. 55).

On July 26, 1990, President George H. W. Bush signed into law the Americans with Disabilities Act (ADA). The definition of *disability* under the ADA is "a physical or mental impairment which substantially limits one or more of the major life activities of the individual" (p. 2). A major life activity includes functions such as caring for oneself, standing, lifting, reaching, seeing, hearing, speaking, breathing, learning, and walking. This significant legislation has extended civil rights protection to millions of Americans with disabilities. The first part of the law, effective in January 1992, mandated accessibility to public accommodations. In July 1992, the second part of the law went into effect, requiring employers to make reasonable accommodations in hiring people with disabilities (Merrow & Corbett, 1994).

Thus, the ADA legislation makes it illegal to discriminate on the basis of a disability in the areas of employment, public service, public accommodations, transportation, and telecommunications. This statute provides the foundation on which all facets of society will be free of discrimination, including the healthcare system. Therefore, we can expect to find people with disabilities in every setting in which nurses practice, such as schools, clinics, hospitals, nursing homes, workplaces, and private homes. Persons with a disability will expect nurses and other healthcare professionals to provide appropriate instruction adapted to their special needs.

The Nurse Educator's Roles and Responsibilities

The role of the nurse in teaching those who are disabled continues to evolve, as more than ever before, clients expect and are expected to assume greater responsibility as self-care agents. Here, the focus is on wellness and strengths—not limitations—of the individual. It is interesting to note that *Healthy People 2010* includes a chapter on the health of people with disabilities. This reinforces the significant emphasis placed on providing care for individuals and their families (U.S. Department of Health and Human Services, 2000).

Families are increasingly becoming involved in their disabled members' rehabilitation efforts, and individuals with disabilities are expecting and demanding to be a part of community life. Because of the complex needs of this special population group, the nurse's role, out of necessity, must be an integral part of an interdisciplinary team effort with other health professionals such as nurses, physicians, social workers, physical therapists, psychologists, and occupational and speech therapists. In addition, the nurse educator has the responsibility to work in concert with clients and their family members to assess learning needs, design appropriate educational inter-

ventions, and promote an environment conducive to learning (Diehl, 1989). We must become aware of the tangible barriers to learning that exist as well as the interventions and technologies that are available to help special populations overcome those barriers (Cunningham, 2001; Edwards, 2000).

Application of the teaching–learning process is intended to promote adaptive behaviors in clients that support their optimal recovery and a return to life within the community. Emphasis on the various components of the learning process may differ depending on the disability, but it often requires changes in all three domains—cognitive, affective, and psychomotor.

Prior to teaching, assessment is always the first step in determining the needs of clients with respect to the nature of their problems, the short- and long-term consequences of their disability, the effectiveness of the coping mechanisms they employ, and the type and extent of sensorimotor, cognitive, perceptual, and communication deficits they experience. The nurse must determine the extent of the clients' knowledge with respect to their disability, the amount and types of new information needed to effect changes in behavior, and the clients' readiness to learn. At this initial stage, it is imperative that the nurse educator not only obtain feedback from them, but also use assessment skills of observation, testing, and interviewing of family members and significant others as well as taking into account the findings of the healthcare team.

Diehl (1989) outlines the following questions to be asked when determining the disabled person's readiness to learn:

1. Do the individual and family members demonstrate an interest in learning by requesting information or posing ques-

tions in an effort at problem solving or determining their needs?

2. Are there barriers to learning such as low literacy skills, vision impairments, or hearing deficits?

3. If sensory or motor differentiation exists, is the client willing and able to use supportive devices?

4. What learning style best suits the client in processing information and applying it to self-care activities?

5. Is there congruence between the goals of the client and family?

6. Is the environment conducive to learning?

7. Does the client value learning new information and skills as a means to achieve functional improvement?

Prerequisite to the role of the nurse as teacher and provider of care is the nursing responsibility to serve as a mentor to patients and family in coordinating and facilitating the multidisciplinary services required to assist disabled persons in attaining optimal functioning. The family and significant others, as the disabled person's support system in the community, must be invited right from the very beginning to take an active part in learning information as it applies to assisting with self-care activities for their loved ones.

Types of Disabilities

The disabilities affecting millions of Americans can be categorized into two major types: mental and physical. These disabilities may have a neurological, physiological, or cognitive basis, can affect thinking processes, and may involve sensorimotor/neuromuscular functioning. These disabilities may result from an injury, disease,

heredity, or congenital defect. The following seven categories have been chosen for discussion because they are common: (1) sensory deficits, (2) learning disabilities, (3) developmental disabilities, (4) mental illness, (5) physical disabilities, (6) communication disorders, and (7) chronic illness. Included within each category are the specific teaching strategies that should be used to meet the needs of the learner who has a particular disability.

Sensory Deficits

Sensory deficits include problems with using one or more of the five senses—auditory, visual, tactile, olfactory, and gustatory. Emphasis will be placed on hearing and visual impairments because they are the two most common sensory losses that have an impact on a person's ability to learn.

Hearing Impairments

People with impaired hearing—both the deaf and the hard of hearing—have a complete loss or a reduction in their sensitivity to sounds. Strong (1996) explains that "[the word] 'deaf' with a lowercase 'd' is used to refer to the physical condition of hearing loss, whereas 'Deaf', with an uppercase 'D' is used to refer to special collectives and attitudes arising out of interaction among people with hearing losses. The distinction was first made by Woodward (1972) and is standard in most of the literature on sociocultural aspects of deafness" (p. xi). *Hearing impairment* is a term used to describe any type of hearing loss, the etiology of which may be related to either conductive or sensorineural problems resulting from congenital defect, trauma, or disease.

Approximately 28 million Americans have a hearing impairment. Hearing loss affects about

17 in 1,000 children under age 18. Incidence increases with age. About 314 in 1,000 people over 65 years old have hearing loss and 40–50% of people 75 years and older have hearing loss (NIDCD, 2005). For those who are deaf, "being a recipient of health care services is similar to being in a foreign country without fluency in the native language" (Harrison, 1990, p. 113).

Regardless of the degree of hearing loss, any person with a hearing impairment faces communication barriers that interfere with efforts at patient teaching (Stock, 2002). Hearing loss poses a very real communication problem because deaf and hearing-impaired individuals also may be unable to speak or have limited verbal abilities and often have poor vocabularies. This is especially true for adults who are prelingually deaf—that is, they have been deaf since birth or early childhood. They and speakers of other languages share many of the same problems in learning English.

In many families with deaf children, American Sign Language (ASL) is used in the home and is the first language for these children. For other children who are raised in an environment where Deaf culture predominates, ASL is the medium of social communication among peers, which reinforces English as a second language. Most, if not all, of these children have difficulty achieving native-like fluency in English.

It is clear that individuals who are deaf will have different skills and needs depending on the type of deafness and how long they have been without a sense of hearing. For those who have been deaf since birth, they will not have had the benefit of language acquisition. As a result, they may not possess understandable speech and may have limited reading and vocabulary skills as well. Most likely, their primary modes of communication will be sign language and lipreading.

If deafness has occurred after language has been acquired, deaf people may speak quite understandably and have facility with reading and writing and some lipreading abilities. If deafness has occurred in later life, often caused by the process of aging, affected individuals will probably have poor lipreading ability, but their reading and writing skills should be within average range, depending on their educational and experiential background. If aging is the cause of hearing loss, visual impairments also may be a compounding factor. Because vision and hearing are two common sensory losses in the older adult, these deficits pose major communication problems when teaching older clients.

Deaf and hearing-impaired persons, like other individuals, will require health care and health education information at various periods during their life. Although the nurse educator will encounter many differences among people who are deaf, there is one common denominator—deaf individuals will always rely on their other senses for information input, especially their sense of sight. For patient education to be effective, then, communication must be visible.

Because there are several different ways to communicate with a person who is deaf, one of the first things nurse educators need to do is ask clients to identify communication preferences. Sign language, written information, lipreading, and visual aids are some of the common choices. It is true that one of the simplest ways to transfer information is through visible communication signals such as hand gestures and facial expressions. However, this method will not be adequate for any lengthy teaching sessions.

The following modes of communication are suggested as ways to decrease the barriers of communication and facilitate teaching and learning for hearing-impaired patients in any setting:

SIGN LANGUAGE

For most deaf people whose native language is ASL, sign language is often the preferred mode of communication. If you do not know ASL, you need to obtain the services of a professional interpreter. Sometimes a family member or friend of the patient skilled in signing is willing and available to act as a translator during teaching sessions. However, prior to enlisting the assistance of an interpreter, always be certain to obtain the patient's permission because information communicated regarding health issues may be considered personal and private. If the information to be taught is confidential, it is advised that family or friends should not be enlisted as an interpreter. Hiring a certified language interpreter is often the best strategy.

When a nurse is considering the services of an interpreter, the deaf individual should be the one who makes the choice. If a professional interpreter is requested by a deaf patient in a health facility receiving federal funds, it is required by federal law that one be secured (Section 504 of the Rehabilitation Act of 1973, PL 93-112). If the patient cannot provide the names of interpreters, one can contact the state Registry of Interpreters of the Deaf (RID). This registry can provide an up-to-date list of qualified sign language interpreters.

When working with an interpreter, the nurse should stand or sit next to the interpreter. He or she should talk at a normal pace and look and talk directly to the deaf person when speaking.

LIPREADING

One common misconception among hearing persons is that all people who are deaf can read lips. This assumption is potentially dangerous. Only about 40% of English sounds are visible on the lips. Therefore, only a skilled lip-reader will obtain any real benefit from this form of communication (DiPietro, 1979).

If the individual can lip-read, it is not necessary to exaggerate lip movements, because this action will distort the movements of the lips and interfere with interpretation of the words. If lipreading is preferred, speakers must be sure to provide sufficient lighting on their faces and remove all barriers from around the face, such as gum, pencils, hands, and surgical masks. Beards, mustaches, and protruding teeth also present a challenge to the lip-reader. Because less than half of the English language is visible on the lips, one should supplement this form of communication with signing or written materials.

WRITTEN MATERIALS

Written information is probably the most reliable way to communicate, especially when understanding is critical. In fact, nurse educators should always write down the important information as a supplement to the spoken word even when the deaf person is versed in lipreading. Written communication is the safest approach, even though it is time consuming and sometimes stressful.

Nurses should provide printed patient education materials that match the readability level of the audience. When putting information in writing for a client who is deaf, they should keep the message as simple as possible. For instance, instead of writing, "When running a fever, take two aspirin," they might revise the message to read, "For a fever of 100.5°F or more, take two aspirin." Remember that a person with limited reading skills often interprets words literally; therefore, the word *running* could be confusing because it is often used in the context of someone who is running to the store. Visual aids such as simple pictures, drawings, diagrams, models, and the like are also very useful media as a supplement to increase understanding of written materials (see Chapter 7 for guidelines on writing effective printed materials).

Verbalization by the Client

Sometimes clients who are deaf will choose to communicate through speaking, especially if they have established a rapport and a trusting relationship with someone. Often the tone and inflection of the patient's voice will be different than normal speech, so educators must make time for listening carefully. They should listen without interruptions until they become accustomed to the person's particular voice intonations and speech rhythms. Those who still have trouble understanding what a client is saying might try writing down what they hear, which may help them to get the gist of the message.

Sound Augmentation

For those patients who have a hearing loss but are not completely deaf, hearing aids are often a useful device. Clients who have already been fitted for a hearing aid should be encouraged to use it, and it should be readily accessible, fitted properly, turned on, and with the batteries in working order. If the client does not have a hearing aid, with permission of the patient and family, the nurse should make a referral to an auditory specialist, who can determine whether such a device is appropriate for the patient. Only one out of five people who could benefit from a hearing aid actually wear one (NIDCD, 2005).

Another means by which sounds can be augmented is by cupping one's hands around the client's ear or using a stethoscope in reverse.

That is, the patient puts the stethoscope in his or her ears, and the nurse talks into the bell of the instrument (Babcock & Miller, 1994).

If the patient can hear better out of one ear than the other, speakers should always stand or sit nearer to the good ear, using slow speech, providing adequate time for the patient to process the message and to respond, and avoiding shouting, which distorts sounds. It is not necessarily an increase in decibels that makes a difference, but it is the tone, rhythm, articulation, and pace of the words.

Telecommunications

Telecommunication devices for the deaf (TDD) are an important resource for patient education. Television decoders for closed-caption programs are an important tool for further enhancing communication. Caption films for patient education are also available free of charge through Modern Talking Pictures and Services. Under federal law, these devices are considered to be reasonable accommodations for deaf and hearing-impaired persons.

In summary, the following guidelines suggested by Navarro and Lacour (1980) should be applied when using any of the aforementioned modes of communication:

- Nurse educators should:
  - be natural.
  - not be rigid and stiff or attempt to overarticulate speech.
  - use simple sentences.
  - be sure to get the deaf person's attention by a light touch on the arm before beginning to talk.
  - face the patient and stand no more than 6 feet away when trying to communicate.

- Nurse educators must be considerate and refrain from the following:
  - Talking and walking at the same time.
  - Bobbing their head excessively.
  - Talking with their mouth full, while chewing gum, and so forth.
  - Turning their face away from the deaf person while communicating.
  - Standing directly in front of a bright light, which may cast a shadow across their face or glare directly into the patient's eyes.
  - Placing an IV in the hand the patient will need for sign language.

No matter what methods of communication for teaching are chosen, it is important to confirm that health messages have been received and understood. It is essential to validate patient comprehension in a nonthreatening manner. In attempts to avoid embarrassing or offending one another, patients as well as healthcare providers will often acknowledge with a smile or a nod in response to what either one is trying to communicate when, in fact, the message is not understood at all. To ensure that the health education requirements of deaf or hearing-impaired patients are being met, the nurse educator must find effective strategies to communicate the intended message clearly and precisely while at the same time demonstrating acceptance of individuals by making accommodations to suit their needs (Harrison, 1990). Patients who have lived with a hearing impairment for a while usually can indicate what modes of communication work best for them.

Visual Impairments

As stated by Vitale, Cotch, and Sperduto (2006), "Sight is an important indicator of health and quality of life" (p. 2158). The most prevalent condition that results in some degree of visual impairment is myopia (nearsightedness). This refractive error usually can be corrected with eyeglasses or contact lenses. As the population ages and is becoming more racially and ethnically diverse, the rates of myopia have increased in the United States and in the population worldwide. Improving the vision of those individuals with myopia through refractive correction is considered to be an important public health initiative. Correction of this common visual impairment has implications for safety and quality of life by reducing falls, fractures, depression, and car accidents.

A *visual impairment* is defined as some form and degree of visual difficulty and includes both partial and total blindness. In the United States, a person is determined to be legally blind if vision is 20/200 or less in the better eye with correction or if visual field limits in both eyes are within 20 degrees in diameter. Severe visual impairment after correction with glasses is defined as the inability to read newspaper print (Nelson, 1991). People lose their vision and may be rendered legally blind for a variety of reasons, including infections, accidents, poisoning, aging, or congenital degeneration such as retinitis pigmentosa. Most recently, blindness in AIDS patients as a result of infection has been associated with the end stages of this disease.

Visual impairment is especially common among older persons. The American Foundation for the Blind (AFB) estimates there are approximately 10 million blind and visually impaired people in the United States, of whom about 5.5 million are over the age of 65. About 1.3 million Americans are legally blind (AFB, 2007). The four leading eye diseases associated with the aging process are macular degeneration, cataracts, glaucoma, and diabetic retinopathy (**Figure 9–1**).

Figure 9–1 Photo essay on partial sight (low vision).

Major diseases causing serious vision impairment that cannot be corrected with conventional spectacles or lenses are cataract, macular degeneration, glaucoma, and diabetic retinopathy. People who have advanced stages of these diseases have difficulty performing ordinary visual tasks, like reading.

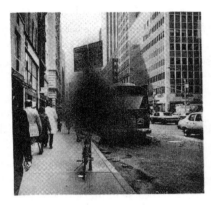 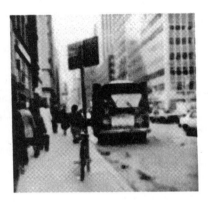

MACULAR DEGENERATION—The deterioration of the macula, the central area of the retina, results in an area of decreased central vision. Peripheral, or side, vision remains unaffected. This is the most prevalent eye disease.

CATARACT—An opacity of the lens results in diminished acuity but does not affect the field of vision. There are no blind spots, but the person's vision is hazy overall, particularly in glaring light.

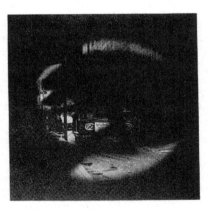 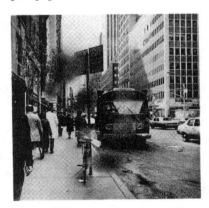

GLAUCOMA—Chronic elevated eye pressure in susceptible individuals may cause atrophy of the optic nerve and loss of peripheral vision. Early detection and close medical monitoring can help reduce complications.

DIABETIC RETINOPATHY—Leaking of retinal blood vessels in advanced or long-term diabetes can affect the macula or the entire retina and vitreous, producing blinding areas.

 The Lighthouse Inc.

Source: Reprinted courtesy of The Lighthouse Inc., New York, New York.

Patients who seem to be legally blind but have not been evaluated by a low-vision specialist should be provided with contact information for these sources: the local Blind Association and the local Commission for the Blind and Visually Handicapped. Patients may require assistance in negotiating the complex system and in obtaining services.

Fortunately, many devices are available to help legally blind persons maximize their remaining vision. Patients who are without sight most likely have had services and are familiar with those adaptations that work best for them. However, depending on patients' situations and the circumstances under which one is teaching, the nurse educator may want to further investigate their background to assure that the most appropriate format and tools for communicating with visually impaired clients are being used.

The following are some tips nurses might find helpful in caring for a blind or visually impaired patient:

- A low-vision specialist can prescribe optical devices such as a magnifying lens (with or without a light), a telescope, a closed-circuit TV, or a pair of sun shields, any of which will enable nurses to adapt their teaching material to meet the needs of their clients.

- Persons who have long-standing blindness have learned to develop a heightened acuity of their other senses of hearing, taste, touch, and smell. When conveying messages, they rely on their auditory and tactile senses as a means to help them assimilate information from their environment. Usually their listening skills are particularly acute; it is not

necessary to shout. Just because they have impaired vision does not mean they cannot hear well.

Unlike a sighted person, the blind cannot attend to nonverbal cues such as hand gestures, facial expressions, and other body language. Those who approach a visually impaired person should always announce their presence, identify themselves, and explain clearly why they are there and what they are doing. Because blind people's memory and recall also are better than the abilities of most sighted persons, educators can use this talent to maximize learning (Babcock & Miller, 1994).

- When explaining procedures, educators should be as descriptive as possible. They should expound on what they are doing and explain any noises associated with treatments or the use of equipment. The patient should be allowed to touch, handle, and manipulate equipment. Instructors should use the patient's sense of touch in the process of teaching psychomotor skills as well as when the client is learning to return demonstrate.

- Because people who are blind are unable to see shapes, sizes, and the placement of objects, tactile learning is an important technique to use when teaching. For example, such patients can identify their medications by feeling the shape, size, and texture of tablets and capsules. Gluing pills to the tops of bottle caps and putting medications in different-sized or -shaped containers will aid them in identifying various medications (Boyd, Gleit, Graham, & Whitman,

1998). In this way, they will be able to be more self-sufficient in following their prescribed regimens. Also, keeping items in the same place at all times will help them independently locate their belongings. Arranging things in front of them in a regular clockwise fashion will facilitate learning to perform a task that must be accomplished in an orderly, step-by-step manner (McConnel, 1996).

- When using printed or handwritten materials, enlarging the print (font size) is typically an important first step for those who have diminished sight.

- Color is a key factor in whether a visually impaired person can distinguish objects. Assessment should be done on the medium in which the client sees better—black ink on white paper or white ink on black paper. Colors and varying hues of color other than black and white are more difficult to discriminate by the older person with vision problems.

- Proper lighting is of utmost importance in assisting the visually impaired to read the printed word. Regardless of the print size and the color of the type and paper used, if the light is insufficient, they will have a great deal of difficulty reading print or working with objects.

- Providing contrast is a very helpful technique. For example, using a dark placemat with white dishes or serving black coffee in a white cup will allow persons with visual problems to better see items in front of them.

- Providing blind people with a template (writing guide) for signing their name or writing checks and addressing envelopes is a way to encourage independence.

- Large-print watches and clocks with either black or white backgrounds are available through a local chapter for the visually handicapped.

- Audiotapes and cassette recorders are very useful tools. Today, many health education texts as well as other printed health information materials are available as talking books and can be obtained through the National Library Service (see Appendix B), or through the state library for the blind and visually handicapped. Also, these services are available for people with other disabilities. In addition, oral instructions can be audiotaped so that information can be listened to as necessary at another time and place. Repetition allows the opportunity for memorization to reinforce learning.

- The computer is a popular and useful tool for this population of learners. Although they are costly, some computers have synthetic speech as well as Braille keyboards.

- Most blind associations have a Braille library, or clients can access appropriate resources for information, such as the National Braille Press (see Appendix B). Local blind associations might print patient education materials in Braille so they can be used by visually impaired learners.

- When assisting the person who is blind to ambulate, one should always use the sighted guide technique; that is, the guide should allow the person to grasp his or her forearm while the guide walks about one half step ahead of the blind person. Another resource person to help with ambulation is an orientation and mobility instructor. These specialists are available in most school districts and the local associations for the blind.

Diabetes education consumes a great deal of a nurse educator's teaching time and presents unique challenges to the nurse. Because of the high incidence of this disease in the American population, diabetic retinopathy is a major cause of blindness. Persons who have lost their sight due to diabetic retinopathy probably have already mastered some of the necessary skills to care for themselves but will need continued assistance. However, it is also possible for visually impaired persons to be diagnosed at a later time with diabetes. In either case, at some point in the course of their lives, these persons will need to learn how to use appropriate adaptive equipment.

In 1993, a task force consisting of representatives from groups of diabetes educators and rehabilitation specialists for the blind developed a document entitled *Adaptive Diabetes Education for Visually Impaired Persons* (ADEVIP). ADEVIP provides consistent practice guidelines for the care of diabetics who are visually handicapped.

Fortunately, there also has been continuous improvement in the equipment used for self-monitoring of blood glucose levels. Easy-to-use monitors with large display screens or voice instructions are available now. Just as several devices for monitoring blood glucose levels have been developed, several nonvisual adaptive devices for measuring insulin are also available. It is evident that the teamwork among these health professionals has led to the development of a variety of useful mechanisms that allow blind diabetic patients the opportunity to care for themselves and achieve both a successful medical outcome and a good rehabilitation outcome (Baker, 1993).

Learning Disabilities

What exactly constitutes a learning disability (LD) has been the subject of a great deal of controversy over the years. Educators and psychologists alike have debated this very issue (Santrock, 2006; Snowman & Biehler, 2006; Vander Zanden, Crandell, & Crandell, 2007; Ysseldyke & Allgozzine, 1983). The Individuals with Disabilities Education Improvement Act (1997) defines *learning disability* as a "disorder in one or more of the basic psychological processes involved in understanding or in using language, spoken or written, that may manifest itself in an imperfect ability to listen, think, speak, read, write, spell or do mathematical calculations" (Learning Disabilities Roundtable, 2005). This definition stands as the accepted working definition for purposes of assessment, diagnosis, and categorization of an array of learning disabilities.

Learning disabilities include such conditions as attention deficit disorders, integrative processing disorders, memory deficits, visual and auditory perceptual disabilities, minimal brain dysfunction, and developmental language problems (NICHCY, 2002). As many as one out of every five people in the United States has a learning disability. Almost 3 million children (ages 6–21) have some form of a learning problem. This represents a substantial increase in just the past few decades in the percentage of children classified as learning disabled—from less than 30% receiving special education in 1977 to over 50% today (Santrock, 2006).

About three to four times as many boys as girls are identified as having a learning disability, but this gender difference is thought to be due to referral bias—more boys are referred for treatment because of their behavior (Santrock, 2006; Vander Zanden et al., 2007). Most children with LD receive special education in school

(NICHCY, 2004), which accounts for about 14% of the total federal education budget of over $360 billion (Vander Zanden et al., 2007).

In the past, a learning disability was thought to be a problem involving only children. Now, however, evidence supports the belief that most individuals do not outgrow the problem (Vander Zanden et al., 2007). Indeed, the rate of learning disabilities in adults is probably similar to the rate in children. The majority of people with learning disabilities have language and/or memory deficits. If the problem is compounded with the stresses and anxieties caused by illness and subsequent hospitalization or the pressures of having to perform in an academic setting, people with learning disabilities find themselves in a situation that is not at all conducive to learning.

Individuals with learning disabilities appear normal and have been found to have at least average, if not superior (gifted), intelligence. In fact, learning disabilities are often labeled the invisible handicap because they do not necessarily result in low achievement. Some very famous and successful people in world history are thought to have had some type of learning disability—artists (Leonardo da Vinci), political leaders (Woodrow Wilson, Winston Churchill, and Nelson Rockefeller), military figures (George Patton), and scientists (Albert Einstein and Thomas Edison) (Vander Zanden et al., 2007). Even though there is a large discrepancy between a learning disabled person's intellectual abilities and his or her performance levels, no cause-and-effect relationship exists. Those who exhibit this discrepancy are not necessarily learning disabled (Santrock, 2006; Vander Zanden et al., 2007). **Table 9–1** lists common myths and corresponding facts about learning disabilities. A person can be of average or above average intelligence, not have any major sensory problems, and still struggle to keep up with

people the same age in learning. Learning disability is not a single disorder but refers to a group of disorders.

The factors that may affect learning in a learning disabled person are memory, language, motor, and integrative processing disabilities. These factors fall under two general headings—input and output disabilities. *Input disabilities*, which refer to the process of receiving and recording information in the brain, include visual perceptual, auditory perceptual, integrative processing, and memory disorders. *Output disabilities*, which refer to the process of orally responding and performing physical tasks, include language and motor disorders.

Although these problems and their associated characteristics are frequently identified in reference to disabled children in particular, many of the characteristics of these problems can apply equally well to an older person who has not been diagnosed as learning disabled until later in adulthood. It is important to remember that a learning disabled individual can experience one type of learning disability or a combination thereof.

Input Disabilities

VISUAL PERCEPTUAL DISORDERS

This type of disability results in an inability or difficulty with reading (dyslexia), writing (dysgraphia), or dealing with numbers (dyscalcula). Dyslexia accounts for the largest percentage of the LD population (Vander Zanden et al., 2007). With dyslexia, letters of the alphabet may be seen in reverse or rotated order—for example, *d* is seen as *b* and *p* as *q* or *g*. Words also may be confused with one another such as *was* being perceived as *saw*.

In addition, the individual may have trouble focusing on a particular word or group of words, taking a general view rather than attending to

---

Table 9–1 MYTHS AND FACTS ABOUT LEARNING DISABILITIES

Myth: Children are labeled "learning disabled" because they can't learn.

Fact: They can learn, but their preferred learning modality must be identified.

Myth: Children who have a learning disability must be spoken to more slowly.

Fact: Those who learn auditorily may become impatient with slower speech and stop listening; those who learn visually would benefit more from seeing the information.

Myth: Children who are learning disabled just have to try harder.

Fact: Telling these children to try harder is a turnoff. They already do try hard.

Myth: Children outgrow their disabilities.

Fact: Children do not outgrow their disabilities. They develop strategies to compensate for and minimize their disabilities.

Myth: Children with learning disabilities should be treated like everyone else.

Fact: That treatment would be unfair; they would not get what they need.

Myth: Nearly all children with learning disabilities are boys.

Fact: Boys are more often referred for proper identification of learning disabilities because they are more overt in acting out their frustrations.

Source: Reprinted from (1991, September/October). *MCN: American Journal of Maternal Child Nursing, 16*(5), pp. 260–263. Greenberg, L. A. (1991). Teaching children who are learning disabled about illness and hospitalization. Used with permission.

specifics, which contributes to reading difficulty (Vander Zanden et al., 2007). Also, there may be a figure ground problem, such that the person is unable to attend to a specific object within a group of objects, such as finding a cup of juice on a food tray. Furthermore, judging distances or positions in space or dealing with special relationships may prove difficult, resulting in the person's bumping into things, being confused about left and right or up and down, or being unable to throw a ball or do a puzzle.

People with visual perceptual deficits tend to be auditory learners. With these individuals, visual stimulation should be kept to a minimum. Visual materials such as pamphlets or books are ineffective unless the content is explained orally or the information is read aloud. If visual items are used, only one item should be given at any one time with a sufficient period in between times to allow for the information to be focused on and mastered.

Because persons with visual perceptual deficits usually learn best through hearing, using CDs and audiotapes (with or without earphones) and verbal instruction are keys in helping them learn. Recall and retention of information can be assessed by oral questioning, allowing learners to express orally what they understand and remember about the content that has been presented.

AUDITORY PERCEPTUAL DISORDERS

This type of disability is characterized by the inability to distinguish subtle differences in sounds—for example, *blue* and *blow* or *ball* and *bell*. There also may be a problem with auditory figure ground, such that the sound of someone speaking cannot be identified clearly when others are speaking in the same room. Auditory lags may occur, whereby sound input cannot be processed at a normal rate. Parts of conversations may be missed unless one speaks at a speed that allows the disabled person enough time to process the information.

During instruction, it is important to limit the noise level and eliminate distractions in the background. Using as few words as possible and repeating them when necessary (using the same words to avoid confusion) are useful strategies. Direct eye contact helps keep the learner focused on the task at hand.

Visual teaching methods such as demonstration–return demonstration, gaming (e.g., puppetry), modeling, and role playing, as well as provision of visual instructional tools such as written materials, pictures, charts, films, books, puzzles, printed handouts, and the computer are the best ways to communicate information. Using hand signs for key words when giving verbal instructions and allowing the learner to have hands-on experiences and opportunities for observation are useful techniques.

Directions for learning via these methods and tools should be in written form. The visual learner may intently watch the instructor's face for the formation of words, expressions, eye movements, and hand gestures. Awareness to these details may have developed as a compensatory strategy to aid comprehension. If the learner does not understand something being taught, he or she may exhibit frustration in the form of irritability and inattentiveness.

Individuals with either visual or auditory perceptual problems often rely on tactile learning as well. They enjoy doing things with their hands, want to touch everything, prefer writing and drawing, engage in physical exploration, and enjoy physical movement through sports activities.

Integrative Processing Disorders

Recording information in the brain requires that the information be organized and processed if it is to be used correctly. An inability to sequence or abstract visual, auditory, or tactile stimuli is characteristic of this type of disability. A child who has difficulty sequencing information may read and understand the word *dog* as *god* because the letters *d*, *o*, and *g* are processed in the incorrect order. Thought sequencing also may progress from the middle to the end rather than normally (i.e., starting at the beginning).

Abstraction is the inability to infer meaning from words or phrases. That is, the specific intended meaning of words or thoughts is misunderstood. For example, a person who has difficulty with abstractions may interpret *window shopping* or *blowing smoke* in the literal rather than the figurative sense (Ysseldyke & Allgozzine, 1983).

Those with an integrative processing disability need specific explanations. Educators should avoid using confusing phrases, puns, or sarcasm with such learners, and they should frequently ask the person to repeat or demonstrate what was learned to immediately clear up any misconceptions.

Short-Term or Long-Term Memory Disorders

Once information is recorded and integrated in the brain, it must be stored and made ready for retrieval. Normally, most people can retrieve information fairly quickly and without much effort from either their short-term or long-term memories. *Short-term memory* refers to information that is remembered as long as one is attending to it—for example, being able to remember what one has been told recently or taking a telephone order and then being able to write it down completely soon after hanging up the phone. Individuals with short-term memory deficits may be unable to recall what they learned an hour before, but they may be able to recall the information at a later point in time. *Long-term memory* consists of information that has been repeated and stored and becomes available whenever one thinks about it, such as being able to remember a telephone number (including one's own) over a long period of time. People with both short- and long-term memory disabilities need brief, frequent, repetitive teaching sessions for constant reinforcement of information.

Output Disabilities

LANGUAGE DISORDERS

There are two types of oral language—spontaneous (initiating a conversation) and demand (asking a question). With spontaneous language, persons select a topic, organize their thoughts, and choose the correct words to express themselves orally. Demand language occurs when someone else starts a conversation and poses questions for another person to answer. In response to demand language, the language disabled person may panic and answer, "Huh?" or "What?" or "I don't know." If the nurse educator detects this response pattern, allowing sufficient time either to process the information received or to formulate a response will reduce barriers to communication as a result of anxiety and frustration.

For persons with either type of language disability, the greatest gift one can give them is time—time to process internal thoughts, to find words, and then to speak for the purpose of initiating a conversation or responding with answers to questions. Patience on the part of the educator will reduce the learner's feelings of embarrassment, anxiety, or frustration.

Although there is no one way to ensure results, the following are some adaptive techniques:

- Provide information on tape, or give a learner the option of responding to questions orally with a tape recorder.
- Use hand signs for key words when giving verbal directions.
- Use hands-on experiences or provide opportunities for observation.
- Highlight important information.
- Use a computer.
- Capitalize on teachable moments.
- Use puzzles.
- Appeal to the major senses—auditory, visual, and tactile.
- Use mnemonics (**Table 9–2**).
- Use a cognitive map (**Figure 9–2**).
- Use an active reading strategy such as SQ3R (skim, question, read, rehearse, revise).

Table 9–2 MNEMONICS

P artner
R esponsible
E nthusiastic
C oach
E valuation
P atience
T eacher
O pen minded
R ole model

Figure 9–2 Diabetes mellitus cognitive map.

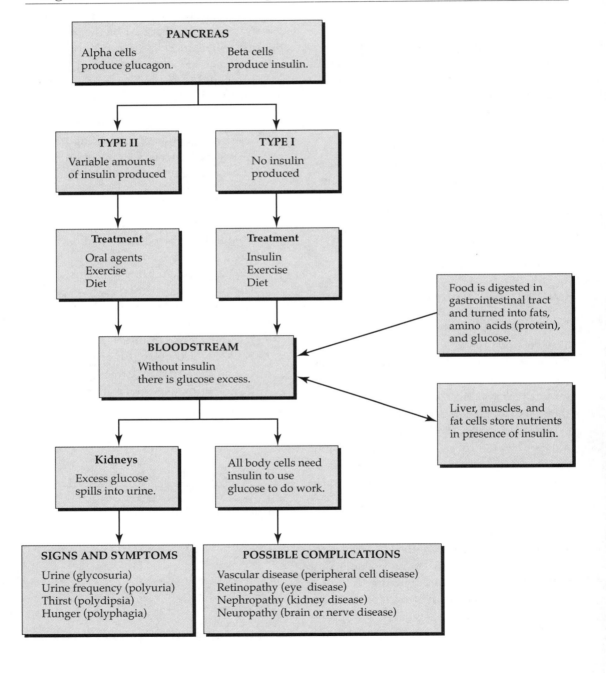

MOTOR DISORDERS

Learning psychomotor tasks will be difficult if the individual has problems with performing gross and fine motor tasks. Often people with this type of disability will avoid such tasks because of inadequate motor skills. For example, they will shy away from using writing as a form of communication because it requires fine motor coordination to accomplish. Instead of forcing them to handwrite, providing a tape or video recorder is a good substitute that allows them to demonstrate their knowledge of information. Depending on the disabled person's auditory and visual strengths, computers, CDs, DVDs, and preprinted materials may prove helpful tools for teaching and learning.

Safety also is always a concern for those with gross motor difficulties because they are prone to clumsiness, stumbling, or falling. The environment should be kept as uncluttered as possible to avoid injury and embarrassment.

Attention Deficit Hyperactivity Disorder

The ability to pay attention is an important prerequisite to success at school, work, and in one's personal life. Any difficulty with attending skills can have an adverse effect on learning. *Attention deficit hyperactivity disorder* (ADHD) is a disability that involves one or more of the characteristics of inattention, hyperactivity, and impulsivity over a period of time (Santrock, 2006). This is an appropriate term to use in such cases when these difficulties are prominent and almost always present in an individual. One in every 20 school-age children have significant difficulty keeping high levels of physical activity under control, are unable to focus or get bored very easily, cannot curb their reactions, and do not think before they act.

Approximately 2 million children between the ages of 6 to 11 are diagnosed with ADHD (Vander Zanden et al., 2007). Boys outnumber girls by at least three to one in incidence of this disorder (Snowman & Biehler, 2006). *Attention deficit disorder residual type* (ADDRET) is a term sometimes used to indicate residual attention deficit disorder (ADD) in older adolescents who were identified as having ADHD at a younger age but who no longer are hyperactive (ADDA, 2006). Approximately 50% of those with ADHD will seem to mature out of this disability at puberty (Kid Source, 2007). However, adults continue to experience this condition although the symptoms are different than they were originally. Either these adults tend to hyperfocus and become quite successful in their careers or they develop antisocial disorders or engage in substance abuse (Vander Zanden et al., 2007).

ADHD affects children with average ability as well as those who are gifted. This problem and other learning disabilities frequently occur together. Often, medication therapy is the treatment of choice for children with ADHD. Before embarking on any educational intervention with these children, educators should have an open discussion with the child and the parents to determine what works best for them. Most older children have been involved in special programs at school that, among other things, help the child use specific learning strategies consistently, which is of primary importance.

Those with ADHD, ADDRET, or ADD tend to be disorganized, poor time managers, and demonstrate sloppy writing skills (Santrock, 2006). Therefore, it is best to provide new information to such patients in a quiet environment, which may necessitate using another place for teaching sessions—a place other than their hospital room. When giving instructions or assigning a task, it helps to give directions one at a time and divide the work into small parts. Instructors should reward achievement and ignore inappropriate behavior. They should eliminate as much distraction as possible and encourage the older child to keep a notebook and to write the instructions down.

In summary, it is important to stress that learning disabled people are not mentally retarded; they just learn differently. They may have one or more disabilities, ranging from mild to severe. The challenge is to determine how the client learns best and then to adapt teaching strategies to meet their preferred style of learning—auditory, visual, or tactile.

The most reliable way to determine what accommodations need to be made in the teaching approach is to ask learning disabled individuals about problems they encounter in processing information and what they find to be the most appropriate instructional methods and tools to help them with learning. In the case of children, questions should be directed to both the child and the parents.

Individuals' strengths and weaknesses with respect to learning can be identified through direct, individualized assessment. An individualized education plan (IEP) can then be developed to promote learning through use of teaching and learning strategies that compensate for or minimize the effect of their disability (Greenberg, 1991; Vander Zanden et al., 2007).

Developmental Disabilities

A large proportion of children with a developmental disability are born with it. Parental response to the birth of a child with a disability is similar to the grieving process experienced by families after the death of a loved one. A typical reaction is, "Why me?" (Fraley, 1992). Shock or disbelief prevails, and when the reality settles in, the family attempts to integrate the child into the family structure. Enormous amounts of time, physical effort, and psychological energy are expended during this difficult period.

The Developmental Disabilities Act of 1978 defined a *developmental disability* as a severe chronic state that is present before 22 years of age and is likely to continue indefinitely (Snowman & Biehler, 2006). It may be caused by either a mental or a physical impairment or by a combination of the two (NICHCY, 2002). The individual who is developmentally disabled has substantial limitations in at least three of the following major life activities: self-care, receptive and expressive language learning, mobility, self-direction, capacity for independent living, and economic self-sufficiency.

In 1975, Public Law (PL) 94-142, the Education of All Handicapped Children Act, mandated state grant money be made available to provide all children with disabilities with a free and appropriate public education. In 1986, PL 99-457 amended the earlier law to provide special funding for educating all eligible preschool children with disabilities, ages 3 through 5, to help states develop early intervention programs for infants and toddlers (birth through age 2), and to require states to use qualified providers of special education and related services. In 1990, PL 101-476 made additional changes to the law, including a name change to Individuals with Disabilities Education Act (IDEA). In 1997, IDEA was again amended to entitle all eligible preschool and school-aged children with disabilities to receive a free and appropriate education, including special education and related services

(Snowman & Biehler, 2006). In the latest update of IDEA, which took effect in 2004, regulations include more specific classifications of developmental disabilities such as autism, emotional disturbance, hearing and visual impairment, traumatic brain injuries, learning disabilities, and mental retardation (Vander Zanden et al., 2007).

Developmental disabilities affect approximately 17% of children younger than 18 years of age (CDC, 2006). The manner in which the mentally retarded are provided services has gone through a major transformation in much the same way that the care of the mentally ill has changed. Mandated early intervention and inclusion have increased the presence of such children and adults in all facets of society, including hospitals and outpatient clinics.

Many nurses are limited in their ability to provide holistic care for this population. Indeed, most nursing staff lack prior experience and often feel uncomfortable caring for those with developmental disabilities. This problem becomes acute when the nurse is faced with trying to help the clients understand particular treatments or tasks. When dealing with children who are developmentally disabled, the real experts in caring and working with them are their parents. It is a wise nurse who invites these parents to participate and assist the nursing staff during their child's hospitalization. However, caution should prevail, as the hospitalization may be the parents' only respite from an arduous care schedule.

Managing the treatment of persons with developmental disabilities accounts for an increasing portion of healthcare practice today. Because developmental disabilities usually are diagnosed during infancy and are likely to last a lifetime, nurses must acquire sensitivity to family issues and learn to be flexible in their approaches to meet the intellectual, emotional, and medical concerns of clients with special needs (Webb, Tittle, & VanCott, 2000).

When planning a teaching intervention, nurses must keep in mind the client's developmental stage, not his or her chronological age. If the child does not communicate verbally, the nurse should note whether certain nonverbal cues, such as gestures, signing, or other symbols, are used for communication purposes. Most children with mental retardation are incapable of abstract thinking. Although the majority can comprehend simple explanations, concrete examples must be given. For example, instead of saying, "Lunch will be here in a few minutes," the nurse could show a clock and point to the time. For children scheduled to have surgery, giving them a surgical mask to play with will help dispel fears they may have when entering the operating room.

Instructors must always remember that facial expression and voice tone are more important than words spoken. They should be sure the family explains any nonverbal cues for a "yes" or "no" response, and then try to ask questions in a manner requiring a "yes" or "no" answer. Nurses should lavish any positive behavior with great praise. They should keep the information simple, concrete, and repetitive, and they should be consistent, but firm, setting appropriate limits. They should be careful not to dominate any teaching session, but let the child actively participate and have a sense of accomplishment. Nurse educators must assign simple tasks with simple directions and show what is to be done, rather than relying on verbal commands. They should give only one direction at a time. A reward system often works very well with such patients. Stickers with familiar childhood characters placed on their bed or pajamas can remind the child of a job well done.

Mental Illness

In the United States, mental disorders are determined based on the *Diagnostic and Statistical Manual of Mental Disorders* (*DSM-IV*). According to the National Institute of Mental Health (NIMH, 2007) and based on the data provided by its large global burden of disease study, mental illness, including suicide, accounts for over 15% of the burden of disease in established market economies, such as the United States. This is more than that caused by *all* cancers.

In the United States, mental disorders affect an estimated 26.2% of Americans ages 18 and older. That is, about one in four adults suffer from a diagnosable mental disorder in any given year. When applied to the U.S. Census Bureau's (2004) residential population estimates for ages 18 and older, this figure translates to 57.7 million people. Mental disorders are the leading cause of disability in the United States and Canada for ages 15–44, and many suffer from more than one type at a given time (NIMH, 2007). These statistics reveal the relative prevalence of mental illness in our society and indicate that nurses will often care for patients with a psychiatric problem as a primary or secondary diagnosis.

Until about 1886, the mentally ill were restrained in iron manacles. With the advent of pharmacotherapy in the 1950s, the life of a person with a mental illness began to change. The discovery of the various neuroleptic and antidepressant drugs was a major contribution to the improved quality of life for the mentally ill. Previously dependent clients were able to live outside of an institution. For the last 25 years, the care of the mentally ill has been moving into community health centers, and clients are spending less time confined to a mental health facility and more time in the community, at work, and at home (Haber, Krainovich-Miller, McMahon, & Price-Hoskins, 1997). The quality of treatments and, therefore, the quality of life for those with mental illness can only improve. It is incumbent upon nurses to examine their own feelings about mental illness so they can enter into a viable teaching–learning relationship.

Although educating clients with mental disorders requires the same basic principles of patient teaching, there are some specific teaching strategies to consider. As with any other nursing intervention, the first step is to begin with a comprehensive assessment. In this case, it is wise to determine whether the consumer has any cognitive impairment or inappropriate behavior as well as to assess the patient's level of anxiety. The emotional threat that a person perceives as a result of a psychiatric disorder may result in an increased anxiety level and subsequently begin a chain of physiological reactions that then decrease his or her readiness to learn (Haber et al., 1997). High anxiety can make learning nearly impossible (Kessels, 2003; Stephenson, 2006). Despite the nurse's best efforts, clients with a mental disorder may not be able to identify their need to learn and may not be sufficiently ready to learn. However, the nurse may not be able to wait for readiness to happen. Therein lies the challenge.

Although persons with mental disorders are able to learn given the right circumstances and strategies, it is important to remember that people with mental illness can experience difficulty in processing information and verbally communicating information. In addition, they may experience decreased concentration and become easily distracted, which can limit their ability to stay on task. Thus, it is very important that the family or significant other participate in the health education of the client. Therefore, they should be included in teaching sessions (Haber et al., 1997).

The following is a summary of three essential strategies that have been successful when teaching people with mental illness (Haber et al., 1997):

1. Teach by using small and brief words, repeating information over and over—use mnemonics, write down important information by placing it on index cards, and use simple drawings or symbols. Be creative.
2. Keep sessions short and frequent. For instance, instead of a 1-hour session, break the learning period into four 15-minute sessions.
3. Involve all possible resources, including the client and his or her family. Actively engage them to help determine the client's learning styles as well as the best way to reinforce content. Consider using computer-assisted instruction, videotapes, and role modeling with clients.

As with any teaching program, it is important to set goals and determine outcomes with the client. The specific behavioral objectives depend on individual learning needs as well as overall learning outcomes. These would include empowering clients to take as much control over their health as possible.

In spite of all the great strides made in the treatment of acute mental illness, the mentally ill person still faces the problem of being stigmatized. Nurse educators should explore teaching strategies that have been successful in the field of mental health. Education programs for the mentally ill are few and far between. Their needs for learning are great, but they are often not given the same opportunities for educational programs as those persons with physical disabilities.

Motivating the patient with a chronic mental illness can be challenging. A certificate of recognition may be given to each patient when he or she completes a program, which can be a powerful motivator. To have a positive effect on the quality of life of the chronically mentally ill, educators must provide useful information. Independence and self-management remain goals for this special population, as with all other populations. Therefore, the nurse educator will need to consider the strategies available from all specialties to meet the challenge of teaching the person with a mental illness.

Physical Disabilities

Spinal Cord Injury

Before 1945, the survival prognosis for people with paraplegia or quadriplegia was very poor. By the 1970s, several regional spinal cord injury centers had been established across the country (Zejdlik, 1992). Catastrophic injuries to the spinal cord affect thousands of people each year. Accidents, falls, violence, and sporting and recreational injuries are the major causes. Annually about 11,000 new cases occur, which is about 40 cases per million population in the United States (Spinal Cord Injury Information Network, 2006). The spinal cord-injured population has benefited directly from these specialized services and from application of advanced technologies (McKinley, Tewksbury, Sitter, Reed, & Floyd, 2004). Not only are people surviving, but they are also living greatly improved lives. For example, today the availability of electric wheelchairs enables people with spinal cord injuries to be much more independent. That mobility, along with the utilization of computer and assistive and adaptive technology, gives those with a spinal cord injury (SCI) much greater quality of life.

The average age of the population of the United States has increased by approximately 8 years since the mid-1970s, and the median age of someone experiencing an SCI has also increased. Today, the average age of a person with such an injury is 38 years. Moreover, the percentage of persons older than 60 years of age at injury has grown from 4.7% prior to 1980 to 11.5% at the turn of the century. However, most SCIs happen to males (77.8%) between the ages of 16 and 30 (Spinal Cord Injury Information Network, 2006).

Residual impairment from spinal cord injury affects all areas of life—physical, social, psychological, vocational, and spiritual. Spinal cord injury is sudden and devastating, both to the injured person and to the family. The adjustment is difficult and continuous. During the rehabilitation phase of hospitalization, all interventions are driven by the goal of independent living. Since this type of injury occurs most frequently in young adult males, the individual and his family are already in the midst of dealing with his need for independence, which is a normal developmental characteristic of the adolescent/young adulthood stage, but now the family will be asked to redefine what are appropriate roles and responsibilities during this developmental period. Fink (1967), a psychologist, described four sequential phases of recovery, which are still relevant today: (1) shock, (2) defensive retreat, (3) acknowledgment, and (4) adaptation. With the shortened

lengths of hospital stay for both critical care and rehabilitation, the newly injured person and family members have less time to reach the adaptation phase of adjustment to a disability before going home, where new and ongoing challenges greet them every day.

Initially, most SCI clients receive comprehensive rehabilitation services at spinal cord injury centers. However, many skills are required to maintain physical and emotional equilibrium over the ensuing months and years. Often the quantity of information to meet self-care needs is overwhelming, and people with spinal cord injuries find themselves plagued with frequent hospital readmissions. The most common physical problems they experience are urinary tract infections and skin breakdown. Very often they possess knowledge and skills to prevent such complications, but it is more a matter of sustaining their motivation and individualizing the approach to make interventions and treatments fit their lifestyle.

Much of the rehabilitation as it relates to patients' functional living is actually done by trial and error. It is wise to remember that adolescents and young adults are particularly concerned about occupational and vocational goals as well as maintaining relationships. Lubkin and Larsen (2006) address the effects of limitations resulting from illness or disability as defining their ability to fulfill these goals.

Before developing strategies that allow learners to cope with a disability, the nurse must consider some common obstacles that are likely to be encountered, not the least of which is readiness to learn. Presenting important health-related information is only half the challenge. The other half is the ability of patients to accept and use the information to change or improve their health status.

Denial is the most frequent obstacle to learning readiness in the young spinal cord-injured patient. Although one object of this denial is often the bowel program, denial frequently reappears whenever any task seems overwhelming. Although denial is a coping mechanism, it is a negative approach that interferes with readiness to learn.

Another obstacle to learning readiness is the lack of physical endurance. This weakness may be especially apparent in the older client. In this situation, it may be prudent to involve a friend or family member to ensure that a relief person will be able to take over when the client's energy level is inadequate.

In her work with rehabilitation patients, Vance (1992) cited role changes related to dependence or independence as an obstacle to learning readiness. In this situation, either clients or caregivers may view the acquisition of new information or skills as a threat to their role as patient or caregiver. For example, it is now possible for a person with quadriplegia to drive. If the client has been transported by a good friend or family member for several years, this new independence may be viewed as a serious threat to his or her role as caregiver.

All too often the need for sharing problems and issues is overlooked. Patients and their families need to have a positive vision of the future, and feelings of isolation can quickly overwhelm them. One way to remedy this problem is by using the group approach to teaching, whereby spinal cord-injured persons who have adjusted to their disability can be included in some of the teaching sessions. In this way, newly injured persons can benefit from the trials and errors of those who have gone before them. It is critical to understand that significant others and children need support throughout this experience,

too. Everyone has to work through the injury at their own pace.

It is imperative that at whatever juncture the nurse educator encounters a person with a spinal cord injury, a careful assessment of the patient's readiness to learn must be carried out first and foremost. Next, the family and, most important, the immediate caregiver, who may or may not be a family member, must be involved. With the appropriate support and knowledge, the client and significant others will be given the opportunity for success in learning and maintaining independence.

Brain Injury

A fall, car accident, gunshot wound, or blow to the head are just a few potential causes of traumatic brain injury. About 1.4 million people sustain a traumatic brain injury (TBI) each year in the United States. Of these, 235,000 are hospitalized and 1.1 million are treated and released from the emergency department (CDC, 2006). TBI includes two specific types: closed head injury, which refers to nonpenetrating injury, and open head injury, which refers to penetrating injury resulting in brain tissue exposure and disruption of normal protective barriers.

Males are about 1.5 times as likely to sustain a TBI. The two age groups at highest risk for the injury are 0–4-year-olds and 15–19-year-olds. Of course, military duty increases the risk of sustaining a TBI (Marchione, 2007). The Centers for Disease Control and Prevention estimates that at least 5.3 million Americans currently have a long-term or lifelong need for help to perform activities of daily living as a result of a TBI (CDC, 2006).

The cognitive deficits that occur depend on the severity and location of the injury and may include poor attention span, slowness in thinking, confusion, difficulty with short-term and long-term memory, distractibility, impulsive and socially inappropriate behaviors, poor judgment, mental fatigue, and difficulty with organization, problem solving, reading, and writing. As might be expected, communication skills will more than likely be an issue.

The treatment of people with severe brain injury is most often divided into three stages:

1. Acute care (in an intensive care unit)
2. Acute rehabilitation (in an inpatient brain-injury rehabilitation unit)
3. Long-term rehabilitation after discharge (at home or in a long-term care facility)

At every stage, there are many hurdles to conquer. Once the injured person's life is assured and the physical condition improves, the patient is discharged from the acute care unit. It is at this point that someone not familiar with traumatic brain injuries might wonder why a person who looks healthy and independent still needs rehabilitation. For this reason, families need to be kept up to date on their loved one's prognosis and progress from the very beginning. Throughout the rehabilitation process, family teaching must be consistent and thoughtful, as most of the residual impairments are not visible, with the exception of the sensorimotor deficits.

The communication, cognitive-perceptual, and behavioral changes may be dramatic. However, the most difficult problem for the family is the recognition that their relative will probably never be the same person again. In fact, personality changes present the biggest burden for the family. Studies have shown that the level of the family stress is directly related to personality changes and the relative's own perception of the symptoms arising from the head injury (Grinspun, 1987).

Although most of the literature deals with the importance of family inclusion during the rehabilitation period, it is clear that brain-injured persons will always need the involvement of their family. Again, the benefits of participation in family groups are immeasurable. Considerable strength is gained from group participation, and learning is accomplished through a friendly, informal approach. Of particular importance for brain-injured persons is the need for unconditional acceptance from their friends and family.

Learning needs for this population center on the issues of client safety and family coping. Safety issues are related to cognitive and behavioral capabilities. Families are faced with a life-changing event and will require ongoing support and encouragement to take care of themselves. Recovery may require several years, and most often the person is left with some form of impairment.

According to the National Center for Injury Prevention and Control (1999), 40% of those hospitalized with a TBI have at least one unmet need for services 1 year after the injury. The most frequent are managing stress and emotional upsets, controlling one's temper, improving one's job skills, and regaining memory and problem solving.

Table 9–3 lists some dos and don'ts for effective teaching of the person with a brain injury.

Communication Disorders

"Communication is a universal process by which human beings exchange ideas, impart feelings and express needs" (Adkins, 1991, p. 74). Communication occurs in a variety of ways, including drama, music, literature, and art. It is

---

Table 9–3 GUIDELINES FOR EFFECTIVE TEACHING OF THE BRAIN-INJURED PATIENT

DO	DON'T
Use simple rather than complex statements.	Stop talking or trying to communicate.
Use gestures to complement what you are saying.	Speak too fast.
Give step-by-step directions.	Talk down to the person.
Allow time for responses.	Talk in the person's presence as though he or she is not there.
Recognize and praise all efforts to communicate.	Give up (instead, seek the assistance of a speech-language pathologist).
Ensure the use of listening devices.	
Keep written instructions simple, with a small amount of information on each page.	

---

verbal and nonverbal, and there are both sending and receiving components.

Stroke, or cerebrovascular accident, is the most common cause of impaired communication. As is true with the other disabilities discussed in this chapter, a stroke is a major crisis for both the person and the family. Many of the strategies discussed for teaching spinal cord injury patients are also applicable to an educational program for the person with a stroke. This discussion will cover some useful strategies appropriate for working with an individual with impaired communication such as aphasia.

On average, every 45 seconds someone in the United States has a stroke (Center of Excellence on Health Disparities, n.d.). In fact, each year about 700,000 people experience a first or recurrent stroke. About 500,000 of these are first attacks (Center of Excellence on Health Disparities, n.d.). Over the course of a lifetime, four out of every five American families will be touched by stroke.

Stroke is the leading cause of disability. Over 4 million Americans are living with the effects of stroke. About one third have mild impairments, another third are moderately impaired, and the remainder are severely impaired (National Stroke Association, 2003).

One of the most common residual deficits of a stroke is a problem with language. Aphasia is a disorder from damage to the language center of the brain. Primary signs of the disorder include difficulty in expression, trouble understanding speech, and difficulty reading and writing. Although seen commonly in adults who have suffered a stroke, aphasia can also result from a brain tumor, infection, head injury, or dementia.

It is estimated that about 1 million people in the United States today suffer from aphasia. The type and severity of the language dysfunction depends on the precise location and the extent of the damaged brain tissue (National Institute for Neurological Disorders and Stroke, 2007). When you prepare to work with someone with aphasia, it is necessary to determine which type it is—expressive or receptive. If the nurse's involvement with the client occurs during the early stage of rehabilitation, the speech-language pathologist would be a good teammate.

The function of language primarily resides in the left hemisphere of the brain. Most often when an injury affects the dominant cerebral hemisphere, which is usually the left, the result is expressive aphasia. About three quarters of the overall population has a dominant left hemisphere. Expressive aphasia occurs when an injury damages the inferior frontal gyrus, just anterior to the facial and lingual areas of the motor cortex, known as Broca's area. Because Broca's area is so near the left motor area, the stroke often leaves the person with right-sided paralysis as well.

Wernicke's area of the brain is located in the temporal lobe and is needed for auditory and reading comprehension. When this area is affected, persons are left with receptive aphasia. Although their hearing is unimpaired, they are nevertheless unable to understand the significance of the spoken word. See **Table 9–4** for different types of aphasia.

Although persons with both types of aphasia are unable to communicate verbally or have difficulty doing so, it does not mean they are intellectually impaired. The inability to communicate verbally is a highly frustrating experience for the patient and caregivers. Speech therapy should be one of the earliest interventions, and the nurse will need to incorporate those strategies into the teaching–learning plan. Every effort must be made to establish communication at some level. Remember, regardless of how severe the communication deficit, it is almost always possible to have stroke patients communicate in some manner and to some extent.

Expressive Aphasia

In the event structured speech therapy is not available, the nursing staff will need to develop its own plan of care. When working with patients who have *expressive aphasia,* the nurse might try having them recall word images, first by naming commonly used objects (e.g., spoons, knives, forks) and then those objects in the immediate environment (e.g., bed, table). Another strategy is having the person repeat words spoken by the nurse. It is wise to begin with simple terms and work progressively to the more complex.

These exercises may be carried out frequently during the day, keeping the sessions short. Most people become tired when sessions are longer than 30 minutes. Often their speech will become slurred, and they will experience mental fatigue. In a following section of this chapter, some helpful information regarding assistive technology is provided. Computers are a wonderful tool to assist patients with expressive aphasia in their efforts to communicate.

Receptive Aphasia

Patients who have *receptive aphasia,* need help establishing a means for nonverbal communication. Facial expressions, gestures, and even pantomime will be effective in conveying messages. Most often, patients are unaware of their impairment and will speak in what seems to them like a correct statement, but on examination the words do not make sense. Nurses should speak more slowly and slightly louder to the person with receptive aphasia, as auditory stimulation seems to be effective. When comprehension and memory span increase, the person will begin to respond appropriately.

Also, aphasic persons have trouble with retention and recall. It seems old personal memories return first and recent events take longer to reappear. "It is a lonely, isolated world for those who cannot communicate with other

Table 9–4 CLINICAL FEATURES OF APHASIA

Type	Involved Anatomy	Expression	Auditory Comprehension	Written Comprehension	Naming	Word/Phrase Repetition	Ability to Write
Broca's (motor, expressive)	Precentral gyrus, Broca's area	Nonfluent, telegraphic, may be mute	Subtle deficits	Subtle deficits	Impaired	Impaired	Impaired
Wernicke's (receptive, sensory)	Superior temporal gyrus	Fluent but content inappropriate	Impaired	Impaired	Severely impaired	Impaired	Impaired
Global (mixed)	Frontal-temporal area	Nonfluent	Severely impaired	Impaired	Severely impaired	Impaired	Severely impaired
Conductive (central)	Arcuate fasciculus	Fluent	Intact	Intact	Impaired	Severely impaired	Impaired
Anomic (amnesic)	Angular gyrus	Fluent	Intact	Intact	Severely impaired	Intact	Subtle deficits
Transcortical sensory (TCSA)	Periphery of Broca's and Wernicke's areas (watershed zone)	Fluent	Impaired	Impaired	Impaired	Intact	Severely impaired
Transcortical motor (TCMA)	Anterior, superior, or lateral to Broca's area	Nonfluent, speech initiation difficult	Intact	Subtle deficits	Impaired	Intact	Impaired

Source: Reprinted by permission from Bronstein, S., Popvich, J. M., & Stewart-Amidei, C. (1991). *Promoting stroke recovery: A research-based approach for nursing.* St. Louis, MO: Mosby-Year Book, Table 11–1.

human beings" (Jennings, 1981, p. 39). As nurses attempt to work with and engage them in a teaching–learning intervention, they must be aware of their own attitudes. The effort to communicate with someone without using their usual speech and language is one of the more frustrating experiences. They should be sure to take time out and reflect on the rewards of assisting the client and family in overcoming this barrier.

Encouragement and explanation when teaching people with aphasia will go a long way in ensuring client participation and recovery. Educators should be sure their teaching sessions are filled with praise and always acknowledge the client's frustration. They should keep distractions to a minimum by turning off the radio and television so that they have the full attention of the client.

Usually extra effort is required by people with aphasia to understand spoken messages. To them it is as if they are trying to comprehend a foreign language. The person may need extra time to process and understand what is being said. It may be especially hard to follow very fast speech like that heard on the radio or television news. Also, the subtleties of language can be easily misinterpreted (e.g., taking the literal meaning for sarcasm or a figure of speech like, "He kicked the bucket").

Difficulty with one or more of these skills may lead to communication breakdowns and frustrating communication for both the person with aphasia and his or her listener (ASHA, 2007a). Sometimes one is able to help the person develop stronger language skills to express himself or herself, such as using gestures and writing rather than speaking. Also, group sessions for teaching and learning allow the patient to practice conversation, as well as listen to others in the group.

Dysarthria

Many people with degenerative disorders, such as Parkinson's disease, multiple sclerosis, and myasthenia gravis also have dysarthria. *Dysarthria* is a problem with the voluntary muscle control of speech. It occurs as a consequence of damage to the central or peripheral nervous system and affects the same muscles used in eating and speaking. The result is unintelligible speech. The type and severity of dysarthria depend on which area of the nervous system is affected (ASHA, 2007b).

Several types of dysarthria exist, including flaccid, spastic, ataxic, hypokinetic, and mixed. Although the incidence of the various types is unknown, this category of communication problems will certainly increase as the medical treatments for the various brain diseases improve and people live longer. Those who do survive will need help in overcoming all the residual social and communication problems.

Currently, Parkinson's disease is managed very well with medication, and there is ongoing research in the medical management of multiple sclerosis and myasthenia gravis. The intervention of a speech-language pathologist may help improve the function of various muscles used for speech. There are also some helpful mechanical devices, such as a prosthetic palate, which is used to control hypernasality.

Another useful tool is sign language, which may be used if the person's arm and hand muscles are unaffected. The nurse should work with the speech-language pathologist to determine whether any of the other nonverbal aids would be appropriate, such as communication boards or a portable electronic voice synthesizer. With the advent of adaptive technologies, the possibilities are limitless.

To improve communication with the dysarthric person, Yorkston et al. (2001) make the following suggestions:

- Control the communication environment by reducing distractions.
- Pay attention to the speaker and watch him or her as he or she talks.
- Be honest and let the speaker know you have difficulty understanding him or her.
- Convey the part of the message that you don't understand so the patient does not have to repeat the entire message.
- If you are unable to get the gist of the message after repeated attempts, ask questions that require a yes or no answer or have the patient write his/her message to you.

Laryngectomy

Cancer of the larynx accounts for approximately 2–5% of diagnosed cancer. More than twice as many men as women are diagnosed. Most cases occur between the ages of 50 and 70 (ASHA, 2007c).

Until recently, esophageal speech was the primary method for speaking after a laryngectomy. Esophageal speech involves taking air into the upper part of the esophagus and adapting its normal sphincters to vibrate like vocal cords. With practice, the new voice sounds quite natural.

Motivation and persistent effort are essential in learning this new kind of speech. Encouragement and support of the family as well as the clients are also critical for success. About 75% of all clients who have their larynx removed acquire some sort of speech therapy, and most people return to work in 1 to 2 months.

Tracheoesophageal speech is a more rapid restoration of speech. The speech is closer to normal in rate and phrasing, and it is more pleasing than that created with an electrolarynx. On the other hand, it means the person must rely on a prosthesis, and the tracheoesophageal fistula may undergo stenosis.

The tracheoesophageal puncture (TEP), which was first successfully performed in 1980, is one of the more popular methods of alaryngeal speech production. It can be performed at the time of the laryngectomy or afterwards. The surgeon creates a connection between the trachea and the esophagus with a small puncture. A small, one-way shunt valve is then inserted into this puncture (**Figure 9–3**). To speak, the person inhales air though the stoma and into the lungs. Then he or she covers the stoma with a finger. Air from the lungs is then directed from the trachea, through the shunt valve, and into the esophagus. The esophagus vibrates, creating a sound for speech that is then shaped into speech sounds in the mouth in the same way it was done before laryngectomy (ASHA, 2007c). During such speech, the stoma needs to be occluded. Education of the person and family includes what to do if the prosthesis comes out.

If an individual is unable to learn esophageal speech in 60 to 90 days after surgery, a speech aid such as a vibrator or an electronic artificial larynx is recommended. This battery-powered, handheld device has a vibrating diaphragm that a person with a laryngectomy presses against the soft tissues of the neck. The newer models permit a more natural type of speech.

As previously noted, many of the people with laryngectomies are older and often have a difficult time adjusting to their new condition. If they are unable to use any of the aforementioned interventions, the nurse needs to be vigilant about preventing silent suffering and social isolation. It is essential that contact with other

Figure 9–3 Tracheoesophageal puncture.

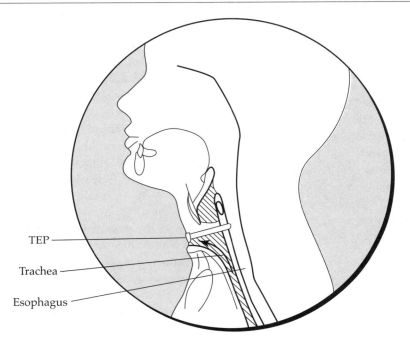

TEP

Trachea

Esophagus

people remain intact. If none of the assistive speech devices work, then other means of nonverbal communication need to be adopted.

Augmentative and alternative communication (AAC) refers to ways (other than speech) that are used to send a message from one person to another. We all use augmentative communication techniques, such as facial expressions, gestures, and writing, as part of our daily lives. In difficult listening situations (a noisy room, for example), we tend to augment our words with even more nonverbal expressions.

People with severe speech or language problems must rely quite heavily on these standard techniques as well as on special augmentative techniques that have been specifically developed

for them. Some of these techniques involve the use of specialized gestures, sign language, or Morse code. Other techniques use communication aids, such as charts, computers, and language boards. On aids such as these, objects may be represented by pictures, drawings, letters, words, sentences, special symbols, or any combination thereof (ASHA, 2007c).

When we are unable to speak naturally, other ways of communicating ideas can be used, such as gestures and sign language. There is a large variety of methods available to a person who has difficulty communicating, whether it be a language/speech disorder or a physical impairment. Many of the AAC methods are electronic, transmitting the communication in response to input from the user. By using an electronic device, an individual can communicate independently.

Losing the ability to communicate through speaking can be an isolating, depressing experience. It is of particular concern in this day and age of increased technology, when it is easy to lose sight of the human touch as the universal means of communication.

Chronic Illness

Lubkin and Larsen (2006) state that chronic illness is the nation's greatest health care problem. In 2004, it was estimated that there were 133 million individuals living with at least one chronic illness. Unlike acute illnesses, which usually have a clearly defined beginning and end, chronic illness is permanent. It is never completely cured and requires the full involvement of its victims. Every aspect of life is affected—physical, psychological, social, economical, and spiritual. Because successful management of a chronic illness is a lifelong process, the development of good learning skills is a matter of survival. Because it is impossible within the confines of this chapter to cover specific teaching strategies for each chronic illness, some general teaching and learning principles will be suggested in the following pages.

The learning process for individuals with a chronic illness is fraught with hills and valleys. There is no cure, little predictability, and much uncertainty. Most illnesses have several phases that affect the educational needs of both the ill person and his or her family. Therefore there is no one approach that will fit each teaching–learning situation.

It is important to be aware of the timing, acuity, and severity of the disease progression. The family's reaction and perception of the chronic illness are also important influences on the teaching–learning process (McCahen, 2006). Families need information and education to deal with the limitations and changes in their loved one's lifestyle.

There is often a conflict between feelings of dependence and the need to be independent. Sometimes the energy and focus of maintaining independence are overwhelming, both physically and emotionally. Often, living with a chronic illness includes a loss and/or change in roles. When people suffer from role loss (e.g., a father who is no longer able to keep his job), their self-esteem also may be affected. If there are lingering issues surrounding the individual's role loss and self-esteem, these need to be addressed, as they are obstacles to readiness to learn.

Controlling symptoms is a major time-consuming activity for those with chronic illnesses. Strauss and others (1984) identified the following eight key problem areas experienced by chronically ill patients and their families:

1. Prevention of medical crises and the management of problems once they occur
2. Control of symptoms
3. Carrying out prescribed regimens and the management of problems attendant with adhering to self-care
4. Prevention of, or living with, social isolation that decreases contact with others
5. Adjustment to changes in the course of the disease, whether it exacerbates or enters remission
6. Normalizing both interactions with others and one's lifestyle
7. Funding (finding the necessary money to pay for treatments or to survive despite partial or complete loss of employment)

8. Confronting attendant psychological, marital, and family problems

When working with a chronically ill person who must manage a complex therapeutic regimen, it is easy to see how the label of noncompliance might enter the assessment. The truth is, the person with a chronic illness requires more than just new information and psychomotor skill to deal with the problems of everyday life. Braden's self-help model: learned response to chronic illness experience, is a middle range nursing theory that proves a framework to describe enabling factors that enhance learning and mediate responses in chronic illness (Lubkin & Larsen, 2006). This model proposes that the learned self-management response, as opposed to a learned helplessness or a passive response to the experience of chronic illness, will assist nurses in developing appropriate teaching interventions.

The Family's Role in Chronic Illness or Disability

Families' reaction and perception of the impact of chronic illness or disability, rather than the illness or disability itself, influence all aspects of adjustment. Families are usually the care providers and the support system for the disabled person, and they need to be included in all the teaching–learning interactions. The literature has documented that family participation does have a profound influence on the success of a client's rehabilitation program.

When assessing the client and family, it is important to note what the family considers high-priority learning needs. Most often it will be related to the caregiver's perceived lifestyle change. A caregiver might ask, "Can I continue working outside?" or "Will I be able to main-

tain my relationships with friends?" It is important that the nurse assist the client and family to identify problems and develop mutually agreed-upon goals. Adaptation is key. Communication between and among family members is crucial. If a family has open communication, the nurse is in a good position to help the family mobilize so as to obtain needed educational and emotional support.

Also the educational process needs to take into consideration the family's strategies for coping with their relative's disability. Without a doubt, the overwhelming nature of chronic illness affects the quality of life not only for the chronically ill person, but for all the family members (Lubkin & Larsen, 2006). In their role as caregivers, they have their own anxieties and fears.

A chronic illness or disability can either destroy or strengthen family unity. Siblings and children of the disabled person may be at a different stage of acceptance. Denial may be present during the initial diagnosis of an illness or disability. Later, as the client and his or her family realize the permanency and the consequences of the situation, the nurse may witness periods of anger, guilt, depression, fear, and hostility. As these feelings dissipate, teaching lessons will need to be readjusted to fit the new circumstances. Flexibility is vital to attaining successful outcomes. Be sure to treat each family member as unique, and recognize that some family members may never fully adjust. Table 9–5 lists some of the most common sources of tension in client and family education.

Nurses need to value their teaching role when they work with the family having a disabled member. Unlike families dealing with an acutely ill member, families with permanently disabled members will have intermittent contact with the healthcare system throughout their lives. Therefore, whenever teaching ses-

Table 9–5 RELIEVING EXTERNAL TENSIONS IN CLIENT AND FAMILY EDUCATION

Problem	Response
FAMILY DYNAMICS	
Client or family member feels overwhelmed	Goal setting: Help family refocus on tasks at hand. Review goals that have been attained to boost morale.
Anxiety and fear of performing complex procedures	Establish an atmosphere of acceptance. Don't be in a hurry. Offer opportunities for talk and questions. Reassure client and family that they have made the right treatment choice.
Emotions associated with chronic or terminal conditions	Provide opportunities to express feelings. Offer referrals to community resources.
Caregiver burnout and illness	Simplify client management where possible (e.g., scheduling drug doses to reduce nighttime treatment). Remain accessible. Remember: When caregiver needs are not being met, resentments increase. Provide information on respite care.
Client fatigue, especially with chronic illness	Help the client identify individual tolerance for tiredness in planning for as much active participation in the family life as possible.
Young clients are frequently overwhelmed by complex emotions about their illness and therapy	Encourage both children and adolescents to use artwork to express their feelings. Suggest support groups. Offer support to parents and siblings who must alter their family lifestyle.
GERIATRIC CONSIDERATIONS	
An increase in the number of drugs taken daily (on average four or more per day) increases the potential for adverse reactions	Use only one pharmacy so that one source keeps track of medications. Continually evaluate all drugs taken for need, safety, compatibility, potential adverse reactions, and expiration dates.
Decreased visual acuity	Use teaching materials with large, bold type. Encourage the use of a magnifying glass.

Source: Adapted by permission from LaRocca, J. C. (1994). *Mosby's home health nursing pocket consultant.* St. Louis, MO: Mosby–Year Book.

sions are required, the families' availability should be a primary consideration. Given adequate support and resources, families with a chronically ill family member can adapt, make adjustments, and live healthy, happy, full lives.

Assistive Technologies

The growth of modern technology has invaded all areas of our lives. Without a doubt, the personal computer has become the technology that has had the greatest impact. Until recently, however, computers have been inaccessible to individuals with a disability. Yet, when assistive technology has been made available, disabled individuals have experienced dramatic changes in their lives. Computers with the appropriate adaptations have liberated people from social isolation and feelings of helplessness and have instilled feelings of self-worth and independence.

Since the enactment of the ADA in 1990, the diversity of the client population cared for by nurses has grown to include more individuals with disabilities in every practice setting. As nurses' understanding of assistive technology is enhanced, so will their ability to advocate, recommend, and assist persons to attain the appropriate equipment and training (Reed & Bowser, 1999). Assistive technology is defined as technological tools (computers and communication devices) available for the disabled that provide access to education, employment, recreation, and communication opportunities that allow them to live as independently as possible (ATA, n.d.). Some examples of assistive technology include, but are not limited to, talking word processors, specialized keyboards, communication devices, arm and wrist supports, amplified telephone handsets, screen magnifiers, and environmental controls (ATA, n.d.).

Assistive technology plays an ever increasing role in our work and daily living activities. Today the possibilities are endless. For instance, issues of the *Journal of Visual Impairment and Blindness,* published by the American Foundation for the Blind and available at http://www.afb.org, advertise several products that are available to the disabled, such as those that read aloud from the computer screen in either human or synthetic speech and a glow-in-the-dark print Braille rubber wristband for children who are visually impaired. As you can imagine, these adaptations are very helpful to anyone who has vision, learning, or cognitive disabilities.

Most people use a combination of systems or devices depending on their needs. The good news is that the mainstream technology is moving in the direction of universal design, which means that it will be available to almost anyone. Technology has the potential to improve the lives of people with disabilities by giving them the tools to become more independent, more productive, and better able to participate in a wide range of life experiences.

People with communication problems, especially those who are unable to speak or whose speech is difficult to understand, can use augmentative and alternative communication devices, such as the computer, to add a whole new dimension or quality to their lives. Technology has already made much of the previously impossible possible and even greater advances can be expected in the future. It is incumbent upon the nurse to know how to help individuals with disabilities locate and access whatever assistive technology is needed to convey health information. This technology might include software programs with closed captioning built in for the hearing impaired or on-screen keyboards that can be accessed with a mouse, trackball, or an illuminated pointer device for someone with fine or gross motor deficits.

Every computer-based solution is the result of a carefully planned, individually determined process. Individuals with a disability are the experts on what works best for them. However, some guidelines should be considered when selecting the best adaptive computer. The best computer solution for individuals with disabilities will allow for independent and effective use. Other criteria include affordability, portability, flexibility, and simplicity of learning. If these criteria are met, then the adaptive computer is probably in compliance with the ADA's reasonable accommodations.

Scherer, Say, Vanbiervleit, Cashman, and Scherer (2005) point out that as available options of assistive technologies have increased, their use has been more widely considered and recommended. It remains a challenging and sometimes complex process to match the person with the right technology. Those with physical, sensory and/or cognitive impairments affecting their ability to use a computer may benefit from a host of adaptive devices (McKinley et al., 2004).

Assistive technology is here to stay. While assistive technology will probably be forever changing, the process for ensuring individualized computer solutions will remain much the same, and the benefits are enormous. It is exciting to reflect on the positive, possibly life-changing effects the personal computer and other telecommunication devices can have on the lives of individuals with a disability. They have the potential of changing what it means to be disabled.

The role of nurse as educator includes a client advocacy component. As client advocate, the nurse can work with the multidisciplinary team, including the assistive technology specialist, to enable special populations to participate in all of life's experiences. Thanks to what assistive technologies will be able to do, more people with disabilities will be among us.

State of the Evidence

As previously noted, for the first time, the United States Surgeon General's Report on Health Promotion and Disease Prevention, *Healthy People 2010,* includes data and health objectives for people with disabilities. This national report is a reflection of almost all accommodations and services, especially health services, available to people with disabilities. This is particularly notable in the area of patient education. It is an unusual nursing text that includes information on how to assist those with disabilities in learning. The *Healthy People 2010* report identifies 207 objectives of care for people with disabilities; however, data regarding those objectives is only available for 88 of the 207 (CDC, 2006).

In a recent search of the literature, one reference (Ravesloot, 2003) provided specific recommendations based on a study of Medicaid beneficiaries. Although the primary goal of the study was not centered on teaching strategies, it nonetheless identified barriers to increased participation in health promotion programs. The investigators determined that the two most problematic barriers to health promotion activities were pain and fatigue. Certainly, this is useful information for nurses when trying to implement a successful teaching plan.

In a recent review of the Cochrane Database of Systematic Reviews (2007), there was a notable lack of research on the topic of disabilities. This review found little or no data on teaching people with disabilities. It is encouraging that there is an emerging base of research for some of the more common disabilities such as traumatic brain injury, learning disabilities, and spinal cord injuries. However, it is apparent that an area in need of further investigation is patient education for people with mental health and other chronic illnesses. One recent review of education for those with schizophrenia, entitled *Psychoeducation for Schizophrenia,* by Pekkala and Merinder (2002) concluded that there seems to be some suggestion that psychoeducation may improve compliance with medication, although the extent of improvement remained unclear. However, the study showed a possibility that psychoeducation has positive effects on a person's overall well-being. This type of study may have implications for nurse educators managing patients with other chronic mental illnesses. Yet, as the review on patients with schizophrenia concluded, "The scarcity of studies made the comparison between efficacy of different formats weak" (Pekkala & Merinder, 2002). Clearly, this is true of the evidence to support and identify specific teaching strategies that would help nurse educators work with a variety of special populations.

Summary

This chapter covered some of the most common disabilities faced by millions of Americans as a result of disease, injury, heredity, aging, and congenital defects. These conditions affect physical, cognitive, or sensory capacities and require behavioral change in one or more of these domains of learning. The nurse educator must be creative, innovative, flexible, and persistent when applying the principles of teaching and learning to meet the needs of these special populations of individuals, their families, and others.

The shock of any disability, whether it occurs at the beginning of life or toward the end, has a tremendous impact on individuals and their families. At the onset and all through the transition and recovery process, the patient and family are met with new information to be learned, as successful habilitation or rehabilitation means acquiring knowledge and applying it to their situation. Inner strength and courage are attributes needed to face each new day, as the effort to live a normal life never ends. The physical, social, emotional, and vocational implications of living with a disability necessitate the nurse as educator to be well prepared to meet any member of this special population right where they are in their struggle to live independently.

REVIEW QUESTIONS

1. How do the terms *habilitation* and *rehabilitation* differ from one another?
2. What are the major causes of disabilities?
3. What questions should be asked by the nurse educator when assessing a disabled person's readiness to learn?
4. What are the two major types of disabilities?
5. What are the seven categories of disabilities?
6. When should the nurse educator enlist the help of a professional interpreter rather than a member of the family when teaching a hearing-impaired person?
7. What are 10 tips you might find helpful in teaching a blind or visually impaired person?
8. What are the four types of input disabilities and the two types of output disabilities?
9. What are the characteristic behaviors of persons with ADHD and the educational interventions that should be used with them for effective teaching and learning?
10. How is the term *developmental disability* defined, and what laws have been enacted to protect children with mental and/or physical impairments?
11. What are the key problem areas experienced by chronically ill patients and their families?
12. How can assistive technology devices improve the quality of life for a person with a disability?

References

Adkins, E. R. H. (1991). Nursing care of the client with impaired communication. *Rehabilitation Nursing, 16*(2), 74–76.

The Alliance for Technology Access (ATA). (n.d.). *Services.* Retrieved June 28, 2007, from http://www.ataccess.org/about/services.html

American Foundation for the Blind (AFB). (2007). Retrieved May 21, 2007, from http://www.afb.org

American Speech-Language-Hearing Association (ASHA). (2007a). *Aphasia.* Retrieved June 28, 2007, from http://www.asha.org/public/speech/disorders/aphasia.htm

American Speech-Language-Hearing Association (ASHA). (2007b). *Dysarthria.* Yorkston, K. Retrieved June 28, 2007, from http://www.asha.org/public/speech/disorders/dysarthria.htm

American Speech-Language-Hearing Association (ASHA). (2007c). *Laryngeal cancer.* Retrieved June 28, 2007, from http://www.asha.org/public/speech/ disorders/LaryngealCancerCauses.htm

Attention Deficit Disorder Association (ADDA). (2006). Retrieved June 19, 2007, from http://www.add.org

Babcock, D. E., & Miller, M. A. (1994). *Client education: Theory and practice.* St. Louis, MO: Mosby.

Baker, S. S. (1993). Teamwork between the health care community and the blind rehabilitation system. *Journal of Visual Impairment and Blindness, 87*(9), 349–352.

Boyd, M. D., Gleit, C. J., Graham, B. A., & Whitman, N. I. (1998). *Health teaching in nursing practice* (3rd ed.). Stamford, CT: Appleton & Lange.

Center of Excellence on Health Disparities. (n.d.). Retrieved September 26, 2007, from http://web.msm.edu/export/stroke_facts.htm

Centers for Disease Control and Prevention (CDC). (2006). Retrieved June 19, 2007, from http://www.cdc.gov/ncbddd/dd/ddsurv.htm

Cunningham, C. (2001, February). Breaking the barriers to math and science for students with disabilities. *Syllabus*, 41–42.

DeLisa, J. A., & Gand, B. M. (Eds.). (1998). *Rehabilitation medicine: Principles and practice.* Philadelphia: Lippincott.

Diehl, L. N. (1989). Client and family learning in the rehabilitation setting. *Nursing Clinics of North America, 24*(1), 257–264.

DiPietro, L. (1979). *Deaf patients, special needs, special responses.* Washington, DC: National Academy of Gallaudet College.

Edwards, P. A. (2000). *The specialty practice of rehabilitation: A core curriculum* (4th ed.). Glenville, IL: Association of Rehabilitation Nurses.

Fraley, A. M. (1992). *Nursing and the disabled: Across the lifespan.* Sudbury, MA: Jones and Bartlett.

Fink, S. L. (1967). Crisis and motivation: A theoretical model. *Archives of Physical Rehabilitation, 48,* 492–597.

Greenberg, L. A. (1991). Teaching children who are learning disabled about illness and hospitalization. *MCN: American Journal of Maternal Child Nursing, 16*(5), 260–263.

Grinspun, D. (1987). Teaching families of traumatic brain-injured adults. *Critical Care Nursing Quarterly, 10*(3), 61–72.

Haber, J., Krainovich-Miller, B., McMahon, A. L., & Price-Hoskins, P. (1997). *Comprehensive psychiatric nursing.* St. Louis, MO: Mosby.

Harrison, L. L. (1990). Minimizing barriers when teaching hearing-impaired clients. *MCN: American Journal of Maternal Child Nursing, 15*(2), 113.

Jennings, S. (1981). Communicating with your aphasic patients. *Journal of Practical Nursing, 31,* 22–23.

Kessels, R. P. C. (2003). Patients' memory for medical information. *Journal of the Royal Society of Medicine, 96,* 212–222.

Kid Source, American Speech-Language-Hearing Association. (2007). Retrieved May 21, 2007, from http://www.kidsource.com/ASHA

LaRocca, J. C. (1994). *Handbook of home care IV therapy.* St. Louis, MO: Mosby–Year Book.

Learning Disabilities Roundtable. (2005, February). Comments and recommendations on regulatory issues under the Individuals with Disabilities Education Improvement Act of 2004. Public Law 108-446, 1-12. Retrieved May 21, 2007, from http://www.cec.sped.org/pdfs/Appendix2004LDRoundtableRecs.pdf

Lubkin, I. M., & Larsen, P. (2006). *Chronic illness* (6th ed.). Sudbury, MA: Jones and Bartlett.

McCahen, C. P. (2006). Client and family education. In I. M. Lubkin & P. Larsen (Eds.), *Chronic illness: Impact and interventions* (6th ed., pp. 351–374). Sudbury, MA: Jones and Bartlett.

Marchione, M. (2007, September 9). *Brain damage plagues thousands of GIs.* Retrieved September 10, 2007, from http://news.aol.com/health

McConnel, E. A. (1996). Clinical do's & don'ts: Caring for a patient with a vision impairment. *Nursing, 26*(5), 28.

McKinley, W., Tewksbury, M., Sitter, P., Reed, J., Floyd, S. (2004). Assistive technology and computer adaptations for individuals with spinal cord injury. *Neuro Rehabilitation, 19,* 141–146. Retrieved from EBSCO host June 15, 2007.

Merrow, S. L., & Corbett, C. (1994). Adaptive computing for people with disabilities. *Computers in Nursing, 12*(4), 201–209.

National Center for Injury Prevention and Control (1999, December). *Traumatic brain injury in the United States: A report to Congress.* Retrieved May 8, 2007, from http://www.cdc.gov/NCIPC/tbi/tbi_congress/tbi_congress.htm

National Dissemination Center for Children With Disabilities (NICHCY). (2004). *Twenty-fourth annual report to Congress.* U.S. Department of Education. Retrieved May 21, 2007, from http://www.nichcy.org/IDEA.htm

National Institute on Deafness and Other Communication Disorders (NIDCD). (2005, August 18). *Fact sheets.* Retrieved May 21, 2007, from http://www.nidcd.nih.gov

National Institute of Mental Health (NIMH). (2007). *Statistics.* Retrieved May 21, 2007, from http://www.nimh.nih.gov/healthinformation/statisticsmenu.cfm

National Institute of Neurological Disorders and Stroke. (2007). *NNDS aphasia information.* Retrieved June

17, 2007, from http://www.ninds.nih.gov/disorders/aphasia/aphasia.htm

National Stroke Association. (2003). *National Stroke Association's complete guide to stroke.* Retrieved May 28, 2007, from http://www.stroke.org/site/DocServer/NSA_complete_guide.pdf

Navarro, M. R., & Lacour, G. (1980). Helping hints for use with deaf patients. *Journal of Emergency Nursing, 6*(6), 26–28.

Nelson, K. (1991). *Projected increase in the prevalence of severe visual impairment among elderly Americans.* New York: American Foundation for the Blind.

Pekkala, E., & Merinder, L. (2002). Psychoeducation for schizophrenia. Cochrane Database of Systematic Reviews, retrieved September 26, 2007, from http://www.cochrane.org/previews/en/ab002831.html

Ravesloot, C. (2003). *Rural disability and rehabilitation research progress report #18.* Retrieved September 26, 2007, from http://rtc.ruralinstitute.umt.edu/health/marketing.htm

Reed, P., & Bowser, G. (1999, November). Assistive technology and the IDEA. *Exceptional Parent, 54*–55, 57–58.

Rehabilitation Act of 1973, PL 93-112, Section 504, retrieved September 26, 2007, from http://www.dol.gov/oasam/regs/statutes/sec504.htm

Santrock, J. W. (2006). *Lifespan development* (10th ed.). Boston: McGraw-Hill.

Scherer, M., Say, C., Vanbiervleit, A., Cashman, L., & Scherer, J. (2005). Prediction of assistive technology use: The importance of personal and psychosocial factors. *Disability & Rehabilitation, 27*(21), 1321–1331. Retrieved through EBSCO host June 15, 2007.

Snowman, J., & Biehler, R. (2006). *Psychology of applied teaching* (11th ed.). Boston: Houghton Mifflin Company.

Spinal Cord Injury Information Network (2006). *Spinal cord injury: Facts and figures at a glance.* Retrieved February 11, 2007, from http://www.spinalcord.uab.edu/show.asp?durki-21446

Stephenson, P. L. (2006). Before teaching begins: Managing patient anxiety prior to providing education. *Clinical Journal of Oncology Nursing, 10*(2), 241–245.

Stock, S. (2002, January 21). When science isn't golden. *Advance for Nurses, 28*–29.

Strauss, A. L., Corbin, J., Fagerhaugh, S., et al. (1984). *Chronic illness and quality of life* (2nd ed.). St. Louis, MO: Mosby.

Strong, M. (1996). *Language learning and deafness.* New York: Cambridge University Press.

U.S. Census Bureau. (2004). Resilient population by sex and age: 2005–2050. *Statistical abstract of the United States.*

U.S. Department of Health and Human Services. (2000). *Healthy People 2010: Understanding and Improving Health* (2nd ed.). Washington, DC: U.S. Government Printing Office.

Vance, J. L. (1992). Learning readiness in rehabilitation patients. *Rehabilitation Nursing, 17*(3), 148–149.

Vander Zanden, J. W., Crandell, T. L., & Crandell, C. H. (2007). *Human development* (8th ed.). Boston: McGraw-Hill.

Vitale, S., Cotch, M. F., & Sperduto, R. D. (2006). Prevalence of visual impairment in the United States. *JAMA, 295*(18), 2158–2163.

Webb, M., Tittle, M., & VanCott, M. (2000). Increasing students sensitivity to families of children with disabilities. *Nurse Educator, 25*(1), 43–47.

Woodward, J. C. (1972). Implications for sociolinguistic research among the deaf. *Sign Language Studies, 1,* 1–7.

Yorkston, K. M., Spencer, K. A., Duffy, J. R., Beukelman, D. R., Golper, L. A., Miller, R. M., et al. (2001). Evidence-based practice guidelines for dysarthria: Management of velopharyngeal function. *Journal of Medical Speech-Language Pathology, 9*(4), 257–273.

Ysseldyke, J., & Allgozzine, B. (1983). LD or not LD: That's not the question! *Journal of Learning Disabilities, 16*(1), 29–31.

Zejdlik, C. D. (1992). *Management of spinal cord injury* (2nd ed.). Boston: Jones and Bartlett.

Part Three

Techniques and Strategies for Teaching and Learning

Chapter 10

Behavioral Objectives

Susan B. Bastable
Julie A. Doody

CHAPTER HIGHLIGHTS

KEY TERMS

- educational objectives
- instructional objectives
- behavioral (learning) objectives
- goal
- objective
- subobjectives
- taxonomy
- cognitive domain
- massed practice
- distributed practice

- affective domain
- psychomotor domain
- transfer of learning
- selective attention
- intrinsic feedback
- augmented feedback
- teaching plan
- learning contract
- learning curve

OBJECTIVES

After completing this chapter, the reader will be able to

1. Identify the differences between goals and objectives.
2. Recognize opposing viewpoints regarding the use of behavioral objectives in education.
3. Demonstrate the ability to write behavioral objectives accurately and concisely using the four components of condition, performance, criterion, and who will do the performing.
4. Cite the most frequent errors made in writing objectives.
5. Distinguish among the three domains of learning.
6. Explain the instructional methods appropriate for teaching in the cognitive, affective, and psychomotor domains.
7. Develop teaching plans that reflect internal consistency between elements.
8. Recognize the role of the nurse educator in formulating objectives for the planning, implementation, and evaluation of teaching and learning.
9. Describe the importance of learning contracts as an alternative approach to structuring a learning experience.
10. Identify the potential application of the learning curve concept to the development of psychomotor skills.

In previous chapters, the characteristics and attributes of the learner with respect to learning needs, readiness to learn, and learning styles have been addressed. Clearly, assessment of the learner is an essential first step in the teaching–learning process. Assessment determines what the learner needs to know, when and under what conditions the learner is most receptive to learning, and how the learner actually learns best.

Before a decision can be made about selecting the content to be taught or choosing the instructional methods and materials to be used to change learner behavior, the educator must first decide what the learner is expected to accomplish. Client needs are determined by identifying the gaps in the learner's knowledge, attitudes, or skills. Identification of needs is a prerequisite to formulating behavioral objectives that serve to guide subsequent planning, implementation, and evaluation of teaching and learning.

Historically, noted educators and education psychologists in the 20th century have developed approaches to writing and classifying behavioral objectives that offer teachers assistance in organizing instructional content for learners functioning at various levels of ability. Mager (1997) has been the primary educator credited with developing a system for writing behavioral objectives that serves to help teachers make appropriate instructional decisions as well as to assist learners in understanding what they need and are expected to know. The underlying principle has been, if one does not know where he or she is going, how will the person know when he or she has arrived?

In addition, the taxonomic system devised by Bloom, Englehart, Furst, Hill, and Krathwohl (1956) for categorizing learning objectives according to a hierarchy of behaviors has been the cornerstone of teaching for almost a half century. This concept of taxonomy, that is, the ordering of these behaviors according to their type and complexity, pertains to the nature of the knowledge to be learned, the behaviors most relevant and attainable for a particular learner or group of learners, and the sequencing of knowledge and experiences for learning.

The skill in preparing and classifying behavioral objectives is a necessary function of the educator's role, whether teaching patients and their families in healthcare settings, teaching staff nurses in in-service and continuing education programs, or teaching nursing students in academic institutions. The importance of understanding the systems of writing and categorizing behavioral objectives for the purpose of specifying learner outcomes is imperative if data yielded from educational efforts are to be consistent and measurable. Additionally, the knowledge and use of these techniques are becoming essential because of the need to quantify and justify the costs of teaching others in an environment characterized by ever-increasing cost-containment pressures.

This chapter examines the importance of behavioral objectives for effective teaching; describes how to write clear and precise behavioral objectives; explores the levels of achievement in the taxonomic hierarchy of cognitive, affective, and psychomotor domains; and outlines the development of teaching plans and learning contracts. All of these elements provide a framework for the successful instruction of the learner.

Types of Objectives

It is important to clarify the meaning of the terms *educational objectives*, *instructional objectives*, and *behavioral* or *learning objectives*. Although often used synonymously, these terms can be distinguished from one another. Educational objectives are used to identify the intended outcomes of the education process, whether in reference to an aspect of a program or a total program of study, that guide the design of curriculum units. Instructional objectives describe the teaching activities and resources used to facilitate effective learning (Morrison, Ross, & Kemp, 2004). Behavioral or learning objectives, on the other hand, make use of the modifiers *behavioral* or *learning* to denote that they are action oriented rather than content oriented, learner centered rather than teacher centered, and outcome focused rather than process focused. Behavioral objectives describe precisely what the learner will be able to do following a learning situation.

Characteristics of Goals and Objectives

The terms *goal* and *objective* are often used interchangeably—albeit incorrectly. A real difference exists between the two terms. This distinction must be clearly understood by nurse educators. Time span and specificity are the two factors that differentiate goals from objectives, and vice versa (Haggard, 1989).

A *goal* is the final outcome of what is achieved at the end of the teaching–learning process. A goal is a statement that describes the ideal or ultimate state of being at some future point in time. Goals are global and broad in nature; they serve as long-term targets for both the learner and the teacher. Goals are the desired outcomes of learning that are realistically achievable in weeks or months. They are considered multidimensional in that a number of objectives are subsumed under or incorporated into an overall goal.

An *objective*, in contrast, is a specific, single, unidimensional behavior. As stated by Anderson et al., "When we teach, we want our students to learn. What we want them to learn as a result of our teaching are our objectives" (2001, p. 3). Objectives are short term in nature and should be achievable at the conclusion of one teaching session or within a matter of a few days following a series of teaching sessions. According to Mager (1997), an objective describes a performance that learners should be able to exhibit before they are considered competent. A behavioral objective is the intended result of instruction, not the process or means of instruction itself. Objectives are statements of specific or short-term behaviors that lead step by step to the more general, overall long-term goal.

Subobjectives also may be written and reflect aspects of a main objective. They too, are specific statements of short-term behaviors that lead to the achievement of the primary objective. Objectives and subobjectives specify what the learner will be able to do as a result of being exposed to one or more learning experiences.

Objectives must be achieved before the goal can be reached. They must be observable and measurable to be able to determine whether they have been met by the learner. Objectives can be thought of as advance organizers, statements that inform the learner of what is expected from a cognitive, affective, or psychomotor perspective to meet the intended outcome (Babcock & Miller, 1994). Objectives are derived from a goal and must be consistent with and related to

that goal. As an analogy, a goal can be thought of as an entire pie, the objectives as individual portions of the pie that make up the goal, and the subobjectives as bite-sized pieces of a single portion of the pie.

Together, objectives and goals form a map that provides directions (objectives) as to how to arrive at a particular destination (goal). For example, a goal might be that a diabetic patient will learn to manage diabetes. To accomplish this goal, which has been agreed on by both the nurse and the patient, specific objectives must be outlined to address changes in behavior such as the need to learn diet therapy, insulin administration, exercise regimens, stress management, and glucose monitoring. The objectives to accomplish the goal become the blueprint for attaining the desired outcomes of learning.

The successful achievement of predetermined objectives is, in part, the result of appropriate instruction. Certainly, many other factors, such as learner motivation and ability to perform, are also key factors to the successful demonstration of specific behaviors before overall competence by the learner can be declared.

If the teaching–learning process is to be successful, the setting of goals and objectives must be a mutual decision on the part of both the teacher and the learner. Both parties must participate in the decision-making process and buy into the immediate objectives and ultimate goals. Involving the learner right from the start in creating goals and objectives is absolutely crucial. Otherwise, time and effort on the part of the educator and the learner may be wasted, because the learner may choose to reject the content if it is deemed from his or her perspective to be unimportant, irrelevant, impractical, or something already known.

Goal and objective setting for any educational experience should be as much a responsibility of the learner as it is of the teacher. Blending what the learner wants to learn with what the teacher has determined that the learner needs to know into a common set of objectives and goals provides for an educational experience that is mutually accountable, respectful, developmental, and fulfilling (Reilly & Oermann, 1990).

Objectives and goals must also be clearly written, realistic, and learner centered. If they do not precisely state what the learner is expected to do in the short and long term, respectively, then there are no clear guideposts to follow nor an obvious end result for which to strive in the learning process. Likewise, if goals and objectives are unrealistic in that they are too difficult to achieve, the learner will become easily discouraged, which dampens motivation and interferes with the ability to comply. For instance, a goal that a patient will maintain a *salt-free* diet is likely to be impossible to accomplish or to adhere to over an extended period of time. Establishing a goal of maintaining a *low-salt* diet, with the objectives of learning to avoid eating and preparing high-sodium foods, is a much more realistic and achievable expectation of the learner.

Also, goals and objectives must be directed to what the learner is expected to be able to do, not what the teacher is expected to teach. Educators must be sure not only that their teaching remains objectives oriented but also that the objectives are learner centered. This approach keeps educators targeted on results, not on the act of teaching. Educators must remember, as Anderson et al. (2001) stated, not all learners will take away the same thing from the same instruction, unless objectives are focused and precisely expressive.

The Debate About Using Behavioral Objectives

Educators have made strong arguments for and against the use of behavioral objectives for teaching and learning. Certainly behavioral objectives are not a panacea for all the problems encountered in the planning, implementation, and evaluation of education (Reilly & Oermann, 1990). The following list, outlined by Arends (1994), Reilly and Oermann (1990); Haggard (1989); Durbach, Goodall, and Wilkinson (1987); and Morrison, Ross, and Kemp (2004), presents some common arguments by educators against using behavioral objectives:

- The understanding by experienced educators of learners' needs is so sophisticated that the exercise of writing behavioral objectives is superfluous.
- The practice of writing specific behavioral objectives leads to reductionism, a format that reduces behavioral processes into equivalents that do not reflect the sum total of the parts.
- Objectives writing is a time-consuming task, requiring more effort for development than is warranted by their effect on an instructional program. That is, the cost benefit does not justify the amount of time required to formulate them.
- The preparation of objectives is merely a pedagogic exercise often expressing the teacher's expectations of the outcome of teaching and precluding the opportunity for learners to seek their own objectives.
- Predetermined objectives, with their emphasis on precise and observable learner behaviors, force teachers and

learners to attend only to specific areas, which stifle creativity and interfere with the freedom to learn and to teach.

- The writing of specific objectives is incompatible with the complex field of study such as nursing because an infinite number of objectives are possible for almost any subject or topic.
- Behavioral objectives are unable to capture the more intricate cognitive processes that are not readily observable and measurable.

The rationale for using behavioral objectives, however, far outweighs the arguments against their use. The following considerations justify the need for writing behavioral objectives (Ferguson, 1998; Morrison et al., 2004). Careful construction of objectives

- Helps to keep educators' thinking on target and learner centered.
- Communicates to others, both learners and healthcare team members alike, what is planned for teaching and learning.
- Helps learners understand what is expected of them so they can keep track of their progress.
- Forces the educator to organize educational materials so as not to get lost in content and forget the learner's role in the process.
- Encourages educators to question their own motives—to think deliberately about why they are doing things and analyze what positive results will be attained from accomplishing specific objectives.
- Tailors teaching to the learner's particular circumstances and needs.
- Creates guideposts for teacher evaluation and documentation of success or failure.

- Focuses attention not on what is taught but on what the learner will come away with once the teaching–learning process is completed.
- Orients both teacher and learner to the specific end result of instruction.
- Makes it easier for the learner to visualize performing the required actions.

Robert Mager (1997), a recognized authority on preparing behavioral objectives, points out three other major advantages to writing explicit objective statements:

1. They provide a sound basis for the selection or design of instructional content, methods, and materials.
2. They provide learners with the means to organize their efforts and activities toward accomplishing the intent of instruction.
3. They allow for a determination as to whether an objective has, in fact, been accomplished.

As Mager (1997) asks, "If you don't know where you're going, how will you know which road to take to get there" (p. 14)? That is, before the educator prepares instruction, before materials and teaching methods are selected, before the means to evaluate learning is chosen, it is important to clearly and concisely state just what the intended results of instruction are to be. To paraphrase Mager's thinking, mechanics do not select repair tools until they know what has to be fixed; surgeons do not choose instruments until they know what operation is to be performed; and builders do not buy construction materials before drafting a blueprint.

Haggard (1989) summarized the following questions that arise if objectives are not always written:

- How will anyone else know what objectives have been set?
- How will the educator evaluate and document success or failure?
- How will learners keep track of their progress?

The writing of objectives is not merely a mechanical task but a synthesizing process. The process of developing behavioral objectives not only helps educators explore their own knowledge, values, and beliefs about the entire spectrum of teaching and learning, but it also encourages them to examine the experiences, values, motivations, and knowledge of the learner. The time and effort expended in writing objectives represent a thoughtful deliberation about the knowledge, attitude, and skill requirements needed by the learner in meeting the desired level of competency.

The educator and learner should work together to compose objectives and goals that focus on what is to be accomplished in the short and long run. This process provides direction that helps the educator and learner identify

- The time that will be needed for teaching and learning.
- The clues as to how the learner best acquires information.
- The teaching methods that will work most effectively.
- The best ways to evaluate the learner's progress.

In addition, the process of stating well-written objectives encourages the educator to seriously contemplate what is worth teaching and what is worth spending time to accomplish. Also, the process can serve to highlight the value of an existing instructional program and provide the basis for improving a current teaching plan. Thus, the mutual setting of objectives and goals is considered by many educators to be the initial, most important consideration in the education process (Haggard, 1989; Mager, 1997).

Writing Behavioral Objectives

Well-written behavioral objectives give learners very clear statements about what is expected of them and assist teachers in being able to measure learner progress toward achieving outcomes of learning. Over the past 3 decades, Robert Mager's (1997) approach to writing behavioral objectives has been widely accepted among educators. His message to educators is that for objectives to be meaningful, they must precisely, clearly, and very specifically communicate the teacher's instructional intent (Arends, 1994).

According to Mager (1997), the format for writing concise and useful behavioral objectives includes the following three important characteristics:

1. *Performance:* Describes what the learner is expected to be able to do or perform to demonstrate the kinds of behaviors the teacher will accept as evidence that objectives have been achieved. Activities performed by the learner may be visible, such as writing or listing, or invisible, such as identifying or recalling.
2. *Condition:* Describes the testing situation, resources, assistance, or constraints under which the behavior will be observed or completed or the performance is expected to occur.
3. *Criterion:* Describes how well, with what accuracy, or within what time frame the learner must be able to perform for the

behavior to be considered acceptable; the standard, quality level, or amount of performance defined as satisfactorily demonstrating mastery. It is the level of competence that a learner must achieve.

The aforementioned three characteristics translate into the following questions: (1) What should the learner be able to do? (2) Under what conditions should the learner be able to do it? (3) How well must the learner be able to do it?

A fourth component must also be included; it should describe the *who* to ensure that the behavioral objective is learner centered. For education in health care, the learner may be the patient, family members or significant others of the patient, staff nurses, or student nurses.

Thus, behavioral objectives are statements that communicate under particular conditions *who* will *do what* under *what conditions* and *how well* (Cummings, 1994). The more complete the statements of objectives, the better the objectives will serve to communicate exactly what is expected of the learner and what is the intent of instruction. To link the behavioral objectives together, the following four steps are recommended:

1. Identify the testing situation (*condition*).
2. Identify who will perform (*the learner*).
3. State what the learner will demonstrate (*performance*).
4. State how well the learner will perform (*criterion*).

For example: "Following a 20-minute teaching session on hypoglycemia (*condition*), Mrs. Smith (*the learner*) will be able to identify (*performance*) three out of four major symptoms of low blood sugar (*criterion*)."

An easy way to remember the four elements that should be in a behavioral objective is to follow the ABCD rule proposed by Heinich, Molenda, Russell, and Smaldino (2001):

A—audience (who)
B—behavior (what)
C—condition (under what circumstance)
D—degree (how much; to what extent)

Table 10–1 outlines the four-part method of objective writing. **Table 10–2** gives samples of well-written and poorly written objectives.

It is important to note, however, that there are really two accepted approaches to writing behavioral objectives, depending on the audience of learners. Reilly and Oermann (1990) distinguish between what are known as specific behavioral objectives and general behavioral objectives. With both types of objectives, the learners and the behaviors to be learned must be clearly stated. The difference between the two types of objectives lies in the desirability of including the conditions of learning and the criteria for the level of performance expected.

Specific behavioral objectives are close-ended statements that incorporate the condition and criterion for learning, which make them more prescriptive and predictive for the measurement of outcomes. This relatively linear format for writing specific behavioral objectives is an asset to help focus the learning process on a step-by-step basis, especially when a low-level skill is the intended outcome. For example, when teaching a patient to test blood glucose levels or teaching a nurse a new procedural protocol for a dressing change, the writing of specific behavioral objectives is preferred.

General behavioral objectives, which do not include the condition or criterion for learning, are open-ended statements that lend themselves to be used in evaluating higher cognitive skills. This format is more appropriate for stating outcomes

Table 10–1 THE FOUR-PART METHOD OF OBJECTIVE WRITING

Condition (Testing Situation)	Who (Identify Learner)	Performance (Learner Behavior)	Criterion (Quality or Quantity of Mastery)
Without using a calculator	the student	will solve	5 out of 6 math problems
Using a model	the staff nurse	will demonstrate	the correct procedure for changing sterile dressings
Following group discussion	the patient	will list	at least two reasons for losing weight
After watching a video	the caregiver	will select	high-protein foods with 100% accuracy

of an academic program, when knowledge of the learner is not expected to be just an accumulation of designated parts, but rather an integration and synthesis of broader concepts and theories over time. As such, the writing of general behavioral objectives is more compatible when teaching nurses in a staff development program or nursing students in a course within a professional program of study. It allows teachers to be more creative in teaching and accommodates acceptable

Table 10–2 SAMPLES OF WRITTEN OBJECTIVES

WELL-WRITTEN OBJECTIVES

After watching a demonstration on suctioning, the staff member will be able to correctly suction a tracheostomy tube using aseptic technique.

Following a class on hypertension, the patient will be able to state three out of four causes of high blood pressure.

On completing the reading materials provided on the care of a newborn, the mother will be able to express any concerns she has about caring for her baby after discharge.

POORLY WRITTEN OBJECTIVES

The patient will be able to prepare a menu using low-salt foods (*condition and criterion missing*).

Given a list of exercises to relieve low back pain, the patient will understand how to control low back pain (*performance not stated in measurable terms, criterion missing*).

The nurse will demonstrate crutch walking postoperatively to the patient (*teacher-centered*).

variations in the learner that foster the creative expression of ideas and knowledge.

It is important to recognize the existence of and distinction between these two types of behavioral objectives. In this chapter, however, the focus will be on writing specific behavioral objectives appropriate for the learning of particular skill sets by patients and staff.

Performance Words with Many or Few Interpretations

When writing behavioral objectives using the format suggested by Mager (1997), the recommendation is to use precise action words (verbs as labels, known as verbals) that are open to few interpretations when describing learner performance.

An objective is considered useful only when it clearly states what a learner must demonstrate for mastery in a knowledge, attitude, or skill area. A performance verb (verbal) describes what the learner is expected to do. A performance may be overt, visible, or audible—for example, the learner is able to *list*, to *write*, to *state*, or to *walk*. These performances are directly observable. A performance also may be invisible—for example, the learner is able to *identify*, to *solve*, to *recall*, or to *recognize*. Any performance, visible/audible or invisible, described by a doing word is measurable.

If a word is used to describe something a learner can *be*, then it is not a *doing* word but rather a *being* word. Examples of being words, known also as abstractions, are to *understand*, to *know*, to *enjoy*, or to *appreciate* (Mager, 1997). Understanding, knowing, enjoying, and appreciating are considered abstract states of being and cannot be directly measured but merely inferred from performances. Therefore, verbs

that signify an internal state of thinking, feeling, or believing should be avoided because they are difficult to measure or observe.

It is impossible to identify all behavioral terms that may be used in objective writing. The important thing to remember in selecting verbs (verbals) to describe performance is that they must be specific, observable or measurable, and action oriented. As stated by Anderson et al. (2001), if the teacher is able to describe the behavior to be attained, it will be easily recognized when the learning has occurred. The lists in **Table 10–3** give examples of verbals that, on the one hand, are too broad, ambiguous, and imprecise to evaluate, and, on the other hand, are specific and relatively easy to measure (Gronlund, 1985 and 2004).

Common Mistakes When Writing Objectives

In formulating behavioral objectives, there are a number of common pitfalls that can easily be made by the novice as well as by the seasoned educator. The most frequent errors in writing objectives are:

- To describe what the instructor rather than the learner is expected to do.
- To include more than one expected behavior in a single objective (avoid using the compound word *and* to connect two verbs—e.g., the learner will select *and* prepare).
- To forget to include all four components of condition, performance, criterion, and who will do the performing.
- To use terms for performance that are subject to many interpretations, not action oriented, and difficult to measure.

Table 10–3 VERBALS WITH MANY OR FEW INTERPRETATIONS

Terms with Many Interpretations (Not Recommended)	Terms with Few Interpretations (Recommended)	
to know	to apply	to explain
to understand	to choose	to identify
to appreciate	to classify	to list
to realize	to compare	to order
to be familiar with	to contrast	to predict
to enjoy	to construct	to recall
to value	to define	to recognize
to be interested in	to describe	to select
to feel	to demonstrate	to state
to think	to differentiate	to verbalize
to learn	to distinguish	to write

Source: Adapted from Gronlund, N. E. (1985). *Stating objectives for classroom instruction* (3rd ed.). New York: Macmillan; and Gronlund, N. E. (2004). *Writing instructional objectives for teaching and assessment* (7th ed.). Upper Saddle River, NJ: Pearson Merrill, Prentice-Hall.

- To write an objective that is unattainable given the ability level of the learner.
- To write objectives that do not relate to the stated goal.
- To clutter an objective by including unnecessary information.
- To be too general so as not to clearly specify the expected behavior to be achieved.

In summary, if you use the SMART rule, it is easy to create effective objectives for different audiences in diverse settings. This objective-setting process is shown in **Table 10–4**.

Taxonomy of Objectives According to Learning Domains

A *taxonomy* is a mechanism used to categorize things according to how they are related to one another. "A taxonomy is a special kind of framework in which categories lie along a continuum" (Anderson et al., 2001, p. 4). For example, biologists use taxonomies to classify plants and animals based on their natural characteristics.

In the late 1940s, psychologists and educators became concerned about the need to develop

Table 10–4 Writing SMART Objectives	
Specific	Be specific about what is to be achieved (i.e., use strong action verbs, be concrete).
Measurable	Quantify or qualify objectives by including numeric, cost, or percentage amounts or the degree/level of mastery expected.
Achievable	Are your objectives attainable?
Realistic	Are resources available to achieve objectives (i.e., personnel, facilities, equipment)?
Timely	When will the objectives be achieved (i.e., within a week, a month, by the day of patient discharge, before a new staff member completes orientation)?

Source: Adapted from Glenn M. Parker Associates, Inc. (2000). *Team workout.* Amherst, MA: HRD Products.

a system for defining and ordering levels of behavior according to their type and complexity (Reilly & Oermann, 1990). Bloom et al. (1956) and Krathwohl, Bloom, and Masia (1964) developed a very useful taxonomy, known as the *taxonomy of educational objectives*, as a tool for systematically and logically classifying behavioral objectives. This taxonomy, which became widely accepted as a standard aid for planning as well as evaluating learning, is divided into three broad categories or domains—cognitive, affective, and psychomotor.

Inherent in the concept of taxonomy is the notion that although these three domains of cognitive, affective, and psychomotor learning are described as existing as separate entities, they are, in fact, interdependent and can be experienced simultaneously. Humans do not possess thoughts, feelings, and actions in isolation of one another and typically do not compartmentalize learning. For example, the affective domain influences the cognitive domain and vice versa; the processes of thinking and feeling influence psychomotor performance and vice versa (Menix, 1996).

In the taxonomy of educational objectives, the objectives in each domain are ordered in a taxonomic form of hierarchy. Behavioral objectives are classified into low, medium, and high levels with simple behaviors listed first (designated by numbers 1.0 or 2.0), followed by behaviors of moderate difficulty (designated by numbers 3.0 and 4.0), and the more complex behaviors listed last (designated by numbers 5.0 or 6.0). Subobjectives are listed under the main objective and are designated by numbers that range between whole numbers (e.g., 2.1, 2.2, 2.3, etc.). Inherent in the concept of hierarchy is the serial structure that learners must successfully achieve behaviors at the lower levels of the domains before they are able to adequately learn behaviors at the higher levels of the domains.

The Cognitive Domain

The *cognitive domain* is known as the thinking domain. Learning in this domain involves the acquisition of information and addresses the development of the learner's intellectual abilities, mental capacities, understanding, and thinking processes (Eggen & Kauchak, 2001).

Objectives in this domain are divided into six levels, each specifying cognitive processes ranging from the simple (knowledge) to the more complex (evaluation), as listed and described by Bloom et al. (1956) in **Table 10–5**.

EXAMPLES OF BEHAVIORAL OBJECTIVES IN THE COGNITIVE DOMAIN

Analysis level: After reading handouts provided by the nurse educator, the family member will calculate the correct number of total grams of protein included on average per day in the family diet.

Synthesis level: Given a sample list of foods, the patient will devise a menu to include foods from the four food groups (dairy, meat, vegetables and fruits, and grains) in the recommended amounts for daily intake.

Table 10–6 lists verbs commonly used in writing cognitive-level behavioral objectives.

TEACHING IN THE COGNITIVE DOMAIN

A variety of teaching methods and tools exist for the primary purpose of developing cognitive abilities. The methods most often used to stimulate learning in the cognitive domain include lecture, one-to-one instruction, and self-instruction activities such as computer-assisted instruction (see Chapter 11). Verbal, written, and visual tools are

---

Table 10–5 LEVELS OF COGNITIVE BEHAVIOR

Knowledge (1.00–1.99): Ability of the learner to memorize, recall, define, recognize, or identify specific information, such as facts, rules, principles, conditions, and terms, presented during instruction.

Comprehension (2.00–2.99): Ability of the learner to demonstrate an understanding or appreciation of what is being communicated by translating it into a different form or recognizing it in a translated form, such as grasping an idea by defining it or summarizing it in his or her own words (knowledge is a prerequisite behavior).

Application (3.00–3.99): Ability of the learner to use ideas, principles, abstractions, or theories in particular and concrete situations, such as figuring, writing, reading, or handling equipment (knowledge and comprehension are prerequisite behaviors).

Analysis (4.00–4.99): Ability of the learner to recognize and structure information by breaking it down into its constituent parts and specifying the relationship between parts (knowledge, comprehension, and application are prerequisite behaviors).

Synthesis (5.00–5.99): Ability of the learner to put together parts and elements into a unified whole by creating a unique product that is written, oral, pictorial, and so on (knowledge, comprehension, application, and analysis are prerequisite behaviors).

Evaluation (6.00–6.99): Ability of the learner to judge the value of something, such as an essay, design, or action, by applying appropriate standards or criteria (knowledge, comprehension, application, analysis, and synthesis are prerequisite behaviors).

Table 10–6 COMMONLY USED VERBS ACCORDING TO DOMAIN CLASSIFICATION

COGNITIVE DOMAIN

Knowledge: choose, circle, define, identify, label, list, match, name, outline, recall, report, select, state

Comprehension: describe, discuss, distinguish, estimate, explain, generalize, give example, locate, recognize, summarize

Application: apply, demonstrate, illustrate, implement, interpret, modify, order, revise, solve, use

Analysis: analyze, arrange, calculate, classify, compare, conclude, contrast, determine, differentiate, discriminate

Synthesis: categorize, combine, compile, correlate, design, devise, generate, integrate, reorganize, revise, summarize

Evaluation: appraise, assess, conclude, criticize, debate, defend, judge, justify

AFFECTIVE DOMAIN

Receiving: accept, admit, ask, attend, focus, listen, observe, pay attention

Responding: agree, answer, conform, discuss, express, participate, recall, relate, report, state willingness, try, verbalize

Valuing: assert, assist, attempt, choose, complete, disagree, follow, help, initiate, join, propose, volunteer

Organization: adhere, alter, arrange, combine, defend, explain, express, generalize, integrate, resolve

Characterization: assert, commit, discriminate, display, influence, propose, qualify, solve, verify

PSYCHOMOTOR DOMAIN

Perception: attend, choose, describe, detect, differentiate, distinguish, identify, isolate, perceive, relate, select, separate

Set: attempt, begin, develop, display, position, prepare, proceed, reach, respond, show, start, try

Guided response mechanism and complex overt response: align, arrange, assemble, attach, build, change, choose, clean, compile, complete, construct, demonstrate, discriminate, dismantle, dissect, examine, find, grasp, hold, insert, lift, locate, maintain, manipulate, measure, mix, open, operate, organize, perform, pour, practice, reassemble, remove, repair, replace, separate, shake, suction, turn, transfer, walk, wash, wipe

Adaptation: adapt, alter, change, convert, correct, rearrange, reorganize, replace, revise, shift, substitute, switch

Origination: arrange, combine, compose, construct, create, design, exchange, reformulate

---

Source: Adapted from Gronlund, N. E. (1985). *Stating objectives for classroom instruction* (3rd ed.). New York: Macmillan; and Gronlund, N. E. (2004). *Writing instructional objectives for teaching and assessment* (7th ed.). Upper Saddle River, NJ: Pearson Merrill, Prentice-Hall.

all particularly successful in supplementing the teaching methods (see Chapter 12) to help learners master cognitive content. For example, the effectiveness of using interactive video as an instructional tool to increase knowledge of core concepts in mental health by nursing home staff, as reported by Rosen, Mulsant, Kollar, Kastango, Mazumdar, and Fox (2002) and Green et al. (2003), found streaming video to be a useful instructional tool to improve the efficiency in cognitive learning by nursing students.

Cognitive skills can be gained by exposure to all types of educational experiences, including the instructional methods used primarily for affective and psychomotor learning. Cognitive knowledge, however, is an essential prerequisite for the learner to engage in other educational activities such as group discussion or role playing. Otherwise, what results is pooled ignorance. For example, clients cannot adequately learn through group discussion if they do not possess an accurate and at least basic knowledge level of the subject at hand to draw on for purposes of discourse. Participating in a group discussion experience is not the same thing as engaging in a brainstorming session. Brainstorming does not necessarily require prior knowledge of information about issues or problems to be explored.

Cognitive domain learning is the traditional focus of most teaching. In education of patients, nursing staff, and students, emphasis remains on the sharing of facts, theories, concepts, and the like. Cognitive processing—that is, the means through which knowledge is acquired—often takes precedence over psychomotor skill development and the learning of affective behaviors (Ellis, 1993). Perhaps this emphasis has occurred because educators typically feel more confident and more skilled in being the giver of information rather than being the facilitator and coordi-

nator of learning. Lecture and one-to-one instruction are the most often used methods of teaching. Both of these instructional approaches, when taught in a typical fashion, are directed almost exclusively at the cognitive domain.

With respect to cognitive learning, how much time for practice is necessary to influence the short-term and long-term retention of factual information? Cognitive scientists have been exploring the allocation of practice time to the learning of new material. Generally, research findings indicate that learning distributed over several sessions leads to better memory than information learned in a single session.

This phenomenon has been described by Willingham (2002) as the "spacing effect." That is, learning information all at once on one day, which is known as *massed practice,* is much less effective for remembering facts than learning information over successive periods of time, which is known as *distributed practice.* Massed practice, similar to what is commonly identified as cramming, might allow the recall of information for a short time, but evidence strongly supports that distributed practice is very important in forging memories that last for years.

The effect of spreading out learning over time is very clear. The average person exposed to distributed practice remembers 67% better than people getting massed training. That is, spacing the time allocated for learning significantly increases memory. The longer the delays between practice sessions, the greater and more permanent is the learning. In fact, if learning is distributed over time, not only does this spacing effect hold, but it becomes even more robust.

This evidence, when applied to the education of patients, staff nurses, or student nurses, strongly suggests the need to allocate time for the acquisition of knowledge. Such scientific findings explain, for example, why teaching a patient on the day of discharge from the hospital is ineffective.

The Affective Domain

The *affective domain* is known as the feeling domain. Learning in this domain involves an increasing internalization or commitment to feelings expressed as emotions, interests, beliefs, attitudes, values, and appreciations. Whereas the cognitive domain is ordered in terms of complexity of behaviors, the affective domain is divided into categories that specify the degree of a person's depth of emotional responses to tasks. The affective domain includes emotional and social development goals. As stated by Eggen and Kauchak (2001), educators use the affective domain to help learners realize their own attitudes and values.

Although nurse educators recognize the need for individuals to learn in the affective domain, constructs such as attitudes, beliefs, and values cannot be directly observed but can only be inferred from words and actions (Maier-Lorentz, 1999). Educators tend to be less confident and more challenged in writing behavioral objectives for the affective domain because it is difficult to develop easily measurable objectives and evaluation of learning outcomes is based on inferences of someone's observed behavior (Morrison et al., 2004).

Competencies in the affective domain relate to the development of a value system. Behavior is guided by notions held by an individual and society as to what is considered good and right. Thus affective competencies involve moral reasoning and ethical decision making. For staff nurses, competency in the affective domain is required to intervene with clients in a humanistic and caring manner.

Reilly and Oermann (1990) differentiate between the terms *beliefs*, *attitudes*, and *values*. *Beliefs* are what an individual perceives as reality; *attitudes* represent feelings about an object, person, or event; and *values* are operational beliefs that guide actions and ways of living. Maier-Lorentz (1999), acknowledging the difficulty in writing and measuring specific objectives in the affective domain, presents a rating scale to evaluate learning outcomes for a gerontological nursing in-service program that measures beliefs, attitudes, and values of staff using a Likert scale.

Objectives in the affective domain are divided into five categories, each specifying the associated level of affective responses as listed and described by Krathwohl et al. (1964), in **Table 10–7**.

EXAMPLES OF BEHAVIORAL OBJECTIVES IN THE AFFECTIVE DOMAIN

Receiving level: During a group discussion session, the patient will admit to any fears he may have about needing to undergo a repeat angioplasty.

Responding level: At the end of one-to-one instruction, the child will verbalize feelings of confidence in managing her asthma using the peak flow tracking chart.

Characterization level: Following a series of in-service education sessions, the staff nurse will display consistent interest in maintaining strict hand-washing technique to control the spread of nosocomial infections to patients in the hospital.

Table 10–6 lists verbs commonly used in writing affective-level behavioral objectives.

TEACHING IN THE AFFECTIVE DOMAIN

A variety of teaching methods have been found to be powerful and reliable in helping the learner

---

Table 10–7 LEVELS OF AFFECTIVE BEHAVIOR

Receiving (1.00–1.99): Ability of the learner to show awareness of an idea or fact or a consciousness of a situation or event in the environment. This level represents a willingness to selectively attend to or focus on data or to receive a stimulus.

Responding (2.00–2.99): Ability of the learner to respond to an experience, at first obediently and later willingly and with satisfaction. This level indicates a movement beyond denial and toward voluntary acceptance, which can lead to feelings of pleasure or enjoyment as a result of some new experience (receiving is a prerequisite behavior).

Valuing (3.00–3.99): Ability of the learner to regard or accept the worth of a theory, idea, or event, demonstrating sufficient commitment or preference to be identified with some experience seen as having value. At this level, there is a definite willingness and desire to act to further that value (receiving and responding are prerequisite behaviors).

Organization (4.00–4.99): Ability of the learner to organize, classify, and prioritize values by integrating a new value into a general set of values, to determine interrelationships of values, and to harmoniously establish some values as dominant and pervasive (receiving, responding, and valuing are prerequisite behaviors).

Characterization (5.00–5.99): Ability of the learner to integrate values into a total philosophy or worldview, showing firm commitment and consistency of responses to the values by generalizing certain experiences into a value system or attitude cluster (receiving, responding, valuing, and organization are prerequisite behaviors).

Source: Krathwohl, D. R., Bloom, B. J., & Masia, B. B. (1964). *Taxonomy of educational objectives: The classification of educational goals. Handbook II: The affective domain.* New York: David McKay.

---

acquire elements of the affective domain. Role modeling, role playing, simulation gaming, and group discussion sessions are examples of instructional methods that can be used to prepare nursing staff and students as well as patients and their families to incorporate values and to explore attitudes, interests, and feelings in the process of developing affective behaviors.

Nurse educators have been encouraged to attend to the needs of the whole person by recognizing that learning is subjective and values driven (Schoenly, 1994). For practicing nurses, affective learning is especially important because they are constantly faced with ethical issues and value conflicts (Tong, 2007). In addition, our increasingly pluralistic society requires nurses to respect the racial and ethnic diversity in the population groups served by healthcare providers (Reilly & Oermann, 1990). Advancing technology also places nurses in advocacy positions when patients, families, and other healthcare professionals are constantly grappling with treatment decisions. In turn, patients and family members are faced with making moral and ethical choices as well as learning to internalize the value of complying with prescribed treatment regimens and incorporating health promotion and disease prevention practices into their daily lives.

The environment in which teaching and learning take place is important to the successful achievement of affective behavioral outcomes. A trusting relationship and an open, empathetic, accepting attitude by the educator toward clients are necessary to secure client interest and involvement in learning. Staff nurses' beliefs, attitudes, and values significantly influence their affective behavior and, thus, the quality of nursing care they deliver. A nurse's personal value system must coincide with the values of the nursing profession when teaching staff nurses in the affective domain (Maier-Lorentz, 1999). Three American Nurses Association documents, *Code of Ethics for Nurses With Interpretive Statements* (2001), *Standards of Clinical Nursing Practice* (2004), and *Nursing's Social Policy Statement* (2003), provide educators with sources of professional values.

Unfortunately, adequate weight is not usually given to teaching in the affective domain. The educator's focus more often emphasizes cognitive processing and psychomotor functioning with little time set aside for exploration and clarification of learner feelings, emotions, and attitudes (Ellis, 1993; Morrison et al., 2004; Rinne, 1987).

Schoenly (1994) examined affective teaching strategies that can be used to assist learners in acquiring affective domain behaviors. Once appropriate objectives and an accepting climate have been established, the following educational interventions can be selected and implemented:

> *Questioning:* Although the lecture method is usually identified with helping the learner gain cognitive skills, the technique of careful questioning during the lecture process can assist in meeting objectives in the affective domain. Affective questioning increases interest and motivation to learn about feelings, values, beliefs, and attitudes regarding a topic under study. Low-level affective questions are directed at stimulating learner awareness and responsiveness to a topic, midlevel affective questioning assists in determining the strength of a belief or the internalization of a value, and high-level affective questioning probes for information about the depth of integration of a value.

> *Case study:* This method can assist the learner in developing problem-solving and critical-thinking skills through exploration of participant attitudes, beliefs, and values. Using learning groups with the reader assuming the role of a key player in the situation (nurse, family member, patient) rather than as a neutral observer will help in eliciting affective behavioral responses.

> *Role playing:* This method provides an excellent opportunity to practice new behaviors and explore feelings, attitudes, and values; to problem solve; and to resolve personal problems associated with human circumstances. Role playing allows the learner to walk in someone else's shoes, but without the actual risk, thereby gaining empathy for the reality of another's situation. Being an observer during role playing can sensitize the learner to the phenomenon, while active participation in role playing energizes the learner to attend and respond to the phenomenon under consideration.

> *Gaming:* Games that are controlled by the participants and have flexible rules are more appropriate for accomplishing affective behavioral objectives than games that are characterized by structured roles and

have specific rules, which are better for cognitive learning. Gaming promotes active involvement of the learner in goal-directed, but not necessarily competitive, activities. Debriefing following gaming is an important aspect of the technique to provide an opportunity for learners to understand how attitudes, beliefs, and values from the gaming experience can be applied and incorporated into everyday life.

Group discussion: This method provides an opportunity for clarifying personal values as well as exploring social values and moral issues. Value clarification involves identifying and sharing personal values for the purpose of increasing self-awareness and self-discovery. Values inquiry involves investigating the value systems of various ethnic groups. Both approaches provide the chance for in-depth learning of affective behaviors.

The affective domain encompasses three levels that govern attitudes and feelings:

- The intrapersonal level includes personal perceptions of one's own self, such as self-concept, self-awareness, and self-acceptance.
- The interpersonal level includes the perspective of self in relation to other individuals.
- The extrapersonal level involves the perception of others as established groups.

All three levels are important in affective skill development and can be taught through a variety of methods specifically geared to affective-domain learning.

Affective learning is a part of every educational experience, even though the primary focus for learning may be on either the cognitive or the psychomotor domain. Learner feelings or emotions cannot help but be aroused to some extent when exposed to new and different educational experiences (Bucher, 1991). In fact, Morrison et al. (2004) suggest that attitudinal development, such as receptivity, cooperation, and motivation, can even precede successful learning in other domains.

Without a doubt, learning is a multidimensional process that can occur in all three domains simultaneously, formally or informally, and in structured or unstructured settings. Evaluation of learning is just as complex a process. However, evaluation of affective behavior is more difficult than determining cognitive and psychomotor skill acquisition, because affective behaviors are not usually overt and clearly observable. Rather, these behaviors are less tangible and more challenging to measure. Bucher (1991) and Maier-Lorentz (1999) suggest using the Likert scale as a means of discovering learner attitudes relative to particular learning experiences.

The Psychomotor Domain

The *psychomotor domain* is known as the skills domain. Learning in this domain involves acquiring fine and gross motor abilities with increasing complexity of neuromuscular coordination to carry out physical movement such as walking, handwriting, manipulation of equipment, or carrying out a procedure. Psychomotor skill learning, according to Reilly and Oermann (1990), "is a complex process demanding far more knowledge than suggested by the simple mechanistic behavioral approach" (p. 81). However, according to Eggen and Kauchak (2001), "while intellectual abilities enter into each of the psychomotor tasks, the primary focus is on the development of manipulative skills rather than on the growth of intellectual capability" (p. 17).

Thus, for development of psychomotor skills to take place, there must be integration of the other two domains of learning as well. The affective component conveys recognition of the value or worth of the skill being learned; the cognitive component relates to knowing the principles, relationships, and processes in carrying out the overt physical movement. Although all three domains are involved in demonstrating a psychomotor competency, the psychomotor domain can be examined separately and requires different teaching approaches and evaluation strategies (Reilly & Oermann, 1990). In contrast to the cognitive and affective domains, psychomotor skills are easy to identify and measure because they include primarily overt movement-oriented activities that are relatively easy to observe.

Psychomotor learning, including perceptual-motor tasks, can be classified in a variety of ways (Dave, 1970; Harrow, 1972; Moore, 1970; Simpson, 1972). Simpson's system seems to be the most widely recognized as relevant to client teaching. Objectives in this domain, according to Simpson (1972), are divided into seven levels as listed and described in **Table 10–8**.

EXAMPLES OF BEHAVIORAL OBJECTIVES IN THE PSYCHOMOTOR DOMAIN

Guided response level: After watching a 15-minute video on the procedure for self-examination of the breast, the client will perform the exam on a model with 100% accuracy.

Set level: Following demonstration of proper crutch walking, the patient will attempt to crutch walk using the correct three-point gait technique.

Table 10–6 lists verbs commonly used in writing psychomotor-level behavioral objectives.

Another taxonomic system for psychomotor learning proposed by Dave (1970) is also based on behaviors that include muscular action and neuromuscular coordination. Reilly and Oermann (1990) suggest that this taxonomy allows teachers to acknowledge the multivariant characteristics of psychomotor behavior and to focus on the orderly process of neuromuscular development over time of student nurses in academic programs. They support this taxonomy to measure competence in performance within educational programs because it stresses accuracy over speed. Also, Dave's system recognizes that levels of skill attainment can be achieved and refined over a period of months due to the infrequency of students using certain skills in practice. Objectives in this domain, according to Dave (1970), are divided into five levels as seen in **Table 10–9**.

These taxonomic criteria for the development of psychomotor skill competency suggest that accuracy should be stressed before the speed at which a skill is acquired (Reilly & Oermann, 1990). The levels of psychomotor behavior, no matter which taxonomic system is used, require the general and orderly steps of *observing, imitating, practicing*, and *adapting*.

TEACHING OF PSYCHOMOTOR SKILLS

When teaching psychomotor skills, it is important for the educator to remember to keep skill instruction separate from a discussion of principles underlying the skill (cognitive component) or a discussion of how the learner feels about carrying out the skill (affective component). Psychomotor skill development is very egocentric and usually requires a great deal of concentration as the learner works toward mastery of a skill.

It is easy to interfere with psychomotor learning if the teacher asks a knowledge (cognitive) question while the learner is trying to focus on

Table 10–8 LEVELS OF PSYCHOMOTOR BEHAVIOR

Perception (1.00–1.99): Ability of the client to show sensory awareness of objects or cues associated with some task to be performed. Cues relevant to a situation are attended to, symbolically translated, and selected to guide action, gain insight, and receive feedback. This level involves reading directions or observing a process with attention to steps or techniques inherent in a process.

Set (2.00–2.99): Ability of the learner to exhibit readiness to take a particular kind of action, such as following directions, through expressions of willingness, sensory attending, or body language favorable to performing a motor act (perception is a prerequisite behavior).

Guided response (3.00–3.99): Ability of the learner to exert effort via overt actions under the guidance of an instructor to imitate an observed behavior with conscious awareness of effort. Imitating may be performed hesitantly but with compliance to directions and coaching (perception and set are prerequisite behaviors).

Mechanism (4.00–4.99): Ability of the learner to repeatedly perform steps of a desired skill with a certain degree of confidence, indicating mastery to the extent that some or all aspects of the process become habitual. The steps are blended into a meaningful whole and are performed smoothly with little conscious effort (perception, set, and guided response are prerequisite behaviors).

Complex overt response (5.00–5.99): Ability of the learner to automatically perform a complex motor act with independence and a high degree of skill, without hesitation and with minimum expenditure of time and energy; performance of an entire sequence of a complex behavior without the need to attend to details (perception, set, guided response, and mechanism are prerequisite behaviors).

Adaptation (6.00–6.99): Ability of the learner to modify or adapt a motor process to suit the individual or various situations, indicating mastery of highly developed movements that can be suited to a variety of conditions (perception, set, guided response, mechanism, and complex overt response are prerequisite behaviors).

Origination (7.00–7.99): Ability of the learner to create new motor acts, such as novel ways of manipulating objects or materials, as a result of an understanding of a skill and developed ability to perform skills (perception, set, guided response, mechanism, complex overt response, and adaptation are prerequisite behaviors).

Source: Simpson, E. J. (1972). The classification of educational objectives in the psychomotor domain. In M. T. Rainer (Ed.), *Contributions of behavioral science to instructional technology: The psychomotor domain* (3rd ed.). Englewood Cliffs, NJ: Gryphon Press, Prentice-Hall.

the performance (psychomotor response) of a skill. For example, while a staff member is learning to suction a patient, it is not unusual for the teacher to ask, "Can you give me a rationale for why suctioning is important?" or "How often should suctioning be done for this particular patient?" As another example, while the patient is learning to self-administer parenteral medication, the teacher may simultaneously ask the patient to cognitively respond to the question, "What are the actions or side effects of this medication?" or "How do you feel

---

Table 10–9 DAVE'S LEVELS OF PSYCHOMOTOR LEARNING

Imitation (1.0–1.99): At this level, observed actions are followed. The learner's movements are gross, coordination lacks smoothness, and errors occur. Time and speed required to perform are based on learner needs.

Manipulation (2.0–2.99): At this level, written instructions are followed. The learner's coordinated movements are variable, and accuracy is measured based on the skill of using written procedures as a guide. Time and speed required to perform vary.

Precision (3.0–3.99): At this level, a logical sequence of actions is carried out. The learner's movements are coordinated at a higher level, errors are minimal and relatively minor. Time and speed required to perform remain variable.

Articulation (4.0–4.99): At this level, a logical sequence of actions is carried out. The learner's movements are coordinated at a high level, and errors are limited. Time and speed required to perform are within reasonable expectations.

Naturalization (5.0–5.99): At this level, the sequence of actions is automatic. The learner's movements are coordinated at a consistently high level, and errors are almost nonexistent. Time and speed required to perform are within realistic limits, and performance reflects professional competence.

---

about injecting yourself?" These questions demand cognitive and affective responses during psychomotor performance.

Although a teacher frequently intervenes with questions in the midst of a learner's performing, it is definitely an inappropriate teaching technique. What the educator is doing, in fact, is asking the learner to demonstrate at least two different behaviors at the same time. This technique can result in frustration and confusion, and ultimately it may result in failure to achieve any of the behaviors successfully. Questions related to the cognitive or affective domain should only be posed *before* or *after* the learner practices a psychomotor skill (Oermann, 1990).

In psychomotor skill development, the ability to perform a skill is not equivalent to having learned or mastered a skill. Performance is a transitory action, while learning is a more per-

manent behavior that follows from repeated practice and experience (Oermann, 1990). The actual mastery of a skill requires practice to allow the individual to repeat the performance time and again with accuracy, coordination, confidence, and out of habit. Practice does make perfect, and so repetition leads to perfection and reinforcement of the behavior.

The riding of a bicycle is a perfect example of the difference between being able to perform a skill and having mastered or learned that skill. When one first attempts to ride a bicycle, movements tend to be very jerky, and the performance requires a great deal of concentration. Once the skill is learned, bicycle riding becomes a smooth, automatic operation that requires minimal attention to the details of fine and gross motor movements acting in concert to allow the learner to achieve the skill of riding a bicycle.

Some behaviors that are mastered do not require much reinforcement, even over a long period of disuse, whereas other behaviors, once mastered, need to be rehearsed or relearned to perform them at the level of skill once achieved. The amount of practice required to acquire any new skill varies with the individual, depending on many factors. Oermann (1990) and Bell (1991) have addressed some of the more important variables:

Readiness to learn: The motivation to learn affects the degree of perseverance exhibited by the learner in working toward mastery of a skill.

Past experience: If the learner is familiar with equipment or techniques similar to those needed to learn a new skill, then mastery of the new skill may be achieved at a faster rate. The effects of learning one skill on the subsequent performance of another related skill is known as *transfer of learning* (Gomez & Gomez, 1984). For example, if someone already has experience with downhill skiing, then learning cross-country skiing should come more easily and with more confidence because the required coordination and equipment are similar. To use an example in teaching healthcare skills, if a family member already has experience with aseptic technique in changing a dressing, then learning to suction a tracheostomy tube using sterile technique should not require as much time to master.

Health status: Illness state or other physical or emotional impairments in the learner may affect the time it takes to acquire or successfully master a skill.

Environmental stimuli: Depending on the type and level of stimuli as well as the learning style (degree of tolerance for certain stimuli), distractions in the immediate surroundings may interfere with skill acquisition.

Anxiety level: The ability to concentrate can be dramatically affected by how anxious someone feels. Nervousness about performing in front of someone is particularly a key factor in psychomotor skill development. High anxiety levels interfere with coordination, steadiness, fine muscle movements, and concentration levels when performing complex psychomotor skills. It is important to reassure learners that they are not necessarily being tested during psychomotor skill performance. Reassurance and support reduce anxiety levels related to the fear of not meeting expectations of themselves or of the teacher.

Developmental stage: Physical, cognitive, and psychosocial stages of development all influence an individual's ability to master a movement-oriented task. Certainly, a young child's fine and gross motor skills as well as cognitive abilities are at a different level than those of an adult. The older adult, too, will likely exhibit slower cognitive processing and increased response time (needing longer time to perform an activity) than younger clients.

Practice session length: During the beginning stages of learning a motor skill, short and carefully planned practice sessions and frequent rest periods are valuable techniques to help increase the rate and success of learning. These techniques are thought to be effective because they help prevent physical fatigue and restore the learner's attention to the task at hand.

Performing motor skills is not done in a vacuum. The learner is immersed in a particular environmental context full of stimuli. Learners must select those environmental influences that will assist them in achieving the behavior (relevant stimuli) and ignore those that interfere with a specific performance (irrelevant stimuli). This process of recognizing and selecting appropriate and inappropriate stimuli is called *selective attention* (Gomez & Gomez, 1984).

Motor skills should be practiced first in a laboratory setting to provide a safe and nonthreatening environment for the novice learner. Gomez and Gomez (1987) suggest also arranging for practice sessions to be done in the clinical or home setting to expose the learner to actual environmental conditions. This technique is known as open skills performance learned under changing and unstable environments.

In addition, research findings indicate that progress in mastery of a psychomotor skill can be accomplished just as effectively through self-directed study as with teaching in a structured laboratory situation (Love, McAdams, Patton, Rankin, & Roberts, 1989). Yoder (1993) found that computer-assisted interactive video instruction (CAIVI) resulted in a greater amount of transfer of cognitive learning than did linear video for the performance of psychomotor skills in a clinical setting. Yoder reported that the following three types of transfer learning occur: (1) self-transfer (repetition of learning), (2) near transfer (occurs in situations that are very similar), and (3) far transfer (occurs in situations that are very different). Application of psychomotor skills in the clinical arena is a type of far transfer.

More recently, Miracle (1999) summarized research findings on educational strategies and innovations for teaching psychomotor skills to nursing students and suggested that the limited and mixed findings of research studies warrant further investigation on methods to teach kinesthetic skills. In any event, contact with the teacher during practice sessions is an important element for successful psychomotor learning. Although educator workload necessitates finding cost-effective and time-efficient ways to teach skill development, mediated instruction should not be used as a substitute, only a supplement, for instructor input (Baldwin, Hill, & Hanson, 1991).

In addition to using demonstration and return demonstration, mediated instruction, and self-directed study as teaching methods for psychomotor learning, mental imaging (also known as mental practice) has surfaced as a viable alternative for teaching motor skills. Research indicates that learning psychomotor skills can be enhanced through use of imagery. Mental practice is similar to the type of practice athletes use when preparing to perform in a sports competition (Bachman, 1990; Doheny, 1993; Eaton & Evans, 1986; Miracle, 1999).

Another hallmark of psychomotor learning is the type and timing of the feedback given to learners. Psychomotor skill development allows for immediate feedback such that learners have an immediate idea of the results of their performance. During skill practice, learners receive *intrinsic feedback* that is generated from within the self, giving them a sense of or a feel for how they have performed. They may sense that they either did quite well or that they felt awkward and need more practice. In addition, the teacher has the opportunity to provide *augmented feedback* by sharing with learners an opinion or conveying a message through body language about how well they performed (Oermann, 1990). The immediacy of the feedback, together with the self-generated and teacher-supplemented feedback, makes this a unique feature of psychomotor learning. Performance checklists, which can serve as guides for teaching and learning, are also an effective tool for evaluating the level of skill performance.

An important point to remember is that it is all right to make mistakes in the process of teaching or learning a psychomotor skill. If the teacher makes an error when demonstrating a skill or the learner makes an error during return demonstration, this is the perfect teaching opportunity to offer anticipatory guidance: "Oops, I made a mistake. Now what do I do?" Unlike cognitive skill development, where errorless learning is the objective, in psychomotor skill development a mistake made represents an opportunity to demonstrate how to correct an error and to learn from the not-so-perfect initial attempts at performance. The old saying, "You learn by your mistakes," is most applicable to psychomotor skill mastery.

The spacing of practice time, which has been found to improve the likelihood that learners will remember new facts as described by Willingham (2002) under the cognitive domain section of this chapter, seems to apply to the learning of simple motor skills as well. However, to what degree this spacing effect positively influences the acquisition of complex skills is still not well understood. Willingham (2004) also addresses the value of sustained practice when learning a new psychomotor skill. In fact, he describes the necessity for practice to be repeated beyond the point of perfection if skill learning is to be long lasting, automatic, and achieved with a high level of competence.

Thus learning is a very complex phenomenon. It is clear that the cognitive, affective, and psychomotor domains, although representing separate behaviors, are to some extent interrelated. Movement-oriented activities require an integration of related knowledge and values (Morrison et al., 2004; Oermann, 1990). For example, the performance of a psychomotor skill requires a certain degree of cognitive knowledge or understanding of information, such as the scientific principles underlying a practice or why a skill is important to carry out. Also, there is an affective component to performing the movement dimension for the psychomotor behavior to be integrated as part of the learner's overall experience and ability to attain the ultimate goal of independence in self-care or practice delivery.

Development of Teaching Plans

After mutually agreed-upon goals and objectives have been written, it should be clear what the learner is to learn and what the teacher is to teach. A predetermined goal and related objectives serve as a basis for developing a teaching plan.

Organizing and presenting information in the format of an internally consistent teaching plan require skill by the nurse educator. A *teaching plan* is a blueprint for action to achieve the goal and the objectives that have been agreed upon by the educator and the learner. In addition to the goal and objectives, it also should include purpose, content, methods and tools, timing, and evaluation of instruction. The teaching plan should clearly and concisely identify the sequencing of these various elements of the education process.

The three major reasons for constructing teaching plans are:

1. To force the teacher to examine the relationship among the steps of the teaching process to ensure a logical approach to teaching, which can serve as a map

for organizing and keeping instruction on target.

2. To communicate in writing and in an outline format exactly what is being taught, how it is being taught and evaluated, and the time allotted for accomplishment of the behavioral objectives. If this is done, not only is the learner aware of and able to follow the action plan, but, just as importantly, other healthcare team members are informed and can contribute to the teaching effort with a consistent approach.

3. To legally document that an individual plan for each learner is in place and is being properly implemented. Also, the existence of current teaching plans is essential evidence required by healthcare agencies and organizations to satisfy mandates for institutional accreditation.

Teaching plans can be presented in a number of different formats to meet institutional requirements or the preference of the user, but all parts must be included for the teaching plan to be considered comprehensive and complete. A teaching plan should consist of the following eight basic elements (Ryan & Marinelli, 1990):

1. The purpose
2. A statement of the overall goal
3. A list of objectives (and subobjectives, if necessary)
4. An outline of the related content
5. The instructional method(s) used for teaching the related content
6. The time allotted for the teaching of each objective
7. The instructional resources (materials/tools and equipment) needed
8. The method(s) used to evaluate learning

A sample teaching plan format is shown in **Figure 10–1**. This format is highly recommended because the use of columns allows the educator, as well as anyone else who is using it, to see all the parts of the teaching plan at one time. Also, this format provides the best structure for determining if a relationship is apparent among all the elements of a plan. Internal consistency is the major criterion for judging the integrity of a teaching plan.

When constructing a teaching plan, the educator must be certain that above all else, internal consistency exists within the plan (Ryan & Marinelli, 1990). A teaching plan is said to be internally consistent when all of its eight parts are related to one another. Adherence to the concept of internal consistency requires that the domain of learning of each objective must be consistently reflected across each of the elements of the teaching plan, from the purpose all the way through to the end process of evaluation. The following example is adapted from Ryan and Marinelli's self-study module, *Developing a Teaching Plan*:

If the educator has decided to teach to the psychomotor domain, then the goal, objectives and subobjectives, related content, and so on should be reflective of the psychomotor domain.

Purpose: To provide the client with the information necessary for monitoring blood glucose.

Goal: The client will demonstrate the ability to test for blood glucose on a regular basis.

Objective: Following a 20-minute teaching session, the client will be able to use a reagent strip, Chemstrip bG, to determine blood glucose level with 100% accuracy.

Subobjective: The client will be able to assemble all equipment necessary to test

Figure 10–1 Sample teaching plan.

PURPOSE: GOAL:					
Objectives and Subobjectives	**Content Outline**	**Method of Instruction**	**Time Allotted** (in min.)	**Resources**	**Method of Evaluation**

for blood glucose using a reagent strip without assistance.

In the example, the purpose, goal, objective, and subobjective are reflective of the psychomotor domain, and, thus, the content, instructional method(s), instructional resource(s), time allotment, and evaluation method(s) should be appropriate to the psychomotor domain as well. This ensures internal consistency of the plan.

The decision about the number and types of objectives (reflecting one or more domains of learning) that should be included in a teaching plan must be made prior to developing the plan. If the purpose and goal are written for the accomplishment of a skill set that includes more than one domain, then the teaching plan should include one or more objectives for each domain. Important also is that the content, method(s) of teaching, and method(s) of evaluation should flow across the plan in parallel with each objective and be appropriate for accomplishing the domain of learning in each objective (see **Figure 10–2**). Thus in the overall design of the teaching plan, internal consistency requires that all elements must match whatever domain(s) of learning has/have been selected.

In addition to determining the type (domain) of the objective to be achieved, another aspect of internal consistency identified by Ryan and Marinelli (1990) that must be considered is related to the complexity of each objective. The educator must determine the detail of the content to be taught depending on the data obtained during assessment of the learner. The client's readiness to learn, learning needs, and learning style, must be taken into consideration when deciding the amount and depth of information to be taught. For example, the focus for teaching a low-level learner would be to con-

centrate on the need to know information. This would ensure that a skill can be performed safely without overwhelming the learner. By comparison, a high-level learner can handle and may desire additional nice to know information.

Whoever the client may be, the content to be taught for each objective must be directly related to the type and complexity of that objective. If subobjectives are included in the plan, then the same rule applies; that is, the content to be taught for each subobjective must be directly related to that subobjective.

The method of instruction chosen also should be appropriate for the type and level of content being taught. If, for example, the purpose is to teach a client to self-administer medication from an asthma inhaler (psychomotor domain), then the primary method of teaching that best helps with psychomotor skill development should be chosen, such as demonstration and return demonstration. Conversely, if the objective is to impart knowledge of what constitutes a low-fat diet (cognitive domain), then lecture and programmed instruction are appropriate teaching methods.

The time set aside for the teaching and learning of each objective and subobjective also must be specified. How much time is needed for instruction and acquisition of a skill depends on learner attributes, the type and complexity of the behavior, the depth of content, and the resources to be used to supplement teaching and assist with learning. Ideally, each patient teaching session should be no more than 15 to 20 minutes in length and certainly no more than 30 minutes. Audiences of staff nurses and nursing students can tolerate longer sessions. In this period of time, one or more objectives may be accomplished or partially accomplished. Additional teaching sessions may be required for the learner to attain expected outcomes.

Figure 10–2 Completed teaching plan for self-administration of insulin.

PURPOSE: To provide patient with information necessary for self-administration of insulin as prescribed

GOAL: The patient will be able to perform insulin injections independently according to treatment regimen

Objectives	Content Outline	Method of Instruction	Time Allotted (in min.)	Resources	Method of Evaluation
Following a 20-minute teaching session, the patient will be able to:					
Identify the five sites for insulin injection with 100% accuracy (cognitive)	Location of five anatomical sites Rotation of sites	1:1 instruction	2	Anatomical chart	Post-testing
Demonstrate proper techniques according to procedure for drawing up insulin from a multidose vial (psychomotor)	Accepted technique according to procedure Reading syringe unit dose markings	Demonstration Return demonstration	5	Alcohol sponges Sterile SQ needles and insulin syringes Multidose vial of sterile water	Observation of return demonstration
Give insulin to self in thigh area with 100% accuracy (psychomotor)	Procedure for injecting insulin SQ at 90° angle using aseptic technique	Demonstration Return demonstration	10	Human model SQ needle and syringe Multidose vial of sterile water Alcohol sponges	Observation of return demonstration
Express any concerns about self-administration of insulin (affective)	Summarize common concerns Exploration of feelings	Discussion	3	Video Written handouts	Question and answer

The resources to be used, which refer to instructional materials and equipment needed for teaching, should appropriately match the content and teaching methodology. If the purpose is to teach breast self-examination, for example, then written or audiovisual materials or an anatomical model of the breast would be useful instructional tools. It is also important for the educator to keep in mind what resources would be an appealing, comfortable, and convenient medium for the learner. A variety of resources may be necessary to maintain the learner's attention and to serve as reinforcers of information. An important consideration is the literacy level of the learner. Giving a low-literate person technical reading materials will merely frustrate and confuse the learner and defeat the plan for teaching. Conversely, it is possible that giving too simple material to a highly literate person may lead to boredom and inattention to instruction.

Finally, the method of evaluation should match the type and complexity of learning that is to be achieved. For example, if the learner is expected to be able to state, list, or circle (or some other low-level cognitive performance term) the three most important symptoms of a heart attack, then the evaluation method that appropriately tests that knowledge must be chosen. Evaluation methods must measure the desired learning outcomes to determine if and to what extent the learner achieved the expectations for learning.

In summary, just as with a nursing care plan, all elements of a teaching plan need to hang together. Figure 10–2 is a good example of a plan that adheres to all the rules of construction. The goal is reflective of the purpose, the objectives depend on and are derived from the goal, the instructional content depends on and is appropriate to meet the objectives, the teaching

methodology depends on and is related to the content, and so forth.

If, for instance, content outlined in a teaching plan is not related to any of the objectives, then the content is either unnecessary or another objective must be written as a basis for including the extra content. Likewise, if a teaching plan has no content relative to a particular stated objective or subobjective, then additional content must be included or the objective or subobjective eliminated, if necessary.

Also, during the teaching process, if the learner indicates in some way an interest in or demonstrates a need for knowing more than an original plan addressed, then the plan should be revised accordingly. Whether a plan is adhered to or revised, it must, above all else, reflect internal consistency (see Appendix C for additional samples of completed teaching plans).

Use of Learning Contracts

The concept of learning contracts is a relatively new but increasingly popular approach to teaching and learning that can be implemented with any audience of learners—patients and their families, nursing staff, or nursing students. Learning contracts are "based on the principle of the learners being active partners in the teaching–learning system, rather than passive recipients of whatever it is that the teacher thinks is good for them" (Atherton, 2005, p. 1).

In the strictest sense, a contract is a formal legal agreement governing the terms of a transaction over a specified period of time between two or more parties (O'Reilly, 1994). In education, a *learning contract* is defined as a written (formal) or verbal (informal) agreement between the teacher and the learner that delineates specific teaching and learning activities that are to occur within a certain time frame. A learning contract is a mutually negotiated agreement, usually in the form of a written document drawn up by the teacher and the learner, that specifies what the learner will learn, the resources needed, how learning will be achieved and within what time allotment, and the criteria for measuring the success of the venture (Keyzer, 1986; Knowles, Holton, & Swanson, 1998; McAllister, 1996).

Inherent in the learning contract is the existence of some type of reward for upholding the contractual agreement (Wallace & Mundie, 1987). For patients and families, the reward may be recognition of their success in mastery of a task that facilitates moving closer to independence in self-care and a higher quality of life. For staff nurses, the reward might be having the privilege granted to practice in a chosen setting or at an advanced level. For nursing students, the reward might result in being allowed continued progression through a program of study. Rewards may be tangible, such as a certificate or award in recognition of successful attainment of an outcome; or intangible, such as outward praise from the teacher or an intrinsic sense of satisfaction in accomplishing a predetermined goal.

Contract learning has been introduced in education as an alternative, innovative approach to structuring a learning experience that embodies the principles of adult learning (Knowles et al., 1998). The origin of contract learning is derived from humanistic theory that acknowledges the person as an autonomous being whose efforts are continuously aimed at self-determination and self-actualization. The central view of the humanistic educational theory is that knowledge is a process, not a product (Mazhindu, 1990). As such, according to Kreider and Barry (1993), contract learning emphasizes how a body of knowledge will be acquired (process plan), not how a body of knowledge will be transmitted (content plan).

Learning contracts are considered to be an effective teaching strategy for empowering the learner because they emphasize self-direction, mutual negotiation, and mutual evaluation of established competency levels. A number of terms have been used to describe this approach, such as *independent learning, self-directed learning,* and *learner-centered* or *project-oriented learning* (Chan & Chien, 2000; Lowry, 1997; Waddell & Stephens, 2000).

Knowles et al. (1998) describe the purpose of using learning contracts, the steps to developing a learning contract, and the guidelines for the implementation of learning contracts. Years of research on adult learners have revealed time and again that "what adults learn on their own initiative, they learn more deeply and permanently than what they learn by being taught" (p. 211).

The imposed structure of traditional education—that is, telling learners the objectives they need to work toward, what resources they are to use, how and when to use those resources, and how their accomplishments will be evaluated—conflicts with the psychological need by adults to be self-directing. Being told what, how, and when to learn something may lead to resistance, apathy, or withdrawal by the learner. This does not mean that adult learners do not need guidance or that they do not want structure or specifics, but rather that they often desire flexibility for learning and they want to be involved in decision making when it comes to planning, implementation, and evaluation of their learning.

Learning contracts stress shared accountability for learning between the teacher and the learner. The method of contract learning actively involves the learner at all stages of the teaching–learning process, from assessment of learning needs and identification of learning resources to the planning, implementation, and evaluation of learning activities.

Because learning contracts are a unique way of presenting information to the learner and are the essence of an equal and cooperative partnership, they challenge the traditional teacher–client relationship through a redistribution of power and control. Allowing learners to negotiate a contract for learning shifts the control and emphasis of the learning experience from a traditionally teacher-centered focus to a learner-centered focus. Active involvement of the learner increases feelings of commitment and fosters accountability for self-directed learning (Knowles et al., 1998; Wallace & Mundie, 1987).

The purpose of learning contracts is to encourage active participation by the learner, improve teacher–client communication, and enhance learner expressiveness and creativity. Learning contracts, whether formal or informal, can be used to facilitate personal development of the learner.

In the case of staff and student nurses, this approach to learning can enhance professional development as well. As stated by Waddell (1998), "the use of learning contracts empowers the students to learn on their own, reflect on their strengths and weaknesses, choose learning activities which best match their learning styles, use resources effectively to promote their learning, and self-evaluate" (p. 1).

Learning contracts serve as a vehicle for fulfilling the internal needs of the learner and the external needs of an organization (Keyzer, 1986; Knowles, 1990). Learners have an opportunity to change behavior and reach their human potential through an approach that fosters choice and growth-promoting independence

and allows for self-paced learning. Clearly defined expectations reduce learner anxiety, decrease frustration, increase levels of personal satisfaction, encourage the development of self-directed learning habits, increase the rate and quality of learning, and provide a defined basis for evaluation of the learner (Waddell, 1998).

Learning contracts also can be used to facilitate discharge of patients to the home setting. In complex cases involving the care of a patient by a large number of multidisciplinary team members, a contract provides cohesion and an excellent communication tool between the patient, family caretakers, and the healthcare team (Cady & Yoshioka, 1991).

Components of the Learning Contract

A complete learning contract includes the following four major components (Knowles, 1990; Wallace & Mundie, 1987):

1. *Content*—specifies the precise behavioral objectives to be achieved. Objectives must clearly state the desired outcomes of learning activities. Negotiation between the educator and the learner determines the content, level, and sequencing of objectives according to learner needs, abilities, and readiness.

2. *Performance expectations*—specify the conditions under which learning activities will be facilitated, such as instructional strategies and resources.

3. *Evaluation*—specifies the criteria used to evaluate achievement of objectives, such as skills checklists, care standards or protocols, and agency policies and procedures of care that identify the levels of competency expected of the learner.

4. *Time frame*—specifies the length of time needed for successful completion of the objectives. The target date for completion should reflect a reasonable period in which to achieve expected outcomes depending on the learner's abilities and circumstances.

In addition to these four components, it is important to include the terms of the contract. Role definitions describe the teacher–learner relationship with respect to clarifying the expectations and assumptions about the roles each will play. The educator is responsible for coordinating and facilitating all phases of the contract process. In the case of nursing staff and student nurse learning, the educator plays a major role in the selection and preparation of preceptors and acts as a resource person for both the learner and the preceptor. (See **Figure 10–3** for a sample learning contract.)

Steps to Implement the Learning Contract

Knowles et al. (1998) and Knowles (1990) described the steps involved in developing a learning contract with any adult learner. Wallace and Mundie (1987) also outlined the steps to implement a learning contract, although they

Figure 10–3 Sample learning contract.

Name of Learner: _____

Name of Educator: _____

Name of Preceptor (if applicable): _____

Date of Contract Negotiated: _____

Terms of Contract: _____

_____

Objectives	Activities	Evaluation	Target Date	Completion Date
Lists cognitive, affective, and psychomotor behaviors mutually agreed on and intended to be achieved	Lists teaching–learning strategies and resources to be used to achieve the objectives	Lists the criteria to be used to measure learning demonstrated	Lists a realistic time frame for achievement of expected outcome(s)	Specifies the dates that each objective is accomplished

Signatures: _____ (Learner) _____ (Educator) _____ (Preceptor)

specifically addressed the implementation of contract learning with regard to the orientation of new staff nurses. The following steps apply to establishing and carrying out a learning contract for any type of learner:

Step 1 *Determine specific learning objectives.* Encourage the learner to identify his or her learning needs and what the learner wants to be able to do within an allotted time frame.

Step 2 *Review the contracting process.* It is vital that learners have a complete understanding of what contract learning is all about as well as their role in the process. Because learning contracts have not been widely used until recently, most people are unfamiliar with this teaching–learning strategy.

Step 3 *Identify the learning resources.* Introduce the learner to instructional resources available, such as self-study materials and audiovisual tools.

Step 4 *Assess the learner's competency level and learning needs.* The entire process of negotiation of a contract is based on the learner's current abilities and learning needs. The educator initiates the assessment of the learner and collects data primarily through interview, observation, and pretesting to formulate objectives.

Step 5 *Define roles.* Before planning learning experiences and negotiating a contract, the roles of the learner and the educator must be clearly established regarding expectations of each.

Step 6 *Plan the learning experiences.* Determine the content, learning resources to be used, the skills that must be demon-strated, and the amount of time to pursue learning through assisted study or self-study to meet the predetermined objectives.

Step 7 *Negotiate the time frame.* Based on appropriate sequencing of behaviors, from simplest to most complex, establish a target date for completion of each objective.

Step 8 *Implement the learning experience.* Take into consideration individual variations in the level of ability to do self-directed study and any other variables that may play a factor in completion of the specified learning activities. For patients, progress in learning may be influenced by changes in their health status. For staff nurses, the constant pressures of providing patient care services may place constraints on the time available for educational activities. For any learner, the education process is influenced by readiness to learn and how well the information to be learned is organized and communicated.

Step 9 *Renegotiate.* The type and level of complexity of behavioral objectives and the target dates set forth for accomplishing these objectives may be renegotiated at any point along the continuum of the learning experience to meet the needs of the learner. Adults may change their notions about what they want to learn, how they want to learn it, and how long it will take to achieve objectives, so they should be encouraged to revise their contract as it is being carried out.

Step 10 *Evaluate.* Periodic (formative) and final (summative) evaluation of the learner's progress and the actual learning experience itself is a shared responsibility between the learner and the educator.

Preestablished performance criteria, agreed on prior to the initiation of the learning process, serve as the means to ascertain achievement of outcomes based on predetermined and prenegotiated behavioral objectives.

Step 11 *Document.* Evidence of achievement of learning objectives is determined jointly by the learner and the educator (and preceptors if used for nursing staff and students). When an objective is satisfactorily met according to written performance expectations, each party signs

the date completed in the appropriate column. (See **Figure 10–4** for an example of a completed learning contract.)

The Concept of Learning Curve

Learning is an active process in which learners attempt to make sense of information that ultimately results in a change in behavior. Specifically, the concept of the *learning curve* has historically been used only to describe how long it takes for a

Figure 10–4 Completed learning contract.

Objectives	Activities	Evaluation	Target Date	Completion Date
Improve time management and organizational skills to increase productivity by 20%	Read articles and books on topic Interview three managers on how to organize work and manage time Observe a productive colleague for one day, noting techniques used	Report on knowledge acquired Performance of productivity observed with feedback from observer		

Name of Learner: _____
Name of Educator: _____
Name of Preceptor (if applicable): _____
Date of Contract Negotiated: _____
Terms of Contract: Employee will increase work efficiency at place of employment by 20% within 2 months

Source: Adapted from Knowles, N. S., Holton, E. F., & Swanson, R. A. (1998). *The definitive classic in adult education and human resource development* (3rd ed., p. 245). Houston, TX: Gulf Publishing.

learner to acquire a psychomotor skill. As such, it also implies the level of difficulty in achieving an outcome related to simple and complex motor skill development.

Recently, the term *learning curve* has been applied more loosely, albeit incorrectly, to the time it takes someone to learn anything new, including cognitive and affective behaviors. It is a misnomer to use the term in describing learning of any behavior other than psychomotor. Research findings only support the use of this term in relation to psychomotor learning.

Although the learning curve concept has great potential for understanding psychomotor skill development when teaching patients, staff nurses, or nursing students, a thorough search of the nursing literature reveals no documentation whatsoever that this concept has ever been applied to skill practice. Only in the last few years has reference been found in the medical literature to describe the application of this concept to the learning of surgical and other invasive techniques (Gawande, 2002). Medicine is just beginning to realize the usefulness of the learning curve concept in determining how long it takes for physicians to become competent in performing procedures using new technologies, such as simulators, laparoscopes, or robotic instruments (Eversbusch & Grantcharov, 2004; Flamme, Stukenborg-Colsman, & Wirth, 2006; Hernandez et al., 2004).

To understand the learning curve concept as it relates to the process of teaching and learning, one must refer to educational psychology literature. Cronbach (1963) defined the learning curve, specifically related to psychomotor skill development, as "a record of an individual's improvement made by measuring his ability at different stages of practice and plotting his scores" (p. 297).

The learning curve (also sometimes referred to as the experience curve) is a phenomenon that can be applied to the analysis of learning that occurs by any individual or groups of individuals. The concept of learning curve has been adopted by business and industry to measure employee productivity. It has a direct effect on cost of labor, the time it takes to manufacture a product or deliver a service, the quality of the product or service, and the pricing of goods and services. The concept has been broadened to be used in other fields of activities, as the cost of doing repetitive tasks generally decreases as experience is gained. For example, Kratzer (1995) reported on a study measuring the effectiveness of mentoring beginning teachers in their first year of practice. She concluded that the mentorship model offers a way to accelerate the learning curve of new teachers as well as to increase their longevity in the profession.

McCray and Blakemore (1985) note that the learning curve "is basically nothing more than a graphic depiction of changes in performance or output during a specified time period" (p. 5). A learning curve shows the relationship between practice and performance of a psychomotor skill and provides a concrete measure of the rate at which one or more people learn a task. In many situations, evidence of learning (improvement) follows a very productive and predictable pattern.

The theoretical learning curve is a schematic used to summarize many features of psychomotor skill acquisition, which, according to Cronbach (1963), is divided into six stages (see **Figure 10–5**):

1. *Negligible progress:* Initially very little improvement in score is detected. This prereadiness period is when the learner

Figure 10–5 A schematic learning curve.

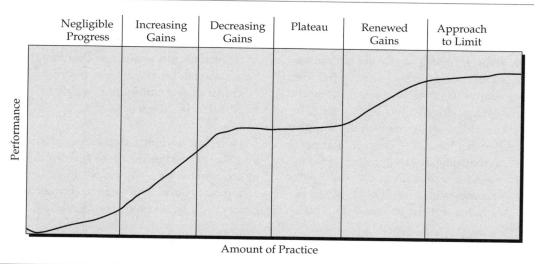

Source: Adapted from Cronbach, L. J. (1963). *Educational psychology* (2nd ed., p. 299). New York: Harcourt, Brace, & World.

is not ready to perform the entire task, but relevant learning is taking place, such as developing attention, manipulation, and perceptual skills. This period can be relatively long in young children who are developing physical and cognitive abilities, as well as in older adults who may have difficulty in making key discriminations.

2. *Increasing gains:* The rate of learning increases as the learner grasps the essentials of the task. Scores rise rapidly as the learner becomes aware of cues to attend to, goals to attain, or ways to effectively organize responses. Motivation may account for rapid gains when the learner has interest in the task, receives approval from others, or

experiences a sense of pride in discovering the ability to perform.

3. *Decreasing gains:* The rate of improvement slows. In this period of refinement, the slowing of task mastery is inevitable as practice does not produce such steep gains. Learning occurs in smaller increments of response as the learner incorporates changes by using cues to smooth out performance.

4. *Plateau:* No substantial gains are made. This leveling off period is characterized by a negligible rate of progress in level of performance but further gains are possible. During this stage, the learner is making small adjustments, such as modifying subskills, reducing dependence on mediators, and correcting responses to more

remote cues. Plateaus are not observed in all instances, and the very idea of a period of no progress is considered false. Gains in skills can occur even though overall performance scores remain stable.

5. *Renewed gains:* The rate of performance again rises if further gains are possible. If additional progress can be made after the plateau period has ended, it usually is due to growth in physical development, renewed interest in the task, a response to challenge, or the drive for perfection.

6. *Approach to limit:* Progress at this point becomes negligible. The ability to perform has reached its potential. That is,

no matter how much more someone practices a skill, he or she is incapable of doing any better. The limit is a hypothetical stage only because there is never certainty that a learner cannot improve further. Just as with an Olympic athlete who has broken a world record, he or she may at some point be able to exceed his or her top score.

Individual learning curves are characterized by irregularity (see **Figure 10–6**) and are often unlike the smooth theoretical curve. Fluctuations in performance can be attributed to changes in such factors as focus, interest, energy, ability, situa-

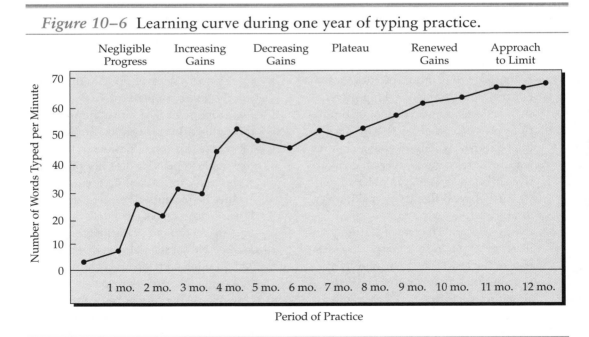

Figure 10–6 Learning curve during one year of typing practice.

Source: Adapted from Cronbach, L. J. (1963). *Educational psychology* (2nd ed., p. 303). New York: Harcourt, Brace, & World.

tional circumstances, or favorable/unfavorable conditions for learning (Barker, 1994; Cronbach, 1963; Gage & Berliner, 1998). The learning curve can be skewed by the reliability of the performance. As stated by Atherton (2005, p. 1), "any novice can get it right occasionally (beginner's luck), but it is consistency which counts and the progress of learning is often assessed on this basis." As Atherton further elaborates, it is incorrect to use the cliché "steep learning curve" to imply that something is difficult to learn. In fact, just the opposite is true. As a learner practices a difficult skill, the line rises slowly, not quickly, over time. This means the steepness of the curve actually refers to the demands of the task—how many trials it takes as well as, in reality, how long it takes to master a skill—rather than the description of the process itself. In other words, a steep, short learning curve indicates that the learner was able to master a skill rapidly and easily.

Nursing research on application of the learning curve concept to the teaching and learning of psychomotor skills by patients, nursing staff, and nursing students must be conducted. Such studies would help educators to improve their understanding of the normal or expected pattern and pace of learning, assist them in recognizing the multitude of variables that affect the length of time and the ease or difficulty for any given learner to achieve an intended outcome, and aid them in choosing appropriate educational interventions based on evidence of the different stages of practice required by the learner for improvement in skill development. Research could answer such questions in patient and staff education as the following:

- Can a learning curve be shortened given the characteristics of the learner, the situation, or the task at hand?

- Why is the learning curve steeper, more drawn out, or more irregular for some learners than for others?
- Can we predict the learning curves of our patients or nursing staff and students depending on their educational or experiential backgrounds?
- How many times does a particular skill need to be practiced to improve competency and ensure consistency of performance?
- What can we do from an educational standpoint to influence the pace and pattern of learning that may result in earlier or more complete achievement of expected outcomes?
- How can the learning curve concept be applied to improve staff performance, thereby increasing work satisfaction and productivity, decreasing costs of care, and improving the quality of care?

These are just a few of the questions that research could attempt to answer to provide evidence as a basis for practice changes in approaches to teaching and learning by the nurse educator.

The implications of applying the learning curve concept to patient teaching and staff and student education are many. Perhaps one key benefit to understanding this concept is to realize that the pattern and pace of learning is irregular, not linear and even as once supposed. The learning of any task is often rapid after an initial slow start, inevitably decreases, then reaches a plateau, and then increases again, until a limit is reached when likely no more significant improvement in mastery of a skill can be achieved. Understanding this phenomenon will help educators adjust their expectations or deal with their frustrations when different paces and patterns of learning occur in individuals as they attempt to master any psychomotor skill.

Awareness that learning is not linear and that the amount of practice needed to improve performance is variable can also be shared with learners to reduce their expectations and frustrations when mastering a skill. For example, a patient who is undergoing rehabilitation to learn how to walk again following a stroke or injury may easily become discouraged with the progress he or she is making toward the achievement of a goal. This may happen because gains in the learning may slow down or the patient may experience a time at the beginning or in the middle of the curve when he or she seems not to be learning at all. Educators can realistically support the learner if they understand the pace and pattern of skill development.

State of the Evidence

Nurse educators require not only knowledge and experience to effectively teach various audiences of learners, but they also need the clinical evidence to prove their teaching methods and interventions are actually effective. Evidence should be based on up-to-date research to help guide the nurse in the delivery of evidence-based care. The nurse should identify the types of information needed in particular situations and be competent in accessing the appropriate databases to obtain the information and research necessary to carry out all aspects of the educator role. "This leads to an increased awareness for the need for appropriate information to provide best care, solve an identified clinical problem, or facilitate a change in practice" (Pierce, 2005, p. 236).

Plenty of evidence establishes the value and utility of behavioral objectives for teaching and

learning. Also, numerous research studies in the psychology literature have substantiated the framework, known as the taxonomic hierarchy, for categorizing behaviors (cognitive, affective, and psychomotor) according to type (domain) and complexity (level of difficulty). Furthermore, a body of knowledge on how to develop internally consistent teaching plans using these behavioral objectives for the purpose of legally documenting and properly implementing individual plans of care for patient education is available. These plans are mandated according to expectations set forth by accrediting bodies of healthcare agencies and organizations.

Although the use of learning contracts is a relatively new concept, evidence has been forthcoming by educational psychologists based on developmental research indicating the needs of adult learners for independent, self-directed, problem-centered, and participatory learning. However, the concept of the learning curve, although superficially and widely adopted as a term used by educators, has not been well defined or well explored for its theoretical application to teaching and learning in the health professions. Little evidence exists on its reliability and validity in patient and nursing education for psychomotor skill acquisition. It is clearly apparent more research needs to be conducted to prove that the learning curve concept is a useful principle for nurse educators to incorporate into the process of teaching and learning.

Summary

The major portion of this chapter focused on differentiating goals from objectives, preparing accurate and concise objectives, classifying objectives according to the three domains of learning, and the teaching of cognitive, affective, and psychomotor skills using appropriate instructional interventions. The writing of behavioral objectives as to type and complexity is fundamental to the education process. Goals and objectives serve as a guide to the educator in the planning, implementation, and evaluation of teaching and learning.

Assessment of the learner is a prerequisite to formulating objectives. Prior to selecting the content to be taught and the methods and materials to be used for instruction, there must be a clear understanding of what the learner is expected to be able to do. Appraisal should be based on a mutual determination between the educator and the client as to what needs to be learned, under what conditions learning can best occur, and the teaching and evaluation methods most preferred. Objectives setting must be a partnership effort by the learner and the educator for any learning experience to be successful and rewarding in the achievement of expected outcomes.

This chapter also outlined the development of teaching plans and learning contracts. Teaching plans provide the blueprint for organizing and presenting information in a coherent manner. Above all else, a teaching plan must reflect internal consistency of its parts. Learning contracts are an innovative and unique alternative to structuring a learning experience based on adult learning principles. Contracts are designed to provide for self-directed study, thereby encouraging active involvement and accountability on the part of the learner. The communication of desired behavioral outcomes and the mechanisms for accomplishing behavioral changes in the learner are essential elements in the decision-making process with respect to both teaching and learning.

The concept of learning curve is applicable to the process of teaching and learning. It must be explored from a research perspective to yield findings for the practice of evidence-based teaching.

REVIEW QUESTIONS

1. What is the difference between the terms *educational*, *instructional*, and *behavioral* or *learning objectives*?
2. What two major factors distinguish goals and objectives from one another?
3. What are the definitions of the terms *goal* and *objective*?
4. Why do some educators argue against the use of behavioral objectives?
5. What five reasons justify the importance of writing clear and concise statements of expected behaviors?
6. What are the four components that should be included in every written behavioral objective?
7. What eight mistakes are commonly made when writing behavioral objectives?
8. What are the three domains of learning?
9. Which levels of behavior, according to the taxonomic form of hierarchy, are considered the most simple and the most complex in the cognitive, affective, and psychomotor domains?
10. Why is it important for the educator to remember to keep psychomotor skill instruction separate from the cognitive and affective components of skill development?
11. What five factors or variables influence the amount of practice required to learn any new skill?
12. What are the eight basic components of a teaching plan?
13. Why are learning contracts an increasingly popular approach to teaching and learning?
14. What are the four major components of a learning contract?
15. Why is the concept of the learning curve an important consideration in teaching and learning for psychomotor skill development?

References

American Nurses Association. (2001). *Code of ethics for nurses with interpretative statements*. Washington, DC: Author.

American Nurses Association. (2003). *Nursing's social policy statement*. Washington, DC: Author.

American Nurses Association. (2004). *Standards of clinical nursing practice*. Washington, DC: Author.

Anderson, L. W., Krathwohl, D. R., Airasian, P. W., Cruikshank, K. A., Mayer, R. E., Pintrich, P. R., et al. (2001). *A taxonomy for learning, teaching, and assessing* (Rev. ed.). New York: Longman.

Arends, R. I. (1994). *Learning to teach* (3rd ed.). New York: McGraw-Hill.

Atherton, J. S. (2005). *Learning contracts*. Retrieved October 31, 2006, from http://www.learningandteaching.info/teaching/learningcontracts.htm

Babcock, D. E., & Miller, M. A. (1994). *Client education: Theory and practice*. St. Louis: Mosby–Year Book.

Bachman, K. (1990). Using mental imagery to practice a specific psychomotor skill. *Journal of Continuing Education in Nursing, 21*(3), 125–128.

Baldwin, D., Hill, P., & Hanson, G. (1991). Performance of psychomotor skills: A comparison of two teaching strategies. *Journal of Nursing Education, 30*(8), 367–370.

Barker, L. M. (1994). *Learning and behavior: A psychobiological perspective.* New York: Macmillan College Publishing Company.

Bell, M. L. (1991). Learning a complex nursing skill: Student anxiety and the effect of preclinical skill evaluation. *Journal of Nursing Education, 30*(5), 222–226.

Bloom, B. J., Englehart, M. S., Furst, E. J., Hill, W. H., & Krathwohl, D. R. (1956). *Taxonomy of educational objectives: The classification of educational goals. Handbook 1: Cognitive domain.* New York: David McKay.

Bucher, L. (1991). Evaluating the affective domain. *Journal of Nursing Staff Development, 7*(5), 234–238.

Cady, C., & Yoshioka, R. S. (1991). Using a learning contract to successfully discharge an infant on home total parenteral nutrition. *Pediatric Nursing, 17*(1), 67–70, 74.

Chan, S. W., & Chien, W.-T. (2000). Implementing contract learning in a clinical context: Report on a study. *Journal of Advanced Nursing, 31*(2), 298–305.

Cronbach, L. J. (1963). *Educational psychology* (2nd ed.). New York: Harcourt, Brace, & World.

Cummings, C. (1994). Tips for writing behavioral objectives. *Nursing Staff Development Insider, 3*(4), 6, 8.

Dave, R. (1970). *Psychomotor levels in developing and writing objectives.* Tucson, AZ: Educational Innovators Press.

Doheny, M. O. (1993). Mental practice: An alternative approach to teaching motor skills. *Journal of Nursing Education, 32*(6), 260–264.

Durbach, E., Goodall, R., & Wilkinson, K. (1987). Instructional objectives in patient education. *Nursing Outlook, 35*(2), 82–83, 88.

Eaton, S. L., & Evans, S. B. (1986). The effect of nonspecific imaging practice on the mental imagery ability of nursing students. *Journal of Nursing Education, 25*(5), 193–196.

Eggen, P. D., & Kauchak, D. P. (2001). *Strategies for teachers teaching content and thinking skills* (4th ed.). Boston: Allyn and Bacon.

Ellis, C. (1993). Incorporating the affective domain into staff development programs. *Journal of Nursing Staff Development, 9*(3), 127–130.

Eversbusch, A., & Grantcharov, T. P. (2004). Learning curves and impact of psychomotor training on performance in simulated colonoscopy: A randomized trial using virtual reality endoscopy trainer. *Surgical Endoscopy, 18*(10), 1514–1518.

Ferguson, L. M. (1998). Writing learning objectives. *Journal of Nursing Staff Development, 14*(2), 87–94.

Flamme, C. H., Stukenborg-Colsman, C., & Wirth, C. J. (2006). Evaluation of the learning curves associated with uncemented primary total hip arthroplasty depending on the experience of the surgeon. *H/P International, 16*(3), 191–197.

Gage, N. L., & Berliner, D. C. (1998). *Educational Psychology* (6th ed.). Boston: Houghton Mifflin.

Gawande, A. (2002, January 28). The learning curve. Annals of medicine. *The New Yorker*, pp. 52–61.

Gomez, G. E., & Gomez, E. A. (1984). The teaching of psychomotor skills in nursing. *Nurse Educator, 9*(4), 35–39.

Gomez, G. E., & Gomez, E. A. (1987). Learning of psychomotor skills: Laboratory versus patient care setting. *Journal of Nursing Education, 26*(1), 20–24.

Green, S. M., Voegeli, D., Harrison, M., Phillips, J., Knowles, J., Weaver, M., et al. (2003). Evaluating the use of streaming video to support student learning in a first-year life sciences course for student nurses. *Nurse Education Today, 23,* 255–261.

Gronlund, N. E. (1985). *Stating objectives for classroom instruction* (3rd ed.). New York: Macmillan.

Gronlund, N. E. (2004). *Writing instructional objectives for teaching and assessment.* (7th Ed.). Upper Saddle River, NJ: Pearson Merrill Prentice-Hall.

Haggard, A. (1989). *Handbook of patient education.* Rockville, MD: Aspen.

Harrow, A. J. (1972). *A taxonomy of the psychomotor domain: A guide for developing behavioral objectives.* New York: David McKay.

Heinich, R., Molenda, M., Russell, J., & Smaldino, S. (2001). *Instructional methods and technologies for learning* (7th ed.). Englewood Cliffs, NJ: Prentice Hall, Inc.

Hernandez, J. D., Bann, S. D., Munz, Y., Moorthy, K., Datta, V., Martin, S., et al. (2004). Qualitative and quantitative analysis of the learning curve of a simulated surgical task on the da Vinci system. *Surgical Endoscopy, 18*(3), 372–378.

Keyzer, D. (1986). Using learning contracts to support change in nursing organizations. *Nurse Education Today, 6*(8), 103–108.

Knowles, M. (1990). *The adult learner: A neglected species* (4th ed.). Houston, TX: Gulf Publishing Company.

Knowles, M. S., Holton, E. F., & Swanson, R. A. (1998). *The definitive classic in adult education and human resource development* (3rd ed.). Houston, TX: Gulf Publishing.

Krathwohl, D. R., Bloom, B. J., & Masia, B. B. (1964). *Taxonomy of educational objectives: The cassification of educational goals. Handbook II: The affective domain.* New York: David McKay.

Kratzer, C. C. (1995, April). *Reflective practice in a community of beginning teachers: Implementing the STEP program.* Paper presented at the annual meeting of the American Educational Research Association, San Francisco, CA.

Kreider, M. C., & Barry, M. (1993). Clinical ladder development: Implementing contract learning. *Journal of Continuing Education in Nursing, 24*(4), 166–169.

Love, B., McAdams, C., Patton, D. M., Rankin, E. J., & Roberts, J. (1989). Teaching psychomotor skills in nursing: A randomized controlled trial. *Journal of Advanced Nursing, 14*(11), 970–975.

Lowry, M. (1997). Using learning contracts in clinical practice. *Professional Nurse, 12*(4), 280–283.

Mager, R. F. (1997). *Preparing instructional objectives* (3rd ed.). Atlanta, GA: Center for Effective Performance.

Maier-Lorentz, M. M. (1999). Writing objectives and evaluating learning in the affective domain. *Journal for Nurses in Staff Development, 15*(4), 167–171.

Mazhindu, G. N. (1990). Contract learning reconsidered: A critical examination of implications for application in nurse education. *Journal of Advanced Nursing, 15*(1), 101–109.

McAllister, M. (1996). Learning contracts: An Australian experience. *Nurse Education Today, 16*(3), 199–205.

McCray, P., & Blakemore, T. (1985). *A guide to learning curve technology to enhance performance prediction in vocational evaluation.* Menomonie, WI: Research and Training Center, Stout Vocational and Rehabilitation Institute, School of Education and Human Services, University of Wisconsin–Stout.

Menix, K. D. (1996). Domains of learning: Interdependent components of achievable learning outcomes. *Journal of Continuing Education in Nursing, 27*(5), 200–208.

Miracle, D. J. (1999). Teaching psychomotor skills in simulated learning labs. In K. R. Stevens and V. R. Cassidy (Eds.), *Evidence-based teaching: Current research in nursing education* (pp. 71–103). Sudbury, MA: Jones and Bartlett.

Moore, M. R. (1970). The perceptual-motor domain and a proposed taxonomy of perception. *Audio Communications Review, 18,* 379–413.

Morrison, G. R., Ross, S. M., & Kemp, J. E. (2004). *Designing effective instruction* (4th ed.). Hoboken, NJ: John Wiley & Sons, Inc.

Oermann, M. H. (1990). Psychomotor skill development. *Journal of Continuing Education in Nursing, 21*(5), 202–204.

O'Reilly, D. (1994). Communication and effective learning: Negotiated study and learning contracts. *Nursing Times, 90*(9), i–viii.

Parker, G. M. Associates, Inc. (2000). *Team workout.* Amherst, MA: HRD Products.

Pierce, S. T. (2005). Integrating evidence-based practice into nursing curricula. In M. H. Oermann and K.T. Heinrich (Eds.), *Annual review of nursing education strategies for teaching, assessment, and program planning* (3rd ed., pp. 233–248). New York: Springer Publishing Company.

Reilly, D. E., & Oermann, M. H. (1990). *Behavioral objectives: Evaluation in nursing* (3rd ed.). Pub. No. 15–2367. New York: National League for Nursing.

Rinne, C. (1987). The affective domain: Equal opportunity in nursing education. *Journal of Continuing Education in Nursing, 18*(2), 40–43.

Rosen, J., Mulsant, B. H., Kollar, M., Kastango, K. B., Mazumdar, S., & Fox, D. (2002). Mental health training for nursing home staff using computer-based interaction video: A 6-month randomized trial. *Journal of the American Medical Directors Association, 3*(5), 291–296.

Ryan, M., & Marinelli, T. (1990). *Developing a Teaching Plan.* Unpublished self-study module, College of Nursing, State University of New York Health Science Center at Syracuse.

Schoenly, L. (1994). Teaching in the affective domain. *Journal of Continuing Education in Nursing, 25*(5), 209–212.

Simpson, E. J. (1972). The classification of educational objectives in the psychomotor domain. In M. T. Rainier (Ed.), *Contributions of behavioral science to instructional technology: The psychomotor domain* (3rd ed.). Englewood Cliffs, NJ: Gryphon Press, Prentice-Hall.

Tong, R. (2007). *New perspectives in health care ethics: An interdisciplinary and crosscultural approach.* Upper Saddle River, NJ: Pearson Education, Inc.

Waddell, D. L. (1998). Facilitating independent study through learning contracts. *National Student Nurses' Association Dean's Notes, 19*(5), 1–3.

Waddell, D. L., & Stephens, S. (2000). Use of learning contracts in a RN-to-BSN leadership course. *Journal of Continuing Education in Nursing, 31*(4), 179–184.

Wallace, P. L., & Mundie, G. E. (1987). Contract learning in orientation. *Journal of Nursing Staff Development, 3*(4), 143–149.

Willingham, D. T. (2002, Summer). Allocating student study time: "Massed" versus "distributed" practice. *American Educator*, 37–39, 47. Washington, DC: American Federation of Teachers.

Willingham, D. T. (2004, Spring). Practice makes perfect—but only if you practice beyond the point of perfection. *American Educator,* 31–33, 38.

Yoder, M. E. (1993). Computer use and nursing research: Transfer of cognitive learning to a clinical skill: Linear versus interactive video. *Western Journal of Nursing Research, 15*(1), 115–117.

Chapter 11

Instructional Methods and Settings

Kathleen Fitzgerald

CHAPTER HIGHLIGHTS

Instructional Methods
  Lecture
  Group Discussion
  One-to-One Instruction
  Demonstration and Return Demonstration
  Gaming
  Simulation
  Role Playing
  Role Modeling
  Self-Instruction Activities

Selection of Instructional Methods
Evaluation of Instructional Methods
Increasing Effectiveness of Teaching
  Techniques to Enhance the Effectiveness
    of Verbal Presentations
  General Principles for All Teachers
Instructional Settings
  Sharing Resources Among Settings
State of the Evidence

KEY TERMS

- ❑ instructional strategy
- ❑ instructional method
- ❑ lecture
- ❑ group discussion
- ❑ one-to-one instruction
- ❑ demonstration
- ❑ return demonstration
- ❑ gaming
- ❑ simulation
- ❑ role playing
- ❑ role modeling
- ❑ self-instruction
- ❑ skill inoculation
- ❑ instructional setting
- ❑ healthcare setting
- ❑ healthcare-related setting
- ❑ nonhealthcare setting

OBJECTIVES

After completing this chapter, the reader will be able to

1. Define the term *instructional method*.
2. Explain the various types of instructional methods.
3. Describe how to use each method effectively.
4. Identify the advantages and limitations of each method.
5. Discuss the variables that influence the selection of the various methods.
6. Recognize techniques to enhance teaching effectiveness.
7. Explain how to evaluate instructional methods.
8. Classify instructional settings according to the primary purpose of the organization or agency in which the nurse functions as educator.

After an excellent presentation, you might have heard someone comment, "Now, there is a born teacher!" This comment would seem to indicate that effective teaching comes automatically. In reality, teaching effectively is a learned skill. Development of this skill requires knowledge of the educational process, including the instructional methods to use with different audiences in a variety of settings.

Stimulating and effective educational experiences are designed, not accidental. *Instructional strategy* is the overall plan for a teaching–learning experience that involves the use of one or several methods of instruction to achieve the desired learning outcomes (Rothwell & Kazanas, 2004).

An *instructional method* is the way information is taught that brings the learner into contact with what is to be learned. Some examples of methods are lecture, group discussion, one-to-one instruction, demonstration and return demonstration, gaming, simulation, role playing, role modeling, and self-instruction mod-

ules. Instructional materials or tools, on the other hand, are the objects or vehicles to transmit information that supplement the act of teaching. Books, videos, and posters are examples of materials and tools used as adjuncts to communicate information. It is important to draw this distinction between the terms *instructional methods* and *instructional materials* because they often are used interchangeably by educators and not dealt with as distinctly separate entities, which they should be when planning an educational activity.

This chapter will review the types of instructional methods available and consider how to choose and use them most efficiently and effectively. In doing so, the advantages and limitations of each method, the variables influencing the selection of various methods, and the approaches for evaluating the methods will be identified to improve the delivery of instruction. Because the nurse is expected to teach many different audiences in all types of situations and circumstances, examples will be provided throughout this chapter in the application of these instructional methods to enhance teaching and learning experiences. Settings in which the nurse educator functions also will be highlighted.

Instructional Methods

There is no one perfect method for teaching all learners in all settings. Neither can any approach change behavior in all three domains for learning. Whatever the method chosen, it will usually be most effective if used in conjunction with other instructional techniques and tools to optimize learning. The importance of selecting appropriate methods to meet the needs of learners should not be underestimated.

The nurse educator functions in a vital role of facilitator by providing guidance and support for learning (Musinski, 1999). Even though a teacher may rely on one method predominantly, that single method is rarely adhered to in a pure fashion and is often a combination of various methods. For example, the lecture may be used as the primary format, with opportunities for question and answer periods and short discussion sessions being interspersed throughout the lecture period.

Decisions about which methods to use must be based on a consideration of such major factors as:

- Audience characteristics (size, diversity, learning style preferences)
- Educator's expertise
- Objectives of learning
- Potential for achieving learning outcomes (acquisition, retention, and recall)
- Cost effectiveness
- Instructional setting
- Evolving technology

These many variables are addressed in the following review of the instructional methods available for teaching and learning.

Lecture

Lecture can be defined as a highly structured method by which the teacher verbally transmits information directly to groups of learners for the purpose of instruction. It is one of the oldest and most often used approaches to teaching.

The word lecture comes from the Latin term *lectura,* which means "to read." The lecture method has been much maligned in recent years because in its purest form, the lecture format allows for only minimal exchange between the teacher and the learner. Also, critics of the lecture method have expressed particular concern about the passive role of learners (DeYoung, 2003).

Nevertheless, if a lecture is well organized and delivered effectively, it can be a very useful method of instruction (Bain, 2004; Bartlett, 2003). The lecture format can demonstrate patterns, highlight main ideas, or present unique ways of viewing information, such as introducing an agency's mission statement to new nursing staff orientees or explaining diabetes mellitus to a group of lay people. The lecture should not be employed, however, to give people the same information that they could read independently at another time and place. It is the lecturer's expertise, both in theory and experience, that can substantially contribute to the learner's understanding of a subject.

The lecture is an ideal way to provide foundational background information as a basis for subsequent group discussions. Also, it is a means to summarize data and current research findings not available elsewhere (Boyd, Gleit, Graham, & Whitman, 1998). In addition, the lecture can be easily supplemented with handout materials and other audiovisual aids. **Table 11–1** summarizes the main advantages and limitations of the lecture method of instruction.

Lecturing is an acquired skill learned over time, and it is a more complex task than commonly thought (Young & Diekelmann, 2002). Specific strategies exist to strengthen the effectiveness of a lecture (Cantillon, 2003). Each lecture should include an introduction, body, and conclusion.

INTRODUCTION

During the introduction phase of a lecture, learners should be presented with an overview of the behavioral objectives pertinent to the lecture topic, along with an explanation as to why these objectives are significant. The use of set, the open-

---

Table 11–1 MAJOR ADVANTAGES AND LIMITATIONS OF LECTURE

ADVANTAGES

- An efficient, cost-effective means for transmitting large amounts of information to a large number of people at the same time and within a relatively reasonable time frame.

- Useful to demonstrate patterns, highlight main ideas, summarize data, and present unique ways of viewing information.

- An effective approach for cognitive learning, especially at lower levels of the cognitive domain.

- Useful in providing foundational background information as a basis for subsequent learning, such as group discussion.

- Easily supplemented with handout materials and other audiovisual aids to enhance learning.

LIMITATIONS

- Largely ineffective in influencing affective and psychomotor behaviors.

- Does not provide for much stimulation or participatory involvement of learners.

- Very instructor centered, and thus the most active participant is frequently the most knowledgeable one—the teacher.

- Does not account for individual differences in background, attention span, or learning style.

- All learners are exposed to the same information regardless of their cognitive abilities, learning needs, or stages of coping.

- The diversity within groups makes it challenging, if not impossible, for the teacher to reach all learners equally.

ing to a presentation, can engage attention and focus the group on the speaker, which gets learners ready to listen. This technique of set captures attention, clarifies goals and objectives, motivates the learner, and demonstrates the relevance of the content in a way that can stimulate the interest of learners in the subject. As an example, prior to a lecture on creative problem solving, each member of the audience can be asked to solve a puzzle that requires them to think in a different manner (Kowalski, 2004). Learners' attention can also be engaged by conducting an informal survey or stating the objectives as questions that will be answered during the body of the lecture.

If the occasion is one of a series of lectures, the lecturer needs to make a connection with the overall subject and the topic being presented as well as its relationship to previous topics covered and the lectures that will follow. And lastly, the lecturer should establish a rapport with the audience by letting his or her personality shine through and by using humor, if appropriate.

BODY

The next portion of the lecture involves the actual delivery of the content related to the topic being addressed. Careful preparation is needed so that the important aspects are covered in an organized, accurate, logical, cohesive, and interesting manner. Examples should be used throughout to enhance the salient points, but extraneous facts and redundant examples should be avoided so as not to reduce the impact of the message. Because the lecture format tends to be a passive approach to learning, the instructor can enhance the effectiveness of the presentation by combining it with other instructional methods, such as discussion or question and answer sessions, to enhance active learner participation.

Use of audiovisual materials, such as a video, overhead projections, or PowerPoint slides, can also add variety to a lecture. The widespread availability of computer software programs makes it easy to enhance a presentation, but lecturers should adhere to the following general guidelines (Evans, 2000):

- Do not put all content on slides, but include only the key concepts to supplement the presentation.
- Use the largest font possible.
- Do not exceed 25 words per slide.
- Choose colors that provide a high level of contrast between background and text if presenting in a large room with bright lights.
- Use graphics for presenting large amounts of numerical data.
- Do not overdo the use of action figures, which can be very distracting to the audience.
- Make sure that all audiovisual equipment is functional, and the instructor should know how to use it to avoid a technical malfunction that will be disconcerting for both lecturer and audience.

Nervous or inexperienced lecturers should practice first before a mirror, a video camera, or a colleague. They should outline just the key points of their presentation on index cards, overhead projections, or slides. They can use this summary information to elaborate on the topic by giving examples and further explanations. Reading a printed copy of the entire presentation word for word is exceedingly boring and is a sure way to turn off the audience. Also, instructors should vary their presentation style and tone of voice to avoid monotony and move around the stage or room. Demonstrating enthusiasm, expertise, and interest in the topic will capture and hold the group's attention. Finally, they should be sure to keep within the time allotted. Lectures of long duration will result in loss of attention and boredom on the part of the learner.

Conclusion

If a lecture has not exceeded the prescribed time, the instructor can avoid having it end abruptly without a wrap-up. This final section of the lecture format is reserved to summarize the information provided in the presentation. At this juncture, review the major concepts presented. Try to leave some leeway for questions and answers. Lecturers who are using a microphone in a large group should be sure to repeat the questions asked so the rest of the audience can hear them and understand the response. If time runs short, the instructor will be able to answer only a few queries, but he or she should invite immediate follow-up by meeting with interested individuals alone or in a smaller group or by suggesting relevant readings.

Although the lecture method is considered efficient and cost effective, the effort put into design and delivery should not be determined just by calculating the teacher–learner ratio of contact hours. Other factors must be taken into account, such as teacher preparation time, how often the same material needs to be repeated to different audiences, and follow-up time required to individualize learning and evaluate outcomes.

With the advent of networking technology, the lecture can be delivered to even a wider variety of learners in locations far away from one another. Distance learning is an ideal way to maximize resources and to transmit current information. The cost and time of travel no longer needs to be incurred for the audience to meet face-to-face with an expert.

Group Discussion

Group discussion, by definition, is a method of teaching whereby learners get together to exchange information, feelings, and opinions with one another and with the teacher. As a commonly employed instructional technique, this method is learner centered as well as subject centered. Group discussion is an effective method for teaching in both the affective and cognitive domains.

Group size, a major consideration in group teaching, should be determined by the purpose or task to be accomplished (Boyd et al., 1998). Group size can vary somewhat but discussion is most effective with relatively small groups because more learners can take an active role (DeYoung, 2003). For patient education, 2–20 members with an average of 10 has been recommended as the most desirable size (Tang, Funnell, & Anderson, 2006).

Preset behavioral objectives should be the focus when using this method. These objectives guide the achievement of the learning outcomes for the interaction and should be presented at the beginning of each session. Careful adherence to them will prevent the discussion from becoming an aimless wandering of ideas or a forum for the strongest group member to expound on his or her opinions and feelings. The teacher's role is to act as a facilitator to keep the discussion focused and to tie important points together. The instructor must be well versed in the subject matter to field questions, to move the discussion along in the direction intended, and to give appropriate feedback.

Teacher involvement and control of the process vary with the needs of the group members. Group discussion requires the teacher to be able to tolerate less structure and organization than other methods such as lecture or one-to-one instruction. The group must have some knowledge of the content before this method can be effective; otherwise, the discussion will be based on pooled ignorance. For example, a group of staff with a significant amount of practical knowledge and expertise may need little input while they work out a complex patient problem. A new group of patients or family members with little understanding of a topic will need to access information directly from the teacher or another source before they can meaningfully participate in problem solving integral to the discussion process.

The teacher's responsibility is to make sure that every member of the group has interpreted information correctly, because failure to do so will lead to conclusions based on faulty data. For this reason, patient groups need to be pre-screened. While diversity within a group is beneficial, a large range in literacy skills, states of anxiety, and experiences with acute and chronic conditions may lead to difficulty in meeting any one member's needs.

Abruzzese (1996) suggested some learning techniques as good vehicles for active learning that require preparation by staff prior to the group discussion activity. For example, debates offer teams with opposing views the opportunity to present each side of an issue and help staff consider others' perspectives. Seminars can be designed so that each member reads an assignment and considers questions prior to the discussion so that all learners can actively participate. The case study approach offers an opportunity to thoroughly become acquainted with a patient situation before discussing

patient needs and identifying health-related problems. Another example of the creative use of this teaching method with staff is arranging a panel presentation by patients coping with a specific disease or problem. Following the panel, a group session is most beneficial, in particular, for affective learning. This was found to be a useful approach to breaking down the negative stereotypes of persons living with AIDS on the part of some healthcare workers (Peters & Connell, 1991).

Carkhuff (1996) addressed the reflection-on-action technique for work groups as learning groups to develop the critical thinking skills of nursing staff in the workplace. The educator facilitates staff, critically analyzing their actions and determining if there is an alternative to their action. It is helping learners learn to learn.

It is important for the teacher to maintain the trust of the group. Everyone must feel safe and comfortable enough to express his or her point of view. Harsh or sarcastic treatment resulting in insults breaks down the relationship between the teacher and the learners as well as relationships among learners, which creates an environment unsuitable for learning. One helpful approach is to tell the group at the beginning of the session that the goal is to hear from all members by asking for their input and points of view during the discussion period. Persons who digress should be requested to hold questions that can be handled privately until the end of class because these inquiries are important but unique to their circumstances.

Respectful attention and tolerance toward others should be modeled by the teacher and required of all group members. Of course, this consideration does not preclude correcting errors or disagreements. A clear message must be given stating that while personal opinions may be debatable, the inherent value of what each member has to say and the member's right to participate is guaranteed.

Teaching people in groups rather than individually allows the teacher to reach a number of learners at the same time. The group discussion method is economically beneficial from a time-efficiency perspective when compared with educating each learner individually. With healthcare costs rising, this method should be considered as an efficient and effective method to teach simultaneously a number of individuals who have similar learning needs, such as information to prepare for childbirth or cardiac bypass surgery. Oermann (2003) reported that a group of patients in a waiting room of an ambulatory care center were educated via a videotape about glaucoma, which was then followed by group interaction with a nurse to discuss key points and answer questions. This approach led to higher satisfaction with the education received during their visit.

Discussion is effective in assisting learners to identify resources and to internalize the topic being discussed by helping them to reflect on its personal meaning (Brookfield & Preskill, 1999). Through group work, members share common concerns and receive reinforcement from one another. The idea that everyone is in the same boat or if one person can do it, so can the others serves to stimulate motivation for learning as a result of peer support.

Group discussion has proved particularly helpful to patients and families dealing with chronic illness. This method is most effective during the accommodation stage of psychological adjustment to chronic illness, because the interactions reduce isolation and foster identification with others who are in similar circum-

stances (Fredette, 1990). Discussion in a group offers members a forum for them to share information for cognitive growth as well as an opportunity to learn self-efficacy. This increase in confidence levels of patients and families enhances their ability to handle an illness (Lorig & Gonzalez, 1993).

Group process informs people about how to respond to situations, improve their coping mechanisms, and explore ways to incorporate needed changes into their lives. Group self-management education for people with diabetes has been found in some instances to be not only more cost effective but to result in greater treatment satisfaction and to be slightly better in supporting lifestyle changes (Tang et al., 2006).

Table 11–2 highlights the main advantages and limitations of group discussion as a method of instruction.

It must be noted that third-party reimbursement for some types of group patient education programs may be difficult to obtain when the traditional fee-for-service payment system is not in place. However, these programs may be economically valuable in preventing hospitalization or reducing time in acute care. Documenting these benefits based on measurable outcomes can justify the importance of group discussion as a cost-effective method of instruction.

One-to-One Instruction

One-to-one instruction involves delivering information specifically designed to meet the needs of an individual learner. It is an opportunity for both the teacher and the learner to communicate knowledge, ideas, and feelings primarily through oral exchange, although nonverbal messages can be conveyed as well. This method should never be a lecture delivered to an audience of one to meet the teacher's goals. Instead, the experience

---

Table 11–2 MAJOR ADVANTAGES AND LIMITATIONS OF GROUP DISCUSSION

ADVANTAGES

- Enhances learning in both the affective and cognitive domains.

- Is both learner centered and subject centered.

- Stimulates learners to think about issues and problems.

- Encourages members to exchange their own experiences, thereby making learning more active and less isolating.

- Provides opportunities for sharing of ideas and concerns.

- Fosters positive peer support and feelings of belonging.

- Reinforces previous learning.

LIMITATIONS

- One or more members may dominate the discussion.

- Easy to digress from the topic, which interferes with achievement of the objectives.

- Shy learners may refuse to become involved or may need a great deal of encouragement to participate.

- Requires skill to tactfully redirect learners who digress or dominate without losing their trust and that of other group members.

- Particularly challenging for the novice teacher when members do not easily interact.

- More time consuming for transmission of information than other methods such as lecture.

- Requires teacher's presence at all sessions to act as facilitator and resource person.

---

should actively involve the learner and be based on his or her unique learning needs.

One-to-one instruction can be tailored to meet objectives in all three domains of learning. It begins with an assessment of the learner and the mutual setting of objectives to be accomplished. As part of the assessment process, it is very important to determine if any problem behaviors such as smoking exist and at which stage of change the person is with respect to

dealing with such behaviors. Once this is determined, educational interventions can be tailored to that stage (Prochaska, DiClemente, Velicer, & Rossi, 1993). The stages of change model (as described in Chapter 6) is generalizable across a broad range of behaviors, including but not limited to smoking cessation, weight control, avoidance of high-fat diets, safer sex, and exercise initiation (Prochaska et al., 1994). The following describes how nurse educators can focus their interactions to help a learner through the stages of change (Saarmann, Daugherty, & Riegel, 2000):

- *Precontemplation stage*—provide information in a nonthreatening manner so that the learner becomes aware of the negative aspects or consequences of his/her behavior.
- *Contemplation stage*—support decision making for change by identifying benefits, considering barriers to the change, and making suggestions for dealing with these obstacles.
- *Preparation stage*—support a move to action by contracting with the learner in establishing small, realistic, and measurable goals, providing information on effective ways to achieve the desired change, and giving positive reinforcement.
- *Action stage*—encourage constant practice of the new behavior to instill commitment to change by pointing out the benefits of each step achieved, providing rewards and incentives, and assisting the learner to monitor his or her behavior through the implementation of such strategies as keeping a food diary.
- *Maintenance stage*—continue encouragement and support to consolidate the new behavior and prevent relapses.

For example, the patient with a chronic problem such as obesity will need to consider the options available for weight control and then an action plan he thinks can be accomplished can be designed. His confidence level can be assessed by asking on a scale of 0–10 how certain he is of achieving this goal. A score of seven or higher makes it more likely he will be successful (Lorig, 2003).

Mutual goal setting is a very important first step to be undertaken between the teacher and the learner. Contracting, which clearly spells out the roles and expectations of both teacher and learner, is one effective way to facilitate mutual goal setting. Contracts should be written in specific terms and evaluated by both participants (see an explanation of learning contracts in Chapter 10).

Whenever teaching is done on a one-to-one basis, instructions should be specific and time should be given for an immediate response from the learner followed by direct feedback from the teacher. Allowing learners the opportunity to state their understanding of information gives the teacher an opportunity to evaluate the extent of learning. Also, communicating to learners what further information is forthcoming allows them to connect what they have just learned with what they will be learning. For example, the nurse teaching a patient about hypoglycemia might say, "Now that you understand what causes low blood sugar, we will talk about how to tell when you have it and what to do if you experience it after discharge."

The process of one-to-one instruction involves moving learners from repeating the information that was shared to applying what they have just learned. In the preceding example regarding hypoglycemia, the nurse might offer the learner a hypothetical situation similar to what the patient might experience given his lifestyle and have him work through how to respond to it. In this type of one-to-one exchange, a potentially threatening situation can be presented in a nonthreatening manner (Boyd et al., 1998). For instance, the instructor might ask a busy executive who has diabetes how he would respond to feeling shaky and sweaty at 2:00 p.m. on a day when a meeting runs late and he misses lunch.

Be sure to clearly state that scenarios like this are not a test but rather a "dress rehearsal" for life situations. You can change the scenarios with further questioning to help learners plan how they could prevent such occurrences in the future. This technique gives learners a chance to use the information at a higher cognitive level and provides an opportunity for the nurse educator to evaluate their learning in a safe environment.

With the one-to-one method of instruction, questioning is an excellent technique. It encourages learners to be active participants in the learning process and gives the instructor important feedback on their progress. Questions can be matched with the behavioral objectives to be achieved. For example, to determine a patient's knowledge level in the cognitive domain, the instructor might ask "What is the next step that you should take?" For the higher level of synthesis in the cognitive domain, the nurse educator might ask a staff nurse to plan for how he or she would respond to an angry family member (Abruzzese, 1996).

Questioning should not be interpreted by the learner as a test of knowledge but rather as a way to exchange information and stimulate thinking. However, two problems can occur with questioning. Questions can be so ambiguous that the learner does not know what the question is, or they can contain too many facts to process effectively (House, Chassie, & Spohn, 1990). The instructor should watch the learner's nonverbal reactions and rephrase the question if he or she detects either of these problems. If the learner seems confused, it is helpful to state that perhaps the question was not clear. This technique will guard against the learner feeling guilty or becoming discouraged if a question was incorrectly answered.

Also, it is important to give learners time to process information and respond to your ques-

tions. Sometimes teachers are uncomfortable waiting in silence for an answer or are impatient and attempt to correct an answer before learners complete their responses. Questioning will be ineffective as a technique when learners are not given enough time to process information. Preliminary interruption may further interfere with a learner's thinking abilities and create a tense atmosphere.

Many nurse educators conduct individualized teaching of other nurses or student learners in the clinical setting. Clinical instruction is not a discrete instructional method but rather can be an extension of one-to-one teaching in a very complex setting for experiential learning. A variety of methods other than one-to-one instruction can be used, such as role modeling, demonstration, return demonstration, and group discussion. However, one-to-one instruction very well may be involved as a teaching approach during new employee orientation, student preceptorship, or a continuing staff education activity. The learner is singularly guided in the actual practice setting and each learning experience requires specific objectives, known to both the instructor and the learner, that are tailored to meet the individual's needs. A performance-based development system was designed to determine a newly hired nurse's competency (del Bueno, Griffin, Burke, & Foley, 1990). This structured assessment of an individual's abilities is completed before initiating clinical experiences. Very focused clinical activities can then be planned with the staff nurse, nurse educator, and clinical manager to optimize experiences for learning.

Preceptors who assume clinical teaching roles are usually expert clinicians but may not necessarily be expert teachers. If this is the case, in order to carry out their roles effectively, they will need to be taught how to be educators through workshops and coaching sessions. One-to-one instruction has many strengths as a teaching method, but it also has its drawbacks. Table 11–3 summarizes the major advantages and limitations of this method.

From an economic standpoint, one-to-one instruction is a very labor-intensive method and should be well tailored to make the expense worthwhile in terms of achieving learner outcomes. One-to-one teaching of patients and families is often an inefficient approach to learning because the educator is reaching only one person at a time. Clinical teaching of students and continuing education for staff are vital for professional development, but they are costly endeavors when carried out on a one-to-one basis. Also, orientation of new staff is a significant expense to an institution or agency in terms of payroll dollars and short-term nonproductivity of the employee being oriented (del Bueno et al., 1990).

Demonstration and Return Demonstration

It is imperative to begin this discussion by making a clear distinction between demonstration and return demonstration. *Demonstration* is done

---

Table 11–3 MAJOR ADVANTAGES AND LIMITATIONS OF ONE-TO-ONE INSTRUCTION

ADVANTAGES

- The pace and content of teaching can be tailored to meet individual needs.

- Ideal as an intervention for initial assessment and ongoing evaluation of the learner.

- Good for teaching behaviors in all three domains of learning.

- Especially suitable for teaching those who are learning disabled, low literate, or educationally disadvantaged.

- Provides opportunity for immediate feedback to be shared between the teacher and the learner.

LIMITATIONS

- The learner is isolated from others who have similar needs or concerns.

- Deprives learners of the opportunity to identify with others and share information, ideas, and feelings with those in like circumstances.

- Can put learners on the spot because they are the sole focus of the teacher's attention.

- Questioning may be interpreted by the learner as a technique to test their knowledge and skills.

- The learner may feel overwhelmed and anxious if the educator makes the mistake of cramming too much information into each session.

by the teacher to show the learner how to perform a particular skill. *Return demonstration* is carried out by the learner in an attempt to perform a task with cues from the teacher as needed. These two methods require different abilities by both the teacher and the learner. In particular, they are effective in teaching psychomotor domain skills. However, both also may be used to enhance cognitive and affective learning, such as when helping a staff member develop interactive skills for crisis intervention or assertiveness training.

Prior to giving a demonstration, the teacher should inform learners of the purpose of the procedure, the sequential steps involved, the equipment needed, and the actions expected of them. Equipment should be tested before use to ensure that it is complete and in working order. For the demonstration method to be employed effectively, the learners must be able to clearly see and hear the steps being taught. Therefore, the demonstration method is best suited to teaching individuals or small groups. A large screen or multiple screens for video presentations of demonstrations can allow larger groups to participate.

Watching a demonstration can be a passive activity for learners, whose role is to observe the teacher presenting an exact performance of a required skill. The demonstration can be enhanced if the teacher slows down the pace of performing the demonstration, exaggerates some of the steps (de Tornyay & Thompson, 1987) or breaks lengthy procedures into a series of shorter steps. In the process of demonstrating a skill to either nurses or patients, it is important to explain why each step needs to be carried out in a certain manner (DeYoung, 2003; Lorig, 2003).

Demonstration allows for mental rehearsal of procedures (Haggard, 1989). The performance should be flawless, but it is important that the educator take advantage of a mistake to show how errors can be handled. If an error does occur, it may serve to increase rapport with the learners and allow them to relax, knowing mistakes do happen and can be corrected. However, too many mistakes disrupt the mental image that the learners are forming.

When demonstrating a psychomotor skill, if possible, the nurse educator should work with the exact equipment that the learner will be expected to use. This consideration is particularly important for novice learners. For instance, the patient or family member who is learning to administer tube feedings at home will be anxious and frustrated if taught with one type of pump in the hospital when another type is used after discharge. Often the learner is too inexperienced to see the skill pattern and instead will treat handling of each pump as a separate task. The seasoned staff nurse, on the other hand, will find it easier to transfer what is already known about tube feeding pumps if called on to learn to use a newly purchased pump from a different manufacturer.

Return demonstration should be planned to occur as close as possible to when the demonstration was given. Learners may need reassurance to reduce their anxiety prior to beginning of the performance because the opportunity for return demonstration may be viewed by them as a test. This may lead them to believe they are expected to carry out the expectation of a perfect performance the very first time around. Once a learner recognizes that the teacher is a coach and not an evaluator, the climate will be less tense and the learner will be more comfortable in attempting to practice a new skill. Stress the fact that it is expected that the initial performance will not be perfect.

In addition, allowing the learner to manipulate the equipment before being expected to use it may help to reduce anxiety levels. Some patients may experience an increased sense of unease when faced with learning a new skill because they identify the need to learn a skill in relation to their illness. For example, a young woman learning to care for a venous access device may be very anxious because her diagnosis of cancer has necessitated the need for this device.

When the learner is giving a return demonstration, the teacher should remain silent except for offering cues when necessary or briefly answering questions. Learners may be prompted by a series of pictures or coached by a partner with a checklist. The first time patients return a demonstration they may need a significant amount of coaching. Instructors should limit their help to coaching and not doing the task for the patients. The next time they practice, the instructor should observe and coach only if needed (Lorig, 2003). Also, instructors should avoid casual conversations or asking questions because they merely serve to interrupt the learner's thought processes and interfere with efforts to focus on mentally imprinting the procedure while performing the task.

Breaking the steps of the procedure into small increments will give the learner the opportunity to master one sequence before attempting the next. Praising the learner along the way for each step correctly performed will reinforce behavior and give the learner confidence in being able to successfully accomplish the task in its entirety. Emphasis should be on what to do, rather than on what not to do.

Practice should be supervised until the learner is competent enough to perform steps accurately. It is important that the initial skill pattern be correct before allowing for independent practice. To ensure safety, high-risk skills should be performed first on a model prior to actual clinical application.

Learners will need a varying amount of practice to become competent, but once they have acquired the skill, they can then practice on their own to increase speed and proficiency. The value of practice should not be underestimated. For a new skill to become automatic and long lasting, repeated practice beyond the point of mastery is essential (Willingham, 2004). However, if a task is similar to one performed before, the time required to master a skill will be less. For example, a critical care nurse will probably need little practice with a new IV pump that is like other kinds already mastered. In contrast, a patient learning for the first time to manipulate a pump for home IV therapy may need many practice sessions.

Return demonstration sessions should be planned close enough together so that the learner does not lose the benefit of the most recent practice session. As with demonstration, the equipment for return demonstration needs to exactly match that used by the instructor and expected to be used by the learner. Learners also will require help in compensating for individual differences. For instance, if you are right-handed and the learner is left-handed, sitting across from each other during instruction would be more helpful than sitting adjacent to one another. The person with difficulty seeing the increments on a syringe may need a magnifying device to facilitate accurate performance of a skill.

A summary of the advantages and limitations of demonstration and return demonstration can be found in **Table 11–4**.

Perhaps the biggest drawbacks to demonstration and return demonstration are the expenses

---

Table 11–4 MAJOR ADVANTAGES AND LIMITATIONS OF DEMONSTRATION AND RETURN DEMONSTRATION

ADVANTAGES

- Especially effective for learning in the psychomotor domain.

- Actively engages the learner through stimulation of visual, auditory, and tactile senses.

- Repetition of movement and constant reinforcement increases confidence, competence, and skill retention.

- Provides opportunity for overlearning to achieve the goal.

LIMITATIONS

- Requires plenty of time to be set aside for teaching as well as learning.

- Size of audience must be kept small to ensure opportunity for practice and close supervision.

- Equipment can be expensive to purchase and replace.

- Extra space and equipment is needed for practicing certain skills.

- Competency evaluation requires 1:1 teacher–student ratio.

---

associated with these methods. Group size must be kept small to ensure that each learner is able to visualize the procedures being performed and to have the opportunity for practice. Individual supervision is required during follow-up practices. Furthermore, the cost of obtaining, maintaining, and replacing equipment is significant and also must be calculated.

There are some ways, however, to reduce the cost of these methods. If, for example, the audience is comprised of a homogeneous group of health professionals who need yearly CPR review, demonstration can be done via videotape. Also, return demonstration can initially be performed with a partner supervising the competency of the skill. Nevertheless, the final evaluation of staff competency must be carried out by an expert to ensure the accuracy of learning. In addition, expenses can be reduced by reusing equipment if it will not interfere with the accuracy, safety, or completeness of the demonstration/return demonstration.

Gaming

Gaming is an instructional method requiring the learner to participate in a competitive activity with preset rules. The goal is for the learners to win a game by applying knowledge and rehearsing skills previously learned. Games can be simple or they can be more complex to challenge the learner's ability to use higher order problem-solving and critical-thinking strategies. These activities do not have to reflect reality, but they are designed to accomplish educational objectives. This instructional method is primarily effective for improving cognitive functioning but can also be used to enhance skills in the psychomotor domain and to influence affective behavior through increased social interaction (Robinson, Lewis, & Robinson, 1990). Games connect theory to experience for nurses without any risk to patient safety (Henry, 1997).

Games can be placed anywhere in the sequence of a learning activity (Joos, 1984)—as a device to conduct a needs assessment, introduce a topic, check learner progress, or summarize information. However, some games may require prerequisite knowledge for the learner to participate effectively and, therefore, may require a prior session of teaching before the game can be played (Henry, 1997). For purposes of a needs assessment, Rowell and Spielvogle (1996) used an infection-control game to determine whether a knowledge deficit among staff was contributing to rising rates of methicillin resistant *Staphylococcus aureus* (MRSA). The staff members were asked to identify violations of infection-control practices in a mock isolation room. Participants completed and turned in an answer sheet, then proceeded to an answer station. Not only did staff have an opportunity to test themselves and correct wrong information, but participants also provided information that was helpful in planning future education programs.

Games can be designed for a single individual, such as puzzles, or for activities participation by a group of players. For gaming activities that involve multiple participants, the teacher's role is that of a facilitator. At the beginning of a game, the learners need to be told the objectives and the rules. Any materials required to play a game are distributed, and the various teams are assigned. Once the game starts, the teacher needs to keep the flow going and interpret the rules. The game should be interrupted as seldom or as briefly as possible so as not to disturb the pace (Joos, 1984).

When the game is completed, winners should be rewarded. Prizes do not have to be expensive because their main purpose is to acknowledge achievement of learners in a public manner (Robinson et al., 1990). At the finish of the game, the teacher should conduct a debriefing session focusing on educational content and evaluating the gaming experience. Learners should be given a chance to discuss what they learned, ask questions, receive feedback regarding the outcome of the game, and offer suggestions for improving the process.

Games may be either purchased or designed. Well-known commercial games such as Trivial Pursuit, bingo, Monopoly, or Jeopardy have the advantage in that their formats can be modified, the equipment is reusable for different topics, and many players already have familiarity with the rules of the games. Word searches, crossword puzzles, treasure hunts, and card and board games also are flexible in format and can be developed inexpensively and with relative ease. Be sure to test any games prior to widespread use. Some examples of games are: a word search puzzle for foods (**Figure 11–1**) known to elevate serum potassium that is appropriate for use by patients with end-stage renal disease (Robinson et al., 1990); Emergency Pursuit, which has content related to emergency situations that staff might encounter on a medical-surgical unit (Schmitz, MacLean, & Shidler, 1991); and a sacred cow contest for nursing students that generates their interest in examining the evidence base for selected nursing practices (Leake, 2004). Computer games, although much more expensive, are becoming increasingly available and are a popular option for many learners.

Figure 11–1 Sample word search game for patients.

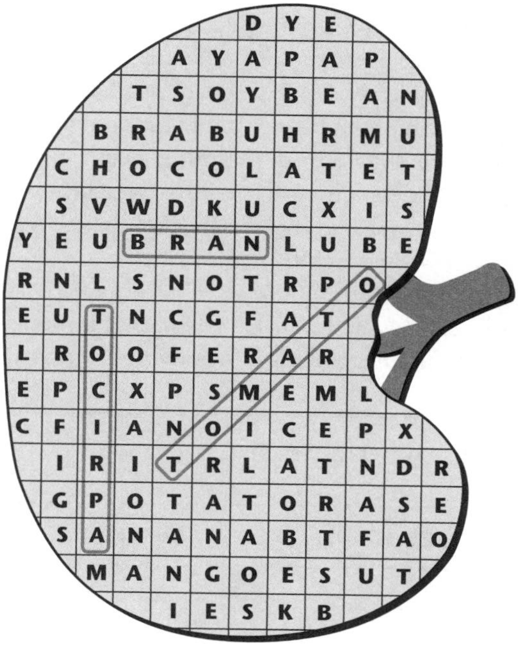

Source: Robinson, K. J., Lewis, D. J., & Robinson, J. A. (1990). Games: A way to give laboratory values meaning. (1990, August). *ANNA Journal, 17*(4), 307. Reprinted with permission of the American Nephrology Nurses Association, publisher.

Computer games, also referred to as *edutainment* (educational software disguised in a game format), introduce content or involve the process of competition in the application of strategies for decision making toward attaining a goal. They are an enjoyable and effective way to teach specific cognitive, psychomotor, and affective skills (Green & Brightman, 1990). The Game Show Presenter, software that is now available to educators to create many types of games, can be accessed at http://www.almorale.com.

Gaming is a method particularly attractive to children, who enjoy the challenge of learning through play-like activity. Lieberman (2001) described an interactive video game designed for people ages 8–16 years with Type 1 diabetes. This game modeled the daily challenges of self-care, and participants were told to play the game as much or as little as they wished. By the end of the 6-month trial, there was a 77% drop in diabetes-related urgent care as well as an increase in self-efficacy in communication with parents about diabetes and in self-care related to diabetes.

Lewis, Saydak, Mierzwa, and Robinson (1989) designed a game suitability checklist that remains relevant today in determining if gaming is a viable alternative to meet the objectives for learning (**Figure 11–2**).

It is particularly important to remember that games, whether purchased or self-developed, must serve the purpose of helping the learner accomplish the predetermined behavioral objectives. Are people learning while they are having fun? Bays and Hermann (1997) tested students who learned the same content but through two different methods. One group was taught with gaming and the other with lecture. A posttest showed no significant difference in scores between the two groups. Lieberman (2001) reported that children and adolescents improved their self-care after engaging in interactive games related to smoking prevention, asthma, and diabetes.

The advantages and limitations of the gaming method are outlined in **Table 11–5**.

Economic considerations include either the cost of purchasing a game or the time taken by the instructor to design, test, and update the gaming material. Also, some types of games require the educator to be present as facilitator each time that they are played.

Simulation

Simulation is a method whereby an artificial or hypothetical experience that engages the learner

Figure 11–2 Game suitability checklist.

GAME SUITABILITY CHECKLIST		
Criteria	**Yes**	**No**
• Does the game meet the program objectives?	_____	_____
• Can the game be completed within the time allotted?	_____	_____
• Is the size and layout of the room conducive to the game?	_____	_____
• Will the available participants meet the minimum number required for the game?	_____	_____
• Do staff members have the time and interest to design or adapt games? If not, are funds available to purchase games?	_____	_____
• If the game requires equipment or supplies, are they readily available?	_____	_____
a. Are resources or funds available to design or purchase needed materials?	_____	_____
b. Does the game require replacement of materials following each use?	_____	_____
• Does the game require preparation or cleanup time?	_____	_____

Source: Lewis, D. J., Sayjack, S. J., Mierzwa, I. P., & Robinson, J. A. (1989). Gaming: A teaching strategy for adult learners. *Journal of Continuing Education in Nursing, 20,* 80–84. Reprinted with permission from *The Journal of Continuing Education in Nursing.*

Table 11–5 MAJOR ADVANTAGES AND LIMITATIONS OF GAMING

ADVANTAGES

- Games are fun with a purpose.

- Retention of information is promoted by stimulating learner enthusiasm and increasing learner involvement.

- Easy to devise or modify for individual or group learning.

- Adds variety to the learning experience.

- Excellent for dull or repetitious content that must be periodically reviewed.

LIMITATIONS

- Creates a competitive environment that may be threatening to some learners.

- Group size may need to be kept small for participation by all learners.

- Requires more flexible space for teamwork than a traditional conference room or classroom.

- Potentially higher noise level may require special space accommodations.

- Requirements may be more physically demanding than many other methods.

- Some learners may not be able to participate if they are restricted by a disability.

---

in an activity that reflects real-life conditions but without the risk-taking consequences of an actual situation is created (Rystedt & Lindstrom, 2001). To some extent, an overlap exists between the methods of gaming, simulation, and role playing because all three instructional approaches require learners to engage in experiential learning. Simulation allows participants to make decisions in a safe environment, witness the consequences, and evaluate the effectiveness of their actions (DeYoung, 2003; Lyons & Milton, 1999). A follow-up discussion with learners after use of these experiential methods is important to facilitate their analysis of the experience.

When planning a simulation, it is most effective if the learning experience is made to resemble real life as much as possible but in a nonthreatening way. The activity should challenge the decision-making ability of the learner by imposing time constraints, providing realistic levels of tension, and using actual equipment or other important features of the environment in which the specific skill will be performed. For example, a scenario could be developed to help parents of a baby prevent sudden infant death syndrome (SIDS) by working through a situation in which a monitor signals respiratory difficulty in their infant. As another example, a staff nurse along with other team members are expected to make a rapid assessment and intervene with accuracy, coordination, and speed in caring for a chest trauma victim in a simulated emergency room setting.

These simulations can be created for the purpose of determining whether the learner has the necessary skills to perform the activity correctly. Simulation should always be followed by a debriefing session that includes a discussion of events that happened during the experience, the decisions made, the actions taken, the consequences of the choices, the possible alternatives, and suggestions for improvement in skill performance. Simulations provide the opportunity for anticipatory learning (Abruzzese, 1996; Lyons & Milton, 1999).

There are many types of simulations, including the following:

- Written simulations use case studies about real or fictitious situations and the learner must respond to these scenarios. Staff nurses, for example, are asked to describe how they would handle a personnel communication problem on a unit or manage a physiologically complex patient in the critical care environment.

- Clinical simulations can be set up to replicate complex care situations, such as a mock cardiac arrest. An experienced nurse is a buddy or a coach for the inexperienced nurse who is running the code. This simulation allows the novice to practice these skills in a nonthreatening situation with immediate feedback. Participants reported that this simulation helped them validate their thinking and allowed for ongoing thinking out loud in formulating questions they might otherwise not have asked (Cuda, Doerr, & Gonzalez, 1999).

- Model simulations are frequently used to teach a variety of audiences. For

instance, a nurse may be taught to change a dressing on a model. An effective and economical method to teach certain noninvasive skills is to ask a peer, instructor, or trained individual to act as a patient. Standard patients—people trained to act as patients—were found to be a more effective method of simulation to teach fundamentals to nursing students than lectures and laboratory practice with a model (Yoo & Yoo, 2003).

An exciting new technology is high-fidelity whole-body patient simulators, such as Sim-Man, that reproduce in a sophisticated, lifelike manner the cardiovascular, respiratory, urinary, and neurological systems. Some models even have the ability to respond to selected drugs. However, this resource is still limited by the high cost of this technology (Lupien & George-Gay, 2001).

- Computer simulations are in use in learning laboratories to mimic situations whereby information as well as feedback is given to learners in helping them to develop decision-making skills (Lyons & Milton, 1999; Turner, 2007).

Although the learning laboratory is a commonplace teaching environment for nursing students on college campuses and has been used in the last 15 years to update the skills of nurses reentering the workforce (Wood, 1994), these simulated experiences are not yet widely available to train patients or family providers in self-care skills due to lack of space and the high cost of simulators. In the future, simulation with high-tech, portable equipment could revolutionize patient education.

Simulated experiences for the learner should be followed with actual experiences as soon as possible. Simulation is never exactly the same as the real thing to prepare the learner. Therefore, the learner will need help with the transfer of skills acquired in a simulated experience to the actual situation. Virtual reality technology, still in its infancy in healthcare settings, has the potential to narrow the distance even more between simulation and real life for the education of patients, nursing students, and staff (Turner, 2007).

Simulation can be made more cost effective by reuse of supplies. **Table 11–6** summarizes the main strengths and drawbacks of the simulation method of instruction.

Role Playing

Role playing is a method by which learners participate in an unrehearsed dramatization. They are asked to play assigned parts of a character as they think the character would act in reality. This method is a technique to arouse feelings and elicit emotional responses in the learners. It is used primarily to achieve behavioral objectives in the affective domain. Unlike simulation, which teaches learners mastery of skills for application to their own real-life situations, role playing is a method that teaches learners real-life situations to develop understanding of other people (Redman, 2007). For example, a nurse attending an education program on sensory disabilities will be given the experience of wearing special glasses to see how it feels to function with impaired vision.

The responsibility of the teacher is to design a situation with enough information for learners to be able to assume the role of someone else without actually giving them a script to follow. Occasionally, people are assigned to play them-

---

Table 11–6 MAJOR ADVANTAGES AND LIMITATIONS OF SIMULATION

ADVANTAGES

- Excellent for psychomotor skill development.

- Enhances higher level problem-solving and interactive abilities in the cognitive and affective domains.

- Provides for active learner involvement in a real-life situation with consequences determined by variables inherent in the situation.

- Guarantees a safe, nonthreatening environment for learning.

LIMITATIONS

- Can be expensive.

- Very labor intensive in many cases.

- Not readily available to all learners yet.

selves to rehearse desired behavior, or the educator takes a part to act as a positive role model for the learners. Most often, however, the teacher designates members in a group to play a particular character, and then they pretend to be that person for the duration of the exercise. Participants do and say things that they perceive the actual person would do, say, and feel.

The purpose is to help learners see and understand a problem through the eyes of others. In other words, it gives them a chance to walk in someone else's shoes. For example, children may use role playing with puppets to explore their responses to such illnesses as asthma (Ramsey & Siroky, 1988). Role playing also has been used to teach cultural competence by having a learner assume the role of a patient from another culture. This "patient" interacts with another learner who models a nurse displaying potentially inappropriate cultural responses. After the role play, a third learner can then explain the important cultural characteristics and why the "nurse's" responses were inappropriate and insensitive (Shearer & Davidhizar, 2003). When professional caregivers take the place of patients, this role reversal helps to sensitize staff to the care they deliver.

For role playing to be employed effectively, the teacher must be sure that the group has attained a comfort level that allows each member to feel secure enough to participate in a dramatization. This method should never be used with learners in the beginning of a group session encounter. Members need time to establish a rapport with one another as well as with the instructor, or else learners may feel embarrassed or self-conscious about playing a part. All members of the group should be given an assignment to ensure that they are actively involved in the teaching–learning experience.

Those who are actual participants need to be informed about the role they are to portray so they can effectively develop the appropriate actions. Those who are designated as observers require specific instructions about what to attend to during the role-playing session.

Role playing is best done in small groups so that all learners can serve as either players or as observers. Active participation by learners is particularly important during a postactivity discussion or debriefing session. Because this method is most effective for learning in the affective domain, all participants need to discuss how they felt and share what they observed to gain insight into their understanding of interpersonal relationships and their reactions to role expectations or conflicts.

Role playing can be used in conjunction with other instructional methods, but such a combination requires careful planning as to the sequential placement of this strategy and the important points to be captured during the dramatization period. See **Table 11–7** for a summary of the main advantages and limitations of role playing.

Role Modeling

The use of self as a role model is often overlooked as an instructional method. Learning from *role modeling* is called identification and emanates from learning and developmental theories such as Bandura's social learning theory and Erickson's psychosocial stages of development, which explain how people acquire new behaviors and social roles (Snowman & Biehler, 2006; Vander Zanden, Crandell, & Crandell, 2007). This method primarily achieves behavior change in the affective domain.

Nurse educators have many opportunities to demonstrate behaviors they would like to instill

---

Table 11–7 Major Advantages and Limitations of Role Playing

ADVANTAGES

- Opportunity to explore feelings and attitudes.

- Potential for bridging the gap between understanding and feeling.

- Narrows the role distance between and among clients and professionals.

LIMITATIONS

- Limited to small groups.

- Tendency by some participants to overly exaggerate their assigned roles.

- A role part loses its realism and credibility if played too dramatically.

- Some participants may be uncomfortable in their roles or unable to develop them sufficiently.

---

in learners, whether they be patients, family members, nursing staff, or students. The competency with which the educator performs a skill, the way he or she interacts with others, the personal example he or she sets, and the enthusiasm and interest he or she conveys about a subject or problem all can influence learners' motivation levels and the extent to which they successfully perform a desired behavior.

Behavior is regulated by the social norms and professional expectations that specify what is considered to be appropriate and inappropriate behavior. Role conflict can arise when one's past behavior patterns are incompatible or different from another role one must assume (Vander Zanden et al., 2007). Nurse educators can teach students and staff new behaviors by consistently setting examples and living the standards of the nursing profession. "Actions speak louder than words" is a popular saying relevant to the use of self as a role model (de Tornyay & Thompson, 1987).

See **Table 11–8** for a summary of the advantages and limitations of this method of instruction.

Self-Instruction Activities

Self-instruction is a method used by the teacher to provide or design instructional activities that guide the learner in independently achieving the objectives of learning. Each self-study module usually focuses on one topic, and the hallmark of this format is independent study. The self-instruction method is effective for learning in the cognitive and psychomotor domains, where the goal is to master information and apply it to practice. Self-study also can be an effective adjunct for introducing principles and step-by-step guidelines prior to demonstration of a psychomotor skill.

This method is sometimes difficult to identify as a singular entity because of the variety of terms used to describe it, such as *mini-course, self-instructional package, individualized learning*

Table 11–8 MAJOR ADVANTAGES AND LIMITATIONS OF ROLE MODELING

ADVANTAGES

- Influence attitudes to achieve behavior change in the affective domain.
- Positive role models have the potential to instill socially desired behaviors.

LIMITATIONS

- Requires rapport between the role model and the learner.
- Negative role models have the potential to instill unacceptable behaviors.

---

activities, and *programmed instruction.* For the purposes of this discussion, the term *self-instruction* will be used, and it is defined as a self-contained instructional activity that allows learners to progress by themselves at their own pace (Abruzzese, 1996).

Self-instruction modules come in a variety of forms including, but not limited to, work books, study guides, work stations, videotapes, Internet modules, and computer programs. They are specifically designed to be used independently. The teacher serves as a facilitator/resource person to provide motivation and reinforcement for learning. This method requires less teacher time to give information, and each session with the learner is intended to meet individual needs.

Some learners and teachers resist the self-instructional method because it appears to depersonalize the teaching–learning process (de Tornyay & Thompson, 1987). This is not necessarily true. Communication can still occur between the teacher and the learner, but the focus of instruction is different. The amount of time for direct interaction is more limited than with other methods of teaching such as lecture, group discussion or one-to-one instruction. This method adheres to the principles of adult education whereby the learner assumes responsibility for learning and is self-directed.

A self-instruction module is carefully designed to achieve preset objectives by bringing learners from diverse knowledge and skill backgrounds to a similar level of achievement prior to undertaking the next step in a series of learning activities. As examples, during orientation to an agency, there may be a self-study module on pharmacology prior to staff nurses' attending mandatory medication administration classes; a self-instructional activity can be made available to educate all staff on new infection-control practices in an agency; and patients can learn breast self-examination or cardiopulmonary resuscitation techniques by using specifically prepared self-study materials. Self-instruction modules should be tested with a small group before use with larger groups to confirm their suitability for the intended learners (Schmidt & Fisher, 1992).

Modules can be made readily accessible to learners along with any resources that are needed to complete the self-study program. Each self-instruction module needs to contain the following elements:

- **An introduction and statement of purpose,** which generally include a table of contents, the terminal objectives, the intent of the module, and directions for its use.
- **A list of prerequisite skills** that the learner needs to have to use the module.
- **A list of behavioral objectives,** which are clear and measurable statements describing which skills the learner is expected to acquire on completion of the unit.
- **A pretest** to diagnostically determine whether the learner needs to proceed with the module. Some learners may demonstrate mastery in the pretest and can move on to the next module. Other learners will get a sharper focus on their areas of weakness and may decide to seek additional preparation prior to beginning the module.
- **An identification of resources and learning activities,** which specifies the equipment needed, such as videotapes, slides, or written materials, and outlines the actual learning activities that will be presented. Objectives are given to direct the learner, followed by material presented in small units of discrete information called frames. The total length of a well-designed module is kept relatively short so as not to dampen the motivation to learn.

How the material is presented will vary with the objectives and the resources available. For example, information may be given via programmed instruction or through a series of readings. This can be followed by a video presentation of a relevant case study with the requirement that the learner write a response to what has been read and observed.

- **Periodic self-assessments** to provide feedback to the learner throughout the module. The user is frequently able to do periodic self-assessments prior to moving on to the next unit. This allows the learner to decide whether the previous information has been processed sufficiently enough to progress further.
- **A posttest** to evaluate the learner's level of mastery in achieving the objectives. If learners are aware that a posttest needs to be completed, this requirement encourages them to pay attention to the information. Keeping a record of final outcomes is helpful in both staff and patient education as documentation of competency, as proof that standards were met, and for the purpose of planning for continuing education.

Self-instruction represents an attractive alternative to traditional classroom and group learning methods in the rapidly changing healthcare environment. Hospitals and community agencies are not able to release staff in large numbers for continuing education programs that are rigidly timed. This constraint conflicts with the need to share information on the newest advances and documentation of continuing competence of staff. Self-instruction modules are excellent choices for annual training updates in selected topics or skills that require periodic review to determine competency (Markiewicz & Wells, 1997; O'Very, 1999).

The Internet also offers some continuing education self-instruction modules. Nurse practitioners have the advantage of being educated about numerous problems and issues in primary care with interactive, realistic case studies. E-mail to and from faculty can facilitate communication (Hayes, Huckstadt, & Gibson, 2000).

See **Table 11–9** for a list of major advantages and limitations of this method of instruction.

Self-instruction modules have been found to be cost effective because they are designed to be used by large numbers of individuals with minimal and infrequent revisions. It may be less time consuming and more efficient to purchase, rather than produce, a self-instruction module if the information presented in a commercial product is appropriate for the target audience. Computer-assisted instruction (CAI) is an individualized method of self-study using computers to deliver

an educational activity. CAI allows learners to proceed at their own pace with immediate and continuous feedback on their progress as they respond to a software program. Most computer programs assist the learner in achieving cognitive domain skills (DeYoung, 2003). The computer is a reliable, attentive, and tolerant drill and practice partner (Green & Brightman, 1990). CAIs offer consistent presentation of material and around-the-clock accessibility. They are a time-efficient and effective instructional method that reduces student–teacher ratios (McAlindon & Smith, 1994). This instructional method not only saves time but also accommodates different types of learners. It allows slow learners to repeat lessons as many times as necessary, while learners

---

Table 11–9 MAJOR ADVANTAGES AND LIMITATIONS OF SELF-INSTRUCTION

ADVANTAGES

- Allows for self-pacing.

- Stimulates active learning.

- Provides opportunity to review and reflect on information.

- Frequent feedback is built in.

- Indicates mastery of material accomplished in a particular time frame.

LIMITATIONS

- Limited with learners who have low literacy skills.

- Not appropriate for learners with visual and hearing impairments.

- Requires high levels of motivation.

- Not good for learners who tend to procrastinate.

- May induce boredom if this method is overused with a population with no variation in the activity design.

familiar with material can skip ahead to more advanced material (DeYoung, 2003). There is concern that computer instruction depersonalizes the learning process (DeYoung, 2003). However, CAIs should not be taken to mean that the teacher is unavailable for guidance in learning. Even though this technology simply delivers content, it allows more time for the nurse educator to concentrate on the personal aspects of individual reinforcement and ongoing assessments of learning. CAIs have been used with good patient acceptance for both preoperative and postoperative instruction on joint replacement (Tibbles, Lewis, Reisine, Rippey, & Donald, 1992) and precolposcopy education (Martin, Hoffman, & Kaminski, 2005). Because CAI requires self-motivation, this instructional method may not be adequate for learners who have an external locus of control and who need human interaction to learn best (Poston, 1993).

Selection of Instructional Methods

The process of selecting an instructional method requires a prior determination of the behavioral objectives to be accomplished and an assessment of the learners who will be involved in achieving the objectives. Also, consideration must be given to available resources such as time, money, space, and materials to support learning activities. The teacher is also an important variable in the selection and effectiveness of a method. **Table 11–10** summarizes the general characteristics of instructional methods.

Teachers are at different levels on the novice-to-expert continuum, and how seasoned they are influences their choices of instructional methods. An expert skilled at facilitating small-group discussion may be a novice in the design and selection of games. A nurse may be an expert clinician but have only limited experience and effectiveness in the teaching role. Nurses are expected to teach but may not have adequate time, inclination, energy, or capability for developing the quality and variety of instruction necessary. Teaching is a skill that can be developed in formal academic settings, in continuing education programs, or through guidance by an expert peer mentor.

Teachers are likely to focus on a particular method because it is the one they feel most comfortable using without considering all the criteria for selection. There is no one right method, because the best approach depends on many variables, such as the audience, the content to be taught, the setting in which teaching and learning are to take place, and the resources available. Nevertheless, the ideal method for any given situation is the one that best suits the learner's needs, not the teacher's.

A novice should begin instruction with very familiar content so that he or she can focus on the teaching process itself and feel more confident in trying out different techniques and instructional materials. He or she should ask questions of learners and peers in the evaluation process to ascertain whether the method chosen was appropriate for accomplishing the behavioral objectives and meeting the needs of different learners in terms of their learning styles and readiness to learn.

Narrow (1979) emphasized the importance of periodically examining one's role as a teacher and assessing the factors of energy, attitudes, knowledge, and skills, which influence the priority one assigns to teaching and the ability to teach effectively. The following is a summary of her suggestions.

Table 11–10 GENERAL CHARACTERISTICS OF INSTRUCTIONAL METHODS

Methods	Domain	Learner Role	Teacher Role	Advantages	Limitations
Lecture	Cognitive	Passive	Presents information	Cost effective Targets large groups	Not individualized
Group discussion	Affective Cognitive	Active—if learner participates	Guides and focuses discussion	Stimulates sharing ideas and emotions	Shy or dominant member High levels of diversity
One-to-one instruction	Cognitive Affective Psychomotor	Active	Presents information and facilitates individualized learning	Tailored to individual's needs and goals	Labor intensive Isolates learner
Demonstration	Psychomotor Cognitive	Passive	Models skill or behavior	Preview of exact skill/behavior	Small groups needed to facilitate visualization
Return demonstration	Psychomotor	Active	Individualizes feedback to refine performance	Immediate individual guidance	Labor intensive to view individual performance
Gaming	Cognitive Affective	Active—if learner participates	Oversees pacing Referees Debriefs	Captures learner enthusiasm	Environment too competitive for some learners
Simulation	Cognitive Psychomotor	Active	Designs environment Facilitates process Debriefs	Practice reality in safe setting	Labor intensive Equipment costs
Role playing	Affective	Active	Designs format Debriefs	Develops understanding of others	Exaggeration or under-development of role
Role modeling	Affective Cognitive	Passive	Models skill or behavior	Helps with socialization to role	Requires rapport
Self-instruction	Cognitive Psychomotor	Active	Designs package Gives individual feedback	Self-paced Cost effective Consistent	Procrastination Requires literacy

At any given point in time, the teacher's energy level will be influenced by both psychological and physical factors, such as the amount of satisfaction derived from work, the demands and responsibilities of his or her professional and personal life, and his or her state of health. Feelings toward the learner also influence the enthusiasm the teacher brings to the teaching–learning situation. Nurse educators who feel drawn to the learners because they find them interesting or are concerned or anxious about their situation will find teaching to be a satisfying experience. If, on the other hand, the learners are demanding or display inappropriate behavior, teachers may feel negatively toward them and find the teaching–learning encounter more difficult and less fulfilling. Educators can develop the ability to accept individuals without necessarily approving of their behavior.

Another factor to consider is one's comfort with and confidence in the nature of the subject matter to be taught. Those who find certain content to be stressful to teach because of a lack of relevant knowledge or skills can increase their understanding of the subject and relieve their stress and apprehension with additional study and practice, allowing them to function more effectively in the teaching role.

Those who have difficulty communicating with learners about what they may consider sensitive material, such as sexual behavior, mental illness, abortion, birth defects, disfigurement, terminal illness, and the like, should examine their own feelings, seek support from colleagues, and use resources to help create an effective teaching approach. If the teaching–learning process is to be a partnership, not only is it crucial to assess the learner but it is equally important that the nurse educator assesses himself or herself as the teacher. Often teachers fail to take into account their own circumstances and needs.

Evaluation of Instructional Methods

An important aspect of evaluating any instructional program is to assess the effectiveness of the method. Was the choice selected as effective, efficient, and appropriate as possible? There are five major questions that will help to decide which method to choose or if the method selected should be revised or rejected:

1. **Does the method help the learners to achieve the stated objectives?**
   This question is the most important criterion for evaluation—if the method does not facilitate accomplishing the objectives, then all the other criteria are unimportant. Examine how well matched the method is to the learning domain of the predetermined objectives. Will the method expose learners to the necessary information and training to learn the desired behaviors?

2. **Is the learning activity accessible to the learners who have been targeted?**
   Accessibility includes such issues as when information is presented, the location and setting in which teaching takes place, and the availability of resources and equipment to deliver the message. Patients and family members need programs to be offered at suitable times and accessible locations. For example, childbirth preparation classes scheduled during the daytime hours likely would not be convenient for expectant couples who are working.

3. **Is the method efficient given the time, energy, and resources available in relation to the number of learners the educator is trying to reach?**

To teach large numbers of learners, one will have to choose a method that can accommodate groups, such as lecture, discussion sessions, or role playing, or a method that can reach many individuals at one time, such as the use of various self-instructional formats.

4. **To what extent does the method allow for active participation to accommodate the needs, abilities, and style of the learner?**

   Active participation has been well documented as a way to increase interest in learning and the retention of information. Evaluate how active learners want to be or are able to be in the process of gaining knowledge and skills. No one method will satisfy all learners, but adhering to one method will exclusively address the preferred style of only a segment of your audience.

5. **Is the method cost effective?**

   It is vital to examine the cost of educational programs to determine whether similar outcomes might be achieved by using less costly methodologies. In this era of cost containment, employers and insurers want their monies invested in patient programs that yield the best possible outcomes at the lowest price as measured in terms of preventing illness and injury, minimizing the severity and extent of illness, and reducing the length of hospital stays and readmissions. Healthcare agencies want the best staff nurse performance with the most reasonable use of resources and the least amount of time taken away from actual practice.

Increasing Effectiveness of Teaching

Excellent teachers have one thing in common—a passion to keep improving their abilities. One does not arrive at being an expert teacher. The drive toward excellence is an ongoing process that continues throughout the teacher's entire professional life. What constitutes creative teaching? The following are techniques, not listed in any particular order, that nurse educators can use to enhance the effectiveness of verbal presentations. In addition, some general principles for teaching that can be used by all teachers are also put forth (Brookfield, 2006; Cunningham & Baker, 1986; Freitas, Lantz, & Reed, 1991; Irvin, 1996; Musinski, 1999; Narrow, 1979; Parrott, 1994; Phillips, 1999).

Techniques to Enhance the Effectiveness of Verbal Presentations

PRESENT INFORMATION ENTHUSIASTICALLY

The teacher who comes across as invested in the material excites the learner to identify with the subject at hand. No matter how well a lesson is planned or how clearly it is presented, if it is delivered in a dry and dull monotone, it will likely fall on deaf ears.

The teacher should try to vary the quality and pitch of his or her voice, use a variety of gestures and facial expressions, change position if necessary to make direct and frequent eye contact with everyone in the group, and demonstrate an ardent interest in the topic to attract and fascinate an audience. The enthusiastic teacher is aware that an energetic attitude is contagious and enticing. However, one must exercise caution in overusing body language and overt actions because mannerisms can be distracting and can adversely affect learning.

INCLUDE HUMOR

Many teachers use humor as a technique to grab, arouse, and maintain the attention of the learner. Appropriate humor can help establish a rapport with learners by humanizing the teacher. Humor does not necessarily require the teacher to tell jokes, and joke telling should not be attempted if this is not a skill one possesses. Furthermore, the teacher should avoid making someone the object of humor if it results in a put-down.

Humor establishes an atmosphere that allows for human error without embarrassment and encourages freedom and comfort to explore alternatives in the learning situations. Humor is a means to reduce anxiety when dealing with sensitive material, to provide poignant examples of everyday life experiences, and to reinforce information.

EXHIBIT RISK-TAKING BEHAVIOR

Effective teachers are willing to develop exercises in which many variables can lead to any number of possible outcomes. They use this technique to encourage learners to reach their own conclusions about controversial issues. Regardless of the outcome, the teachers should be prepared to deal with uncertainty. Exercises that allow learners freedom to experiment and express their ideas focus more on the process than on the result.

DELIVER MATERIAL DRAMATICALLY

Effective teachers seek ways to engage the learner emotionally by using surprise, controlled tension, or ploys. The teacher uses strategies that connect the educational material directly to the learner's life experiences so that information is made more understandable and relevant. Learners may be asked to participate in simulations, games, or role playing to act out a part, live an experience, or test their capacities. These activities involve the learner and can leave a profound, lasting impression that can be recalled vividly and can be drawn upon when faced with a real situation. This technique engages learners by arousing their emotions.

CHOOSE PROBLEM-SOLVING ACTIVITIES

Whether the learners are staff members or patients, the nurse educator must recognize that learners need to be immersed in activities to help them develop problem-solving skills. In today's world, professionals must have the ability to identify both patient and system problems by searching and sorting data, uncovering problems, and finding solutions. Increasingly, they are expected to work with interdisciplinary teams to determine and implement solutions to healthcare problems. Learning activities must be designed to help these nursing staff members and students develop critical-thinking and collaborative skills.

Patients, especially those with chronic conditions, also need problem-solving skills to know how to respond to changes demanded by their condition. What should they do differently on a sick day, or what constitutes an emergency? Patients and families need more than just low-level cognitive information to make adjustments in their lives. The teacher must therefore devise and orchestrate opportunities that challenge learners to critically analyze situations as well as support the learner in exploring possible alternative situations.

SERVE AS A ROLE MODEL

Educators should constantly seek new information by keeping abreast of current research, theories, and issues in clinical practice for application relevant to the teaching situation. Expanding one's own knowledge base gives credence to what is taught and gains the confidence of learners in the teacher's expertise. A commitment to lifelong learning transmits an important value to others of their need for continuous personal or professional development.

Educators are seen as credible role models when they are actively engaged in scholarly activities, are experienced in the field, and have advanced credentials to teach complex skills. The believability of a role model is greatly affected by the values displayed and the congruence demonstrated between what the teacher says and does (Babcock & Miller, 1994). If the learners regard the behavior of the creative teacher as desirable, they will likely imitate that behavior, which they perceive as eliciting positive effects.

USE ANECDOTES AND EXAMPLES

The creative teacher uses stories and examples of incidences and episodes to illustrate points. Anecdotes, whether amusing, alarming, sad, or anger provoking, are valuable in driving a point home, clarifying a topic under discussion, or helping someone better relate to an issue. The teacher can reinforce the learning principle that simple representations can assist the learner to grasp complex ideas by using examples relevant to past experiences and the knowledge base of learners that help them identify and connect in a concrete way with the material being taught.

USE TECHNOLOGY

Innovative teachers use technology to broaden and add variety to the opportunities for teaching and learning. They continue to increase the level of their own skills by taking advantage of the advances in technology to introduce and

coach others in new ways of learning. They recognize that the sophisticated use of technology is a primary skill that will be needed for educational programs of the future.

The use of different types of technology assists the teacher in helping learners meet their individual needs and styles of learning. Technology has the potential for making the teaching–learning process more convenient, accessible, and stimulating. Effective teachers must be future oriented. A mastery of technological skills assures their ability to teach in innovative and eclectic ways to prepare students for learning in the 21st century.

General Principles for All Teachers

GIVE POSITIVE REINFORCEMENT

Educational research is replete with examples of the effects of positive reinforcement on learning. Acknowledging ideas, actions, and opinions of others by using words of praise or approval, such as "That's a good answer," "I agree with you," and "You have a very good point," or using nonverbal expressions of acceptance, such as smiling, nodding, or a reassuring pat on the back, will encourage learners to participate more readily or try harder to improve their performance. Rewarding even a small success can instill satisfaction in the learner. Reproval, on the other hand, will dampen motivation and cause learners to withdraw. Positive reinforcers, in the form of recognition, tangible rewards, or opportunities, should closely follow the desired behavior. The clearer the correlation between the desired behavior and the reward, the more meaningful the reinforcement will be (see Chapter 3 on learning theories).

A powerful incentive is to ask learners to share their experiences with others. In a group, it is important to recognize the contributions of each member rather than focus primarily on the more aggressive learner or high achiever. What constitutes positive reinforcement for one individual may not suffice for another, as rewards are closely tied to value systems.

The quantity of reinforcement also will vary in its effectiveness from one individual to another. A small amount of praise can have a strong effect on the learner who is not used to succeeding, whereas significant praise may be relatively ineffective for a consistently high achiever. In addition, the effects of reinforcement are transitory. An incentive that works for a learner at one time may not work well at another time.

PROJECT AN ATTITUDE OF ACCEPTANCE AND SENSITIVITY

The ease with which teachers conduct themselves, the willingness to receive and answer questions, the simple courtesies extended, and the responsiveness demonstrated toward an audience are all actions that set the tone for a friendly, warm, and receptive atmosphere for learning. If the teacher exhibits self-confidence and self-respect, the learner in turn will feel comfortable, confident, and secure in the learning environment. If the teacher comes across as believable, trustworthy, considerate and competent, he or she helps to put the audience at ease, which serves as an invitation for them to learn. When teachers exercise patience and sensitivity with respect to age, race, culture, and gender, this projects an acceptance of others, which serves to establish a rapport and opens up the avenues of communication for the sharing of ideas and concerns.

People will learn better in a comfortable and supportive environment. Not only is it important that the physical environment be conducive

to learning, but the psychological climate should also be respectful of learners and focused on their need for an atmosphere of support and acceptance. Educators must have a clear view of their role as facilitators and expert coaches and avoid acting as controlling disseminators of information.

BE ORGANIZED AND GIVE DIRECTION

Excellent discussions, meaningful experiences in role playing, or successful attempts at self-study are examples of teaching that will not happen by accident. They are the result of hours of skilled preparation, careful planning, and organization, which allow the learner to stay focused on the objectives. Material should be logically organized, objectives clearly defined and presented up front, and directions given in a straightforward, specific, and easily understood manner.

Instructional sessions should be relatively brief so as not to overload the learner with too much detail and extraneous content. Need-to-know information should take precedence over the nice-to-know information to ensure that enough time is allotted for the essentials.

Regardless of the method of instruction used, the attention span of the learner waxes and wanes over time, and what is learned first and last is retained the most (Ley, 1972). Audiovisual materials selected to supplement various methods of teaching should clarify or enhance a message. Advance organizers should be used to structure information and assist the learner in identifying the subject to be presented and in what order.

ELICIT AND GIVE FEEDBACK

Feedback should be a reciprocal process. It is a strategy to give information to the learner as well as to receive information from the learner. Both the teacher and the learner need to seek information about the quality of their performance. Feedback should be encouraged during and at the end of each teaching–learning encounter as well as at the completion of an educational program. It can take the form of either verbal or nonverbal responses to a situation.

Feedback that learners receive can be subjective or objective. Subjective data, whether physiological or psychological, come from within the learners themselves. People sense how they are reacting to a situation. Internally, they usually know how well they performed or how they feel by their own responses, such as fatigue, anxiety, disinterest, or satisfaction. Learners are able to compare their own performance to what they expect of themselves or what they think others expect of them.

Objective data come to the learners from the teacher, who measures their behavior based on a set of standards or criteria and who gives them an opinion on the progress they have made. To get feedback, the learner might ask, "How well did I do?" "Am I on track?" "Did I do all right?" or "What do you think?"

Feedback to the teacher is equally important because the effectiveness of teaching depends to a great extent on the learners' reactions. Whether positive or negative, verbal or nonverbal, feedback enables the teacher to determine if he or she should maintain or modify his or her approach to teaching. Feedback indicates whether to proceed, take time to review or explain, or cease instruction altogether for the moment.

The teacher should be direct in eliciting feedback from the learners by asking questions such as "Did I answer your questions?" "Is this clear?" "Do you need me to explain it further?" or "What more can I help you with?" The teacher should also be sensitive to nonverbal expressions such as a nod, a smile, a look of bewilderment, or a frown indicating an understanding or lack thereof.

Feedback is neutral unless it is compared with established norms, preset criteria, or past behavior. How much someone learned, for example, is meaningless unless compared to what the person knew previously or how the person stacks up against other learners under similar conditions.

Feedback, either positive or negative, is needed by both the learner and the teacher. Praise reinforces behavior and increases the likelihood the behavior will continue. Constructive criticism tends to redirect behavior to conform with expected norms. Labeling someone's personality as cooperative, smart, stubborn, unmotivated, or uncaring is harmful, but it is helpful to label someone's performance to give that person specific information for improving, correcting, or continuing the behavior.

Use Questions

Questioning is one of the means for both the teacher and the learner to elicit feedback about performance. If the educator is skillful in the use of questioning, it serves multiple purposes in the teaching–learning process. Questions help to clarify or substantiate concepts, assess what the learner already knows about the topic, stimulate interest in a new subject, or evaluate the learner's mastery of the predetermined objectives.

Babcock and Miller (1994) identified three types of questions that can be used to elicit different types of answers:

1. Factual or descriptive questions begin with words such as *who, what, where,* or *when* and asks for recall-type responses

from the learner. Factual questions such as "Which foods are high in fat?" or "Whom should you call if you run out of medication?" elicit straightforward facts. Descriptive questions take a more open-ended approach, such as "What kinds of exercise do you get daily?" "What problems do you have with activities of daily living?" or "What are the signs and symptoms of infection?" These questions require a more detailed and organized response from the learner.

2. Clarifying questions ask for more information and help the learner to convey thoughts and feelings. Such questions might include "What do you mean when you say . . . ?" or "I'm not sure I understand exactly what you are expressing."

3. High-order questions require more than memory or perception to answer. They ask the learner to make inferences, establish cause and effect, or compare and contrast concepts. Examples include "Why does a low-salt diet help to control blood pressure?" or "What do you think will happen if you don't take your medication?" or "What do you see as the advantages and disadvantages in following the treatment plan?"

After asking questions, a period of silence may occur. This can be uncomfortable for both the teacher and the learner. Anxiety over silence may be reduced by encouraging the learner to think about the answer before responding. In a group, this strategy also allows all participants to have a chance to think through their responses to the questions, which gives them the opportunity to make more thoughtful and deliberate responses.

Questioning helps the teacher appropriately pace the material being presented. Also, answers to questions allow the educator to arrive at an evaluative judgment as to the progress the learner is making in the achievement of the behavioral objectives.

KNOW YOUR AUDIENCE

The effectiveness of teaching will be severely limited when the choice of instructional method is based on the interest and comfort level of the teacher and not on the assessed needs of the learner. Teachers must use methods that match the topic rather than their personality.

Most teachers have a preferred style of teaching and tend to rely on that approach regardless of the content to be taught. Skilled teachers adapt themselves to a teaching style appropriate to the subject matter, setting, and various styles of the learners. Flexibility is their hallmark in tailoring the instructional design to the unique needs of each population of learners. They should be willing to use a variety of teaching methods to provide the best possible experience for achievement of objectives.

USE REPETITION AND PACING

Repetition, if used with discretion, is a technique that strengthens learning. It reinforces learning by aiding in the retention of information. If overused, repetition can lead to boredom and frustration because the teacher is repeating what is already understood and remembered. If used deliberately, it can assist the learner in focusing on important points and keep the learner on track.

Repetition is especially important when presenting new or difficult material. The opportunity for repeated practice of behavioral tasks is called *skill inoculation*. Repetition can take the form of a simple reminder, a review of previously learned material, or the continued practice of a skill. Assessing the learner's understanding will help one to use repetition effectively.

Pacing refers to the speed at which information is presented. Some self-instruction methods of teaching, such as programmed instruction, allow for individualized pacing so that learners can proceed at their own speed, depending on their abilities and style of learning. Other methods of group learning require the teacher to take command of the rate at which information is presented and processed.

Many factors determine the optimal rate of teaching, such as the following:

- Previous history with learning
- Attention span
- The domain in which learning is to take place
- The learner's eagerness and determination to obtain a reward or attain a goal
- The degree of progress in learning
- The learner's ability to cope with frustration and discomfort

Keeping in touch with the audience will help the teacher to pace his or her teaching. It should be slow enough for assimilation of information, yet fast enough to maintain interest and enthusiasm.

SUMMARIZE IMPORTANT POINTS

Summarizing information at the completion of the teaching–learning encounter gives a perspective on what has been covered, how it relates to the objectives, and what you expect the learner to have achieved. Summarizing also reviews key ideas to instill information in the mind and helps the learner to see the parts of a whole. Closure should be used at the end of one lesson before proceeding to a new topic. Summary reinforces retention of information. It provides feedback as to the progress made, thereby leaving the learner with a feeling of satisfaction with what has been accomplished.

Instructional Settings

Traditionally, the primary focus of nursing practice has been on the delivery of acute care in hospital settings. In recent years, however, the practice of nursing in community-based settings has experienced tremendous growth. The reasons for the shift in orientation of nursing practice from inpatient care sites to outpatient sites relate to the trends affecting the nation's healthcare system as a whole. These trends include public and private reimbursement policies, changing population demographics, advances in healthcare technology, an emphasis on wellness care, and increased consumer interest in health. In response to these trends, the domains of nursing practice have broadened to include a greater emphasis on the delivery of care in community settings such as homes, clinics, health maintenance organizations (HMOs), physicians' offices, public schools, and the workplace.

With the increased focus on prevention, promotion, and independence in self-care activities, today's newly emerging healthcare system mandates the education of consumers to a greater extent than ever before. Opportunities for client teaching have become increasingly more varied in terms of the types of clients encountered, their particular learning needs, and the settings in which healthcare teaching occurs. Because health education has become an increasingly important responsibility of nurses in all practice environments, it is important to acknowledge the various settings where clients, well or ill, are consumers of health care.

Instructional settings are classified according to the relationship health education has to the primary purpose of the organization or agency that provides health instruction. An *instructional setting* is defined as any place where nurses engage in teaching for disease prevention, health promotion, and health maintenance and rehabilitation. An *instructional setting* is any environment in which health education takes place to provide individuals with learning experiences for the purpose of improving their health or reducing their risk for illness and injury. Three types of settings for the education of clients have been identified:

1. A *healthcare setting* is one in which the delivery of health care is the primary or sole function of the institution, organization, or agency. Hospitals, visiting nurse associations, public health departments, outpatient clinics, extended-care facilities, health maintenance organizations, physician's offices, and nurse-managed centers are examples of organizations whose primary purpose is to deliver health care. Health education is an integral aspect of the overall care delivered within these settings. Nurses function to provide direct patient care, and their role encompasses the teaching of clients as part of that care.

2. A *healthcare-related setting* is one in which healthcare-related services are offered as a complimentary function of the agency. Examples of this type of setting include the American Heart Association, the American Cancer Society, and the Muscular Dystrophy Association. These organizations provide client advocacy, conduct health screenings and self-help groups, distribute health education information and materials, and support research on disease and lifestyle issues for the benefit of consumers within the community. Education on health promotion, disease prevention, and improving the quality of life for those who live with a particular illness is the key function of nurses within these agencies.

3. A *nonhealthcare setting* is one in which health care is an incidental or supportive function of an organization. Examples of this type of setting include businesses, industries, schools, and military and penal institutions. The primary purpose of these organizations is to produce a manufactured product or offer a non-health-related service to the public. Industries, for example, are involved in health care only to the extent of providing health screenings and nonemergent health coverage to their employees through a health office within their place of employment, making available instruction in job-related health and safety issues to meet Occupational Safety and Health Administration (OSHA) regulations, or providing opportunities for health education through wellness programs to reduce absenteeism or improve employee morale.

Classifying instructional settings in which the nurse functions as teacher provides a frame of reference through which to better understand the interrelationship between the components of the organizational climate, the target audience, and the resources within the environment influencing the educational tasks to be accomplished. The role and functioning of the nurse is affected differently by these components in each of the identified settings.

Nurses must recognize the numerous opportunities available for the teaching of those who are currently or potentially consumers of health care. Given that teaching is an important aspect of healthcare delivery and given the fact that nurses are functioning as teachers in a multitude of settings, they encounter clients of differing ages and at various stages along the wellness-to-illness continuum. Wherever and whenever teaching takes place, nurses need to recognize the importance of consciously applying the principles of teaching and learning to these encounters for maximum effectiveness in helping clients to attain and maintain optimal health.

Sharing Resources Among Settings

Professional nurses involved in client health education should use available opportunities to share resources among the three identified settings (**Figure 11–3**). Many already perform this service as printed or audiovisual materials are borrowed, rented, or purchased for small fees from area institutions, organizations, or agencies; nurse educators from healthcare or health care-related settings are contracted for or voluntarily provide health education programs to small and large groups in other healthcare, healthcare-related, or non-healthcare settings; and nurses from each category of setting collaborate on individual client situations or on major community health projects.

Figure 11–3 Types of instructional settings for health education.

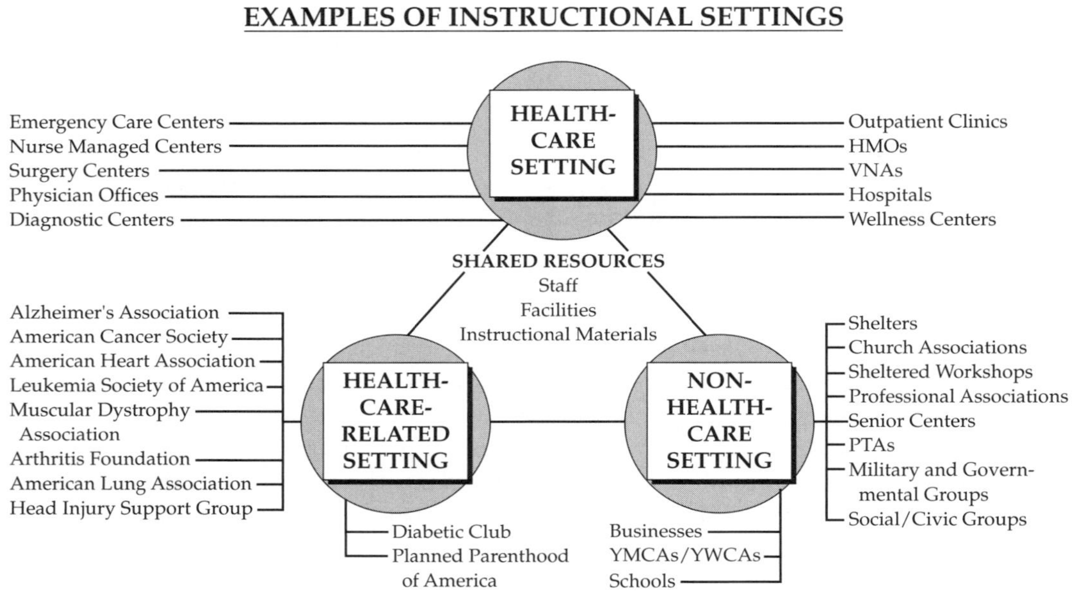

EXAMPLES OF INSTRUCTIONAL SETTINGS

The nurses from each of these settings can establish a health education committee in their community to coordinate health education programming, ensure effective use of all resources, and reduce duplication of efforts. The members of this committee can develop standardized health education content, delineate roles and services for each of the instructional settings, and share resources to provide a well-planned, comprehensive community program of health education for a wide spectrum of clients.*

State of the Evidence

Patient education is very complex. Patients present with a wide variety of chronic and acute illnesses, financial resources, developmental stages, cultural values, reading abilities, learning styles, motivation levels, and social support. Nursing students and staff differ widely on their educational and experiential backgrounds and are also influenced by generation gaps. This reality makes it difficult to generalize the results of research studies. Also it is difficult in some of the literature to analyze the cause and effect relationship between the instructional method used and the outcomes achieved. This, in turn, becomes more challenging when the goal is to compare studies.

Cooper, Booth, Fear, and Gill (2001) critically reviewed 12 meta-analysis studies concerning patient education for people with chronic diseases where the treatment regime required behavior change. The question they asked concerned what type of educational interventions can actually produce the most benefit for these patients. The determination of effects by type of educational intervention was hampered by inadequate descriptions of the interventions. Another problem was the fact that the interventions comprised more than one educational method. Their findings were that effect by educational approach could not be differentiated. Some evidence suggested that didactic and psychosocial strategies produced smaller outcome effects than a combination of behavioral, cognitive, and affective therapies.

Deakin, McShane, Cade, and Williams (2005) systematically reviewed 11 studies of group-based, patient-centered educational programs for people with Type 2 diabetes to assess the effects on clinical, lifestyle, and psychosocial outcomes. This review provided evidence that group-based diabetes education programs for adults with Type 2 diabetes resulted in improvements in glycated hemoglobin, fasting blood glucose and diabetes knowledge when monitored at 4–6 months and at 12 months.

In addition, they recommend more research on the theoretical model underpinning the educational programs. Some of the studies suggested that group education is more effective if based on adult learning principles, patient empowerment, and participation. The authors also comment on the need for more research to determine if this type of program is appropriate for all ethnic backgrounds. Cost effectiveness was included under their implications for future research, which is an especially important factor to be considered in the current healthcare environment.

The difficulty with measuring the effectiveness of different methods of instruction is that many studies do not make a distinction between instructional methods and instructional materials (tools), such as the study conducted by Dougal and Gonterman in 1999. Instead the authors

---

* With appreciation to Virginia E. O'Halloran, EdD, RN, for her contribution to information on instructional settings in this chapter.

treat them as one and the same and therefore the studies' findings cannot be compared nor applied as evidence in this chapter that deals exclusively with methods of instruction.

There are many empirical studies and expert reviews on the effectiveness of the various instructional methods available to teach different patient and staff populations, and selected reports are discussed in this chapter. Further research needs to be conducted on specific populations in relation to effectiveness of instructional methods for teaching them about specific topics they need to learn. For example, what is the most effective and efficient method to teach healthcare consumers about important safety behaviors for optimal self-care management?

Summary

This chapter has presented an in-depth review of the various instructional methods and compared the advantages and limitations of each approach. Also, the instructional settings in which teaching takes place was also briefly addressed.

Emphasis was given to the importance of taking into account the learner characteristics, behavioral objectives, teacher characteristics, and available resources prior to selecting or designing any of the vast array of methods at the teacher's disposal. In many instances, guidelines were put forth to assist nurse educators in planning and developing their own instructional activities. In addition, the major questions to be considered when evaluating the effectiveness of instructional methods were assessed in detail. Finally, techniques to enhance verbal presentations and some general principles to increase effectiveness of all methods of instruction were discussed.

What must be stressed are the inherent qualities of each method and the fact that no one method is better than another. The effectiveness of any method depends on the purpose for and the circumstances under which it is used. Nurses in the role of educators are urged to take an eclectic approach to teaching by avoiding reliance on any one particular method. Varying teaching approaches or using them in combination with one another can assist in accomplishing the objectives for learning while meeting the different needs and styles of each and every learner. Multisensory stimulation is best for increasing the acquisition of skills and the retention of information. Research regarding patient and staff education is increasing. It is imperative that nurse educators demonstrate a willingness to make decisions on choosing and using instructional methods based on the evidence that is emerging about the most effective ways to teach in relation to learner and situational variables.

REVIEW QUESTIONS

1. How is the term *instructional method* defined?
2. What are the advantages and limitations of each instructional method?
3. Which instructional methods are most effective in encouraging active participation by the learner?
4. Which instructional methods are best for learning cognitive skills? Psychomotor skills? Affective skills?
5. What variables influence the selection of any method of instruction?
6. What major questions should a teacher ask himself or herself when evaluating the effectiveness of an instructional method? Which question is the most important criterion for evaluation?
7. What is the difference between factual/descriptive questions, clarifying questions, and high-order questions?
8. What are the techniques that teachers can use to enhance the effectiveness of teaching?
9. Are teachers born or made? Explain.
10. What are the three classifications of instructional settings?

References

Abruzzese, R. S. (1996). *Nursing staff development: Strategies for success* (2nd ed.). St. Louis, MO: Mosby-Year Book.

Babcock, D. E., & Miller, M. A. (1994). *Client education: Theory and practice.* St. Louis, MO: Mosby-Year Book.

Bain, K. (2004, April 9). What makes great teachers great? *The Chronicle of Higher Education*, B7–B9.

Bartlett, T. (2003, May 9). Big, but not bad. *The Chronicle of Higher Education*, 35–38.

Bays, C., & Hermann, C. (1997). Gaming versus lecture discussion: Effects on students' test performance. *Journal of Nursing Education, 36*(6), 292–294.

Boyd, M. D., Gleit, C. J., Graham, B. A., & Whitman, N. I. (1998). *Health teaching in nursing practice: A professional model* (3rd ed.). Stamford, CT: Appleton and Lange.

Brookfield, S. D. (2006). *The skillful teacher: On technique, trust, and responsiveness in the classroom.* San Francisco, CA: Jossey-Bass.

Brookfield, S. D., & Preskill, S. (1999). *Discussion as a way of teaching: Tools and techniques for democratic classrooms.* San Francisco: Jossey-Bass.

Cantillon, P. (2003, Feb. 22). ABC of learning and teaching in medicine: Teaching large groups. *British Medical Journal, 326,* 437–440.

Carkhuff, M. H. (1996). Reflective learning: Work groups as learning groups. *The Journal of Continuing Education in Nursing, 27*(5), 209–214.

Cooper, H., Booth, K., Fear, S., & Gill, G. (2001). Chronic disease patient education: Lessons from meta-analyses. *Patient Education and Counseling, 44,* 107–117.

Cuda, S., Doerr, D., & Gonzalez, M. (1999). Using facilitators in mock codes: Recasting the parts for success. *Journal of Continuing Education in Nursing, 30*(6), 279–283.

Cunningham, M. A., & Baker, D. (1986). How to teach patients better and faster. *RN, 49*(9), 50–52.

de Tornyay, R., & Thompson, M. A. (1987). *Strategies for Teaching Nursing* (3rd ed.). New York: Wiley.

Deakin, T., McShane, C. E., Cade, J. E., Williams, R. D. R. R. (2005). Group based training for self-management strategies in people with Type 2 diabetes mellitus. *Cochrane Database of Systematic Reviews,* Issue 2, Art. No.: CD003417. DOI: 10.1002/14651858. CD1858.CD003417.pub2.

del Bueno, D. J., Griffin, L. R., Burke, S. M., & Foley, M. A. (1990). The clinical teacher as a critical link in competence development. *Journal of Nursing Staff Development, 6,* 135–138.

DeYoung, S. (2003). *Teaching strategies for nurse educators.* Upper Saddle River, New Jersey: Prentice Hall.

Dougal, J., & Gonterman, R. (1999). A comparison of three teaching methods on learning and retention. *Journal for Nurses in Staff Development, 15*(5), 205–209.

Evans, M. (2000). Polished, professional presentation: Unlocking the design elements. *Journal of Continuing Education in Nursing, 31*(5), 213–218.

Fredette, S. L. (1990). A model for improving cancer patient education. *Cancer Nursing, 13,* 207–215.

Freitas, L., Lantz, J., & Reed, R. (1991). The creative teacher. *Nurse Educator, 16*(1), 5–7.

Green, P., & Brightman, A. J. (1990). *Independence day: Designing computer solutions for individuals with disabilities.* Allen, TX: Apple Computer.

Haggard, A. (1989). *Handbook of patient education.* Rockville, MD: Aspen.

Hayes, K., Huckstadt, A., & Gibson, R. (2000). Developing interactive continuing education on the Web. *Journal of Continuing Education in Nursing, 31*(5), 199–203.

Henry, J. M. (1997). Gaming: A teaching strategy to enhance adult learning. *The Journal of Continuing Education in Nursing, 28,* 231–234.

House, B. M., Chassie, M. B., & Spohn, B. B. (1990). Questioning: An essential ingredient in effective teaching. *Journal of Continuing Education in Nursing, 21,* 196–201.

Irvin, S. M. (1996, May/June). Creative teaching strategies. *The Journal of Continuing Education, 27*(3), 108–114.

Joos, I. R. M. (1984). A teacher's guide for using games and simulation. *Nurse Educator, 9*(3), 25–29.

Kowalski, K. (2004). The use of set. *The Journal of Continuing Education in Nursing, 35*(2), 56–57.

Leake, P. Y. (2004, November/December). Teaming with students and a sacred cow contest to make changes in nursing practice. *The Journal of Continuing Education in Nursing, 35*(6), 271–277.

Lewis, D. J., Saydak, S. J., Mierzwa, I. P., & Robinson, J. A. (1989). Gaming: A teaching strategy for adult learners. *Journal of Continuing Education in Nursing, 20,* 80–84.

Ley, P. (1972). Primacy, rated importance, and recall of medical statements. *Journal of Health and Social Behavior, 13,* 311–317.

Lieberman, D. (2001). Management of chronic pediatric diseases with interactive health games: Theory and research findings. *Journal of Ambulatory Care Management, 24*(1), 26–38.

Lorig, K. R. (2003). Taking patient ed to the next level: Patients with chronic illnesses need more than traditional patient education. They need you to help them develop the self-management skills that they'll use for the rest of their lives. *RN, 66*(12), 35–44.

Lorig, K., & Gonzalez, V. M. (1993). Using self-efficacy theory in patient education. In B. Gilroth (Ed.), *Managing hospital-based patient education* (pp. 327–337). Chicago: American Hospital Publishing.

Lupien, A., & George-Gay, B. (2001). High fidelity patient simulation. In A. Lowenstein, & M. Bradshaw (Eds.), *Fuszard's innovative teaching strategies in nursing* (3rd ed., pp. 134–148). Gaithersburg, MD: Aspen.

Lyons, J., & Milton, J. (1999). Recognizing through feeling: A physical and computer simulation based on educational theory. *Computers in Nursing, 17*(3), 114–119.

Markiewicz, T., & Wells, N. (1997). Mundanatories no more. *Journal of Continuing Education in Nursing, 28*(2), 88–90.

Martin, J. T., Hoffman, M. K., & Kaminski, P. F. (2005). NPs vs. IT for effective colposcopy patient education. *The Nurse Practitioner, 30*(4), 52–57.

McAlindon, M. N., & Smith, G. R. (1994). Repurposing videodiscs for interactive video instruction: Teaching concepts of quality improvement. *Computers in Nursing, 12,* 46–56.

Musinski, B. (1999). The educator as facilitator: A new kind of leadership. *Nursing Forum, 34*(1), 23–29.

Narrow, B. (1979). *Patient teaching in nursing practice: A patient and family centered approach.* New York: Wiley.

Oermann, M. H. (2003). Effects of educational intervention in waiting room on patient satisfaction. *Journal of Ambulatory Care Management, 26*(2), 150–158.

O'Very, D. (1999). Self-paced: The right pace for staff development. *Journal of Continuing Education in Nursing, 30*(4), 182–187.

Parrott, T. E. (1994). Humor as a teaching strategy. *Nurse Educator, 19*(3), 36–38.

Peters, F. L., & Connell, K. M. (1991). Incorporating the affective component into an AIDS work shop. *Journal of Continuing Education in Nursing, 22*, 95–99.

Phillips, L. D. (1999). Patient education: Understanding the process to maximize time and outcomes. *Journal of Intravenous Nursing, 22*(1), 19–35.

Poston, I. (1993). How to develop computer assisted instruction programs. *Nursing & Health Care, 14*, 344–349.

Prochaska, J., DiClemente, C., Velicer, W., & Rossi, J. (1993). Standardized, individualized, interactive, and personalized self-help programs for smoking cessation. *Health Psychology, 12*(5), 399–405.

Prochaska, J., Velicer, W., Rossi, J., Goldstein, M., Marcus, B., Rakowski, W., et al. (1994). Stages of change and decisional balance for 12 problem behaviors. *Health Psychology, 13*(1), 39–46.

Ramsey, A. M., & Siroky, A. S. (1988). The use of puppets to teach school age children with asthma. *Pediatric Nursing, 14*, 187–190.

Redman, B. K. (2007). *The practice of patient education: A case study approach* (10th ed.). St. Louis: Mosby Elsevier.

Robinson, K. J., Lewis, D. J., & Robinson, J. A. (1990). Games: A way to give laboratory values meaning. *American Nephrology Nurses Association Journal, 17*(4), 306–308.

Rothwell, W. J., & Kazanas, H. C. (2004). *Mastering the instructional design process: A systematic approach* (3rd ed.). San Francisco: Pfeiffer.

Rowell, S., & Spielvogle, S. (1996). Wanted: "A few good bug detectives." A gaming technique to increase staff awareness of current infection control practices. *Journal of Continuing Education in Nursing, 27*(6), 274–278.

Rystedt, H., & Lindstrom, B. (2001). Introducing simulation technologies in nurse education: A nursing practice perspective. *Nurse Education in Practice, 1*(3), 134–141.

Saarmann, L., Daugherty, J., & Riegel, B. (2000). Patient teaching to promote behavior change. *Nursing Outlook, 48*(6), 281–287.

Schmidt, K. L., & Fisher, J. C. (1992). Effective development and utilization of self-learning modules. *Journal of Continuing Education in Nursing, 23*, 54–59.

Schmitz, B. D., MacLean, S. L., & Shidler, H. M. (1991). An emergency pursuit game: A method for teaching emergency decision making skills. *Journal of Continuing Education in Nursing, 22*, 152–158.

Shearer, R., & Davidhizar, R. (2003). Using role play to develop cultural competence. *Journal of Nursing Education, 42*(6), 273–276.

Snowman, J., & Biehler, R. (2006). *Psychology Applied to Teaching*. Boston: Houghton Mifflin Company.

Tang, T. S., Funnell, M. M., & Anderson, R. M. (2006). Group education strategies for diabetes self-management. *Diabetes Spectrum, 19*(2), 99–105.

Tibbles, L., Lewis, C., Reisine, S., Rippey, R., & Donald, M. (1992). Computer assisted instruction for preoperative and postoperative patient education in joint replacement surgery. *Computers in Nursing, 10*, 208–211.

Turner, B. (2007). Embracing simulation and virtual reality. *Duke Nursing Magazine, 2*(1), 22–23.

Vander Zanden, J. W., Crandell, T. L., & Crandell, C. H. (2007). *Human Development* (8th ed.). Boston: McGraw-Hill.

Willingham, D. T. (2004, Spring). Practice makes perfect: But only if you practice beyond the point of perfection. *American Educator, 31–33*, 38.

Wood, R. Y. (1994). Use of the nursing simulation laboratory in reentry programs: An innovative setting for updating clinical skills. *Journal of Continuing Education in Nursing, 25*, 28–31.

Yoo, M. S., & Yoo, I. Y. (2003). The effectiveness of standardized patients as a teaching method for nursing fundamentals. *Journal of Nursing Education, 42*(10), 444–448.

Young, P., & Diekelmann, N. (2002). Learning to lecture: Exploring the skills, strategies, and practices of new teachers in nursing education. *Journal of Nursing Education, 41*(9), 405–412.

Chapter 12

Instructional Materials

Diane S. Hainsworth

CHAPTER HIGHLIGHTS

KEY TERMS

- instructional materials
- characteristics of the learner
- characteristics of the media
- characteristics of the task
- delivery system
- realia
- illusionary representations
- symbolic representations
- replica
- analogue
- symbol
- audiovisual materials

OBJECTIVES

After completing this chapter, the reader will be able to
1. Differentiate between *instructional materials* and *instructional methods*.
2. Identify the three major variables (learner, task, and media characteristics) to be considered when selecting, developing, and evaluating instructional materials.
3. Cite the three components of instructional materials required to effectively communicate educational messages.
4. Discuss general principles applicable to all types of media.
5. Identify the multitude of audiovisual tools—both print and nonprint materials—available for patient and professional education.
6. Describe the general guidelines for development of printed materials.
7. Analyze the advantages and disadvantages specific to each type of instructional medium.
8. Evaluate the type of media suitable for use depending on such variables as the size of the audience, the resources available, and the characteristics of the learner.
9. Identify where educational tools can be found.
10. Critique tools for value and appropriateness.
11. Recognize the supplemental nature of media's role in patient and staff education.

Whereas instructional methods are the approaches used for teaching (as described in Chapter 11), *instructional materials* are the vehicles by which information is communicated. Often these terms are used interchangeably and are frequently referred to in combination with one another as teaching strategies and techniques. But instructional methods and instructional materials are not one and the same, and a clear distinction can and should be made between them. Instructional methods are the way information is taught. Instructional materials, which include print and nonprint media and the accompanying hardware and software needed for delivery, are the adjuncts used to enhance teaching and learning.

Instructional materials, also known as tools and aids, are mechanisms or objects to transmit information that are intended to supplement, rather than replace, the act of teaching and the role of the teacher. These modes by which information is shared with the learner often are not considered in depth, and yet instructional materials represent an important, complex component of the educational process. Given the numerous factors impacting on both the teacher and the learner, such as the increase in staff workloads, the decrease in patient lengths of stay, the increase in patient acuity, the alternative settings in which education is now delivered, and the shrinking resources for educational services, it is imperative that the nurse educator understand the various types of audio and visual media available to efficiently and effectively complement teaching efforts.

Instructional materials provide the nurse educator with tools to deliver messages creatively, clearly, accurately, and in a timely fashion. They

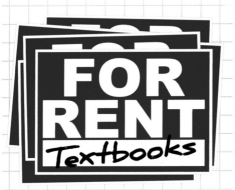

RENT
NOW

SAVE 50%*
OR MORE

RENT·A·TEXT

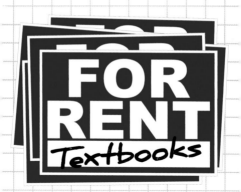

RENT NOW

SAVE 50%* OR MORE

help the teacher reinforce information, clarify abstract concepts, and simplify complex messages. Multimedia resources serve to stimulate a learner's senses as well as add variety, realism, and enjoyment to the teaching/learning experience. They have the potential to assist learners not only in acquiring knowledge and skills but also in retaining more effectively what they learn. As you will see, research indicates that audiovisual materials do, indeed, facilitate teaching and learning.

This chapter provides a systematic overview of the process for selecting, developing, implementing, and evaluating instructional materials. Various types of audio and visual media are examined with an eye to matching them to the particular characteristics of learners, the specific topics to be taught, and the variable situations and settings for teaching and learning. The advantages and disadvantages of each of the media types will be discussed. Although the choice of instructional materials often depends on availability or cost, whichever tools are selected should enhance achievement of expected learning outcomes.

This chapter is intended to inform nurse educators about various media options that will allow them to make informed choices regarding appropriate instructional materials that fit the learner, that affect the motivation of the learner, and that accomplish the learning task. Whether nurses educate patients and their families, staff nurses, or nursing students, the same principles apply in making decisions about the type of materials selected for instruction.

General Principles

Before selecting or developing media from the multitude of available options, you should be aware of the following general principles regarding the effectiveness of audiovisual tools:

- The teacher must be familiar with the media content before a tool is used.
- Print and nonprint materials do change learner behavior by influencing a gain in cognitive, affective, and/or psychomotor skills.
- No one tool is better than another in enhancing learning. The suitability of any particular medium depends on many variables.
- The tools should complement the instructional methods.
- The choice of media should be consistent with subject content and match the tasks to be learned to assist the learner in accomplishing predetermined behavioral objectives.
- The instructional materials should reinforce and supplement—not substitute for—the educator's teaching efforts.
- Media should match the available financial resources.
- Instructional aids should be appropriate for the physical conditions of the learning environment, such as the size and seating of the audience, acoustics, space, lighting, and display hardware (delivery mechanisms) available.
- Media should complement the sensory abilities, developmental stages, and educational level of the intended audience.
- The message imparted by instructional materials must be accurate, valid, authoritative, up to date, state of the art, appropriate, unbiased, and free of any unintended messages.
- The media should contribute meaningfully to the learning situation by adding and diversifying information.

Choosing Instructional Materials

Many important variables must be considered when selecting instructional materials. The role of the nurse educator goes beyond the dispensing of information only; it also involves skill in designing and planning for instruction. Learning can be made more enjoyable for both the learner and the teacher if the educator knows what instructional materials are available, as well as how to choose and use them so as to enhance the teaching–learning experience.

Knowledge of the diversity of instructional tools and their appropriate use will enable the teacher to make education more interesting, challenging, and effective for all types of learners. With current trends in healthcare reform, educational strategies to teach patients, in particular, will need to include instructional materials for health promotion and illness prevention among well persons, as well as instructional materials for health maintenance and restoration for ill persons.

Making appropriate choices of instructional materials depends on a broad understanding of three major variables: (1) characteristics of the learner, (2) characteristics of the media, and (3) characteristics of the task to be achieved (Frantz, 1980). A useful mnemonic for remembering these variables is LMAT: *L*earner, *M*edia, and *T*ask, which is derived from the last letter of the word instructiona*l* and the first three letters of the word *mat*erials.

1. *Characteristics of the learner:* Many variables are known to influence learning. Therefore, it is important to know your audience so as to choose media that best suit the needs and abilities of various learners. You must consider sensorimotor abilities, physical attributes, reading skills, motivational levels (locus of control), developmental stages, learning styles, and cultural backgrounds.

2. *Characteristics of the media:* A wide variety of media, print and nonprint, are available to enhance methods of instruction for the achievement of objectives. Print materials are the most common form through which the information is communicated, and nonprint media include a full range of audio and visual possibilities. Since no single medium is most effective, the educator should be flexible in considering a multimedia approach to complement methods of instruction.

3. *Characteristics of the task:* Identifying the learning domain (cognitive, affective, and/or psychomotor) and the complexity of those behaviors that are required, based on the predetermined behavioral objectives, defines the tasks to be accomplished.

The Three Major Components of Instructional Materials

Depending on the instructional methods used to communicate information, decisions also will have to be made regarding the media potentially best suited to assist with the process of teaching and learning. The delivery system (Weston & Cranston, 1986), content, and presentation (Frantz, 1980) are the three major components of media that should be kept in mind when selecting print and nonprint materials for instruction.

Delivery System

The *delivery system* includes both the software (physical form of the materials) and the hardware used in presentation of information. For instance, the educator giving a lecture might choose to embellish the information being presented using a delivery system, such as PowerPoint slides (software), and a computer (hardware). The content on DVDs (software), in conjunction with DVD players (hardware), and CD-ROM programs (software), in conjunction with the computer (hardware) are other examples of delivery systems.

The choice of the delivery system is influenced by the size of the intended audience, the pacing or flexibility needed for delivery, and the sensory aspects most suitable to the audience. More recently, the geographical distribution of the audience is a significant influence on choice of delivery systems, given the popularity of distance education modalities.

Content

The content (intended message) is independent of the delivery system and is the actual information being communicated to the learner, which might focus on any topic relevant to the teaching/learning experience. When selecting media, the nurse educator must consider several factors:

- the accuracy of the information being conveyed. Is it up-to-date, reliable, and authentic?
- the appropriateness of the medium to convey particular information. Audiotapes and printed pamphlets, for example, can be very appropriate tools for sharing information to change behavior in the cognitive or affective domain but not ideal for skill development in the psychomotor domain. Videos, as well as real equipment for demonstrations and return demonstrations, are much more effective tools for conveying information relative to learning psychomotor behaviors.
- the appropriateness of the readability level of materials for the intended audience. Is the content written at a literacy level suitable for the learner's reading and comprehension abilities? The more complex the task, the more important it is to write clear, simple, succinct instructions enhanced with illustrations, and that the content can be understood by the learner (see Chapter 7).

Presentation

Weston and Cranston (1986) state that the form of the message, in other words, how information is presented, is the most important component for selecting or developing instructional materials. However, a consideration of this aspect of the media is frequently ignored. They describe the form of the message as occurring along a continuum from concrete (real objects) to abstract (symbols).

REALIA

Realia applies to the most concrete form of stimuli that can be used to deliver information. For instance, an actual woman demonstrating breast self-examination is the most concrete example of realia. Because this form of presentation might be less acceptable for a wide range of teaching situations, the next best choice would be a mannequin. This model, analogous to a human figure, has many characteristics that simulate reality, including size and three-dimensionality, but without being the true figure that may very well cause embarrassment for the learner. The message is less concrete, yet using an imitation of a person as an instructional medium allows for an accurate presentation of information with near-maximal stimulation of the learners' perceptual abilities. Further along the continuum of realia is a video presentation of a woman performing breast self-examination. The learner could still learn accurate breast self-examination this way, but the aspect of dimensionality is absent. The message becomes less concrete and more abstract.

ILLUSIONARY REPRESENTATIONS

The term *illusionary representations* applies to a less concrete, more abstract form of stimuli to deliver a message, such as moving or still photographs, audiotapes projecting true sounds, and real life drawings. Although many realistic cues, including dimensionality, are missing from this category of instructional materials, the advantages of illusionary media are that they can offer learners a variety of real-life visual and auditory experiences to which they might otherwise not have access or exposure due to such factors as location or expense. For example, pictures of how to stage decubitus ulcers or audiotapes on how to discriminate between normal and abnormal lung sounds, although more abstract in form, do to some degree resemble or simulate realia.

SYMBOLIC REPRESENTATIONS

The term *symbolic representations* applies to the most abstract types of messages, yet they are the most common form of stimuli used for instruction. They include numbers and letters of the alphabet, symbols that are written and spoken as words, that are employed to convey ideas or represent objects. Audiotapes or oral presentations, graphs, written texts and handouts, posters, blackboards, and whiteboards on which to display words and images are vehicles to deliver messages in symbolic form. The chief disadvantage of symbolic representations stems from their lack of concreteness. For that reason, their use should be limited to more sophisticated learners and may be inappropriate as instructional materials for very young children, learners from different cultures, learners with significant literacy problems, and individuals with cognitive and sensory impairments.

When making decisions about which tools to select in order to best accomplish teaching objectives, the nurse educator should carefully consider these three media components. The various delivery systems available, the content or message to be conveyed, and the form in which information will be presented must be taken into account when choosing from a wide range of print and audiovisual options. Remember, no one type of media is suitable for all audiences in promoting acquisition and retention of information. Most importantly, the function of instructional materials is to supplement, complement, and support the educator's teaching efforts for the successful achievement of learner outcomes.

Types of Instructional Materials

Written Materials

Handouts, leaflets, books, pamphlets, brochures, and instruction sheets are the most widely employed and most accessible type of media used for teaching. Although printed materials have been described as "frozen language" (Redman, 2007, p. 34), they are, nonetheless, the most common form of teaching tool because of the distinct advantages they provide to enhance teaching and learning.

The greatest virtues of written materials are that they are:

- Available to the learner as a reference for reinforcement of information when the nurse educator is not immediately present to answer questions or clarify information.
- Widely used at all levels of society, so this type of media is acceptable and familiar to the public.
- Easily obtainable through commercial sources, usually at relatively low cost and on a wide variety of subjects, for distribution by educators.
- Provided in convenient forms, such as pamphlets, which are portable, reusable, and do not require software or hardware resources.
- Are becoming more widely available in languages other than English due to the recognition of significant cultural and ethnic shifts in the general population.
- Suitable to a large number of learners who prefer reading as opposed to receiving messages in other formats.
- Flexible in that the information is absorbed at a speed controlled by the reader.

The disadvantages of printed materials include the facts that:

- Written words are the most abstract form in which to convey information.
- Immediate feedback on the information presented may be limited.

- A large percentage of materials are written at too high a level for reading and comprehension by the majority of patients (Doak, Doak, Friedell, & Meade, 1998).
- They are inappropriate for persons with visual or cognitive impairment.

COMMERCIALLY PREPARED MATERIALS

A wealth of brochures, posters, pamphlets, and patient-focused texts is currently available from commercial vendors. Whether they enhance the quality of learning is an important question for nurse educators to consider when trying to evaluate these products for content, readability, and presentation. Commercial products may or may not be produced in collaboration with health professionals, which raises the question of how factual the information may be. For example, materials prepared by pharmaceutical companies or medical supply companies might not be free of bias. Several factors must be considered when reviewing printed materials that have been prepared commercially, including the following:

- Who produced the item? Evidence should make it clear if input was provided by healthcare professionals with expertise in the subject matter.
- Can the item be previewed? The educator should have an opportunity to examine the accuracy and appropriateness of content to ensure that the information needed by the target audience is provided.
- Is the price of the teaching tool consistent with its educational value? Getting across an important message effectively may justify a significant cost outlay,

especially if the tool can be used with large numbers of learners. However, simple printed instruction sheets may do the job just as well at less expense and can provide the educator with the ability to update the information on a frequent basis.

The main advantages of using commercial materials is that they are readily available and can be obtained in bulk for free or at a relatively low cost. An educator would need to spend hours researching, writing, and copying materials to create informational materials of equal quality and value.

The disadvantages of using commercial materials include issues of cost, accuracy and adequacy of content, and readability of the materials. Some educational booklets are expensive to purchase and impractical to give away in large quantities to learners. Also, the actual utility of commercially prepared instructional materials must be evaluated because the level of readability might very well be inappropriate for the majority of members in the targeted audience, and the content might not completely and accurately cover all the information that the learners need to know.

INSTRUCTOR-COMPOSED MATERIALS

Educators may choose to write their own instructional materials for the purpose of cost savings or the need to tailor content to specific audiences.

Advantages to composing your own materials are many (Brownson, 1998; Doak et al., 1998). By writing your own materials, you can tailor the information to:

- Fit your own institution's policies, procedures, and equipment.

- Build in answers to those questions asked most frequently by your patients.
- Highlight points considered especially important by your team of physicians or other healthcare professionals.
- Reinforce specific oral instructions that clarify difficult concepts.

Doak et al. (1998) outlined specific suggestions for tailoring information to help patients want to read and remember the message and to act on it. These authors defined tailoring as personalizing the message so that the content, structure, and image fit an individual patient's learning needs. For example, they suggested techniques to tailor information, such as writing the patient's name on the cover, and opening a pamphlet with a patient and highlighting the most important information as it is verbally reviewed. In another example, Feldman (2004) described successful use of child care checklists that had simple line drawings (no more than two to a page) coupled with brief written descriptions that led parents step-by-step through specific care tasks, such as bathing a baby. Audiotapes also accompanied these pictures and simple instructions. Additional studies have supported the efficacy of tailored instruction over nontailored messages in achieving reading, recall, and follow-through in health teaching (Campbell et al., 1994; Skinner, Strecher, & Hospers, 1994).

There are, of course, disadvantages to composing your own materials. You need to exercise extra care to ensure that materials are well written and laid out effectively, which can be a time-consuming endeavor. Although nurse educators are expected to enhance their methods of teaching with instructional materials, few have ever had formal training in the development and application of written materials. Many tools written by patient educators are too long, too detailed, and composed at too high a level for the target audience. Doak, Doak, and Root (1996), and Brownson (1998) suggest the following guidelines to ensure the clarity of self-composed printed education materials:

- Make sure the content is accurate and up to date.
- Organize the content in a logical, step-by-step fashion so learners are being informed adequately but are not overwhelmed with large amounts of information. Avoid giving detailed rationales because they may unnecessarily lengthen the written information. Prioritize the content to address only what learners need to know. Content that is nice to know can be addressed orally on an individual basis.
- Make sure the information succinctly discusses the what, how, and when. Follow the KISS rule: keep it simple and smart. This can best be accomplished by putting the information into a question-and-answer format or by dividing the information into subheadings according to the nature of the content.
- Regardless of format, avoid medical jargon whenever possible, and define any technical terms in layman's language. Sometimes it is important to expose patients to technical terms because of complicated procedures and ongoing interaction with the medical team, so careful definitions can minimize misunderstandings. Be consistent with the words you use.
- Find out the average grade in school completed by the targeted patient pop-

ulation, and write the patient education materials two to four grade levels below that level. For individuals who are non-literate, pictographs can increase recall of spoken medical instruction (Houts et al., 1998; Kessels, 2003). Follow the guidelines in Chapter 7 for decreasing reading level.

Always state things in positive, not negative, terms. Never illustrate incorrect messages. For example, depicting a hand holding a metered-dose inhaler in the mouth not only incorrectly illustrates a drug delivery technique (Weixler, 1994) but reinforces that message by its visual impact alone. **Figure 12–1** illustrates the correct way to use an inhaler and reinforces a positive message.

In addition to the guidelines for clarity and completeness in constructing written materials, format and appearance are equally important in motivating learners to read the printed word. If the format and appearance are too detailed, learners will feel overwhelmed, and instead of attracting the learners, you will discourage and repel them (see **Figure 12–2**). To avoid common pitfalls in writing good instructional tools, see Chapter 7 on how to write effective printed materials.

EVALUATING PRINTED MATERIALS

When evaluating printed materials, the following considerations should be kept in mind.

Nature of the Audience What is the average age of the audience? For instance, older adults tend to prefer printed materials that they can read at their leisure. Lengthy materials may be less problematic for older learners, who frequently have enough time and patience for reading educational materials. Children, on the other hand, like short printed materials with many illustrations.

Figure 12–1 Diagram illustrating proper technique for inhaler use.

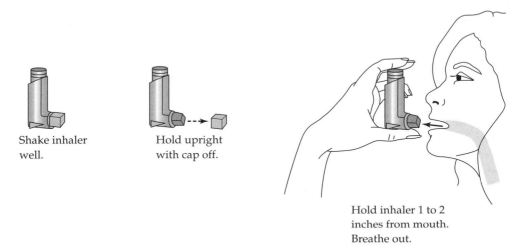

Shake inhaler
well.

Hold upright
with cap off.

Hold inhaler 1 to 2
inches from mouth.
Breathe out.

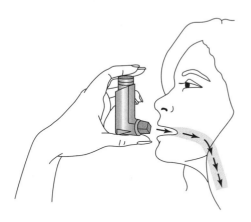

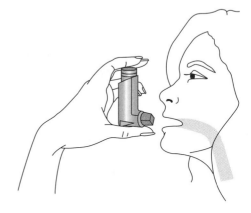

Press down on inhaler. Breathe
in slowly (3 to 5 seconds).

Hold breath 10 seconds,
then repeat puffs.

Also, what is the preferred learning style of the particular audience? Printed materials with few illustrations are poorly suited to patients who not only have difficulty reading but also do not like to read. Representations of information in the form of graphs and charts can be included with the content of printed materials for those who are visual and conceptual learners.

In addition, does your audience have any sensory deficits? Vision deficits are common with

Figure 12–2 Inadequate versus adequate appearance and formatting.

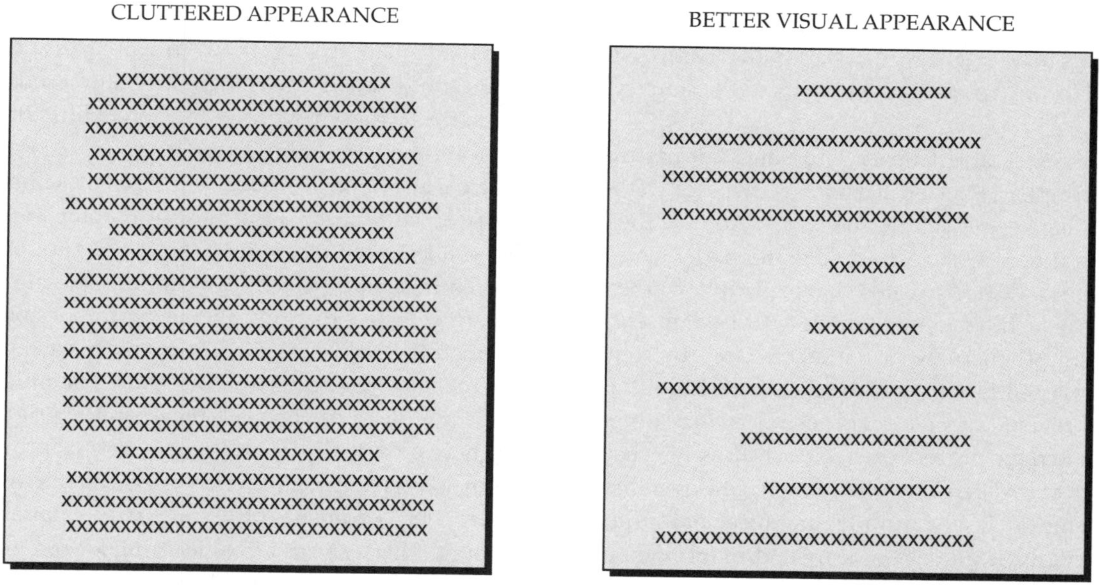

CLUTTERED APPEARANCE BETTER VISUAL APPEARANCE

older adult patients, and short-term memory may be a problem for comprehension. Having materials that can be reread at their own convenience and pace can reinforce earlier learning and minimize confusion over treatment instructions. To accommodate those individuals with vision impairments, use a large typeface and lots of white space, separate one section from another with ample spacing, highlight important points, and use black print on white paper.

Literacy Level Required The effectiveness of patient education materials for helping the learner accomplish behavioral objectives can be totally undermined if the materials are written at a level beyond the comprehension of the learner. The Joint Commission (formerly known as the Joint Commission on Accreditation of Healthcare Or-

ganizations) mandates that health information must be presented in a manner that can be understood by patients and family members. This requirement underscores the importance of screening potential educational tools to be used as adjuncts to various teaching methods. A number of formulas (e.g., Fog, SMOG, Flesch, Fry) are available for determining readability (see Chapter 7 and Appendix A).

Linguistic Variety Available Linguistic variety refers to choices of printed materials in different foreign languages. These may be limited because duplicate materials in more than one language are costly to publish and not likely to be undertaken unless the publisher anticipates a large demand. The growth of minority populations in the United States has promoted increasing attention to the need for non-English language teaching materials. Regional differences exist, so there may be more availability of Asian-language materials on the West Coast and more Spanish-language materials in the Southwest and Northeast than in other parts of the country.

Brevity and Clarity   In education, as in art, simpler is better. Remind yourself of the KISS rule: keep it simple and smart. Address the critical facts only. What does the patient need to know? Choose words that explain how; the why can be filled in by a lecture or discussion. Include simple pictures that illustrate step by step the written instructions being given. **Figure 12–3** provides a good example of a clear, easy-to-follow instructional tool used to teach an asthma patient how to determine when a metered-dose inhaler is empty. Using simple graphics and minimal words, it guides the learner through the procedure with very little room for misinterpretation and is suitable for a wide range of audiences.

Layout and Appearance   The appearance of written materials is crucial in attracting learners' attention and getting them to read the information. If a tool has too much wording, with inadequate spacing between sentences and paragraphs; small margins; and numerous pages, the learner may find it much too difficult and too time consuming to read.

Doak et al. (1996) point out that allowing plenty of white space is the most important step that can be taken to improve the appearance of written materials. This means double spacing, leaving generous margins, indenting important points, using bold characters, and separating key statements with extra space. Inserting a graphic in the middle of the text can break up the print and may be visually appealing, as well as providing a mechanism for reinforcing the narrative information. Redman (2001) states that pictorial learning is better than verbal learning for recognition and recall. For topics that lend themselves to concrete explanations, this is especially true.

Figure 12–3 Examples of a clear, easy-to-follow instructional tool for an asthma patient.

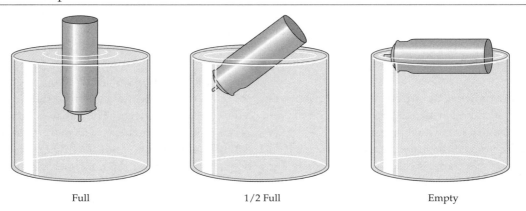

Full   1/2 Full   Empty

An example used earlier in this chapter is teaching the psychomotor task of using a metered-dose inhaler (see Figure 12–1). Also included are simple step-by-step instructions written in the active voice (see **Figure 12–4**).

Opportunity for Repetition   Written materials can be read later, again and again, to reinforce your teaching when you are not there to answer questions. Thus, it is an advantage if materials are laid out in a simple question-and-answer format. Questions demand answers and this format allows patients to find information easily for repeated references. If you are writing your own materials, also be mindful of the need to keep information current, and update it for changing patient populations.

Concreteness and Familiarity   Using the active voice is more immediate and concrete. For example, "Shake the inhaler very well three times" is more effective than "The inhaler should be shaken thoroughly" (see Figure 12–4). Also,

the importance of using plain language instead of medical jargon cannot be overemphasized. Inadequate patient understanding of common medical terms used by healthcare providers is a significant factor in noncompliance with medical regimens. A number of studies have indicated that patients understood medical terms at a much lower rate than health professionals expected (Estey, Musseau, & Keehn, 1994; Lerner, Jehle, Janicke, & Moscati, 2000).

In summary, instructor-designed or commercially produced printed instructional materials are widely used for a broad range of audiences. They vary in literacy demand levels and may be found written in several languages. **Table 12–1** summarizes their basic advantages and disadvantages.

Demonstration Materials

Demonstration materials include many types of nonprint media, such as models and real equipment, as well as displays, such as posters, diagrams, illustrations, charts, bulletin boards, flannel boards, flip charts, chalkboards, photo-

Figure 12–4 Example of instructions written in the active voice.

STEPS FOR CORRECT INHALER TECHNIQUE

1. Shake the inhaler very well three times.
2. Remove cap and hold inhaler upright.
3. Hold the inhaler 1 to 2 inches from your mouth.
4. Tilt your head back slightly and breathe out fully.
5. Press down on the inhaler and start to breathe in slowly.
6. Breathe in slowly and deeply (3 to 5 seconds) to pull the medicine down into your lungs.
7. Hold your breath for 10 seconds to keep the medicine in your lungs.
8. Take a few normal breaths.
9. Repeat puffs by following steps 1–8 again.

Table 12–1 BASIC ADVANTAGES AND DISADVANTAGES OF PRINTED MATERIALS

Advantages	Disadvantages
Always available	Impersonal
Rate of reading is controllable by the reader	Limited feedback; absence of instructor lessens opportunity to clear up misinterpretation
Complex concepts can be explained both fully and adequately	Passive tool
Procedural steps can be outlined	Highly complex materials may be overwhelming to the learner
Verbal instruction can be reinforced	Literacy skill of learner may limit effectiveness
Learner is always able to refer back to instructions given in print	

graphs, and drawings. All represent unique ways of communicating messages to the learner. These aids primarily stimulate the visual senses but can combine the sense of sight with touch and sometimes even smell and taste. From these various forms of demonstration materials, the educator can choose one or more to complement teaching efforts in reaching predetermined objectives. Just as with written tools, these aids must be accurate and appropriate for the intended audience. Ideally, these media forms bring the learner closer to reality and actively engage him or her in a visual and participatory manner. As such, demonstration tools are useful for cognitive, affective, and psychomotor skill development. The major forms of demonstration materials—models and displays—will be discussed in detail.

MODELS

Models are usually three-dimensional instructional tools that allow the learner to immediately apply knowledge and psychomotor skills by observing, examining, manipulating, handling, assembling, and disassembling objects while the teacher provides feedback (Rankin & Stallings, 2001). In addition, these demonstration aids encourage learners to think abstractly and give them the opportunity to use many of their senses (Boyd, Gleit, Graham, & Whitman, 1998). Whenever possible, the use of real objects and actual equipment is preferred, but a model is the next best thing when the real object is not available, accessible, or feasible, or is too complex to use.

The three specific types of models used for teaching and learning, as differentiated by Babcock and Miller (1990), are:

- Replicas, associated with the word *resemble*
- Analogues, associated with the words *act like*
- Symbols, associated with the words *stands for*

A *replica* is a facsimile constructed to scale that resembles the features or substance of the original object. The dimensions of the reproduction may be decreased or enlarged in size to make demonstration easier and more understandable. A replica of the DNA helix is an excellent example of a model used to teach the complex concept of genetics. Replicas can be examined and manipulated by the learner to get an idea of how something looks and works. They are excellent for teaching psychomotor skills because they give the learner an opportunity for active participation through hands-on experience. Not only can the learner assemble and disassemble parts to see how they fit and operate, but the pace of learning can also be controlled by the learner.

Replicas are used frequently by the nurse educator when teaching anatomy and physiology. Models of the heart, kidney, ear, eye, joints, and pelvic organs, for example, allow the learner to get a perspective on parts of the body not readily viewed without these teaching aids. Resuscitation dolls are a common type of replica used to teach the skills of CPR. Breast self-examination is another topic best taught to wide audiences through the use of a model. Learners who regularly refresh their skills using demonstration models as instructional tools are more likely to maintain regular and effective use of the technique than learners who do not (Pinto, 1993). Using inanimate objects first is a technique educators can use to desensitize learners before doing invasive procedures on themselves or other human beings. Instructional models have been found to be effective in reducing fear and enhancing acceptance of certain procedures (Cobussen-Boekhorst, Van Der Weide, Feitz, & DeGier, 2000). Teaching a diabetic how to draw up and inject insulin can best be accomplished by using a combination of real equipment and replicas. Patients first draw up sterile saline in real syringes, then practice injecting oranges, and progress to a model of a person before actually injecting themselves. Sometimes, preliminary use of a video before starting to directly handle equipment may be helpful if learners are very anxious about performing various procedures. For lessons aimed at psychomotor learning, skills checklists can be used as a mecha-

nism for evaluating the accuracy of return demonstrations. Simulation laboratories use this evaluation method frequently. For example, a demonstration day for nurses might have stations for chest tube care, artery catheter placement, exchange transfusion, metabolic screening and rhythm strips, and code arrest. Using various models, demonstration days offer a chance to provide hands-on practice to new staff nurses as well as an annual review of seasoned nurses.

The second type of model is known as an *analogue* because it has the same properties and performs like a real object. Unlike replicas, analogue models are effective in explaining and representing dynamic systems. Mechanical devices such as extracorporeal and dialysis machines are good examples. Although they do not look like the actual anatomy of a person, these pieces of artificial equipment perform similar physiological functions of the heart, lungs, and kidneys. Another popular analogue is a computer model depicting how the human brain functions.

The third type of model is a *symbol*, which is used frequently in teaching situations. Words, mathematical signs and formulas, diagrams, cartoons, stick figures, and traffic signs are all examples of symbolic models that convey a message to the receiver through imaging, convention, or association. International signs, for example, convey a familiar and understandable message to individuals of multilingual or multicultural backgrounds. However, abbreviations and acronyms common to healthcare personnel, such as NPO, PRN, and PO, should be avoided when interacting with consumers because they are likely to be unfamiliar with these abbreviations.

The advantage of models is that they can adequately replace the real object, which may be too small, too large, too expensive, too complex, unavailable, or inappropriate for use in a teaching/learning situation. A vast array of models can be purchased from commercial vendors at varying prices (some for free) or improvised by the teacher. Models do not need to be expensive or elaborate to get concepts and ideas across (Rankin & Stallings, 2001). In particular, models enhance learning by:

- Allowing learners to practice acquiring new skills without being afraid of compromising themselves or others.
- Stimulating active learner involvement.
- Providing the opportunity for immediate testing of psychomotor and cognitive behaviors.
- Receiving instant feedback from the instructor.
- Appealing to the kinesthetic learner who prefers the hands-on approach to learning.

In terms of their disadvantages, some models may not be suitable for the learner with poor abstraction abilities or for visually impaired audiences, unless each individual is given the chance to tangibly appraise the object using other senses. Also, some models can be fragile, very expensive (like the Sim-Man or Sim-Baby used to teach assessment skills), bulky to store, and difficult to transport. Unless models are very large, they cannot be observed and manipulated by more than a few learners at any one time. However, this drawback can be overcome by using team teaching and by creating different stations at which to arrange a replica for demonstration purposes (Babcock & Miller, 1994).

DISPLAYS

Chalkboards, white marker boards, posters, flip charts, bulletin boards, and flannel boards are examples of displays found in almost any educational setting. As they are two-dimensional objects, they are useful tools for a variety of teaching purposes to convey simple or quick messages and to clarify, reinforce, or summarize information on important topics and themes. Although they have been referred to as static instructional tools due to the fact that they are often stationary (Haggard, 1989), some can be portable and most are alterable. As demonstration materials, these tools can effectively achieve behavioral objectives by vividly representing the essence of relationships between subjects or objects. The chalkboard and flip charts and the more modern white marker board are particularly versatile in delivering information. These board devices are most useful in formal classes, group discussions, or during brainstorming sessions to spontaneously make drawings or diagrams (with contrasting colored chalk or markers) or to jot down ideas generated from participants while the educator is in the process of teaching. Information can be added, corrected, or deleted quickly and easily while the learners are actively following what you are doing or saying. Such tools are excellent in promoting participation, keeping the learners' attention on the topic at hand, and noting and reinforcing the contributions of others. Flexible and handy, they provide opportunities for the teacher, in an immediate and direct fashion, to organize data, integrate ideas, perform on-the-spot problem solving, and compare and contrast various points of view. Unlike some other types of visuals, these display tools can allow learners to see parts of a whole picture while assisting the teacher in filling in the gaps.

The following are important guidelines suggested by Babcock and Miller (1994) for instructors using chalkboards and white marker boards:

- Be sure writing is legible and discernible.
- Step aside and face the audience after putting notations on the board to maintain contact with the audience.

- Allow learners time to copy the message.
- Enlist a good note taker to capture a creative design or record an idea before the board is erased.

In particular, the following are some advantages of displays as teaching tools:

- They are a quick way to attract attention and get an idea across.
- Most are flexible, easily modified, and reusable.
- Many are portable and easily assembled or disassembled.
- They stimulate interest or ideas in the observer.
- They are effective for influencing cognitive and affective behaviors.

Some of the disadvantages of displays include the following:

- They may take up a lot of space.
- They can be time consuming to have prepared, and for that reason tend to be used again and again, which increases the risk of their becoming outdated.
- They are unsuitable for large audiences if information is to be viewed simultaneously.
- Limited amounts of information can be included at one time.
- They are ineffective for teaching psychomotor skills.
- They may become too cluttered when too much information is placed on them.
- They may be ignored if they are posted too long, are overused, or are poorly arranged.
- If permanently mounted, they cannot be transported.
- The symbolic nature of the message may be misunderstood, which is a problem that underscores their importance as supplements to learning.

POSTERS

Although they are a type of display material, posters are being addressed separately because they have become an increasingly unique, popular, and important educational tool. Essentially hybrids of print and nonprint media, they heavily employ the written word along with graphic illustrations. Posters are a legitimate and reasonable alternative to more direct, formal presentations for conveying information (Duchin & Sherwood, 1990; Flournoy, Turner, & Combs, 2000; Moneyham, Ura, Ellwood, & Bruno, 1996; Thurber & Asselin, 1999). As a visual supplement to oral instruction of patients and families in various clinical settings, posters are being increasingly accepted as an effective tool to educate staff and students at continuing education meetings and research conferences. Posters can serve as an independent source of information or in conjunction with other instructional methods and materials. Some critics view the poster as a passive instructional medium, but this conjecture can easily be disputed. Inherent in the design, the message conveyed by a well-constructed poster is brief, constant, and interactive with the audience (Duchin & Sherwood, 1990). Because the primary purpose of a poster is visual stimulation, it is meant to attract attention (Flournoy et al., 2000). Effective posters leave a mental image long after they are seen. This mental image is a cue to the viewer to remember the message being delivered. Much like a bumper sticker you see on a car in front of you while driving, effective poster displays can potentially leave lasting impressions that are easily recalled at some future date. **Figure 12–5** is an excellent example.

Figure 12–5 Example of an effective poster for AIDS awareness.

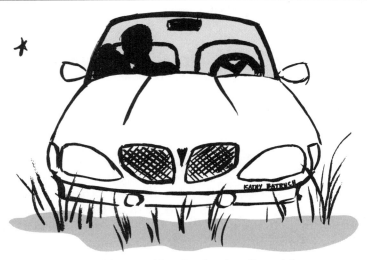

**Last night Jennifer had a fatal accident.
She just doesn't know it yet.**

The advantages of posters are that they can be used as a cognitive stimulator, as a way to reinforce and synthesize information, and as an ongoing instructional resource. Their value derives from the repetition, individual pacing, and availability of the message across various settings (Bach, McDaniel, & Poole, 1994; Duchin & Sherwood, 1990; Hayes & Childress, 1999; Thurber & Asselin, 1999). Posters serve as an important teaching tool to help bring about a change of behavior by adding knowledge, reinforcing skills, or appealing to attitudes. By forcing content brevity and using eye-catching imagery, a message can be disseminated quickly and simultaneously to a large audience in a variety of settings. Posters also can be used with individuals and small groups to transmit or reinforce information with or without the teacher present. In addition, they are rel-

atively inexpensive and easy to produce. With practice, and with the availability of today's computer technology, an educator can become skilled at creating attractive, impressive posters in an efficient and timely manner. Software programs such as Print Shop Deluxe and PowerPoint are excellent resources to produce professional-looking visuals. The major disadvantage of posters is that the content is static and, therefore, may become quickly dated. Also, if the same poster is kept on display for too long, the potential audience begins to disregard its message.

The key to a poster's effectiveness lies in its planning and design. Bushy (1991) states that "good ideas do not speak for themselves . . . a good poster display cannot rescue a bad idea, but a poor one can easily sink the best idea . . ." (p. 11). She puts forth important aesthetic considerations when preparing and evaluating poster presentations specifically for research purposes. Duchin and Sherwood (1990) and Bach et al. (1994) also provide guidelines for developing attractive, simple, yet effective posters that are still relevant today and include considerations of content, audience needs, and settings. Both Bushy (1991) and Duchin and Sherwood (1990) refer to the application of design elements such as color, spacing, graphics, lettering, and borders required to create presentations that not only catch the eye but also persist in memory. Also, effective imagery can take the form of graphic designs or photographs, and great artistic skill is not required. Simple pictures, such as schematics, outlines, and stick figure drawings, work well and can be created using colored pencils, markers, or construction paper.

The ability of a poster to influence behavior or increase awareness can be greatly enhanced by careful consideration of all of these factors. Because aesthetic appeal is critical in capturing learners' attention, the following tips should be adhered to when making and critiquing a poster for use as a teaching tool (Bach et al., 1994; Bushy, 1991; Duchin & Sherwood, 1990; Haggard, 1989):

- Use complementary (opposite-spectrum) color combinations, taking into account the three color aspects of hue (wavelength of the light spectrum), saturation (purity of color), and value (brilliance of color). Two colors clash when they are close to each other in these three elements.
- One color should make up as much as 70% of the display. No two colors should be used in equal proportions, and a third color should be used only to accent or highlight printed components such as titles, subheadings, or credits.

Too many colors make the design appear cluttered and complicated.

- Because a picture is worth a thousand words, graphics should be used to break up blocks of script or lettering.
- Use simple, high-quality (but not necessarily sophisticated or ornate) drawings or graphics that can be easily interpreted.
- Balance script with white space (or another background color) and graphics to add variety and contrast.
- Use high-quality photographs with colored borders and of different contours, widths, and shapes.
- Convey the message in common, straightforward language, avoiding jargon and unfamiliar abbreviations or symbols.
- Adhere to the KISS principle (keep it simple and smart) when using words to decrease length, detail, and crowding. Simplicity and neatness attract attention.
- Be concise; do not repeat. Include only essential information, but be sure the message is complete.
- Keep objectives in mind for the focus of this display tool.
- Be sure content is current and free of spelling, grammar, and mathematical errors.
- Add textures, if desired, by using a variety of paper and fabrics.
- Make titles catchy and crisp, using 10 words or less (no longer than two lines) and lettering large enough to read from a distance of at least 4–6 feet.
- Letters should be straight and at least 1 inch in height. Avoid using all-capital letters except for very short titles and labels. Use capitals for only the first

letter of each word in titles with more than 2–3 words or with words longer than four to six letters.

- Use a title or introductory statement that orients readers to the subject.
- Logically sequence the written and graphic components.
- Use letter-quality script or laser print instead of dot matrix if using computer-generated type.
- Use arrows, circles, or directional lines to merge the parts to achieve correct focus, flow, sequence, and unity.
- Achieve balance in visual weight on each side by positioning information around an imaginary central axis running vertically and horizontally.
- Handouts can be used to supplement, highlight, and reinforce the messages conveyed by the poster.
- If a poster is to be transported, use durable backboards and overlays (Styrofoam, heavy cardboard, lamination, or acrylic sprays).

Bushy (1991) has devised a 30-item research poster appraisal tool (R-PAT), still relevant today, that further assists nurses in critiquing posters specifically designed for research. This tool can be modified for use in preparing and evaluating posters as tools for educational purposes.

The ability of a poster to influence behavior or expand awareness can be greatly enhanced by careful consideration of its content, intended audience, and design elements. The poster for AIDS awareness (Figure 12–5) is a stunning example. The interaction of the viewer with the message is the key to a poster's success. This AIDS awareness poster and the classic World War I poster "Uncle Sam Wants YOU!" are examples of the element of visceral connection between viewer and message that linger in memory.

Table 12–2 summarizes the basic advantages and disadvantages of demonstration materials.

Audiovisual Materials

Technology has changed the traditional approach to teaching. Nowhere is this shift more evident than in the audiovisual arena. *Audiovisual mate-*

Table 12–2 BASIC ADVANTAGES AND DISADVANTAGES OF DEMONSTRATION MATERIALS

Advantages	Disadvantages
Brings the learner closer to reality through active engagement	Content may be static, easily dated
Useful for cognitive reinforcement and psychomotor skill development	Can be time consuming to make
Effective use of imagery may impact affective domain	Potential for overuse
Many forms are relatively inexpensive	Not suitable for simultaneous use with large audiences
Opportunity for repetition	Not suitable for visually impaired learners or for learners with poor abstraction abilities

rials support and enrich the educational process by stimulating the senses of seeing and hearing, adding variety to the teaching–learning experience, and instilling visual memories, which have been found to be more permanent than auditory memories. Audiovisuals have been known to increase retention of information by combining what we hear with what we see. Technology software and hardware are exceptional aids because many can influence all three domains of learning by promoting cognitive development, stimulating attitude change, and helping to build psychomotor skills.

Because we live in an increasingly technological age, educators have to be aware of what audiovisual tools are available, how tools actually and potentially affect the ability to learn, and how to effectively and efficiently implement the various tools at their disposal. When and to what extent we should use them to augment teaching depends on many variables, not the least of which is the educator's comfort level and expertise in operating these technological devices. Also, it should not be forgotten that some adult learners may have difficulty orienting to the newer modes of learning or some learners may have physical or cognitive limitations that preclude the use of one or more types of audiovisual tools. In a riveting article, Prensky (2001) declared that today's young people are no longer the audiences our educational system was originally designed to teach. A growing number of younger learners have been raised in this present digital technology era, surrounded by and oriented to computers, video games, MP3s, cell phones, and many other electronic devices that are integral to their everyday lives. They are known as digital natives. Many educators, on the other hand, who were not born during this age of technology, have had to

acquire new ways of communicating, somewhat akin to a second language. Prensky refers to them as digital immigrants. The challenge, then, for many educators who have for years spoken a different language, is to adapt to as well as adopt the newest forms of instructional tools to teach natives of the digital age. Digital natives are comfortable with multitasking and receiving information rapidly. Use of hypertext and random access comes naturally. Use of streaming video and interactive computer learning modules, as well as video gaming, is becoming more common. For educators not well versed in the use of digital technologies to assist and supplement instruction, the challenge is ongoing.

As with any teaching aids, major concerns affecting which media you choose will depend on accuracy and appropriateness of content, budgetary resources available for the purchase or rental of software programs and hardware equipment, and the time, money, and expertise needed to introduce new technologies or self-produce audiovisual materials.

Audiovisual materials can be categorized into five major types: projected, audio, video, telecommunications, and computer formats. Computer technology is rapidly altering the ways in which educators share information and interact with students.

PROJECTED LEARNING RESOURCES

This category of media includes overhead transparencies, PowerPoint slides, and other computer outputs that are projected on a screen. These media types are appropriate for audiences of various sizes.

PowerPoint   Microsoft's computer-generated software program, PowerPoint, has replaced conventional slides for instruction. PowerPoint slides are easy to design, economical to produce, and an impressive medium by which to share information with a large or small audience. The program allows for flexibility to make changes in the slides whenever necessary as well as flexibility during the presentation to repeat slides or skip slides to move ahead to other content. PowerPoint slides have many advantages. They are an excellent medium for conveying a message because they are an attractive mode for learning at all ages in a manner that facilitates retention and recall. They can enhance an oral presentation by adding visual dimensions to the narration. Presentations can be burned onto a disc or downloaded from a server for presentation through a portable laptop computer. Digital photographs and graphics can easily be scanned and added into PowerPoint slides. Animation also can be an additional feature. And finally, slides can be personalized or tailored to meet specific audience needs.

The biggest disadvantage is that PowerPoint slides must be shown in low light settings for optimum visibility. A screen and computer/projector setup must be available. PowerPoint presentations can be presented using a flash drive if a computer is provided, but educators may need to bring their own laptop. Issues of compatibility between Windows-based PCs or Macintosh computers need to be taken into consideration.

Careful composition of slides is needed to avoid clutter. Too much detail makes it difficult for the viewer to assimilate. DuFrene and Lehman (2004) provide an elegant four-step process for assisting educators to develop and deliver lively PowerPoint presentations designed to avoid the death by PowerPoint experience for intended audiences. The following suggestions should be adhered to when preparing a PowerPoint slide presentation:

- Illustrate one idea per slide.
- Keep images simple by using clear pictures, symbols, or diagrams. Put long lists of words or complex figures on handouts that supplement the slides.
- Avoid distorted images by keeping the proportion of height to width at 2:3.
- Use large, easily readable, and professional-looking lettering.

Brown (2001) suggests additional important tips on how to employ this innovative tool productively:

- Use this medium to generate interaction between the teacher and the learner rather than as a tool that provides an outline of content to be followed for presenting information only in a traditional lecture format.
- On various slides, leave out some points to be made or ideas that should be included so that the learner must figure out what may be missing. This omission encourages critical thinking by the audience.
- Open a blank slide and type in the main points as they emerge from interactive discussion.
- Use text sparingly on each slide to keep details to a minimum by including no more than six points about any one idea per slide and limiting the word count to approximately six words per point.
- Use contrasting but bold complementary colors so the text of each slide is clearly visible. Be sure the background color is dark enough that the words in print are not washed out.
- Be sure the print size on each slide is large enough for the audience to read

with ease at a distance. The floor test is one simple method to determine appropriate print size. That is, can you clearly read a printout of the slide placed on the floor in front of you when in a standing position?

- Minimize or avoid animated text, sounds, and fancy transitions, which can serve to distract the reader from the message being conveyed.
- Keep unity of design from slide to slide by using a master slide as a template.
- Provide students with handouts of the slides (three slides per page) for purposes of note taking.
- Limit the number of slides to be projected for teaching to no more than one to two slides per minute (not to exceed 60 slides for a one-hour presentation) to avoid including too much content in a given period of time. It is important to provide time for cognitive processing that allows learners to internalize the concepts being presented and to give learners a chance to discuss content and ask questions.

Remember, visuals should enrich the message, not become the message. Overuse of slides may flatten out audience participation, potentially sacrificing rich interactive discussions (DuFrene & Lehman, 2004). Dickerson (2005) reminds us that audiovisual resources are only the tools used by the educator to help achieve teaching objectives. She notes a common complaint that PowerPoint presentations can encourage learners to think only in bullet points and suggests laying out presentations with enough space between bullets for learners to fill in critical information developed during a presentation. For further assistance to the nurse educator, Schrock (2003) provides a very useful set of resource links to assist in getting started using PowerPoint in the classroom, and deWest (2006) addresses both the advantages and disadvantages, as well as best applications for effective use of PowerPoint.

PowerPoint slides must be used judiciously to avoid overuse and abuse of this medium as a tool for effective teaching and learning. PowerPoint slides can readily be converted to overheads, as needed, especially for use in handling unexpected computer mishaps. A prepared presenter should keep this type of backup (DuFrene & Lehman, 2004).

Overhead Transparencies   This medium is still frequently used for teaching in a variety of settings, both in the classroom and for small-group presentations. Since the advent of PowerPoint, however, overheads are used less frequently. Nevertheless, advantages remain for using transparencies and the overhead projector (hardware). As with PowerPoint, large numbers of people can see the projected images at one time, and images can be enlarged for easier viewing. Most importantly, transparencies can be shown in fully lighted rooms, are inexpensive to produce or purchase, diagrams and figures can readily be photocopied and made into transparencies, and multiple transparencies can be laid over one another to illustrate changes in the content or build in progression of an idea.

Among the disadvantages of overhead transparencies are the need for both specialized equipment for projection and the support of verbal feedback. For this reason, they are more conducive for use in a classroom than for purposes of individual self-instruction. Another disadvantage is that it is not easy for the educator to refer back or ahead to a particular transparency, and they are difficult for the presenter to keep in order while he or she is trying to stay focused on a presentation. Also, the projector itself is awkward to transport, and the noise given off by the fan of the machine can be distracting in a small room.

It is essential that finished transparencies be viewed ahead of time for an assessment of their readability, specifically related to the size of the lettering. Usually letters 0.25 inch high or letters that can be read at a distance of 10 feet before projection are sufficient for easy reading. Note also that too much content on an overhead transparency will decrease its efficacy as a teaching tool. Babcock and Miller (1994) recommend the following helpful guidelines for the use of overhead projectors and transparencies:

- Do not block the audience's view of the screen by standing in front of the machine. This common error can best be solved by making a habit of sitting or standing to the side to avoid interference with the projected image.

- Turn the projector off when you have finished referring to the transparency so as to keep the learners' attention on you and away from what is being projected. Constant use of the machine is also distracting because of the fan noise.

- Keep the message on the transparency simple. Use handouts to cover complex information as a supplement to your message.

- Display only one point at a time by masking the rest with a piece of paper if you have listed several ideas on one transparency. This approach allows listeners to focus on what you are saying and gives them time for note taking.

- Use a screen large enough for the audience to read the information projected.

- Use a light-colored blank wall if a screen is unavailable or too small.

- Pull the projector closer or farther away from the screen to change the size of the projection. This requires that the room be large enough to accommodate moving the equipment at a distance far enough away for adequate projection.

- Use tinted film to reduce glare of light.

- Use colored pens to help organize information, to provide contrast to images, or make specific points. Color is known to attract attention and help differentiate information for better retention and recall (Cooper, 1990).

- Use overlays to help illustrate complex or sequential ideas. Note, however, that too many overlays can make the picture fuzzy.

Table 12–3 summarizes the basic advantages and disadvantages of projected learning resources.

AUDIO LEARNING RESOURCES

Audio technology, although it has existed for a long time, has not been used to any great extent for educational purposes until recently. For years, it has been a useful tool for the blind or for those with serious visual or motor impairment. However, with significant advances in audio software and hardware, as well as adopting audio technology for more than purely commercial use, audiotapes, compact discs (CDs), and radio have become more popular tools for teaching and learning. These resources can be used to relay many different types of messages, can help learners who benefit from repetition and reinforcement, and are

Table 12–3 BASIC ADVANTAGES AND DISADVANTAGES OF PROJECTED LEARNING RESOURCES

Advantages	Disadvantages
Most effectively used with groups	Lack of flexibility due to static content for some forms
May be especially beneficial for hearing-impaired, low-literate patients	Some forms may be expensive
Good for teaching skills in all domains	Requires darkened room for some forms
	Requires special equipment for use

well suited for those who enjoy or prefer auditory learning. They are also useful adjuncts for teaching individuals who are illiterate or low literate.

Audiotapes and Compact Discs Cassette tapes and CDs are very popular formats today. Use of these media by educators has been growing. The biggest advantage of cassettes and CDs is their practicality. Compact discs have replaced traditional vinyl records and in many instances are rapidly replacing traditional audiotapes. The major advantage of CDs is their superior fidelity, which does not deteriorate over time. They are small, portable, inexpensive, simple to operate, and easy to prepare or duplicate; required cassette recorders are also inexpensive, and the widespread presence of portable disc players makes CDs a very reasonable alternative. Audiotapes are a powerful tool to augment or reinforce information previously presented in other formats, to receive taped feedback from instructors, or to be exposed to information not easily available or accessible. For example, recorded lung sounds, which allow comparison between normal and abnormal breathing, are available in both cassette and CD form. Audio cassettes on a variety of health topics, from stress reduction to programs on how to quit smoking, can be prepared specifically to meet the needs of

a learner by reinforcing facts, giving directions, or providing support. As an example, Hagopian (1996) describes effective use of audiotapes for increasing knowledge and self-care behaviors of persons undergoing radiation therapy. Naperstek (1993) developed a large line of audiotapes and CDs on guided imagery that are being used by practitioners and patients dealing with illness, surgery, and broad treatment modalities. If the tapes are instructor-made, the learner derives much comfort from hearing the instructor's familiar voice and reassuring words. This tool has been used extensively by Excelsior College, a distance learning nursing degree program, to provide direct feedback to students on the results of their examinations. Information on audiotapes and CDs can be listened to at the leisure of the learner and reviewed as often as necessary. They can be used almost anywhere, such as in the home, office, clinic, or hospital setting, and can be played while simultaneously driving a car or fixing a meal, thus filling in what normally would be considered wasted time. Developing a sizable library of tapes is well within the capability of most instructors thanks to this medium's low cost and easy storage. Pictures, diagrams, and printed handouts can accompany these instructional tools to fit the needs of a variety of learners. The versatility of CDs for application to education is currently growing at a rapid rate in academia and will certainly affect patient and staff education in the near future. As with all technologies over time, the cost is becoming very reasonable, and the hardware availability for healthcare education is rapidly increasing.

The disadvantages of using audiotapes and CDs are few. The biggest drawback is that they address only one sense—hearing—and, therefore, cannot be used by hearing-impaired individuals. Also, some learners may become easily distracted from the information being presented unless they have visuals to accompany the recorded information. There is also no opportunity for interactive feedback between the listener and the speaker. As with any medium, audiotapes and CDs should be used only as supplements to the various methods of instruction.

Radio The radio has tremendously affected all of our lives for many years and is one of the oldest forms of audio technology. Due to its commercial nature and appeal to mass audiences, it has typically been used more for pleasure than for education. In recent years, the medium of radio has been exploited by both public and private radio stations, which have begun airing community service and medical talk shows for public education on health issues. These programs are helpful in delivering a message, and, because of the convenience and popularity of radio as a communication tool, it is a useful vehicle for teaching and learning.

The disadvantage of radio relates to the difficulty of consistently delivering information on major topics to general as well as specific populations. That is, the nurse educator has little control over the variety and depth of topics discussed or how regularly one listens to a program, and the general nature of radio programs is not tailored to meet individual needs. Unlike audiotapes, radio does not allow the opportunity for repetition of information. However, because of its widespread use and versatility, it has the potential for becoming a major source for important and useful healthcare information, especially if air time is funded by private foundations or sponsored by special groups or agencies dedicated to health teaching.

Table 12–4 summarizes the basic advantages and disadvantages of audio learning resources.

Video Learning Resources Videotapes and DVDs, along with camcorders, videotape recorders, DVD recorders, television sets, and

Table 12–4 BASIC ADVANTAGES AND DISADVANTAGES OF AUDIO LEARNING RESOURCES

Advantages	Disadvantages
Widely available	Relies only on sense of hearing
May be especially beneficial for visually impaired, low-literacy patients	Some forms may be expensive
May be listened to repeatedly	Lack of opportunity for interaction between instructor and learner
Most forms very practical, cheap, small, and portable	

computer monitors as electronic devices with which to view them, have become commonplace in homes. Nurse educators are using these resources extensively for teaching in a variety of settings. For example, multimedia streaming video and webinar have satisfied the increasing demand for new ways to educate professional and paraprofessional staff in home care and hospice organizations. Webinar format, which allows for interaction between speaker and participants even though sessions are virtual, and streaming technology, which plays audio and visual files from the Internet, are cost effective, easy to use, time efficient, and available wherever the Internet is accessible (Manny, 2006). In other studies, videotapes for in-service education of CNAs were found to be a potentially powerful medium for learning (Brooks, Renvall, Bulow, & Ramsdell, 2000), and Green et al. (2003) reported significant usefulness of streamed video as a resource to support learning by student nurses in a first-year life science course. Videotapes and DVDs are one of the major nonprint media tools for enhancing patient/family, staff, and student education because tapes can be simultaneously entertaining and educational (Carlson, 2003; Tobolowsky, 2007). Videotape, although a logical technology to use for patient care, has been underexploited. Clark and Lester (2000) conducted a research study on videotape interventions with the older adult population and found this instructional tool to be as effective in changing behaviors as the success videotapes have shown in teaching and learning of adolescents and younger adults.

The major disadvantage of videotapes is that the quality of this medium, like audiotapes, can deteriorate over time. For this reason alone, VHS (the analog version of audio and visual projection combined) is rapidly being replaced by DVDs (digital video discs). DVDs, which incorporate the sound quality of CDs and superior images of video by way of digital technology, have incredible archival qualities similar to CDs that allow for long-term storage and use. The market for this innovative technology has increased as the cost of the software and hardware has become more reasonable.

Originally designed for entertainment purposes only, today these discs are popular with a wide range of audiences in both the fields of higher education and patient/staff education. Healthcare facilities broadcast patient education segments via videotapes and DVDs over in-house televisions. The convenience and flexibility of these instructional tools allow educators to use video learning resources for individual patient teaching situations as well as for large-group instruction.

The usefulness of videotape derives from the combination of color, motion, different angles, and sound that enhances learning through visual as well as auditory senses. The disadvantage of purchased tapes is that they may be beyond the viewers' level of understanding, inappropriate for learner needs, or too long. The technology has become very inexpensive and the ready portability of recorders allows you to capture situations unavailable elsewhere for reinforcement of learning. Williams, Wolgin, and Hodge (1998) have outlined detailed steps for creating educational videotapes. They suggest striving for network-quality production by using the following guidelines:

- Write a script for the program. Rehearse thoroughly.
- For a small budget, a single camera with zoom capacity should be used. A larger budget also may allow employing a professional to edit the final product.

- Consider hiring a video technician on a per hour or per diem basis to yield a quality production in a time-efficient and cost-effective manner. The operator of the recorder needs to be knowledgeable of motion picture technology, such as the use of close-ups, dramatization of situations, and angle effects, which are not in the usual repertoire of many nurse educators.
- Always be mindful of the program's objectives to avoid being seduced by the glamour of the process.
- Keep the program short. The attention spans of learners vary, but the longer the video, the more risk of losing viewer interest. A video that is 5–15 minutes long is ideal.

Videotapes, in particular, are also a good means to capture real-life and practice experience situations. Role modeling of specific behaviors, attitudes, and values also may be demonstrated powerfully through this medium. As an example, Daroszewski and Meehan (1997) and Henderson and Cumming (1997) effectively used videotaped role playing as a staff development strategy. Once scenes are captured on tape, a video can serve as an excellent teaching tool to promote discussion and for analyzing and critiquing behaviors that provide direct feedback to learners in the demonstration or rehearsal of complex interpersonal and psychomotor skills. A study by Hill, Hooper, and Wahl (2000) showed improved performance and learner satisfaction among nursing students using video playback as a learning strategy for enhancing their clinical skills. Similar findings were reported by Winters, Hauck, Riggs, Clawson, and Collins (2003). **Table 12–5** summarizes the basic advantages and disadvantages of video learning resources.

TELECOMMUNICATIONS LEARNING RESOURCES

Telecommunications is a means by which information can be transmitted via television, telephone, related modes of audio and video teleconferencing, and closed-circuit, cable, and satellite broadcasting. Telecommunications devices have allowed messages to be sent to many people at the same time in a variety of places at great distances.

Table 12–5 BASIC ADVANTAGES AND DISADVANTAGES OF VIDEO LEARNING RESOURCES

Advantages	Disadvantages
Widely used educational tool	Viewing formats limited depending on use of VHS or DVD
Inexpensive, for the most part	Some commercial products may be expensive
Uses visual and auditory senses	Some purchased materials may be too long or inappropriate for audience
Flexible for use with different audiences	
Powerful tool for role modeling, demonstration, teaching psychomotor skills	

Television The television, ubiquitous in American homes, has been used for many years as an entertainment tool. Today, there are more televisions than telephones in private residences. The TV is also well suited for educational purposes and has become a popular teaching–learning tool in homes, schools, businesses, and healthcare settings. The power to influence cognitive, affective, and psychomotor behavior is well demonstrated by television commercials, whose messages are simple, direct, and variously repetitive to effectively influence the behavior of intended audiences.

Cable TV is legally obligated to provide public access programming by offering channels for community members and organizations to air their own programs. Health education, if placed on the cable system, can be seen in any home with cable access. The advantage of this international option is that distribution of programs is relatively inexpensive. The disadvantage is that there is no control over who is watching, and this medium cannot serve as an interactive question-and-answer experience unless call-in phone lines are provided.

Closed-circuit TV, on the other hand, allows for education programs to be sent to specific locations, such as patient rooms or staff units. The learner can request a particular program at any given time, much like a guest in a hotel can choose from a variety of movies day and night. This telecommunications technology requires programs to be played intermittently or continuously, with program availability clearly advertised. Because the learner controls program viewing, the nurse educator must follow up to answer questions and determine whether learning has, in fact, occurred. Satellite broadcasting, a much more sophisticated form of telecommunications, can reach far more distant locations and carry a number of programs at any one time. Because of its

expense, not many institutions send health information via this mode, but many receive it. More types of satellite systems are being developed to make this form of communication for educational purposes available on a worldwide basis.

Video teleconferencing for continuing education and staff development is one strategy used for maintaining quality and viability of continuing education programs in a cost-effective manner (Heidenreiter, 1995). In addition, several health networks, such as Lifetime, transmit to cable companies and hospitals.

Telephones It is almost impossible to imagine being without the telephone as a daily tool. Americans have come to depend on it as a fundamental means of communication. It is not surprising, therefore, that the telephone can be used effectively for education. In recognition of this fact, many healthcare associations have begun to provide telephone services with messages about disease treatment and prevention. The American Cancer Society, for example, has established a toll-free number for the public to obtain short taped messages about various types of cancer. Hospitals, too, have set up call-in services about a variety of health-related topics and sources for referral.

The advantage is that these services are relatively inexpensive and can be operated by someone with minimal medical knowledge because the taped message contains the substance of the content. Another advantage is that this type of service is available in most cases around the clock. The disadvantage is that there is no opportunity for questions to be answered directly.

Telecommunications as an instructional tool is becoming increasingly popular and sophisticated. Many hospitals and healthcare agencies have already established hotline consumer information centers, which are staffed by knowledgeable healthcare personnel so that information can be personalized and appropriate feedback can be given on the spot. The poison control hotline is a good example of the use of this medium.

Table 12–6 summarizes the basic advantages and disadvantages of telecommunications learning resources.

Computer Learning Resources

In our technological society, the computer has changed our lives dramatically and has found widespread application in industry, business, schools, and homes. The computer can store large amounts of information and is designed to display pictures, graphics, and text. The presentation of information can be changed depending on user input. Although computer technology is a relatively recent addition to the educational field, it is becoming very common, especially with the rapid increase of computer literacy among students, professionals, and the general public (Rice, Trockel, King, & Remmert, 2004). Computer-assisted instruction (CAI) promotes learning in primarily the cognitive domain (Staib, 2003). Computers are an efficient instructional tool in that the educator has more time to devote to teaching other tasks not usually taught via computer, such as affective and psychomotor skills (Boyd et

al., 1998). More research definitely needs to be done to establish its usefulness to change attitudes and behaviors or promote psychomotor skill development. Retention is improved by an interactive exchange between the learner and the computer, even though the instructor is not actually present. For example, telemedicine technology has been found to be as effective an educational tool as in-person teaching for diabetes control (Izquierdo et al., 2003). However, increasing use of interactive videodisc (IVD) programs show promise in this area (Green, Peterson, Baker, Harper, Friedman, Rubenstein, et al., 2004). Also, Flash-based Web resources, available to educators and students, are free or low-cost, high-quality Internet materials for instruction (Lamb & Johnson, 2006). Macromedia Flash is required for access to such resources, but if it is not already installed in one's computer, it is easily downloaded to run on both Windows and Macintosh platforms with any browser. Three key elements of Flash—animation, interaction, and multimedia—give it great appeal and versatility. QuickTime format also is frequently used for digital video. Smith and Lombardo (2005) describe development of a patient education workshop on CD-ROM that utilized Flash, QuickTime, and Acrobat Reader to provide streaming video clips, audio segments, case studies, and interactive practice activities.

Table 12–6 Basic Advantages and Disadvantages of Telecommunications Learning Resources

Advantages	Disadvantages
TV program distribution is relatively inexpensive to wide audiences Telephone is relatively inexpensive, widely available	Complicated to set up interactive capability Expensive to broadcast via satellite

CAI has many unique advantages. Instruction can be individualized to the learner, lessons can be varied readily, and the learner can control the pace. Without time constraints, the learner can move as quickly or as slowly as desired to master content without incurring penalties for mistakes or performance speed. For instance, many educational computer games are designed to teach a subject at a variety of skill levels. Instructions that will present more problems with increasing complexity to learners at a pace of their own choosing can be selected. The ability of computers to internally change the rules or the format of games makes them endlessly challenging and new to the user. Another advantage of CAI is that an instructor can easily track the level of understanding of the learner because the computer has the ability to ask questions and analyze responses to perform ongoing learner assessment. Computers can be programmed to provide feedback to the educator regarding the learner's grasp of concepts, the speed of learning, and those aspects of learning that need reinforcement. The interactive features of this medium also provide for immediate feedback to the learner. An excellent example of efficacy of CAI is the research conducted on mental health training for long-term staff using computer-based interactive videos (Rosen et al., 2002). These authors partnered with Fox Learning Systems, Inc., a company that specializes in eldercare program development using CD-ROM and e-learning formats (www.foxlearningsystems.com).

Computers are also a valuable instructional tool for those with aphasia, motor difficulties, visual and hearing impairments, or learning disabilities (see Chapter 9 on special populations). Assistive technologies, such as screen readers that convert electronic text to spoken language are available to individuals with learning or visual disabilities.

However, learners with various disabilities are likely to have constant challenges in trying to access computer files, software programs, and Web sites. This is because Web pages are created in the HTML file format. Other common file formats include Adobe Acrobat's portable document format (PDF) and PowerPoint. However, most screen reader programs for PDF files, for example, are limited to computers running the Windows operating system and either do not work on or provide fewer, less powerful features for Macintosh users. Also, most Web-based PowerPoint presentations are of limited use for visually impaired learners using screen readers because the embedded graphics do not translate. Hoffman, Hartley, and Boone (2005) address specific problems of access for those who are disabled and provide an excellent resource list for educators and learners who want more information on organizations and Web sites specializing in assistive technologies. In addition, the Center for Applied Special Technology (CAST) is a nonprofit educational, research, and development organization whose mission is expanding opportunities for individuals with disabilities through the development of innovative, technology-based educational resources and strategies (http://www.cast.org). The reader is encouraged to visit this Web site for further information.

The major disadvantage of CAI is the expense of both the hardware and software, making it infeasible for implementation in some learning situations. In most cases, programs must be purchased because they are too time consuming and too complex for the educator to develop. Even if an educator has programming skills, it can take up to 500 hours to produce 1 hour of instructional material (Boyd et al., 1998). See **Table 12–7** for examples of companies that supply patient education materials.

Table 12–7 SOME EXAMPLES OF INTERNET SITES AND COMPANIES THAT
PROVIDE TECHNOLOGY-BASED PATIENT EDUCATION MATERIALS

Accessible Online Through the Internet (Available to the Public)

GENERAL RESOURCES
- Health Library from EBSCO Publishing—assists hospitals and other medical facilities to enhance their patient education Web sites and services (www.epnet.com).
- Wired.MD (www.wired.md)—provides interactive, online videos
- MedlinePlus (www.medlineplus.gov)—a service of the U.S. National Library of Medicine and the National Institutes of Health
- NIH.gov (www.nih.gov)
- Mayoclinic.org (www.mayoclinic.org)
- WebMD.com (www.webmd.com)
- National Cancer Institutes (www.nci.org)

VIDEOS AND ANIMATIONS
- Wired.MD (www.wired.md)
- HealthLibrary (from EBSCO Publishing; www.epnet.com)
- Pritchett & Hull—uses extensive graphics with a lower reading level in many formats and subjects. Online ordering available at www.p-h.com. Adobe Reader needed.
- Hazelden—emphasis on addiction, recovery, sobriety, and similar health issues. Adobe Reader needed. To locate videos, go to www.hazelden.org/OA_HTML/ibeCCtpSctDspRte.jsp? section=10021 and use Search Bookstore, selecting Videos under All Products.
- Milner-Fenwick Online (www.milner-fenwick.com)—free previews covering most health topics. Many available in Spanish and with closed captioning. Adobe Reader needed.
- MedlinePlus in English (www.medlineplus.gov) and Spanish (www.medlineplus.gov/spanish)— interactive tutorials (need a special Flash plug-in, version 6 or above)
  1. diseases and conditions—specific
  2. tests and diagnostic procedures
  3. surgery and treatment procedures
  4. prevention and wellness, e.g., hypertension—slides with audio
- The PatientChannel—GE Healthcare (www.gehealthcare.com)

Accessible Online Through the Internet (Expanded Applications May Be Available Through the Intranet of Individual Organizations)

PRINT RESOURCES
- Krames on Demand (www.krames.com)—self-care guides in Spanish and English. Publisher of choice for American Heart Association, American Stroke Association, American Lung Association, and National Cancer Institute

---

Table 12–7 (CONTINUED)

- Medications
  1. Micromedex (www.micromedex.com)—medications, diseases, procedures, homecare
  2. Lexi-Comp (www.lexi.com)—medications, diseases, procedures
- McKesson (www.mckesson.com)
- Blackboard (for more information see www.blackboard.com/us/index.Bb and www.delmarlearning.com/healthcare/Index.aspx?cat1ID=HCR)
- ADAM (www.adam.com)
- ExitCare (www.exitcare.com)
- HealthWise (www.healthwise.org)

VIDEO RESOURCES
- Emmi Solutions (www.emmisolutions.com)

VIDEOS—DVD COMPANIES FOR PURCHASING INDIVIDUAL TITLES
- Milner-Fenwick.com—videos, digital media, and print resources for health professionals providing direct care—free previews; most have Spanish language and closed captioning. Most healthcare topics covered.
- Aquarius Health Care Media—all videos have an inspirational message of hope and healing (www.aquariusproductions.com). Award-winning videos and DVDs on disabilities, cancer, caregiving, children, diseases and health, death and dying, end of life, bereavement, and mental health.
- NIMCO (www.nimcoinc.com)
- Professional Medical Organizations—e.g., American Academy of Allergy, Asthma, and Immunology (www.aaaai.org/patients/publicedmat/patient_education_videos.stm)

Another barrier is the lack of computer literacy or comfort level with computers by some learners and even some nurse educators. Lashley (2005) describes the importance of institutional support for faculty development in the use of technology for the successful design and delivery of computer-based instructional methods and materials. Furthermore, in particular, many older adults are computer shy, computer illiterate, or lack easy access to computers even if they are technologically savvy. This situation is beginning to change, however, as computers become more of a household item. Unfortunately, people with reading problems will experience major difficulty making sense of the information on the screen (see Chapter 7 on literacy) and learners with physical limitations, such as arthritis, neuromuscular disorders, pain, fatigue, paralysis, or vision impairment also may find computers challenging to use (see Chapter 9 on special populations). Moreover, it should not be forgotten that the computer is a machine, so the learner is necessarily deprived of the personal, compassionate, one-to-one interaction that only a teacher can provide to facilitate learning. Because of the independent nature of the computer learning experience, the CAI format is not very suitable for nondirected or poorly motivated learners. The tremendous growth of the Internet has opened new doors for learners to gain access to libraries and to direct learning experiences, such as online discussions with educators at great distances. For more information on technology in education, see Chapter 13.

Table 12–8 summarizes the basic advantages and disadvantages of computer learning resources.

Evaluation Criteria for Selecting Materials

Choosing the right tools for patient education calls for judgment on the part of the nurse educator, who must take into consideration the variables of the learner, the task, and the media. Decisions as to which instructional materials are not appropriate depend on the size and characteristics of the audience, the predetermined behavioral objectives to be achieved, and the effectiveness and availability of media resources. Answers to these three variables in combination with one another will result in the selection of different teaching tools by the educator, who is faced with multiple situations and varying circumstances on a daily basis. In particular, the

evaluation of media involves appraising the content, the instructional design, the technical production, and the packaging of any given instructional materials. **Figure 12–6** depicts Discenza's checklist, which continues to be a valid instrument for selecting and evaluating instructional materials.

Printed materials, as the most popular tool available for patient education, require a determination of readability levels. This is an essential factor when selecting print media that will be suitable for a given audience of learners (see Chapter 7 on literacy). **Figure 12–7** is an illustration of the learning pyramid. It depicts an important learning principle that, as extensive research shows, people retain information at a higher rate if they are actively involved in the learning process. The effectiveness of teaching and learning is greatly enhanced when instructional materials are used that stimulate multiple senses and modes of learning.

In making final media selections, ask yourself which material(s) will best support your teaching to achieve the outcomes for your particular audience. Remember that active learner

Table 12–8 BASIC ADVANTAGES AND DISADVANTAGES OF COMPUTER LEARNING RESOURCES

Advantages	Disadvantages
Interactive potential promotes quick feedback, retention of learning	Primarily promotes learning in cognitive domain; less useful in changing attitudes and behaviors or promoting psychomotor skill development
Potential database enormous	
Instruction can be individualized to suit different types of learners or different paces for learning	Both software and hardware are expensive, therefore less accessible to a wide audience
Time efficient	Must be purchased—too complex and time consuming for most educators to prepare
	Limited use for many elderly, low-literate learners, and those with physical limitations

Figure 12–6 A checklist for selecting and evaluating instructional materials.

	Yes	No
A. Content		
Is the content valid?	____	____
Relevant?	____	____
Current?	____	____
Is the purpose of the program stated?	____	____
Are instructional objectives given?	____	____
B. Instructional Design		
Are the ideas and information presented logically?	____	____
Is the format of the program appropriate for the audience?	____	____
Does the instructor actively engage the learner?	____	____
Is there evidence of formative evaluation?	____	____
Is summative evaluation material provided?	____	____
C. Technical Production		
Is the visual material sharply focused and clear?	____	____
Is the image composition clear and uncluttered?	____	____
Is the text legible at the maximum viewing distance?	____	____
Is the audio clear and intelligible?	____	____
Is there any distracting background noise?	____	____
Is the pace of the narration appropriate for the audience?	____	____
D. Packaging		
Is the material available in a format for which equipment is available?	____	____
Is descriptive information provided?	____	____
Is a User's Guide provided?	____	____
Has the instructional material won any awards?	____	____

Source: Discenza, D. J. (1993). A systematic approach to selecting and evaluating instructional material. *Journal of Nursing Staff Development, 9*(4), 198. Reprinted by permission of J.B. Lippincott Company.

involvement is best and realia is best for retention of information. Above all else, remember that instructional materials should be used to support learning only by complementing and supplementing your teaching, not by substituting for it.

State of the Evidence

There is broad recognition of the importance that healthcare practice, including patient, staff, and student education, is based on supporting evidence of efficacy. Rather than perpetuating

Figure 12–7 Learning pyramid: Information retention based on level of active learner involvement.

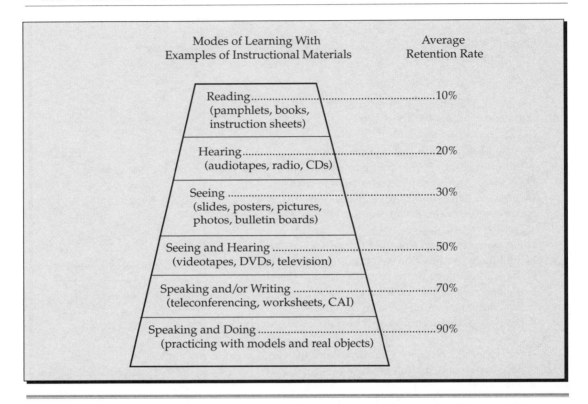

Modes of Learning With
Examples of Instructional Materials

Average
Retention Rate

Reading..10%
(pamphlets, books,
instruction sheets)

Hearing...20%
(audiotapes, radio, CDs)

Seeing 30%
(slides, posters, pictures,
photos, bulletin boards)

Seeing and Hearing 50%
(videotapes, DVDs, television)

Speaking and/or Writing 70%
(teleconferencing, worksheets, CAI)

Speaking and Doing 90%
(practicing with models and real objects)

Source: Adapted from National Training Laboratories. (n.d.). Institute for Applied Behavioral Science, 300 N. Lee Street, Suite 300, Alexandria, VA 22314. 1-800-777-5227.

practices because they have always been done that way, there is more emphasis on demonstrating that learning has occurred and that care has improved by the way in which information has been taught and received. In education, the focus is on both the processes and the outcomes of teaching and learning. This chapter focused on choosing, using, and evaluating instructional materials for patient education, as well as for educating nursing staff and students. Some of the newest studies that validate the usefulness of the different media have been cited within the chapter. It is only within the last few years that research has been conducted to determine the impact of various types of tools on the acquisition, retention, and recall of information and on the satisfaction with learning. The following are examples of research studies exploring the effectiveness of print and nonprint media that stimulate the senses, increase active participation, enhance critical thinking, help with comprehension and memory of information, and make learning easier and more rewarding.

Videotaping and playback have become common strategies to help nursing students and staff improve clinical skills performance. Hill et al. (2000) used skill performance checklists to compare initial performance of venipunctures by registered nurses and student nurses with repeat venipuncture performances after they reviewed and evaluated the videotapes of their initial performance. Results showed that with visual reinforcement of the task, performance improved and learner satisfaction increased. Similar results were found by Winters et al. (2003) in a study with baccalaureate nursing students practicing physical assessment techniques.

As another example of the application of video learning resources, Ruston, Canchola, and Lo (2004) used videotapes of real patient scenarios to trigger discussion in medical ethics courses. These tapes brought to life the experiences and views of persons involved in clinical cases, such as patients, families, nurses, and chaplains. Dramatization of the complexity of ethical dilemmas challenged viewers to engage in thought-provoking exchanges. These authors found support for the idea that videos could be used to increase learning, although locating relevant videos for this purpose was cited as a significant barrier.

Learners with low literacy skills or intellectual disabilities are particularly challenging for nurse educators. Creativity by an educator can often help overcome barriers to teaching and learning. A study by Leiner, Handal, and Williams (2004) compared the effectiveness of printed information about polio vaccination from the CDC with the same message converted into a production of animated cartoons using marketing and advertising techniques. The findings of this study showed that the animated cartoon was more effective in delivering the same message as written instructional materials. In another study, Feldman (2004) described the development, implementation, and evaluation of self-directed learning using pictorial manuals and accompanying audiocassettes to teach basic child-care, health, and safety skills to parents with intellectual disabilities. This study indicated that a significant number of parents with cognitive disabilities were able to improve their parenting skills with these low-cost, low-tech, self-directed materials.

The advent of distance learning via the Internet and various interactive media has begun to blur the lines between instructional methods and instructional materials. It is essential to remember that instructional materials should support learning, not merely *be* the learning experience altogether. With fewer qualified nurse educators and growing numbers of learners, the challenge of meeting the needs of students is a constant pressure. Lashley (2005) described development of an online health assessment course for instruction of RN students, both novices and those returning to pursue baccalaureate education. She employed the Web site to display announcements, provide handouts, and explain assignments. A text and CD-ROM were used for readings and testing. She prepared an instructional video of the physical exam that was digitally streamed onto the Web, which allowed students to readily access it from any site and view it repeatedly as needed.

CD-ROM and DVD versions of this instructional video also were available. The students reported that completing assignments online did not take any longer than the work required in a traditional class, and 80% reported online learning allowed them to work from home or some other location at their own pace. The interactive features of this modality supported and facilitated this educator's ability to teach an effective course. The reader is referred to other studies that illustrate effective use of interactive video and the Internet to support learning (Green et al., 2003; Martin & Klotz, 2001).

Rather than base our teaching strategies on assumptions that one vehicle for instruction is superior to another for learning, research has begun to verify the effectiveness of different tools with a variety of audiences under various circumstances. Much more evidence needs to be uncovered, but it is gratifying that educators are taking steps to undertake such investigations.

Summary

This chapter reviewed the major categories of instructional materials, identified how to select media from a range of possible options based on their advantages and disadvantages, and addressed how to evaluate their effectiveness. Nurse educators are expected to be able to make media choices every day, whether it be to meet the needs of an individual learner or to design a large educational program to satisfy a broader, more diverse group. In this chapter, the importance of considering characteristics of the learner, the media, and the task when choosing instructional materials was emphasized. The supplemental nature of teaching materials was also stressed, as was the need to keep the behavioral objectives in focus when selecting these materials as adjuncts to instruction.

Print media include both commercially prepared and instructor-composed materials. The problem of matching literacy and cognitive levels of learners to printed instructional tools is a relevant concern. The major advantages of printed tools are that they are widely available, patients are able to refer back to these materials for review at any time and at their own pace, and they have potential for reinforcing explanations of complex concepts. Disadvantages include the limited opportunity for learner–educator feedback. For some learners, the readability level and complexity of information may be significant barriers to full utilization of printed tools. The written materials section of the chapter contains several guidelines useful to educators in selecting or developing printed materials appropriate to both the audience and the task.

Demonstration materials include many types of nonprint media, such as models, real equipment, diagrams, charts, flip charts, posters, photographs, and drawings. In particular, they stimulate the senses of sight and touch. They are especially useful for cognitive and psychomotor skill development and may even influence attitudes, feelings, and values in the affective domain. Other advantages include bringing the learner closer to reality through active involvement and the opportunity for repetition. The major disadvantage of demonstration materials is the potential for static content or overuse, as they are often time consuming to prepare and the educator may be reluctant or unable to revise these materials frequently. In addition, these materials are not suitable for simultaneous viewing by large audiences, for visually impaired learners, or for individuals with poor abstraction abilities.

Audiovisual materials make up the fastest growing category of instructional tools. Their ability to stimulate learners' visual and auditory senses enhances their power to actively engage learners and to potentially increase retention of information. Many audiovisual tools can influence all three domains of learning by promoting cognitive development, stimulating attitude change, and helping to build psychomotor skills. The audiovisual materials section of the chapter examined the five major categories of audiovisual tools—projected, audio, video, telecommunications, and computer formats. The discussion included audience appropriateness, expense, and convenience of use. Comprehensive guidelines for selecting and developing audiovisual materials were presented. The principal advantages and disadvantages of the five categories were also described. Learners with low literacy skills may benefit from most categories of these media except computer formats. Audio materials are most appropriate for visually impaired learners, while projected video with captions and computer resources most benefit learners with hearing impairments.

REVIEW QUESTIONS

1. How do instructional materials differ from instructional methods?
2. What are five general principles regarding the effectiveness of audiovisual tools?
3. What are the three major variables to consider when selecting, developing, and evaluating instructional materials?
4. What are the three primary components of media to be kept in mind when evaluating appropriateness of audiovisual materials for instruction?
5. Which instructional materials are examples of illusionary representations?
6. Why are numbers as well as oral and written words known to be the most abstract forms of messages?
7. What factors must be considered when reviewing commercially prepared print materials for use in instruction?
8. What are three of the guidelines to be followed to ensure the clarity of instructor-composed printed education materials?
9. What are some examples of demonstration materials? Of audiovisual materials?
10. What are the major advantages and disadvantages of computer learning resources?
11. Why is it that instructional materials should not be selected before behavioral objectives are determined?

References

Babcock, D. E., & Miller, M. A. (1994). *Client education: Theory and practice*. St. Louis, MO: Mosby–Year Book.

Bach, C. A., McDaniel, R. W., & Poole, M. J. (1994). Posters: Innovative and cost-effective tools for staff development. *Journal of Nursing Staff Development, 10*(2), 71–74.

Boyd, M. D., Gleit, C. J., Graham, B. A., & Whitman, N. J. (1998). *Health teaching in nursing practice: A professional model* (3rd ed.). Stamford, CT: Appleton & Lange.

Brooks, P. A., Renvall, M. J., Bulow, K. B., & Ramsdell, J. W. (2000). A comparison between lecture and videotape inservice for certified nursing assistants in skilled nursing facilities. *Journal of the American Medical Directors Association, 1*(5), 191–196.

Brown, D. G. (2001, March). *Judicious PowerPoint*. Retrieved August 1, 2007, from http://campustechnology.com

Brownson, K. (1998). Education handouts: Are we wasting our time? *Journal of Nurses in Staff Development, 14*(4), 176–182.

Bushy, A. (1991). A rating scale to evaluate research posters. *Nurse Educator, 16*(1), 11–15.

Campbell, M. K., DeVellis, B., Strecher, V. J., Ammerman, A. S., DeVellis, R. S., & Sandler, R. S. (1994). Improving dietary behavior: The effectiveness of tailored messages in primary care settings. *American Journal of Public Health, 84,* 783–787.

Carlson, S. (2003, August 5). Can grand theft auto inspire professors? *The Chronicle of Higher Education*, 1931–1933.

Clark, M. C., & Lester, J. (2000). The effect of video-based interventions on self-care. *Western Journal of Nursing Research, 22*(8), 895–911.

Cobussen-Boekhorst, J. G. L., Van Der Weide, M., Feitz, W. F. J., & DeGier, R. P. E. (2000). Using an instructional model to teach clean intermittent catheterization to children. *BJU International, 85*, 551–553.

Cooper, S. S. (1990). Teaching tips, one more time: The overhead projector. *Journal of Continuing Education in Nursing, 21*(3), 141–142.

Daroszewski, E. B., & Meehan, D. A. (1997). Pain, role play, and videotape: Pain management staff development in a community hospital. *Journal of Nursing Staff Development, 13*(3), 119–124.

deWest, C. F. (2006). Beyond presentations: Using PowerPoint as an effective instructional tool. *Gifted Child Today, 29*(4), 29–39.

Dickerson, P. S. (2005). Nurturing critical thinkers. *Journal of Continuing Education in Nursing, 36*(3), 68–72.

Discenza, D. J. (1993). A systematic approach to selecting and evaluating instructional materials. *Journal of Nursing Staff Development, 9*(4), 196–198.

Doak, C. C., Doak, L. G., Friedell, G. H., & Meade, C. D. (1998). Improving comprehension for cancer patients with low literacy skills: Strategies for clinicians. *CA–Cancer Journal for Clinicians, 48*(3), 151–162.

Doak, C. C., Doak, L. G., & Root, J. H. (1996). *Teaching patients with low literacy*. Philadelphia: J. B. Lippincott.

Duchin, S., & Sherwood, G. (1990). Posters as an educational strategy. *Journal of Continuing Education in Nursing, 21*(5), 205–208.

DuFrene, D. D., & Lehman, C. M. (2004). Concepts, content, construction, and contingencies: Getting the horse before the PowerPoint cart. *Business Communications Quarterly, 67*, 84–88.

Estey, A., Musseau, A., & Keehn, L. (1994). Patient's understanding of health information: A multihospital comparison. *Patient Education and Counseling, 24*, 73–78.

Feldman, M. A. (2004). Self-directed learning of child-care skills by parents with intellectual disabilities. *Infants and Young Children, 17*(1), 17–31.

Flournoy, E., Turner, G., & Combs, D. (2000). Innovative teaching: Read the writing on the wall. *Dimensions of Critical Care Nursing, 19*(4), 36–37.

Frantz, R. A. (1980). *Selecting media for patient education.* TCN/Education for self care. Rockville, MD: Aspen.

Green, M. J., Peterson, S. K., Baker, M. W., Harper, G. R., Friedman, L. C., Rubenstein, W. S., et al. (2004). Effect of a computer-based decision aid on knowledge, perceptions, and intentions about genetic testing for breast cancer susceptibility: A randomized controlled trial. *JAMA, 492*(4), 442–452.

Green, S. M., Voegeli, D., Harrison, M., Phillips, J., Knowles, J., Weaver, M., et al. (2003). Evaluating the use of streaming video to support student learning in a first-year life sciences course for student nurses. *Nurse Education Today, 23*, 255–261.

Haggard, A. (1989). *Handbook of patient education.* Rockville, MD: Aspen.

Hagopian, G. A. (1996). The effects of informational audiotapes on knowledge and self-care behaviors of patients undergoing radiation therapy. *Oncology Nursing Forum, 23*(4), 697–700.

Hayes, S. K., & Childress, D. M. (1999). Fairy tales of storyboarding. *Journal for Nurses in Staff Development, 15*(6), 260–262.

Heidenreiter, T. J. (1995). Using videoteleconferencing for continuing education and staff development programs. *Journal of Continuing Education in Nursing, 26*(3), 135–138.

Henderson, T., & Cumming, B. (1997). An innovative teaching strategy for staff development departments. *Journal of Nursing Staff Development, 13*(4), 183–188.

Hill, R., Hooper, C., & Wahl, S. (2000). Look, learn, and be satisfied: Video playback as a learning strategy to improve clinical skills performance. *Journal for Nurses in Staff Development, 16*(5), 232–239.

Hoffman, B., Hartley, K., & Boone, R. (2005, January). Reaching accessibility: Guidelines for creating and refining digital learning materials. *Interventions in School and Clinic, 40*(3), 171.

Houts, P. S., Bachrach, B., Witmer, J. T., Tringali, C. A., Bucher, J. A., & Localio, R. A. (1998). Using pictographs to enhance recall of spoken medical instructions. *Patient Education and Counseling, 35*, 83–88.

Izquierdo, R. E., Knudson, P. E., Meyer, S., Kearns, J., Ploutz-Snyder, R., & Weinstock, R. S. (2003). A comparison of diabetes education administered through telemedicine versus in-person. *Diabetes Care, 26*(4), 1002–1007.

Kessels, R. P. C. (2003). Patients' memory for medical information. *Journal of the Royal Society of Medicine, 96*, 219–222.

Lamb, A., & Johnson, L. (2006). Flash: Engaging learners through animation, interaction, and multimedia. *Teacher Librarian, 33*(4), 54–56.

Lashley, M. (2005). Teaching health assessment in the virtual classroom. *Journal of Nursing Education, 44*(8), 348–350.

Leiner, M., Handal, G., & Williams, D. (2004). Patient communication: A multidisciplinary approach using animated cartoons. *Health Education Research, 19*(5), 591–595.

Lerner, E. B., Jehle, D. V. K., Janicke, D. M., & Moscati, R. M. (2000). Medical communication: Do our patients understand? *American Journal of Emergency Medicine, 18*(7), 764–766.

Manny, R. (2006, Winter). Multimedia streaming: A big part of the future for CHC [Community Health Care Services Foundation]. *Focus, 3*(1), 1, 4.

Martin, P., & Klotz, L. (2001). Implementing a nursing program via live interactive video: Lessons learned. *Nurse Educator, 26*(4), 187–190.

Moneyham, L., Ura, D., Ellwood, S., & Bruno, B. (1996). The poster presentation as an educational tool. *Nurse Educator, 21*(4), 45–47.

Naparstek, B. (1993). Guided imagery: A technique that engages the imagination in the healing process. *Health Journeys.* [CD]. United Kingdom GlaxoSmithKline.

National Training Laboratories. (ND). *Learning pyramid.* Alexandria, VA: Institute for Applied Behavioral Science. Retrieved January 30, 2007, from http://homepages.gold.ac.uk/polovina/learnpyramid/about.htm

Pinto, B. M. (1993). Training and maintenance of breast self-examination skills. *American Journal of Preventive Medicine, 9*(6), 353–358.

Prensky, M. (2001). Digital natives, digital immigrants. *On the Horizon, 9*(5), 1–6.

Rankin, S. H., & Stallings, K. D. (2001). *Patient education: Principles and practices* (4th ed.). Philadelphia: Lippincott.

Redman, B. K. (2007). *The practice of patient education: A case study approach* (10th ed.). St. Louis, MO: Mosby.

Rice, J., Trockel, M., King, T., & Remmert, D. (2004). Computerized training in breast self-examination: A test in a community health center. *Cancer Nursing, 27*(2), 162–168.

Rosen, J., Mulsant, B. H., Koller, M., Kastango, K. B., Mazumdar, S., & Fox, D. (2002). Mental health training for nursing home staff using computer-based interactive video: A 6-month randomized trial. *Journal of the American Medical Director's Association,* 291–296.

Ruston, D., Canchola, J., & Lo, B. (2004). Use of videos by directors of medical ethics courses. *Journal of Clinical Ethics, 15*(2), 201–208.

Schrock, K. (2003). Software to make you look marvelous. *School Library Journal, 49*(9), 38–39.

Skinner, C. S., Strecher, V. J., & Hospers, H. (1994). Physician's recommendations for mammography: Do tailored messages make a difference? *American Journal of Public Health, 84*, 43–49.

Smith, J. A., & Lombardo, N. (2005). Patient education workshop on CD-ROM: An innovative approach for staff education. *Journal of Nursing Staff Development, 21*(2), 43–46.

Staib, S. (2003). Teaching and measuring critical thinking. *Journal of Nursing Education, 42*(11), 498–508.

Thurber, R. F., & Asselin, M. E. (1999). An educational fair and poster approach to organization-wide mandatory education. *Journal of Continuing Education in Nursing, 30*(1), 25–29.

Tobolowsky, B. F. (2007, March–April). Thinking visually: Using visual media in the college classroom. *About Campus,* 21–24.

Weixler, D. (1994). Correcting metered-dose inhaler misuse. *Nursing, 24*(7), 62–65.

Weston, C., & Cranston, P. A. (1986). Selecting instructional strategies. *Journal of Higher Education, 57*(3), 259–288.

Williams, N. H., Wolgin, C. S., & Hodge, C. S. (1998). Creating an educational videotape. *Journal for Nurses in Staff Development, 14*(6), 261–265.

Winters, J., Hauck, B., Riggs, J., Clawson, J., & Collins, J. (2003). Use of videotaping to assess competencies and course outcomes. *Journal of Nursing Education, 42*(10), 472–476.

Chapter 13

Technology in Education

Deborah L. Sopczyk

CHAPTER HIGHLIGHTS

KEY TERMS

- Information Age
- consumer informatics
- World Wide Web
- Internet
- information literacy
- computer literacy

- asynchronous
- blogs
- digital divide
- e-learning
- m-learning
- distance learning

OBJECTIVES

After completing this chapter, the reader will be able to

1. Describe changes in education that have occurred as a result of Information Age technology.
2. Define the terms *Information Age*, *consumer informatics*, *World Wide Web*, *Internet*, *information literacy*, *computer literacy*, *digital divide*, *blog*, *e-learning*, and *distance learning*.
3. Identify ways in which the resources of the Internet and World Wide Web could be incorporated into healthcare education.
4. Describe the role of the nurse educator in using technology in client and staff education.
5. Recognize the issues related to the use of technology.
6. Discuss the effects that technology has had on professional education for nurses.

Life, as we know it today, was greatly influenced by technological advances of the last century. The birth of the Internet and the World Wide Web, the development of information technology, the wide-scale production of computers, and the development of user-friendly software have had an impact on every aspect of our lives. Some of the most dramatic changes have occurred in the field of education where technology has transformed the way we learn and the way we teach.

Today, students have a world of information at their fingertips. Computers and the Internet have made it possible to get information from anyone, anywhere, anytime, within the blink of an eye. In today's world, virtually all children begin learning on computers when they are in nursery school and are as young as 3 years of age (National Center for Educational Statistics, 2006). This is a very different beginning than that experienced by most adults who grew up in the 20th century.

Educational technologies, once rare and highly desirable resources, have become commonplace. Both the on-site and distance learner now interact in a multidimensional learning environment. Like shiny new toys, educational technologies have captured the imagination of the world. At the same time, they have presented unlimited challenges and opportunities for educators and learners alike.

This chapter explores the challenges and opportunities resulting from the use of technology as they pertain to health, health care, and professional nursing education. The use of technology in education has tremendous potential. Through technology we can increase access, improve educational practices already in place, and create new strategies that transform teaching and learning experiences for nurses and healthcare consumers.

However, technology is not a magic solution that can be implemented without careful planning, monitoring, and evaluation. Although computer-based educational applications have become easier to use and require less technical skill than they did in the past, the decision to use technology as part of an educational program is likely to have significant implications. For example, access, cost, level of support, equipment, process, and outcomes must all be considered.

Technology has incredible power. However, without careful planning, users may find that technology has given them results they had not anticipated or desired. Therefore, the nurse who uses technology to enhance learning must not only have a basic understanding of the technology itself, but he or she must also be able to integrate the technology into a plan that is based on sound educational principles.

This chapter is designed as an introduction to the use of technology in education. Because nurses provide both healthcare and professional education, it will address technology-based resources and strategies appropriate for use with clients and with nurses and other healthcare professionals. Although it is not intended to provide detailed instruction on the mechanics of computers and other types of hardware and software, the chapter will provide a basic overview of the technology involved and implications for the educator and the learner. Chapter 12 discusses the use of audiovisual materials in the classroom. Hence, this chapter will focus primarily on the Internet, the World Wide Web, and computer-based hardware and software applications that can be used to enhance learning with students in the classroom as well as with learners at a distance.

As we begin this chapter, it is important to note that the Internet, the World Wide Web, and computer-based technologies are developing at a rapid pace that is accelerating with each new generation of discoveries and applications (Cetron & Davies, 2001). Because of this phenomenon, consumers are often advised that the computers they buy today are not likely to reflect the state-of-the-art technology of tomorrow. The same caution must be given to readers of books on technology. Given the pace of technology and the development cycle of a textbook, it is impossible to capture all that is new and cutting edge in the world of educational technologies in a textbook. Rather, this chapter is meant to serve as a starting point from which you can begin to investigate the educational technologies and resources available. Ideally, it will generate the interest and skill necessary for you to continue to search for new and exciting ways to integrate technology into your teaching and learning activities.

Health Education in the Information Age

The use of technology in education is a reflection of what is happening on a much larger scale in our communities. Hence, it is useful to think of educational technology within the broader context of the environment in which we live and work. We are in a period of history often referred to as the Information Age. The *Information Age* is a period in time characterized by a change in focus from industry to information. Beginning in the 1970s, improvements in information technology and the decreasing cost of computers suddenly made information more accessible, resulting in a dramatically different world (Finnis, 2003). Although this new access to information may seem insignificant, the impact it has had on global economy, culture, and our way of life have been enormous. New and powerful industries have sprung up and the world very quickly became a much smaller place as it became possible to access people and services from around the world in a blink of an eye and at very low cost.

The demand for technology and for information continues to grow. Twenty-first century adults and children have come to depend upon pocket-sized telephones, media players, and computer-driven devices. If you think about the many ways in which technology has changed the world we live in, it is clear that computers have become more than tools to make life easier—they have become part of our culture.

Computers have also become part of the culture of education. Computers are as common in the educational environment today as chalk and blackboards were in years past. Perhaps the most significant effect computers have on our society and on education are related to their capacity to assist in the collection, management, transportation, and transformation of information at high speed. As a result of this newfound ability to handle information, we have experienced an "information explosion" and as a society we have increased both our use and our production of information of all kinds.

As people living within this information-driven society, we not only benefit from the availability of information but also are challenged to keep up with the information that is bombarding us from all directions. Information and knowledge have become valuable commodities, and the ability to gather and evaluate information efficiently and effectively has become a 21st-century life skill.

How has the Information Age changed health education? Consider the following. As a result of technological advances, the infrastructure to link people around the world to one another, to nurses and other healthcare professionals, and to a vast array of Web-based information exists. Internetworldstats.com (2007), an international Web site that provides comprehensive and current information on Internet usage, reports that in North America alone there are over 230 million Internet users, an increase of 113% between 2000 and 2007. Once a slow and tedious process, connecting to the Internet has become high speed, and over 84 million people in the United States alone report broadband or high-speed Internet access in their homes; this figure is increasing each year (Horrigan, 2006).

As nurses who are providing health and healthcare education, it has never been easier to reach our clients. For the first time, our health and healthcare messages can easily reach beyond local communities to a worldwide audience. Not only can we reach people, but we can also provide interactive learning experiences that extend far beyond what was imaginable in the recent past.

The use of Information Age technology has had such a dramatic influence on health education that a unique and rapidly expanding field of study, consumer informatics (also referred to as consumer health informatics) has emerged. The American Medical Informatics Association (AMIA), one of the principal professional organizations for people working in the field of informatics, has established a consumer informatics working group to advance the field through collaboration and dialogue. This group has developed a definition of *consumer informatics,* which states that it is "a subspecialty of medical informatics which studies from a patient/consumer perspective the use of electronic information and communication to improve medical outcomes and the health care decision-making process" (American Medical Informatics Association, 2007).

Researchers and other professionals in the field of consumer informatics strive to find ways to use technology to strengthen the relationship between client and healthcare provider as well as to use technology to teach and empower clients dealing with issues related to health and wellness. Although much attention has been given to computer-based educational systems, consumer informatics is not restricted to computer-based programs. It includes the study of a wide range of media that can be used to deliver health-related information.

The entire field of consumer informatics is growing rapidly. Many colleges offer courses of study in which healthcare professionals can gain knowledge and skill in using technology to meet the information needs of healthcare consumers. Informaticians and healthcare professionals are conducting research on the use of technology in healthcare education to generate knowledge that will guide future educational endeavors. A review of the literature reveals a growing body of knowledge in the field. Nurses and other healthcare professionals are using this knowledge to guide practice and improve the quality of the education they are providing to their clients.

Despite the rapid growth of technology-based education programs and services, it is important to remember that electronic delivery of health information is still in its infancy. There remain many issues that need to be resolved. One major area of concern is the limited oversight and control over the content that is posted on the Internet and World Wide Web, two of the major vehicles for delivering information to a global audience.

Many people believe that the lack of censorship on the World Wide Web is a freedom of speech issue. However, healthcare professionals are concerned that consumers are making serious healthcare decisions based on information on the Web that has not been reviewed for accuracy, currency, or bias. According to a Pew study (Fox, 2006), 75% of the 85 million Americans who retrieve health-related information from the Web sometimes, hardly ever, or never, check the source or date of the information they are retrieving.

Healthcare education and informatics professionals are working together to develop codes to guide practice and safeguard healthcare consumers who use the educational information and services that are delivered via the World Wide Web and the Internet. For example, the Internet Healthcare Coalition (http://www.ihealthcoalition.org), a not-for-profit group, was founded in 1997 for the purpose of identifying and promoting quality educational resources on the Internet.

One of the organization's most significant accomplishments was the establishment of the *e-Health Code of Ethics*, displayed in six languages on its Web site. The purpose of this code is to ensure confident and informed use of the health-related information found on the Web. The *e-Health Code of Ethics* is based upon the principles of candor, honesty, quality, informed consent, privacy, professionalism, responsible partnering, and accountability that are described in more detail in **Table 13–1**.

Sophisticated technology will continue to make health and healthcare information more accessible and more meaningful to both healthcare consumers and healthcare professionals. Educators in all health disciplines are identifying creative ways to use emerging technology to enhance the teaching–learning process. This trend is reflected in the nursing literature, where an increasing number of articles on uses of technology in professional and patient education can be found.

It is important to note, however, that Information Age technology has done more than alter the way in which we teach. Technology has and will continue to prompt dramatic systemwide changes. These changes will be evident in the roles played by nurses and clients, the relationships they establish, and the environments in which they interact.

Table 13–1 GUIDING PRINCIPLES OF THE *E-HEALTH* CODE OF ETHICS

CANDOR

• Disclose information about the creators/purpose of the site that will help users make a judgment about the credibility and trustworthiness of the information or services provided.

HONESTY

• Be truthful in describing products/services and present information in a way that is not likely to mislead the user.

QUALITY

• Take the necessary steps to ensure that the information provided is accurate and well supported and that the services provided are of the highest quality.
• Present information in a manner that is easy for users to understand and use.
• Provide background information about the sources of the information provided and the review process used to assist the user in making a decision about the quality of the information provided.

INFORMED CONSENT

• Inform users if personal information is collected and allow them to choose whether the information can be used or shared.

PRIVACY

• Take steps to ensure that the user's right to privacy is protected.

PROFESSIONALISM IN ONLINE HEALTH CARE

• Abide by the ethical code of your profession (e.g., nursing, medicine).
• Provide users with information about who you are, what your credentials are, what you can do online, and what limitations may be present in the online interaction.

RESPONSIBLE PARTNERING

• Take steps to ensure that sponsors, partners, and others who work with you are trustworthy.

ACCOUNTABILITY

• Implement a procedure for collecting, reviewing, and responding to user feedback.
• Develop and share procedures for self-monitoring compliance with the *e-Health Code of Ethics.*

Source: Adapted from the Internet Healthcare Coalition. (2000). *e-Health Code of Ethics.* e-Health Ethics Initiative, 2000. Retrieved July 2, 2007, from http://www.ihealthcoalition.org/ethics/ehcode.html

The Impact of Technology on the Teacher and the Learner

Information Age technology has had a significant influence on educators and learners for a number of reasons. Most importantly, access to information bridges the gap between teacher and learner. When information is widely available, it is no longer necessary for the teacher to "find, filter and deliver" content (The Edutech Report, 2006, p. 3). Therefore, the teacher is no longer the person who holds all of the answers or the individual who is solely responsible for imparting knowledge.

Educators in the Information Age are becoming facilitators of learning rather than providers of information and are striving to create collaborative atmospheres in their teaching and learning environments. As information becomes more and more accessible, the need for memorization becomes less important than the ability to think critically. Hence, educators in the Information Age are helping individuals to learn how to refine a problem, to find the information they need, and to critically evaluate the information they find.

Healthcare education can and should follow a similar path. Nurses must structure their approach to healthcare education to be consistent with the needs of Information Age clients. The first step is to reconceptualize the role of the healthcare educator as someone who does more than impart knowledge. The nurse must be prepared to be a facilitator of learning by helping clients to access, evaluate, and use the wide range of information that is available. They must be willing to encourage and support clients in their attempts to seek the knowledge they require.

The nurse must also learn how and when to use technology and remain current as new technology-based tools become available in order to optimize each learning experience. Research studies indicate that this is currently an area that needs improvement. In a study of 454 practicing nurses, Wilbright et al. (2006) found that many nurses only rated themselves as fair to poor in basic information technology skills, such as bookmarking a Web site, conducting a search using Medline or CINAHL, opening more than one computer program at a time, and checking and replying to e-mails. The authors of this study identified the age of nurses as one contributing factor. Consistent with national statistics, they found that the majority of their nurse respondents were between the ages of 35 and 50 and entered the workforce prior to the time when computers became prominent.

In a study of pediatric nurses, Secco et al. (2006) identified additional factors limiting nurses' use of information technology and their ability to develop information literacy skills. These factors included lack of computers with Internet access on clinical units, limited access to bibliographic databases, and lack of time. If nurses are to be effective facilitators of learning in today's world, these problems must be rectified.

The Information Age has been witness to some dramatic changes in the behavior of healthcare consumers, making the role changes discussed earlier inevitable. Technology and the increased accessibility to information it offers have empowered and enlightened healthcare consumers, encouraging them to form new partnerships with their healthcare providers (Kaplan & Brennan, 2001; Shaw et al., 2006). Even those healthcare consumers who are reluctant to assume more responsibility for managing their own health care are moving in that direction as changes in the healthcare delivery system have forced them to assume more active roles. As a result, healthcare consumers in the Information Age are eager to learn about and make use of the many information resources available to them.

Today's healthcare consumers enter the healthcare arena with information in hand. They are prepared to engage in a dialogue with their healthcare providers about their diagnoses and treatments. Surveys of the 113 million healthcare consumers who have gone online to find health information show that the information they found caused them to make decisions about treatment of a condition and made them confident to ask questions of their care provider (Fox, 2006).

Therefore, we can no longer assume that the clients we see in a hospital or clinic have little information other than what we have given them or that they haven't explored the treatment options available to them. Furthermore, we cannot assume that our clients will unquestioningly accept what we tell them. Research studies have shown that twice as many online health information seekers go to the Web after a doctor's visit than before (Rainie, 2003).

Whereas healthcare consumers of the past were often isolated from others with similar diagnoses and were dependent upon healthcare providers for information, today's consumers have the means to access networks of other patients and healthcare providers worldwide. Online support groups, blogs, and discussion groups where healthcare consumers can share experiences are readily available. Consumers who are being treated for healthcare problems can readily find detailed information about their diagnoses, treatments, and prognoses.

Therefore, it is not surprising that the teaching needs of today's healthcare consumers and the expectations they hold for those who will be teaching them are changing. The role of the nurse educator has not been diminished, but it has changed. Nurses must now be prepared not only to use technology in education, but also to help clients access information, evaluate the information they find, and engage in discussions about the information that is available.

In addition to altering the educational needs and expectations of healthcare consumers, the Information Age has made a tremendous impact on professional education. Technology has given rise to a dramatic increase in educational opportunities for nurses and other healthcare providers. Nurses seeking advanced degrees and credentials or continuing education credits can now study at colleges and universities offering distance education programs in a wide range of subject areas.

Computers have made it possible to provide anytime, anywhere access to job training and continuing education. Virtual reality and computer simulation can provide opportunities to learn hands-on skills and develop competencies in areas such as diagnostic reasoning and problem solving. Like consumers, healthcare professionals in the Information Age can use the Internet and the World Wide Web as vehicles for sharing resources and for gaining access to the most current information in their fields of practice.

Strategies for Using Technology in Healthcare Education

The World Wide Web

The technology-based educational resource that is familiar to most people is the World Wide Web. One merely has to turn on a television and hear the commercials for health-related Web sites or hear references to the Web on morning talk shows to appreciate its tremendous influence. A report produced by the Pew Foundation revealed that 113 million adults, or 80% of all American Internet users, have accessed the World Wide Web to obtain health-related information (Fox, 2006).

Healthcare consumers are bombarded with lures to the Web; once there, Web users can find health-related Web sites covering anything from videos of surgical procedures to sites where they can ask questions as well as receive information. The number of healthcare sites on the World Wide Web is difficult to capture with any accuracy, as new sites are being introduced on a daily basis. Nevertheless, there are thousands of health-related Web sites available to consumers offering a wide range of information, products, and services.

It is clear that the World Wide Web is an exceptionally rich educational resource for both professional and consumer use. However, despite people's familiarity with the Web, there is some confusion regarding terminology. Therefore, it may be helpful to clarify some commonly used terms.

The World Wide Web was first conceived by Tim Berners-Lee and Robert Cailliau, two scientists working at a laboratory in Switzerland (livinginternet.com, 2007). From a technical perspective, the *World Wide Web* is a network of information servers around the world that are connected to the Internet. The servers that make up the World Wide Web support a special type of document called a Web page. Web documents or Web pages are written using HTML (hypertext markup language).

In simple terms, the World Wide Web is a virtual space for information. It is almost impossible to track the size of the World Wide Web as there are billions of Web pages in existence with several million new pages being added every month. These Web pages cover a wide range of topics and display a variety of formats including text, audio, graphic, and video.

Links on a Web page allow the user to easily move from one Web page to another with the click of a mouse. A user moves around the World Wide Web by way of a Web browser, a special software program that locates and displays Web pages. Netscape Navigator and Microsoft Internet Explorer are examples of Web browsers.

Search engines and search directories are computer programs that allow the user to search the Web for particular subject areas. Google is an example of a search engine and Yahoo! is an example of a search directory. The Web is so large that any one search engine or directory will cover only a small percentage of the Web pages available (Pandia.com, 2006).

A common misconception is that the World Wide Web and the Internet are two names that describe the same entity. In fact, the World Wide Web and the Internet are related but different. The *Internet* is a huge global network of computers established to allow the transfer of information from one computer to another. Unlike the World Wide Web, which was created to display information, the Internet was created to exchange information.

The World Wide Web resides on a small section of the Internet and would not exist without the Internet's computer network. Conversely, the Internet could exist without the World Wide Web and, in fact, flourished for many years before the World Wide Web was ever conceived. Despite the immense size of both the Internet and World Wide Web, the two are relative newcomers to the world of technology.

The Internet was originally commissioned in 1969 as a program of the Department of Defense. The first experimental version of the World Wide Web was released in the late 1980s (Wikipedia, 2007). Since their inception, both the Internet and World Wide Web have grown dramatically in size and functionality.

Nurses or healthcare consumers need to go no farther than their computers if they wish to learn how to use the Internet or the World Wide Web. Getting into the Internet or the World Wide Web requires a computer with a telecommunication link and software to connect to an Internet service provider (ISP). Once one is connected, it is simple to find a wide range of Web sites devoted to teaching Internet or World Wide Web navigation skills. With a properly worded command (e.g., World Wide Web and tutorial), a search engine will uncover a number of self-paced tutorials designed to teach novice or intermediate users the desired skills. Most search engines even provide guidance in creating commands that will elicit the information needed.

Knowledge of the World Wide Web is critical for nurses who work with and educate healthcare consumers. This is true for the following reasons:

- Nurses can expect to see clients enter the healthcare arena having already searched the Web for information. In fact, a Pew study found that many consumers go to the Web to seek information about a problem they are experiencing in order to help them determine whether it is necessary for them to see a healthcare provider (Rainie, 2003). Therefore, familiarity with the type of information found on the Web will help direct the assessment of clients prior to teaching to identify the needs of the learner and to determine whether follow-up is necessary.

- The World Wide Web is a tremendous resource for both consumer and professional education. To use the Web effectively, nurses must possess information literacy skills and be prepared to teach these same skills to clients, including how to access the information on the Web and how to evaluate the information found.

- The World Wide Web provides a powerful mechanism for nurses to offer healthcare education to a worldwide audience. More and more health organizations are creating Web sites with pages dedicated to presenting healthcare information for consumers. Although nurses may not be responsible for actually creating the HTML document that will be placed on the Web, they may work with the Web site designers to develop the information it contains, evaluate the accuracy of the information presented, and interact with healthcare consumers who access the site.

The World Wide Web is a vital tool for nurses. It is a mechanism for keeping up-to-date on professional and practice issues as well as a resource to be shared with clients. If it is to be used effectively, however, a plan to incorporate the World Wide Web into practice must be set in place.

Healthcare Consumer Education and the World Wide Web

A preteaching assessment of a client in the Information Age must begin with questions about computer use. Despite the widespread use of computers in our society, not everyone has access to a computer or has interest in using a computer. Adults over the age of 65, African Americans, individuals who have less than a high school education, and individuals living in a home without children are less likely to be online than others (Fox, 2005). Therefore, it is important to determine whether a client has a computer in his or her home, has access to the Internet, is knowledgeable about using a computer, and has interest in using a computer to obtain information and resources regarding his or her health care.

If a client does not have a computer but has interest in using one to access resources on the Web, places where he or she may access a computer should be discussed. Libraries, senior centers, and community centers commonly have computers with Internet access for public use and typically offer instruction and assistance for new users.

Clients who use computers should be asked about their use of the Web. A Pew Foundation study revealed that Web users in the United States found information on the Web that did one of the following:

1. Influenced their decisions about how to treat an illness
2. Led them to ask questions
3. Led them to seek a second medical opinion
4. Affected their decision about whether to seek the assistance of a healthcare provider (Fox, 2006)

Because the Web can be so influential, it is important to determine that the information a client has found is accurate, complete, and fully understood. Only 15% of Web users report that they always check the source and date of the information found, and many report feeling overwhelmed, confused, or frightened by the information presented (Fox, 2006).

These findings are not surprising. The World Wide Web contains information designed for both professional and consumer audiences. Healthcare consumers may not have the background necessary to comprehend professional literature and other types of information designed for healthcare professionals. When healthcare consumers do a search on a topic, they will access Web sites designed for them as well as for health professionals. Consumers should not be discouraged from accessing these sites, but nurse educators must help clients find information written for them at their level of readability and comprehension.

The Web also contains information that may be biased, inaccurate, or misleading (Lewis, Gundwardena, & Saadawi, 2005). Many of the health-related Web sites are sponsored by commercial enterprises trying to sell a product. Others contain information posted by nonprofessionals and may be opinion rather than fact based. Because the Web has the potential to change so quickly, it is difficult to regulate. Even Web pages sponsored by physicians, nurses, and university medical centers may contain errors or information that is misleading or difficult to decipher.

Clients may find that the Web has provided too much information, information they are not ready to handle, or information they do not fully understand. For example, a patient newly diagnosed with a serious illness may be overwhelmed with the detailed information found on the Web regarding the course of the disease, prognosis, and treatment. Therefore, it is important to ask clients if they are using the Web to find health-related information and to explore the types of information they have found.

Clients may or may not initially feel comfortable talking about information they have gathered. They may fear health professionals will interpret their research as a lack of trust in the care they receive. Some may be embarrassed to talk about information they do not fully understand. Others may be anxious about how to bring up information that conflicts with what they have been told or how they are being treated.

For these reasons, it is important for nurses to establish early in their relationships with clients that they are interested in talking with them about the information they have gathered from the Web or other resources they have available to them. Clients need to feel that nurses are open to discussing whatever information they find. They need to understand that nurses are a partner in seeking the best information available.

For clients who are being treated for a condition over an extended period of time, it is also important to continue the conversation about their Web searches throughout their treatment. Simply asking "Have you found any interesting information on the Web lately?" will keep the dialogue open and provide the nurse educator with the opportunity to respond to whatever questions or concerns clients may have.

It is advantageous to conduct a teaching session in a place where there is computer access. Having a computer available during a teaching session can accomplish several goals. First, it will provide the nurse educator with the opportunity to review Web-based information with the client. Not only can the nurse introduce Web sites that are relevant to the client's needs, but the nurse can also review some of the sites the client has been using.

By reviewing the Web sites a client has been visiting, nurse educators can begin to determine the type and amount of information to which the client has been exposed, assess the client's knowledge, and identify areas in which the client may have need for further teaching. Nurse educators may also find information that needs further discussion. For example, a client may have visited a Web site that provides distressing information about side effects of treatment, prognosis, or disease progression. Looking at the site together will give the nurse and client the stimulus to talk about what he or she has discovered and do additional teaching if needed.

Another important advantage of reviewing Web sites with a client is that it provides a chance to teach clients *information literacy* skills. There are many definitions of information literacy. Most agree that individuals who are information literate have the following four competencies:

1. The ability to identify the information they need
2. The skills to access the information they need
3. Knowledge of how to evaluate the information they find
4. The ability to use the information they deem valid

Therefore, if clients are going to make use of the vast array of information on the Web, they must be able to identify the questions they need answered, find the information they are looking for, judge whether the information they find is trustworthy, and decide how they will use the information to meet their needs.

Information literacy is different from *computer literacy*. A client who is information literate knows how to find the information needed and can evaluate the information found for accuracy, currency, and bias. A client who is computer literate has the technical skills and knowledge of computers necessary to use contemporary hardware and software and can adapt to new technologies that emerge (Williams, 2003).

Although healthcare consumers may not have the background knowledge to evaluate information to the same extent as a professional, they can be taught some simple steps to develop their information literacy skills and to help them begin to identify which Web sites are useful and which are problematic. These steps include the following:

1. *Reducing a problem or topic to a searchable command that can be used with a search engine or search directory.* If clients do not know how to narrow their topics or problems to a few words, they will be unable to find the information they desire or may be unable to broaden a search to find comprehensive coverage. Once the search command is identified, using a search engine or search directory is easy, especially if the help function available at most sites is used to solve problems.

2. *Categorizing Web pages according to their purpose.* A client should be taught to look for the person or organization responsible for the Web site and then place the Web site into a category reflective of its purpose. For example, the purpose of a site created by a drug manufacturer could be categorized as marketing, sales, or promotion. Other categories could include, but are not limited to, advocacy, promotion, informational/news, personal, or instructional/tutorial.

3. *Identifying sources of potential bias that may influence the content or the manner in which the content is presented.* For example,

an advocacy Web site is likely to present information that favors one side of a debate. A marketing or sales site will have a tendency to include information that is supportive of a particular product or service.

4. *Making a judgment as to the likelihood that the information found on the Web page is accurate and reliable.* Clients can be taught to look for the credentials of authors of reports or articles found on the Web. This helps them to determine whether supportive data are provided, and to look at more than one site to see if they can find similar claims or suggestions. Some of the more reliable health-related Web sites have links to other sites, such that the original site is not the sole source of information on a particular topic.

5. *Making a decision as to the completeness or comprehensiveness of the information presented.* Because clients may not have the background knowledge needed to quickly recognize when information is missing, they should be encouraged to look at more than one site when researching an area of interest. If you know that clients are using the Web to investigate a particular topic, you can help them to identify a list of things they should look for in articles or Web pages addressing the topic.

6. *Determining the currency of the information on a Web page.* Consumers need to know the importance of looking for a creation or modification date or other signs that the information on a Web site is up to date.

7. *Identifying resources to answer questions or verify assumptions made about the content of*

a Web page. If questions arise, healthcare consumers should be encouraged to check out information with their healthcare provider. If the provider does not have the answers or cannot verify assumptions made, he/she can refer the client to other healthcare professionals.

In years past, healthcare consumers were not encouraged to research health topics or to research options, but rather to rely on their healthcare providers for information. There were fears that clients would not understand the information they found or that they would find information they wouldn't be able to handle. Today, we have more confidence in consumers' ability to manage their own health care.

More and more nurses are empowering their clients by teaching and encouraging them to take advantage of the resources at their disposal. Nurses are using a variety of means to expose their clients to the resources on the Web. For example, computers are being placed in waiting rooms set to appropriate Web sites. Also, teaching materials on how to use the Web are being distributed and Web sites are being created for client use. Given concerns about the quality of information available on the Web, some professionals are working together to create trusted Web sites that provide information and resources for specific client populations (Lewis et al., 2005).

There are many reasons why teaching clients where to go on the Web to find information is good practice. Web-based information can be obtained quickly, and the cost of Internet access in the home is minimal, and it is free in libraries and other community service organizations. Many healthcare consumers would benefit from having their questions answered quickly and inexpensively.

For example, families with young children are likely to have frequent questions related to childhood illnesses, growth and development, and behavior problems, and they may not have the time or money to make a visit to the pediatrician. Senior citizens may have questions about the healthcare problems encountered with aging but may have difficulty getting to a healthcare provider because of transportation and financial issues. People with chronic illness may gain some sense of control over their lives when they are able to access information on the Web about their conditions. Healthy people may have many questions but few opportunities to talk with a health provider to get answers.

Even when healthcare consumers do have the opportunity to meet with a healthcare provider, they often leave with unanswered questions. Sometimes they forget to ask, at times they are hesitant to ask, and in today's healthcare delivery system they may not be given sufficient time to ask the many questions that arise when people are dealing with health issues.

In the role of educator, the nurse can teach clients who access the Web to use it more effectively and can be proactive in encouraging others to give it a try. It may be helpful to compile lists of Web sites appropriate to the needs of different client populations. **Table 13–2** provides examples of the various types of Web sites that are available for consumer use. As illustrated in Table 13–2, a variety of types of Web sites exist, from general sites covering a broad range of topics to sites with a specific focus or theme.

In selecting Web sites to share with clients, it is important that the nurse review them carefully. In recent years, multiple rating scales have been developed to assist in the evaluation of such sites. Most scales include criteria that address the accuracy of the content, design, and

Table 13–2 Sample Web Sites for Healthcare Consumers

Title	Sponsor/Author	URL	Description
Medline Plus	National Library of Medicine	http://www.nlm.nih.gov/medlineplus	Example of a government site that provides access to extensive information about specific diseases/conditions, links to consumer health information from the NIH, dictionaries, lists of hospitals and physicians, health information in Spanish and other languages, and clinical trials. There is no advertising on this site.
Aplastic Anemia and MDS International Foundation, Inc.	Aplastic Anemia and MDS International Foundation, Inc.	http://www.aplastic.org	Example of a disease-specific Web site that provides a range of services, including free educational materials and access to a help line where consumer questions will be researched and answered.
MayoClinic.com	Mayo Clinic	http://www.mayohealth.org	Example of a comprehensive hospital site that provides information as well as a variety of interactive tools to help healthcare consumers manage a healthy lifestyle, research disease conditions, and make healthcare decisions. Advertisement helps support this site.
Cancer Net	National Cancer Institute	http://www.nci.nih.gov	Example of a government site devoted to all aspects of cancer. Provides both professional and consumer-oriented information and resources.
Band-aides and Blackboards	Nursing faculty at Fairfield	http://www.lehman.cuny.edu/faculty/jfleitas/bandaides/sitemap.html	Site provides personal rather than factual information about growing up with health problems from the perspectives of kids, teens, and adults.
NetWellness	University of Cincinnati, Ohio State University, and Case Western Reserve University	http://www.netwellness.org	Non profit consumer health Web site that provides high-quality information created and evaluated by medical and health professional faculty at several universities.

aesthetics of the site; disclosure of the authors; sponsors of the site; currency of information; authority of the source; ease of use; and accessibility and availability of the site.

Table 13–3 summarizes the questions that should be asked in evaluating a health-related Web site. Resource lists made up of quality sites will not only serve as references for clients but

---

Table 13–3 Criteria for Evaluating Health-Related Web Sites

ACCURACY

- Are supportive data provided?
- Are the supportive data current and from reputable sources?
- Can you find the same information on other Web sites?
- Is the information provided comprehensive?
- Is more than one point of view presented?

DESIGN

- Is the Web site easy to navigate?
- Is the site Bobby Approved?
- Is there evidence that care was taken in creating the site? Do the links work? Are there typos?
- Is the information presented in a manner that is appropriate for the intended audience?
- Do the graphics serve a purpose other than decoration?

AUTHORS/SPONSORS

- Are the sponsors/authors of the site clearly identified?
- Do the authors provide their credentials?
- Do the authors/sponsors provide a way to contact them or give feedback?
- Do the authors/sponsors clearly identify the purpose of the site?
- Is there reason for the sponsors/authors to be biased about the topic?

CURRENCY

- Is there a recent creation or modification date identified?
- Is there evidence of currency (e.g., updated bibliography reference to current events)?

AUTHORITY

- Are the sponsors/authors credible (e.g., is it a government, educational institution, or healthcare organization site versus a personal page)?
- Are the author's credentials appropriate to the purpose of the site?

also provide examples of the types of sites they should be accessing.

Finally, nurses can create Web sites to bring their healthcare messages to Web users around the world. Table 13–2 provides two examples of Web sites that exemplify the types of roles nurses can play to bring health information to various consumers via the World Wide Web.

Band-aides and Blackboards is a creative site designed by a nurse to facilitate understanding of the problems faced by children growing up with healthcare problems. This site is thought provoking rather than factual. The nurse who created it uses the words and drawings of children and parents to bring a real-life perspective to the thoughts, feelings, and experiences of growing up with illness. Band-aides and Blackboards teaches important messages about not being alone, about ways to solve common problems, and about what really matters to this population.

NetWellness, another site in which nurses play a predominant role, is a very different site than Band-aides and Blackboards. NetWellness is an "electronic consumer health information service developed by the University of Cincinnati Medical Center and more than 35 community partners" (Hern, Weitkamp, Haag, Trigg, & Guard, 1997, p. 316). Developed a number of years ago, NetWellness continues to be a wonderful Web resource for healthcare consumers. Nursing faculty at the University of Cincinnati, Ohio State University, and Case Western University assist in maintaining this site by responding to health consumer questions on the site's Ask the Expert feature and by providing information for the section of the site devoted to hot topics.

Development of a Web site is typically a team effort. In addition to content experts like nurses who provide the material to be included

on the site, Web designers with technical and layout expertise can provide valuable assistance. There are many resources available to healthcare professionals interested in developing Web sites.

For example the Research Based Web Design and Usability Guidelines Web site (http://www. usability.gov/pdfs/guidelines.html) is sponsored by the U.S. Department of Health and Human Services. This resource contains guidelines that can be used in designing health-related Web sites. Not only are the guidelines provided here based on research studies and supporting information from the field, but ratings are also assigned to each guideline according to the strength of the evidence available.

For instance, a guideline that is given a rating of 5 is one that is supported by two or more research studies where hypotheses were tested and the guideline was shown to be effective. A score of 0 indicates that although the guideline may be routinely followed on Web pages, there is no evidence to support its effectiveness.

A number of issues must be considered before engaging in health education via a Web site. Web sites have the potential to reach millions of users over an extended period of time. The healthcare consumers who use the Web have varying levels of sophistication. They may or may not know to check the dates on which the Web site was created and modified. Therefore, it is very important that the information on the site be accurate and updated as often as necessary. Depending on the topics covered, it may be necessary to include a disclaimer about the importance of checking with a healthcare provider.

If the site is interactive and the nurse will be responding to questions submitted by users of the site, liability issues must be carefully considered. Nurses who respond to questions from Web users are providing advice and guidance to people they do not see and cannot assess. Depending on the nature of the site, it may be advisable to include an attorney on the team to provide advice when needed (Hern et al., 1997). It is important to determine if there are relevant legal issues related to practice inherent in the activities of the nurse on the Web site.

Although new technology has opened the door to many new and exciting opportunities, it has also raised many questions about telepractice and licensure. Because technology makes it so much easier than ever before to provide healthcare services to clients across state lines, the provision of nursing, medical, and other types of technology-facilitated healthcare services to clients at a distance has been placed in the spotlight. Multistate licensure and other types of legislation have and will continue to be proposed, and new practice guidelines are likely to be enacted.

Finally, the time commitment required to respond to questions from Web users cannot be underestimated. The nurse educators who respond to questions on NetWellness estimate a time commitment of 20–40 minutes for research and response to each question (Hern et al., 1997). They also suggest that it is important that daily coverage for an interactive Web site be maintained. Healthcare consumers will use the site 24 hours a day, 7 days a week. Therefore, if the site offers interactive features such as Ask an Expert, it is important that questions be answered on a regular basis so that service is not interrupted for long periods of time.

Professional Education and the World Wide Web

The World Wide Web provides unlimited resources for nurses to use in practice and in professional education and development. Web sites provide access to bibliographic databases, continuing education, online journals, and resources for patient teaching and professional practice. Sites established by nursing organizations and publishing companies serve as resource centers where nurses can find a wide range of information and services addressing any number of educational needs.

Many of the informational sites on the World Wide Web provide both consumer and professional education. Some Web sites provide links on the home page directing users to either consumer or healthcare professional resources. Other sites do not attempt to discriminate and allow users to decide whether consumer material or professional literature is more appropriate to their needs.

It is impossible to list all of the educational opportunities for professionals found on the World Wide Web. The Web is constantly changing, with new sites being added and others being removed on a daily basis. **Table 13–4** provides examples of the various types of Web sites that can be used by professional nurses and other healthcare professionals.

The Internet

The World Wide Web is merely a small component of a much larger computer network called the Internet. Although the Internet does not provide the eye-catching Web pages and the multimedia found on the World Wide Web, it does offer a wide range of services, many of which can be used to deliver health and healthcare education to clients. The Internet services most likely to be of interest to nurse educators include those that allow computer-facilitated communication.

While the World Wide Web provides opportunities to send healthcare messages to large

Table 13-4 SAMPLE WEB SITES FOR HEALTHCARE PROFESSIONALS

Title	URL	Sponsor/Author	Description
Medline	http://www.nlm.nih.gov/pubs/factsheets/medline.html	National Library of Medicine	Example of a government site providing access to a bibliographic database containing more than 15 million references to journal articles in the life sciences.
SchoolNurse.com	http://www.SchoolNurse.com	School Nurse Alert	Example of a site devoted to a specialty area of nursing practice.
National Institutes of Health	http://www.nih.gov	U.S. Department of Health and Human Services	Example of a government sponsored site with information as well as links to a broad range of health and professional issues.
AllNursing Schools.com	http://www.allnursingschools.com	All Star Directory, Inc.	An example of a resource database listing the nursing programs offered by subscribing colleges and universities.

groups of people in the form of educational Web pages, the Internet can be used to enhance teaching by enabling individuals to communicate with one another and with groups of people via the computer. E-mail, real-time chat, and e-mail discussion or Usenet newsgroups have all been used to communicate with people about health and health care, some in very creative ways.

E-Mail

Recently, a television commercial was aired depicting a woman who was concerned about all of the unanswered questions she had following a visit to her healthcare provider. The woman in the commercial talked about the lack of time, the questions that she did not think about until after she got home, and her hesitancy to bother her healthcare provider with silly questions. Fortunately, she found a Web site where she could go to get her questions answered.

Although this commercial did not involve a real patient, the message that was conveyed by this fictitious scenario is quite relevant. Despite the best efforts of healthcare professionals to provide needed information to consumers, time, stress, fear, lack of experience, and simple human dynamics may result in clients walking away from a visit to a healthcare provider with incomplete or inaccurate information. Sometimes questions come up only after clients go home and try to follow the instructions they have been given. At other times, they may misunderstand what is being taught or be afraid or hesitant to admit that they do not understand.

Unless there is a mechanism in place for clients to contact the nurse with questions, the client is at risk for making a mistake that may have serious consequences. Simply telling clients to call if they have questions is often inadequate. A call to a busy office or clinic usually results in a call back by the nurse and the patient having to wait by the phone for an answer. Even calling hours can be problematic because they imply that the client is free to call at the designated hour.

E-mail offers a quick, inexpensive way to communicate with clients. It has the advantage of being *asynchronous*. This means that the message can be sent at the convenience of the sender and the message will be read when the receiver is online and ready to read it. Messages can be sent and responded to any time, day or night.

Research has shown that e-mail is universally used among all age groups and is a very popular form of communication among 90% of Internet users (Fox & Madden, 2005). A survey of healthcare consumers revealed that although people in general like to use e-mail, only about 6% actually used e-mail to contact their healthcare provider (Baker, Wagner, Singer, & Bundoff, 2003).

Electronic mail can provide a simple and efficient way to follow up with clients. Nurses, however, are just beginning to recognize its potential. E-mail is a new way of communicating with clients, very different from the face-to-face interaction typically used by nurses.

To date, little has been written in the literature about ways in which nurses have used e-mail to communicate with clients. It should be noted that although there is little information about e-mail in the nursing literature, electronic communication has received much attention in the medical and general health literature.

E-mail is clearly a trend worth watching. In fact, in a discussion of health care in the 21st century, the National Institute of Medicine (2001) proclaimed that both patients and clinicians could benefit from improvements in timeliness through the use of Internet-based communication. Studies suggest that patients are interested in communicating with their healthcare providers via e-mail.

One survey found that one third of online health seekers would consider switching healthcare providers if they could communicate with them via e-mail (Kassirer, 2000).

Physicians and other healthcare providers are beginning to take the steps necessary to offer various electronic communication services, such as e-mail and electronic prescription refills to their patients. However, careful planning is necessary to insure patient privacy (Stone, 2007). The American Medical Association has established guidelines for the use of electronic communication with clients that are helpful for nurses as well. These guidelines are available on the Young Physicians section of the AMA Web site at http://www.ama-assn.org/ama/pub/category/2386.html.

As a form of enhanced communication with clients, e-mail is an approach worthy of further study by nurses. An e-mail message system gives clients who identify questions after leaving a healthcare facility a chance to get answers from a reliable source familiar with their history. Clients who are not sure how to phrase a question or feel rushed when instructions are being given in a clinical setting have a chance to compose their thoughts at home and prepare an e-mail message. Also, from the nurse's perspective, an e-mail message system provides a simple way to check on clients to see whether they understood the instructions they were given and to respond to new questions that have arisen.

In some ways, an e-mail system is preferable to a voice messaging system. For clients who are anxious about asking questions, e-mail allows them all the time they need to gather their thoughts. In addition, clients do not have to remember the answers they are given by the nurse, as the e-mail message provides a written recording of the nurse's response.

In contrast, many voice mail systems are time limited. Clients are sometimes cut off in the middle of a voice message if the message is long or if clients are struggling to make themselves understood. Other clients may hesitate to leave a voice mail in the evening or night hours when they know no one is there to respond. However, by virtue of the way e-mail is designed, clients can feel comfortable sending messages at any time.

An e-mail message system is simple to implement. Client e-mail addresses need to be identified as part of the routine information-gathering process for new clients. Because e-mail addresses are likely to change, they need to be updated, just like telephone numbers, whenever a client visits the office, clinic, or other setting within the healthcare delivery system.

It is a good idea to have more than one person be responsible for responding to e-mail messages, so that questions and concerns can be addressed even when a staff member is away due to vacation or other time out of the office. One way to accomplish this goal is to have messages sent to a mailbox rather than to an individual. Because more than one person can be given access to an electronic mailbox, continuous coverage can be established. If continuous coverage is not provided, it is important that clients know how long they can expect to wait to receive answers to their questions.

E-mail systems can be set up to serve a variety of purposes. If postteaching follow-up is desired, e-mail offers one way for the nurse to initiate contact after the client has left the healthcare delivery system. The nurse can get in touch with the client via e-mail following a teaching session to convey interest in how he or she is doing with a medication regime, treatment, or other types of instructions given.

For example, the e-mail message could stress important points that were made during the teaching session, such as, "Remember to take your pill around the same time every day." Also, an e-mail message could be used to assess the client's understanding of what was taught. For example, a nurse might ask, "What time of day have you decided to give your child his medication?"

Informational resources also can be shared via e-mail by embedding links to Web sites in the e-mail message. In all cases, the nurse should encourage the client to get in touch if questions remain. Any follow-up system will take time and commitment on the part of the organization. Time and resources must be allocated if the system is to work effectively.

An e-mail system can also be established as a mechanism to answer questions and exchange health-related information with clients who have received services at a particular healthcare organization. An e-mail question box can provide simple access to the nurse or other health educator who can serve as a reliable source of information.

For this type of system to work, the e-mail address for the mailbox needs to be widely distributed and easy to remember. For example, a mailbox address such as Questions@RDClinic.org would be easy to remember because it includes the purpose of the mailbox and the name of the organization. The e-mail address can be placed on the bottom of written instructions, teaching materials, appointment cards, and other sources of communication with the client.

A description of the service and instructions for use should also be distributed. For example, it may be helpful for clients to know who will be answering their questions, the types of questions that can be submitted, and the typical response time. Also, it is very important that clients understand that an e-mail message system is not intended to replace a visit or phone call when they need to see or talk with a healthcare provider about an immediate problem.

When sending e-mail messages, it is important to remember that electronic communication differs in several ways from face-to-face communication:

- Electronic communication lacks context. Without cues like facial expressions, tone of voice, and body posture, e-mail messages can appear cold and unfeeling. While emoticons (symbols like smiley faces used to express emotion) are commonly used by people who send e-mail messages, they may not be appropriate for all professional correspondences. However, a carefully constructed e-mail message can convey the intent of the sender.

- Although electronic communication is convenient, it may take longer in that the sender could wait hours or days before the message is received and answered. For this reason, it is very important that an e-mail response to a client question be clear and of sufficient detail so that it does not generate more questions that cannot be answered immediately. Furthermore, urgent issues or messages that need be read or responded to quickly may be inappropriate.

- E-mail messages provide a written record. A printed copy can serve as a handy reference for a client and eliminates any question about what information was shared. However, e-mail messages can also serve as documentation of inaccurate or inappropriate information. When responding to a client question, it is vital that the client's record be reviewed and that the response to the question be accurate and carefully thought out. Copies of the e-mail messages sent to clients should be placed in the client's record.

- Finally, it is important to remember that electronic communication can never be assumed to be private. This reminder is especially important in the era of HIPAA regulations. The health care provider must take steps to insure privacy at both the healthcare facility and the client's computer. It is suggested that clients sign a consent form if health-related information is to be shared via e-mail and that they be given instructions for safe use (American Medical Association, 2007).

Not all information may be appropriate for an e-mail message. For example, it may not be appropriate to send abnormal test results to a patient in electronic form. It is also important that both nurses and clients understand that violations of privacy can occur in many ways. For example, clients who send e-mail messages from work may not be aware of the fact that their messages may be stored on servers and hard drives even after they have been deleted. In some cases, the employer may have legal access to this information (Kassirer, 2000).

E-mail messages can also be easily forwarded. Therefore, the nurse should assume that the client may choose to share a response with others. Privacy also can be insured at healthcare facilities by requiring a password-protected screen saver at all workstations (American Medical Association, 2007).

E-mail communication between nurse and client has tremendous potential to enhance teaching. However, despite the increased use of e-mail among the general population, it is important to remember that not every client has a computer, computer skills, or access to e-mail. A backup system such as voice mail should therefore be made available so that the needs of all clients will be met.

Electronic Discussion Groups

The Internet provides many opportunities for clients and healthcare professionals to participate in electronic discussion groups with other people who share a common interest. In the case of health and healthcare education, common interests can focus on a particular healthcare problem such as cancer, a life circumstance such as death of a spouse, a health interest such as nutrition, or a professional issue such as nursing research.

Although different types of electronic discussion groups are available, all share a common feature—the ability to connect people asynchronously from various locations via computer. People like electronic discussion groups because they are easy to use and are available 24 hours a day. Because electronic discussion involves faceless communication with strangers from all over the world, there is a sense of anonymity even when real names are used.

Electronic discussion groups fall into two main categories: those that distribute mail to individual subscribers and those that post messages in a way that make them accessible to group participants. In the first type of electronic discussion group, messages are sent to the individual. In the second case, the subscriber seeks out the messages that have been posted.

Electronic discussion groups can be structured in many different ways. Some are moderated, whereas others have little or no oversight.

Some electronic discussion groups have thousands of subscribers, whereas others are very small closed groups created for specific purposes.

For the nurse, electronic discussion groups can serve a number of purposes. Electronic discussion groups can be used as a vehicle for teaching or a learning resource to share with clients and other healthcare professionals. The nurse who chooses to create an electronic discussion group can use it to reach large or small groups of healthcare consumers or healthcare professionals from within the immediate vicinity or worldwide.

For example, a number of electronic discussion groups have been created and moderated by nurses as a way to promote networking and information sharing among nurses within a particular specialty area. These groups are open to anyone who is interested and typically have memberships of several hundred people from countries around the world. In comparison, nurses in a hospital or clinic could choose to set up a small private electronic discussion group as a way to facilitate a journal club.

Whether the group is large or small, the asynchronous nature of electronic discussion groups makes it possible for people to communicate with one another despite different time zones and work schedules. And, no matter if the nurse chooses to create an electronic discussion group or uses one already in existence, this form of online communication provides for a creative way to learn and to teach.

Mailing Lists

Automated mailing lists are one of the most common means of setting up an electronic discussion group. With an automated mailing list, people communicate with one another by sharing e-mail messages. The principle by which these groups work is simple. Individuals who have subscribed to the mailing list send their e-mail messages to a designated address, where a software program then copies the message and distributes it to all subscribers. Therefore, when a message is sent to the group, everyone gets to see it.

The most popular of these automated software programs is called "Listserv." In fact, the Listserv program is so commonly used that automated mailing lists are often referred to as "listservs." Other automated programs include Majordomo, Mailbase, and Listproc. Although some minor differences exist between these programs, essentially they all work in the same way.

Although mailing lists are owned or managed by an individual, much of the work involved in running the list is automated by the software program used. Subscribers are given two e-mail addresses to use when interacting with the mailing list: one to use when posting messages to the entire group and another to use for administrative issues such as requests to stop mail for a period of time. Both functions—distributing messages and handling routine requests—are automated and handled by the software program rather than by a person. Subscribers must use the correct address and precisely worded commands when attempting to interact with the list because the computer program cannot problem solve.

Upon enrolling, subscribers are sent directions and a list of properly worded commands that should be used when communicating with the software program. New subscribers are encouraged to save the instructions and refer to them as needed. Despite these precautions, new users frequently make mistakes. It is not uncommon to read messages from frustrated subscribers who cannot stop their mail because they are either posting to the wrong address or failing to use the correct command.

Listservs and other automated mailing groups are wonderful tools for the nurse when used as a means for delivering education to large numbers of people or when shared with clients and colleagues as a learning resource. Mailing lists are easy to use once a user understands how the system works. There are multiple free tutorials available on the Web to help.

With more than 100,000 Listservs and mailing lists available, it is possible to find an online group to cover almost any issue. The quality of the messages is usually very high in both health-related and professional mailing lists. Nurses who choose to create a group rather than to participate in an established one can learn to manage a large or small electronic mailing list without too much difficulty. However, it is helpful for list managers to have either the support of computer professionals in their institution or the knowledge and skill necessary to handle the routine computer issues that arise from time to time.

Listservs or mailing lists can be used effectively as a vehicle for education or information exchange with groups desiring education or information exchange over time. Because mailing lists facilitate group rather than individual communication, they work especially well with groups that are interested in collaborative learning or learning from the experiences of others. Mailing lists designed for professional audiences are good examples. Multiple lists or Listservs are available covering everything from nursing history to nursing research to specific areas of nursing practice. Most lists are quite active, and at any given time, several discussion topics can be addressed by the group. Members post questions, ask advice, and comment on current issues. Relationships between active members are established over time, and group members

come to count on others in the group for their counsel.

For these same reasons, Listservs and other types of automated mailing lists have become popular as mechanisms for online support for health consumers (Fox & Fallows, 2003; Shaw et al., 2006). With the increased use of computers by the general population, an increasing number of people have turned to their computers to access information and resources that can help them deal with their health issues. As a result, the need for electronic discussion groups devoted to particular health problems was identified and online support groups were established.

For example, the Association of Cancer Online Resources, Inc. (ACOR) has been a major player in the move to bring online support to healthcare consumers. This nonprofit organization devoted to assisting people with cancer has established more than 159 different online support groups since 1996, each devoted to a particular type of cancer or cancer-related problem. Its Web page states that ACOR delivers more than 1.5 million messages per week to its subscribers throughout the world (ACOR, 2007). Memberships in the various groups range from about 25 people in the smaller groups to almost 2,000 individuals in the larger groups.

Other individuals and organizations have established similar online groups covering a wide range of healthcare issues. Sometimes groups are started by individuals who have an interest in a particular topic while others are started by professional or advocacy groups interested in providing service to a particular group of people. In addition to the many public groups that have open enrollments, private groups can be established to meet the needs of a group of people associated with a specific healthcare provider or organization.

Online support groups are particularly relevant to a discussion of technology for education. In their study of the categories and themes that emerged from an analysis of the postings in an online support group for colorectal cancer, Klemm, Reppert, and Visich (1998) found that information giving and seeking accounted for a major portion of the messages exchanged in the group. Han and Belcher (2001) surveyed subscribers of an online support group for parents of children with cancer and found that 76% of participants cited information giving and receiving as the main benefit of the online group. A review of the purposes and goals of several online support groups revealed education and information sharing as the reason for starting and maintaining a group.

The emphasis on information sharing in online support groups is not surprising. Many people join online support groups after they or their loved ones have been diagnosed with a serious illness. They come to the support group not only to receive reassurance and encouragement, but also to gather as much information as possible so that they can begin to make necessary decisions about treatment. By joining an online support group, they are turning to people who know what they are going through and who can give practical advice based on real-life experience. The desire to share the most current information is commonly what brings group members together, and a discussion of new treatments and other discoveries found in the literature is commonplace (Han & Belcher, 2001).

Nurses may wish to teach their clients about the benefits of online support groups. If an appropriate group is not available, nurses can start an online support group of their own. Online support groups may be especially helpful to people who find it difficult to leave home because of illness or care responsibilities.

Clients who are unfamiliar with online communication should be reassured that there is no pressure for them to contribute to the discussion and that many people benefit just by reading the comments of others (Klemm et al., 1998). Clients who are insecure about their ability to express themselves in written format may find it helpful to initially compose their messages using a word processor so that they can take the time to think about what they want to say and use the spelling and grammar check function to edit their remarks. Clients who are unsure if an online support group will meet their needs should be encouraged to give one a try. There are no costs involved other than the cost of being online, and there are no obligations to continue. Subscribers can withdraw from a group at any time.

Online support groups have some disadvantages that should be shared with clients who are thinking about joining one. Most people who have participated in a Listserv or other type of mailing list note that the volume of messages received each day can be problematic (Han & Belcher, 2001; Klemm et al., 1998). Some lists report an average of 50 or more messages per day.

Experienced users learn to sort messages and delete the unnecessary or irrelevant ones quickly. Others find requesting that messages be sent in digest form (all messages received in a day are combined and sent in one mailing) helps control the volume of e-mails received. In any case, the daily volume of messages initially can be overwhelming and may present a problem for people with low literacy levels or for people for whom English is a second language.

Clients should also be made aware of the fact that most online groups do not have a professional facilitator. Online groups are often run by someone who is interested in the health problem being discussed either because he or she has the condition or has a family member with the healthcare problem. As a consequence, inaccurate information may be shared and problems with group dynamics may not be addressed.

Although this chapter classifies online support groups as part of the category of automated mailing groups, it should be noted that online support groups take many forms. Many groups use the mailing list or Listserv format described here. Others use a bulletin board format where messages are posted on a site where they can be reviewed by members of the group. Still others maintain a Web site that provides many avenues for communication, including scheduled and unscheduled chats, bulletin boards, mailing lists, and electronic newsletters. Regardless of the format, online support groups provide a mechanism for meeting the teaching and learning needs of many different client populations.

Blogs

One of the newest forms of online communication is blogs. First developed in the late 1990s, *blogs*, or Web logs, are an increasingly popular mechanism for individuals to share information and/or experiences about a given topic. Although sometimes referred to as Web diaries, blogs are much more than that and include images, media objects, and links that allow for public responses (Maag, 2005). Blog entries are viewed in chronological order and are easy to follow.

The number of blogs available on the Web has increased dramatically in recent years. A report of the Pew Internet and American Life Project (Lenhart & Fox, 2006) states that about 12 million Americans have created a blog and another 57 million read blogs on the World Wide Web. Users can find blogs on any given topic using the search engine technorati.com, where more than 71 millions blogs are tracked and rated.

Many of the blogs found on the Web are health related and often tell the story of the creator's experience with a given disease or treatment. For example, a search on technorati.com for blogs on breast cancer revealed over 500 individual breast cancer-related blogs. These blogs covered everything from the stories of cancer survivors and family experiences to information-based blogs describing various breast cancer treatments. Many blog creators provided a picture with a limited or absent biography.

Given the growing popularity of blogs, it is reasonable to assume that healthcare consumers, particularly young people, will turn to blogs for health-related information and support. The Pew Internet and American Life Project Report on Blogging (Lenhart & Fox, 2006) notes that bloggers tend to be young men and women under the age of 30 who use a pseudonym rather than their own name. Most are heavy Internet users. Although some blogs are written by healthcare professionals, most are created by healthcare consumers who have a story to tell. Therefore, it is important to warn clients who are getting information from blogs of the importance of evaluating the content.

Other Forms of Online Discussion

There are many other mechanisms by which online discussion can take place. Although mailing lists and blogs are two of the more common approaches to online discussion, others are worthy of mention. When choosing a method for teaching or exchanging information online, it is important to consider all of the options and select the method that is most appropriate for the content to be delivered and the audience to be targeted.

Online forums, message boards, and bulletin boards are systems that provide a way for people to post messages for others to read and respond to. Online forums, message boards, and bulletin boards are found on Web sites that allow users to post directly to the discussion board rather than indirectly via e-mail. Many people may find this system easier to use.

Although most discussion board-type forums require some system of registration, users can often select a user name of their choosing and e-mail addresses are not displayed. This added privacy is a boon to many people who are reluctant to share their names and e-mail addresses with strangers. Online forums, message boards, and bulletin boards for healthcare consumers and healthcare professionals can be found on many health-related sites on the World Wide Web.

Chat differs from e-mail and the other electronic communication modalities previously discussed in that it provides an opportunity for online conversation to take place in real time. Although chat conversations take the form of text rather than audio, a chat session shares many features with a telephone conference call. In both scenarios, several people from different locations participate in a conversation at the same time. Both allow people to join or leave the session as needed. However, without adequate control systems in place, both chat and teleconferences can experience a number of communication problems, such as multiple ongoing conversations, lack of focus, and periods of silence.

There are many opportunities for clients and healthcare professionals to engage in online chats related to health issues. A search of the World Wide Web will uncover a vast array of scheduled chats where a particular topic is being discussed at a given time as well as ongoing chats where people are invited to stop in at any time to ask questions or engage in conversation with whomever happens to be in the chat room. In addition to public chat rooms, many organizations sponsor chats for their own clients or staff as a way to offer ongoing educational programs or information exchange among groups.

When leading or facilitating a chat group, it is important to plan ahead. The discussion in a chat room can move quickly, and it is very easy to get so involved in the process of chatting that the content to be covered gets lost or forgotten. The following suggestions may help to organize a successful chat session:

- E-mail or post the purpose of the chat session several days in advance. If appropriate, include an agenda, assignments to be completed ahead of time, or other resources that participants will need to prepare for the session.
- Make a list of the discussion points to be covered during the session. The list should be well organized, easy to follow, and placed so that it can be easily seen during the chat. Chat sessions often move so quickly that there is little time for the facilitator to make sense of crumpled or scribbled notes.
- Depending on the topic and the experience of the facilitator, it may be appropriate to limit the number of participants. The larger the group, the more difficult the challenge of running a smooth and productive online chat.

- Sign on to the chat session early and encourage participants to do so as well. You want to be able to handle unexpected problems before the session begins.
- Watch the clock. Time in a busy chat session goes by quickly. If the chat was designed as a question and answer period, it may be helpful to ask people to e-mail important questions ahead of time so they are not forgotten.
- Help the group to follow the conversation taking place. It is easy for chat discussions to become disjointed or off topic. When responding to a question, refer to the query and the person asking it—for example, "Karen asked about pain management. I think . . ." If the group is losing focus, bring the participants back to the agenda and the points being discussed.
- Limit the amount of time spent discussing the detailed questions or concerns of one participant. If someone in the group needs individualized attention, suggest that they e-mail or call you after the chat has ended.
- If appropriate, ask participants who have not participated if they have any questions. Some participants choose not to make comments during a chat, which is acceptable. However, there may be others who were not quick enough to get their comments online and who have questions that need to be asked. A statement such as, "Our conversation moved very quickly tonight so I want to give those who haven't had a chance some time to ask their questions" may slow down the conversation long enough for everyone to have an opportunity to contribute.
- Begin to wrap up the session about 10 minutes before the scheduled end time. Announce that there are 10 minutes left and ask for final questions or comments.

It may also help to prepare participants for the chat experience. Chat sessions can be overwhelming for new users. The following guidelines for chat participation should be shared with clients or colleagues who will be joining a chat session for the first time:

- Allow enough time before the chat starts to download software if it is needed. First-time users are often required to download software, called a chat client, before beginning. This software is typically offered as freeware or shareware on the Internet and is easy to install.
- Be prepared to choose a user name. Participants in public chats with strangers are often advised not to use their real names so as to protect their privacy.
- Keep comments short and to the point. If a user takes a long time to compose a message, the group may have moved on to an entirely new topic by the time the message gets posted.
- Be prepared for chat lingo in public chat rooms. Abbreviations like BTW (by the way) and emoticons [symbols that represent emotions or facial expressions such as ;) for winking] are commonly used.
- Do not worry about typos and grammar. Chat programs do not have spell checks and not everyone is an experienced typist. People who are frequent chat users learn to overlook spelling errors.

Chat works well as an online communication modality for many people. Clients who are homebound or isolated may benefit from having the opportunity to participate in education programs or to receive answers to their questions without leaving home. Likewise, many healthcare professionals would benefit from being able to access professional education that allows real-time discussion and dialogue.

However, some limitations of chat must be considered. Because chat requires that people be online at the same time, scheduling conflicts and time-zone issues result in less accessibility than asynchronous forms of electronic discussion. Due to the fast pace of most chat discussions, it may be difficult for some clients to keep up with the dialogue. Clients with certain disabilities, clients who are ill, and clients with low literacy levels may find it difficult to participate if the group moves along quickly.

The future for electronic communication is exciting. The technology to add audio and video components to online conferencing is available and is becoming more refined and less expensive every day. Chat and other types of conferencing software are also becoming more sophisticated, allowing for more control and greater ease of use.

Issues Related to the Use of Technology

Despite the power of computer and Internet technology to enhance learning, the use of these technologies in healthcare education presents some unique challenges. Think for a moment about the many ways in which healthcare education differs from more traditional classroom education. The characteristics of the learners, the setting, and the access to hardware, software, and technological support are all likely to be different.

Whereas traditional classroom education is likely to take place in a structured setting, healthcare education takes place in a wide range of settings, many of which are unstructured. Students who are part of an educational system are likely to have some access to the hardware, software, and technological support necessary for facilitating technology-based learning. By comparison, access to resources and support varies considerably among healthcare consumers and in healthcare organizations. Students in a classroom also often share many common characteristics related to age and ability, whereas clients in healthcare education programs may cover a wide range of ages, abilities, and limitations. As educators, nurses must be aware of the special issues involved in the use of computer and Internet technology in healthcare education and be prepared to make accommodations as needed.

One of the most widely publicized issues related to the use of computers and Internet technology is that of the *digital divide*, or the gap between those individuals who have access to information technology resources and those who do not. According to a Pew Foundation report, one in five Americans are disconnected; that is, they not only have no Internet access in their homes, they report never having been on the Internet (Fox, 2005).

Studies conducted by the Pew Foundation have found that the factors determining the likelihood that someone will have access to information technology resources are age, income, race or ethnic origin, level of education, and ability (Fox, 2005). These studies revealed that those at risk for limited access included people older than 65, those with household incomes of less than $35,000, African Americans and people of Hispanic descent, adults who did not complete high school, and people with disabilities. In addition, households without children are also not likely to have Internet access.

As a result of the digital divide, many healthcare consumers do not have the resources necessary to gain entry to computer and Internet-based health education programs. Thus, although technology can increase access to healthcare education for some people, educators must be aware that some segments of the population will be denied access if attempts are not made to promote digital inclusion. The first step in promoting digital inclusion is recognizing those groups who are at risk for limited access.

A Pew Foundation study found that although over half of Americans between the ages of 60 and 69 have Internet access, access to the Internet and online activity diminish with age. As little as 22% of adults over the age of 70 go online (Fox, 2006). There are many explanations for these statistics. Older adults are more likely to be retired without employer access to a computer, are less likely to have children in the home who typically bring an enthusiasm and knowledge of computers with them, and may have less disposable income to purchase computer hardware and software.

Despite the statistics, it would be a mistake to discount computer-delivered education as a possibility for the senior population. Research studies have shown that with education and support, older adults enjoy using and learning from computer-based programs (Evangelista et al., 2006; Nahm, Preece, Resnick, & Mills, 2004). Although many older adults have only limited incomes, numerous government and private initiatives are available to provide free or low-cost computer and Internet access for the senior population. While some older adults have physiologic and neurologic problems that make computer use difficult, many other seniors enjoy good health and functionality.

Health and healthcare education are important to senior citizens, and computer- and Internet-based technology holds much promise for this segment of the population. Therefore, it is important that the nurse be prepared to support computer-based learning among older clients. The following interventions may be helpful in encouraging senior citizens to engage in computer-based learning activities:

- *Reinforce principles of ergonomics by making suggestions about equipment and posture that will minimize physical problems related to computer use.* Ergonomics is important for everyone but is especially important for older adults who may have visual problems as well as arthritic changes in the neck, hands, and spine. Proper posture, correct positioning of the keyboard and monitor, adjusted screen colors and font size, a supportive chair, and a reminder to get up and walk around three to four times per hour will help older adults to avoid discouraging physical symptoms that may interfere with computer use.
- *Identify resources that will provide computer access and support in the senior citizen's home community.* Supply seniors with a comprehensive resource list containing places where free computer and Internet access is available, places where computer training is provided for seniors, and contact people who will assist if problems are encountered. In addition to public libraries and community centers, numerous projects nationwide are committed to digital inclusion for all segments of the population, including the older adult population. Many of these projects and resources can be identified on the Web. For example, The

American Association of Retired People (AARP) has a wide range of services designed to promote and support computer use by older adults available on its Web site.

- *Motivate older adults to use a computer by helping them to identify how the computer can meet their needs.* It is important to talk to seniors about their needs and abilities. Find out how they like to learn, what kinds of things they enjoy doing, and what their healthcare needs are. Matching a computer program or Web site to the individual's unique circumstances will encourage computer use. For example, a senior who is caring for a spouse with cancer might appreciate an online support group if he or she enjoys interacting with and learning from the experiences of others. In this way, you will help to generate interest in learning how to use a computer for health education by starting at a place that piques the senior's interest.

- *Create a supportive and nonthreatening environment to teach older adults about using a computer for health education.* Today's seniors did not grow up with computers and may not have confidence in their ability to learn this new skill at this point in their lives. The language of computers may seem foreign to them, so teachers should avoid jargon and define new terms. Teachers should pace their teaching according to the senior learners' responses. Teachers may need to proceed slowly at first and provide opportunities for practice and for reinforcement of skills. They must write the instructions down and go over them

before the teaching session ends so that the senior clients do not go home with unanswered questions.

Computers can open up a whole new avenue of support and information to older adults who are struggling with their own health problems and those of their partners. Seniors who enjoy good health can find resources to help them maintain their health and to become educated healthcare consumers. It is important that older adults be given the same opportunities to take advantage of the Information Age resources that are available to younger clients. The nurse can play a key role in promoting digital inclusion among this segment of the population.

People with disabilities make up another special population that may require additional planning before using technologies in health and healthcare education. Not only are people with disabilities less likely to have computer and Internet access than are members of the general population, but they may also have difficulty using hardware and software. The ability to use a computer without adaptive devices requires the fine motor coordination and mobility necessary to use a mouse and keyboard, the strength to sit and hold the head in an upright position, and the ability to comprehend information presented on the computer screen.

For example, individuals with visual impairments may have difficulty seeing text or graphics on a computer screen or performing tasks on the computer that require hand–eye coordination. When identifying obstacles related to visual impairments, it is important to think broadly and address the wide range of conditions that affect the way we see. Color blindness, which affects approximately 8% of all males and 0.5% of females, can cause significant problems for computer users if the Web site or software used does not display the correct color combinations, if the contrast between background and foreground is inadequate, and if color rather than text is used to convey directions.

Although hearing impairments cause fewer problems for computer users than visual impairments, some accessibility issues nevertheless need to be addressed. An individual with a hearing problem may not be able to hear the sounds that are often used as prompts when a wrong key is struck or when an e-mail message is delivered. Accessibility for individuals with hearing impairments is becoming a bigger issue now that it is easier to send audio signals across the Web and audio messages are becoming more commonplace.

Despite the protections offered by the Americans With Disabilities Act and other federal legislation, accessibility issues on the Web and constraints with hardware and software still exist. Federal legislation outlined in Section 508 of the Workforce Investment Act requires government agencies and institutions receiving government funding to make their Web sites accessible to people with disabilities. However, many Web sites and programs do not fall under this umbrella of protection. Chapter 9 describes potential barriers and specific adaptations that can be employed to assist people who have disabilities to use computers.

Nurses who use the Internet and the World Wide Web to teach also need to consider Web site design when creating or selecting Web sites that might be used by disabled learners. The World Wide Web contains multiple resources that can be used by Web designers or Web users to learn design principles for accessibility. For example, inserting the search command *color blindness* on a search engine will produce Web sites that explain color blindness, illustrate how various types of color blindness affect what might be seen on a Web site, describe good Web design principles for promoting accessibility, and provide tools that can be used to select color combinations that will not create barriers for individuals with color blindness.

Several resources are available to assist Web developers in creating Web sites that meet the needs of people with disabilities. The Web Accessibility Initiative Web site (http://www.w3.org/wai) provides guidelines that are recognized by many as the international standard for accessibility. Another Web site of note is a site created by the Center for Applied Special Technology (CAST). CAST provides a program called "Bobby" to assist Web page authors to identify and correct problems that could make their sites inaccessible to individuals with disabilities. Information on Bobby can be found at the CAST Web site (http://www.cast.org).

Age, disabilities, and other factors that place an individual within the digital divide are also factors that can isolate and diminish access to healthcare resources. Therefore, every effort should be made to help these individuals connect to the wealth of resources that are and can be made available through technology. The nurse can play a vital role in providing the support, education, and advocacy needed to reduce the barriers that still exist for these special groups of people.

Professional Education

From work-site training to higher education, technology is making professional education more accessible and more meaningful for nurses. It is no longer necessary for nurses to quit working or to relocate to earn a higher degree. Technology has contributed to the growth of distance education programs at all levels in nursing. Likewise, technology is making it possible for nurses in the workplace to engage in a variety of continuing education activities designed to keep their practice current, to provide career mobility, and to enhance professional development.

E-Learning

Technology has had such an impact on workforce training that it has given birth to a new industry and a new set of buzz words that define an Information Age approach to staff education. Professional development and training organizations have capitalized on the power of computer technology to provide businesses with learning solutions referred to as *e-learning*, an abbreviation for electronic learning.

Although no consensus of opinion has been reached on a precise definition for the term e-learning, there is some agreement that it involves the use of technology-based tools and processes to provide for customized learning anytime or anywhere. Even though the term e-learning can be applied to any learning that is delivered via technology, it is most commonly used to describe professional development and training programs. Higher education typically uses the phrase *distance learning* to describe academic programs delivered via computers.

The emphasis on e-learning in industry is on outcomes, with the goal of providing an individual with the information or practice opportunities required to perform a task or solve a problem at the point of need. E-learning has the potential to deliver training programs that are cost effective, promote positive patient outcomes, and lead to staff satisfaction. The nature of the work of health care makes workforce training a critical issue, and e-learning appears to have provided a solution to the problem of keeping staff current in a world

where new treatments and new techniques are always on the horizon.

What is the e-learning approach to workforce training in health care? First and foremost, e-learning provides learning opportunities at the point of need. In health care, this statement means that training is available 24 hours a day, 7 days a week. Because the point of need in health care is often related to patient care, e-learning must be structured in a way that it can be delivered on a clinical unit.

Point-of-need training must also be efficient. In this era of nursing shortages and increasing complexity of care, such training must be provided in a way that fits into the schedules of busy healthcare workers. Finally, e-learning in health care must be distributed so that it can be made available to people across any number of environments and situations. Many healthcare organizations have staff in a wide range of settings and locations. A centralized approach to training will not work well if it means that people have to travel to the staff education office for all training programs.

Multiple approaches to e-learning in health care are possible. Examples of some of the features of e-learning products that have proved attractive to healthcare organizations are as follows:

- E-learning training modules can be delivered via the World Wide Web. Web-based products are attractive because they are easily accessed in a variety of environments and situations. A computer workstation can easily fit into a clinical unit, and laptops can be carried into the field.
- E-learning can be delivered in small modules that can be completed in as little as 15 minutes. Many healthcare workers are unable to leave their work

area for long periods of time. However, most can find 15–30 minutes in a given day, particularly if they do not have to leave the unit. Time permitting, staff can complete several modules in one sitting.

- E-learning programs can be customized at a variety of levels: the organization, the staff position, and the individual. Customization personalizes the program and helps to make it relevant to the individual and to the organization.
- E-learning programs can track completion and create a performance report for individual staff members.
- E-learning modules are interactive and reality-based. For example, a patient simulation that allows the participant to manage the care of a virtual patient can be created.

Nurses have many potential roles in the development and implementation of an e-learning program within an institution. As content experts, they may be hired by e-learning companies to create products designed to meet the needs of practicing nurses. Nurses within a healthcare organization may be in a position to work with the e-learning company by customizing the training package purchased and developing a plan for its implementation. Those who use the e-learning system can contribute to the program by completing the modules offered and submitting carefully thought-out evaluations of the products used.

Staff training programs are important to the individual staff members, to the organization, and to the patients served. Every staff member has a responsibility to do what he or she can to ensure the success of the program.

Although early e-learning training programs took the form of computer-based modules, new technologies are emerging. Some of these technologies allow training to take place in real time. Webcasts, or live broadcasts over the Internet, permit audio or video to be transmitted to participants in multiple locations. Webcasts provide a unique mechanism for delivering presentations to users around the globe.

Although webcasts do not allow any type of interaction, they are growing in popularity as a training device for sharing lectures and demonstrations. Webinars, or web conferencing, are similar to webcasts in that they are Internet-based programs; however, webinars do allow for interaction.

Webinars often have two components: a computer-based display, such as a PowerPoint presentation or whiteboard, and a live discussion. Participants can join a Web-based conference via telephone or computer. Webcasts and computer conferencing are relatively new technologies; therefore, price may be an issue for some.

Mobile learning, or *m-learning,* is another new strategy that takes advantage of the many "wireless, mobile, portable and handheld devices" (Traxler, 2007, Introduction, para. 1) that have been developed and widely marketed in recent years (Maag, 2006; Peters, 2007). The word *mobile* refers both to the use of portable technologies such as MP3 players and to the end user, the mobile adult, who can truly learn anytime, any place. Mobile devices can be used for a wide range of activities including accessing course materials, searching the Web, listening to lectures, recording experiences and assignments, and participating in learning-focused games (Peters, 2007).

Although m-learning has great potential, its use is limited at the present time. Cost is a major factor as portable devices are often expensive. However, the popularity of MP3 players, smart phones, and other portable devices, especially among the young, indicate great promise for future use.

Distance Education

As a result of technological advances, distance education for nurses is flourishing in the 21st century (Billings, 2007). This success was not always the case, however. When distance education programs were first introduced, they were quite controversial.

For example, when the Regents External Degree Program was first created in 1974, many people felt that a distance model was inappropriate for nursing education. Today, the Regents External Degree Program, now Excelsior College, is one of the largest nursing programs in the world, with more than 16,000 nursing students enrolled in its associate, baccalaureate, and master's degree programs (Excelsior College, 2007). In 1994, another milestone was reached in nursing education when Duquesne University in Pennsylvania opened the first online distance education program leading to a Ph.D. in nursing.

The Excelsior College and Duquesne University programs represent a mere sample of the many distance education programs in nursing available in the United States today. AllNursingSchools.com, a popular online directory of nursing education programs, lists more than 30 schools across the country offering a wide range of online undergraduate and graduate certificate and degree programs in nursing and specialty areas of practice. This list is far from complete as the number of schools offering distance learning experiences, courses, and totally online programs grows each year.

The term *distance learning* means different things to different people. Online courses, correspondence courses, independent study, and videoconferencing are just a few of the techniques that can be used to deliver education to students studying at a distance. The diversity of distance education programs in the United States reflects the myriad approaches that can be used to meet the needs of students who are separated from the traditional classroom setting. In all cases, distance education means that the teacher and the learner are separated from one another (American Association of Colleges of Nursing Task Force on Distance Technology and Nursing Education, 1999).

A variety of strategies are being used to provide courses to students who are not in the same location as the teacher. However, online courses are growing at such a rapid pace that the Internet is becoming the primary vehicle for delivering distance education (Institute for Higher Education Policy, 2000). Some nursing programs are totally Internet based, whereas others use a combination of on-site and Internet-based courses. Some nursing programs offer hybrid or blended courses that incorporate a mix of classroom instruction and online discussion. It should be noted that online education is not restricted to higher education. Online continuing education programs are also available to nurses from a variety of sources such as their own professional organizations.

Research has shown that distance education provides much more than a flexible approach to learning. Comparisons of students from distance education courses and from traditional classrooms have repeatedly shown that distance education can be a very effective mode for delivering education (Russell, 1998).

However, because distance education and particularly online education are still relatively new phenomena, the education community is still working hard to meet the many challenges associated with educating students who live and work at a distance. Several education organizations have developed guidelines and standards for distance education to assist faculty and to ensure program quality, including the American Council on Education, the National Education Association, the Commission on Higher Education of the Middle States Association of Colleges and Schools, The American Association of Colleges of Nursing, and the Western Interstate Commission on Higher Education (Billings, 2007; Institute for Higher Education Policy, 2000).

Recognizing that distance education involves more than providing coursework, colleges and universities are also attempting to provide the support services necessary to ensure the success of the distance learner. For example, they are establishing online bookstores, online registration processes, virtual libraries, virtual student lounges, and online office hours with faculty.

Given the growth and development of online courses, it is likely that this teaching methodology will be incorporated into health and healthcare education as well. Nurses who are responsible for providing education for clients need to begin thinking about how online courses may fit into their programs. Online courses not only provide learning activities and resources, but also facilitate teacher–learner and learner–learner interactions. Internet-based courses might work very well in areas such as parenting and diabetes education where there is an extended program of instruction and the need for group support.

State of the Evidence

Teaching with technology is not a new concept. Nurses and other educators have been using technology to teach patients and students for many years. However, in the Information Age, the notion of teaching with technology has taken on new meaning. Technology is advancing so quickly that researchers are struggling to keep up with the new products and technology-based strategies that are emerging every day.

There is a large body of research documenting the effects of distance education technologies on student outcomes. One of the classic and most frequently quoted studies on the impact of technology in education was conducted by Thomas Russell. Russell reviewed over 350 studies, reports, dissertations, and papers documenting what he called the "no significant difference phenomenon"; that is, the lack of evidence to support any difference in student outcome for students educated using technology versus traditional methods (Russell, 1998; Young, 2000).

In light of the many new forms of distance education and the numerous research studies that have been conducted in recent years, a Web site has been set up as a companion piece to Russell's work (http://www.nosignificantdifference.org). This Web site provides access to more than 80 years of educational research. The studies included on this site fall into two categories: those that show no difference between traditional and technology-based education and those that show differences in student outcomes based on educational strategy used.

Although not as comprehensive as the studies in higher education, there is a growing body of research on the use of technology in patient education. A review of the literature reveals studies in a broad range of topics including the use of online support groups and the use of computer-based programs for patient education in clinical and home settings. The focus to date has largely been on ways in which clients use technology and the obstacles they face. Most of these studies are small in scope.

Despite a comprehensive body of research on the use of technology in higher education and a growing body of research on patient education, there is much yet to learn, particularly in the area of patient education. Technology is exciting and has many advantages for both consumers and nurses. However, until we can document that it is effective in meeting educational needs, we need to proceed carefully.

Summary

This chapter focused on Information Age technology and its use in healthcare education. Specifically, this chapter discussed ways in which the World Wide Web and the Internet could be used by nurse educators to enhance health and healthcare education for consumers and healthcare professionals. The impact of technology on teachers and learners was addressed, and special considerations for older adults and other client groups were identified. Trends in distance education for nurses were explored.

Information Age technology has the potential to transform health and healthcare education. This powerful tool must be used thoughtfully and carefully, however. Education is about learning, not technology. Technology is merely a vehicle to deliver educational programs and to promote learning. The benefits of technology-based education are numerous, as are the challenges for educators and learners. As nurses, we have a responsibility to learn to use new tools to promote health in our clients and professional growth and development in ourselves. The future looks very bright, and we can help to shape it by continuing to think creatively about how to use technology in education and by participating in research about its effectiveness.

REVIEW QUESTIONS

1. What is the Information Age and how has it influenced education in general, health-care education specifically, and healthcare consumers?
2. What Information Age skills are required by healthcare professionals and healthcare consumers?
3. What are the various standards that have been established to ensure quality on the World Wide Web and access by special populations?
4. What are the ways in which resources on the World Wide Web can be used as a health information resource for healthcare consumers and healthcare professionals?
5. What are the various ways in which the Internet can be used to facilitate electronic communication between and among nurse educators and healthcare consumers? What are the advantages and disadvantages of each?
6. When using computer resources with clients, which segments of the population require special considerations due to limited access or special needs? What are those considerations, and how can they be addressed?
7. What is e-learning, and what advantages does it offer in providing training in health-care settings?
8. How has technology influenced professional and continuing education options for nurses?

References

American Association of Colleges of Nursing. (1999). *Task force on distance technology and nursing education.* Washington, DC: Author.

American Medical Association. (2007). *Guidelines for physician–patient electronic communication.* Retrieved June 15, 2007, from http://www.ama-assn.org/ama/pub/category/2386.html

American Medical Informatics Association. (2007). Retrieved July 2, 2007, from http://www.amia.org

Association of Cancer On-line Resources, Inc. (2007). Retrieved July 3, 2007, from http://www.acor.org

Baker, L., Wagner, T., Singer, S., & Bundoff, K. (2003). Use of the Internet and e-mail for healthcare information. *Journal of the American Medical Association, 289,* 2400–2406.

Billings, D. (2007). Distance education in nursing: 25 years and going strong. *CIN: Computers, Informatics, Nursing, 25,* 120.

Cetron, M. J., & Davies, O. (2001). Trends now changing the world. *The Futurist, 35*(2), 27–40.

The changing role of instructors. (2006). *Edutech Report, 23*(1), 3–7.

Evangelista, L. S., Stromberg, A., Westlake, C., Galstanyan, A., Anderson, N., & Dracup, K. (2006). Developing a Web-based education and counseling program for heart failure patients. *Progress in Cardiovascular Nursing, 21,* 196–201.

Excelsior College. (2007). Retrieved July 17, 2007, from http://www.excelsior.edu

Finnis, J. A. (2003). *Learning in the information age.* Retrieved June 18, 2007, from http://dev.twinisles.com/research/learninfoage.pdf

Fox, S. (2005). *Digital divisons*. Retrieved June 15, 2007, from http://www.pewinternet.org/pdfs/PIP_Digital_Divisions_Oct_5_2005.pdf

Fox, S. (2006). *Online health search. Pew Internet & American life project*. Retrieved June 15, 2007, from http://www.ihep.com/organizations.php3?

Fox, S., & Fallows, D. (2003). *Internet health resources*. Retrieved June 15, 2007, from http://www.pewinternet.org

Fox, S., & Madden, M. (2005). *Data memo: Generations online*. Retrieved June 18, 2007, from http://www.pewinternet.org/pdfs/PIP_Generations_Memo.pdf

Han, H.-R., & Belcher, A. (2001). Computer-mediated support group use among parents of children with cancer—An exploratory study. *Computers in Nursing, 19*(1), 27–33.

Hern, M., Weitkamp, T., Haag, D., Trigg, J., & Guard, J. R. (1997). Nursing the community in cyberspace. *Computers in Nursing, 15*(6), 316–321.

Horrigan, J. B. (2006). *Broad band adoption in 2006. Pew Internet & American life project*. Retrieved June 15, 1007, from http://www.ihep.com/organizations.php3?action=printContentltem&orgid=104&typeID=906&itemID=9230&templateID=1422

Institute for Higher Education Policy. (2000). *Distance learning in higher education*. Retrieved June 1, 2007, from http:www.//ihep.com/organizations.php3?action=printContentltem&orgid=104&typeID=906&itemID=9230&templateID=1422

Internetworldstats.com. (2007). Retrieved July 2, 2007, from http://www.internetworldstats.com

Kaplan, B., & Brennan, P. F. (2001). Consumer informatics: Supporting patients as co-producers of quality. *Journal of the American Medical Informatics Association, 8*(4), 309–315.

Kassirer, J. P. (2000). Patients, physicians and the Internet. *Health Affairs, 19*(6), 115–123.

Klemm, P., Reppert, K., & Visich, L. (1998). A nontraditional cancer support group: The Internet. *Computers in Nursing, 16*(1), 31–36.

Lenhart, A., & Fox, S. (2006). *Bloggers: A portrait of the Internet's new storytellers*. Retrieved June 15, 2007, from http://www.pewinternet.org/PPF/r/186/report_display.asp

Lewis, D., Gundwardena, S., & Saadawi, G. (2005). Caring connection: Developing an Internet resource for family caregivers of children with cancer. *CIN: Computers, Informatics, Nursing, 23*, 265–274.

Livinginternet.com. (2007). *Tim Berners-Lee, Robert Cailliau, and the World Wide Web*. Retrieved June 15, 2007, from http://www.livinginternet.com/w/wi_lee.htm

Maag, M. (2005). The potential use of blogs in nursing education. *CIN: Computers, Informatics, Nursing, 23*, 16–26.

Maag, M. (2006). Podcasting and MP3 players: Emerging technologies. *CIN: Computers, Informatics, Nursing, 24*, 9–13.

Nahm, E., Preece, J., Resnick, B., & Mills, M. (2004). Usability of Web sites for older adults. *CIN: Computers, Informatics, Nursing, 22*, 326–334.

National Center for Educational Statistics. (2006). *Computer and Internet use by students in 2003: Statistical analysis report*. Washington, DC: U.S. Department of Education Institute of Educational Sciences, NCES 2006-065.

National Institute of Medicine. (2001). *Crossing the quality chasm: A new health system for the 21st century*. Washington, DC: National Academy Press.

Pandia.com. (2006). *A short and easy search engine tutorial*. Retrieved June 15, 2007, from http://www.pandia.com/goalgetter

Peters, K. (2007). M-learning: Positioning educators for a mobile connected future. *The International Review of Research in Open and Distance Learning, 8*(2). Retrieved June 15, 2007, from http://www.irrodl.org

Rainie, L. (2003). *The online healthcare revolution and the rise of e-patients and e-caregivers. Pew Internet & American life project*. Retrieved June 15, 2007, from http://www.ihep.com/organizations.php3?actions

Russell, T. L. (1998). *The no-significant difference phenomenon*. Retrieved July 2, 2007, from http://www.nosignificantdifference.org

Schloman, B. (2006). Is it time to visit the blogosphere? *The Online Journal of Issues in Nursing*. Retrieved June 15, 2007, from http://www.nursingworld.org/ojin/infocol/info_21.htm

Secco, L., Woodgate, R., Hodgson, A., Kowalski, S., Plouffe, J., Rothney, P., et al. (2006). A survey study of pediatric nurses' use of information sources. *CIN: Computers, Informatics, Nursing, 24*, 105–112.

Shaw, B. R., Hawkins, R., Aroroa, N., McTavish, F., Pingree, S., & Gustafson, D. H. (2006). An exploratory study of predictors of participation in a computer support group for women with breast cancer. *CIN: Computer, Informatics, Nursing, 23*, 18–27.

Stone, J. H. (2007). Communication between physicians and patients in the era of e-medicine. *New England Journal of Medicine, 356*, 2451–2454.

Traxler, J. (2007). Defining, discussing, and evaluating mobile learning: the moving finger writes and having writ…. [Abstract]. *The International Review of Research in Open and Distance Learning, 8*(2). Retrieved June 15, 2007, from http://www.irrodl.org

Wikipedia. (2007). *History of the Internet*. Retrieved June 15, 2007, from http://en.wikipedia.org/wiki/History_of_the_Internet

Wilbright, W. A., Haun, D., Romano, T. A., Krutzfeldt, T., Fontenot, C., & Nolan, T. (2006). Computer use in an urban hospital. *CIN: Computers, Informatics, Nursing, 24*, 37–43.

Williams, K. (2003). Literacy and computer literacy: Analyzing the NCRs being fluent with information technology. *Journal of Literacy and Technology, 3*(1). Retrieved June 15, 2007, from http://www.literacyandtechnology.org/v3n1/williams.htm

Young, J. (2000). Scholar concludes that distance ed is as effective as traditional instruction. *The Chronicle of Higher Education*. Retrieved July 2, 2007, from http://chronicle.com/free/2000/02/2000021001u.htm

Chapter 14

Evaluation in Healthcare Education

Priscilla Sandford Worral

CHAPTER HIGHLIGHTS

KEY TERMS

OBJECTIVES

After completing this chapter, the reader will be able to

1. Define the term *evaluation*.
2. Discuss the relationships among evaluation, evidence-based practice, and practice-based evidence.
3. Compare and contrast evaluation and assessment.
4. Identify the purposes of evaluation.
5. Distinguish between five basic types of evaluation: process, content, outcome, impact, and program.
6. Discuss characteristics of various models of evaluation.
7. Describe similarities and differences between evaluation and research.
8. Assess barriers to evaluation.
9. Examine methods for conducting an evaluation.
10. Select appropriate instruments for various types of evaluative data.
11. Identify guidelines for reporting results of evaluation.
12. Describe the strength of the current evidence base for evaluation of patient and nursing staff education.

Evaluation is the process that can provide evidence that what we do as nurses and as nurse educators makes a value-added difference in the care we provide. *Evaluation* is defined as a systematic process by which the worth or value of something—in this case, teaching and learning—is judged.

Early consideration of evaluation has never been more critical than in today's healthcare environment, which demands that practice is based upon evidence. Crucial decisions regarding learners rest on the outcomes of learning. Can the patient go home? Can the nurse provide competent care? If education is to be justified as a value-added activity, the process of education must be measurably efficient and must be measurably linked to education outcomes. The outcomes of education, for the learner and for the organization, must be measurably effective.

Evaluation is a process within a process—a critical component of the nursing process, the decision-making process, and the education process. Evaluation is the final component of each of these processes. Because these processes are cyclical, evaluation serves as the critical bridge at the end of one cycle that provides evidence to guide direction of the next cycle.

The sections of this chapter follow the steps in conducting an evaluation. These steps include (1) determining the focus of the evaluation, including use of evaluation models; (2) designing the evaluation; (3) conducting the evaluation; (4) determining methods of analysis and interpretation of data collected; (5) reporting results of data collected; and (6) using evaluation results.

Each of these aspects of the evaluation process is important, but all of them are meaningless if the results of evaluation are not used to guide future action in planning and carrying out educational interventions. In other words, the results of evaluation provide practice-based evidence to support continuing an educational intervention as is or revising that intervention to enhance learning.

Evaluation, Evidence-Based Practice, and Practice-Based Evidence

Evidence-based practice (EBP) can be defined as "the conscientious use of current best evidence in making decisions about patient care" (Melnyk & Fineout-Overholt, 2005, p. 6). Most EBP models describe evidence generated from systematic reviews of clinically relevant randomized controlled trials as the strongest evidence upon which to base practice decisions, especially decisions about treatment. Evidence from research is also called *external evidence* because it is intended to be generalizable beyond the particular study setting or sample.

As will be discussed later in this chapter, results of evaluation are not considered external evidence. This is because evaluations are not intended to be generalizable, but are conducted to determine effectiveness of a specific intervention in a specific setting with an identified individual or group. Results of a systematically conducted evaluation, while not considered external evidence, are still important from an EBP perspective. When evidence generated from research is not available, the conscientious use of *internal evidence* is appropriate. Results of a systematically conducted evaluation are one example of internal evidence (Melnyk & Fineout-Overholt, 2005).

Nurses' understanding and use of EBP has evolved and expanded over the past decade. In contrast, the idea of *practice-based evidence* is only beginning to be defined. In the absence of an official or commonly understood definition of practice-based evidence, what might this term mean? Might practice-based evidence—or evidence derived from practice rather than from research—include results of a systematically conducted evaluation? Might practice-based evidence include patients' responses to care delivered on the basis of clinical expertise and an understanding of individual patient values? Might practice-based evidence include results from systematically conducted quality improvement projects?

The results of evaluations, the outcomes of expert-delivered patient-centered care, and the results of quality improvement projects all comprise internal evidence gathered by nurses and other healthcare professionals on an ongoing basis as an integral and important component of professional practice. Intentional recognition of these findings about current practice as a source of evidence to guide future practice requires that we critically think before acting and engage in ongoing critical appraisal during and after each nurse–patient interaction.

Evaluation Versus Assessment

While assessment and evaluation are highly interrelated and are often used interchangeably as terms, they are not synonymous. The process of assessment is to gather, summarize, interpret, and use data to decide a direction for action. The process of evaluation is to gather, summarize, interpret, and use data to determine the extent to which an action was successful.

The primary differences between these two terms are those of timing and purpose. For example, an education program begins with an assessment of learners' needs. From the perspective of systems theory, assessment data might be called the "input." While the program is being conducted, periodic evaluation lets the educator know whether the program and learners are proceeding as planned. After program completion, evaluation identifies whether and to what extent identified needs were met. Again, from a systems theory perspective, these evaluative data might be called "intermediate output" and "output," respectively.

An important note of caution: although an evaluation is conducted at the end of a program, that is a bad time to plan it. Evaluation as an afterthought is, at best, a poor idea and, at worst, a dangerous one. Data may be impossible to collect, be incomplete, or even be misleading. Assessment and evaluation planning should ideally be concurrent activities. Where feasible, the same data collection methods and instruments should be used. This approach is especially appropriate for outcome and impact evaluations, as will be discussed later in this chapter. "If only . . ." is an all too frequent lament, which can be minimized by planning ahead.

Determining the Focus of Evaluation

In planning any evaluation, the first and most crucial step is to determine the focus of the evaluation. The focus then will guide evaluation design, conduct, data analysis, and reporting of results. The importance of a clear, specific, and realistic evaluation focus cannot be overemphasized. Usefulness and accuracy of the results of an evaluation depend heavily on how well the evaluation is initially focused.

Evaluation focus includes five basic components: (1) audience, (2) purpose, (3) questions, (4) scope, and (5) resources (Ruzicki, 1987). To determine these components, ask the following questions:

1. For what **audience** is the evaluation being conducted?
2. For what **purpose** is the evaluation being conducted?
3. What **questions** will be asked in the evaluation?
4. What is the **scope** of the evaluation?
5. What **resources** are available to conduct the evaluation?

The **audience** comprises the persons or groups for whom the evaluation is being conducted (Ruzicki, 1987). These individuals or groups include the primary audience or the individual or group who requested the evaluation, and the general audience, or all those who will use evaluation results or who might benefit from the evaluation. Thus the audience for an evaluation might include patients, peers, a supervisor, the nursing director, the staff development director, the chief executive officer of the institution, or a group of community leaders.

When an evaluator reports results of the evaluation, he or she will provide feedback to all members of the audience. In focusing the evaluation, however, he or she must first consider the primary audience. Giving priority to the individual or group who requested the evaluation will make focusing the evaluation easier, especially if results of an evaluation will be used by several groups representing diverse interests.

The **purpose** of the evaluation is the answer to the question, "Why is the evaluation being conducted?" The purpose of an evaluation might be to decide whether to continue a particular education program or to determine the effectiveness of the teaching process. If a particular individual or group has a primary interest in results of the evaluation, input from that group can clarify the purpose.

An important note of caution: *Why* one is conducting an evaluation is not synonymous with *who* or *what* one is evaluating. For example, nursing literature on patient education commonly distinguishes among three types of evaluations: (1) learner, (2) teacher, and (3) program. This distinction answers the question of who or what will be evaluated and is extremely useful for evaluation design and conduct. Why learner evaluation might be undertaken, for example, is answered by the reason or purpose for evaluating learner performance. Determining teaching or program effectiveness is another example of the purpose for undertaking evaluation.

An excellent rule of thumb in stating the purpose of an evaluation is keep it singular. In other words, one should state, "The purpose is . . . ," not "The purposes are . . . " Keeping the purpose audience focused and singular will help avoid the all-too-frequent tendency to attempt too much in one evaluation.

Questions to be asked in the evaluation are directly related to the purpose for conducting the evaluation, are specific, and are measurable. Examples of questions are "To what extent are patients satisfied with the cardiac discharge teaching program?" and "How frequently do staff nurses use the diabetes teaching reference materials?" Asking the right questions is crucial if the evaluation is to fulfill the intended purpose. As will be discussed later in this chapter, delineation of evaluation questions is both the

first step in selection of evaluation design and the basis for eventual data analysis.

The **scope** of an evaluation can be considered an answer to the question, "How much will be evaluated?" "How much" includes "How many aspects of education will be evaluated?" "How many individuals or representative groups will be evaluated?" and "What time period is to be evaluated?" For example, will the evaluation focus on one class or on an entire program; on the learning experience for one patient or for all patients being taught a particular skill? Evaluation could be limited to the teaching process during a particular patient education class or it could be expanded to encompass both the teaching process and related patient outcomes of learning.

The scope of an evaluation is determined in part by the purpose for conducting the evaluation and in part by available resources. For example, an evaluation addressing learner satisfaction with faculty for all programs conducted by a staff development department in a given year is necessarily broad and long term in scope and will require expertise in data collection and analysis. An evaluation to determine whether a patient understands each step in a learning session on how to self-administer insulin injections is narrow in scope, is focused on a particular point in time, and will require expertise in clinical practice and observation.

Resources needed to conduct an evaluation include time, expertise, personnel, materials, equipment, and facilities. A realistic appraisal of what resources are accessible and available relative to what resources are required is crucial in focusing any evaluation. Someone conducting an evaluation should remember to include the time and expertise required to collate, analyze, and interpret data and to prepare the report of evaluation results.

Evaluation can be classified into different types, or categories, based on one or more of the five components just described. The most common types of evaluation identified include process, content, outcome, impact, and program evaluation. A number of evaluation models that help to clarify differences among these evaluation types as well as how they relate to one another have been developed (Abruzzese, 1992; Haggard, 1989; Koch, 2000; Puetz, 1992; Rankin & Stallings, 2005; Suhayda & Miller, 2006; Walker & Dewar, 2000).

Evaluation Models

Abruzzese (1992) constructed the Roberta Straessle Abruzzese (RSA) evaluation model for conceptualizing, or classifying, educational evaluation into different categories or levels. Although developed in 1978 and derived from the perspective of staff development education, the RSA model remains useful for conceptualizing types of evaluation from both staff development and patient education perspectives. A more recent example of use of the RSA model is given by Dilorio, Price, and Becker (2001) in their discussion of the evaluation of the Neuroscience Nurse Internship Program at the National Institutes of Health Clinical Center.

The RSA model pictorially places five basic types of evaluation in relation to one another based on purpose and related questions, scope, and resource components of evaluation focus (**Figure** 14–1). The five types of evaluation

Figure 14–1 RSA evaluation model.

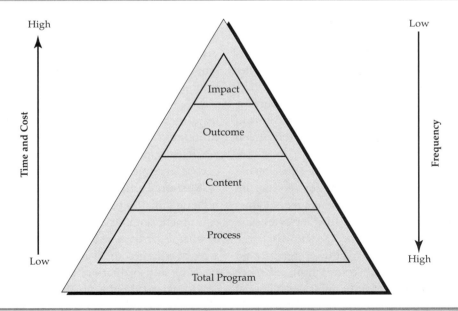

Source: Reprinted by permission of Roberta S. Abruzzese.

include process, content, outcome, impact, and program. Abruzzese described the first four types as levels of evaluation leading from the simple (process evaluation) to the complex (impact evaluation). Total program evaluation encompasses and summarizes all four levels.

Process (Formative) Evaluation

The purpose of *process or formative evaluation* is to make adjustments in an educational activity as soon as they are needed, whether those adjustments be in personnel, materials, facilities, learning objectives, or even one's own attitude. Adjustments may need to be made after one class or session before the next is taught or even in the middle of a single learning experience. Consider, for example, evaluation of the process of teaching a newly diagnosed juvenile insulin-dependent diabetic and her parents how to administer insulin. The nurse might facilitate learning better by first injecting himself or herself with normal saline so they can see someone maintain a calm expression during an injection. If the nurse educator had planned to have the parent give the first injection, but the child seems less fearful, the nurse might consider revising the teaching plan to let the child first perform self-injection.

Process evaluation is integral to the education process itself. It forms an educational activity because evaluation is an ongoing component of assessment, planning, and implementation. As part of the education process, this ongoing evaluation helps the nurse anticipate and prevent problems before they occur or identify problems as they arise.

Consistent with the purpose of process evaluation, the primary question is, "How can teaching be improved to facilitate learning?" The nurse's teaching effectiveness, the teaching process, and the learner's responses are monitored

on an ongoing basis. Abruzzese (1992) described process evaluation as a happiness index. While teaching and learning are ongoing, learners are asked their opinions about faculty, learning/ course objectives, content, teaching and learning methods, physical facilities, and administration of the learning experience. Specific questions could include:

- Am I giving the patient time to ask questions?
- Is the information I am giving in class consistent with information included in the handouts?
- Does the patient look bored? Is the room too warm?
- Should I include more opportunities for return demonstration?

The scope of process evaluation generally is limited in breadth and time period to a specific learning experience such as a class or workshop, yet is sufficiently detailed to include as many aspects of the specific learning experience as possible while they occur. Learner behavior, teacher behavior, learner–teacher interaction, learner response to teaching materials and methods, and characteristics of the environment are all aspects of the learning experience within the scope of process evaluation. All learners and all teachers participating in a learning experience should be included in process evaluation. If resources are limited and participants include a number of different groups, a representative sample of individuals from each group rather than everyone from each group may be included in the evaluation.

Resources usually are less costly and more readily available for process evaluation than for other types such as impact or total program evaluation. Although process evaluation occurs more frequently—during and throughout every learning experience—than any other type, it occurs concurrently with teaching. The need for additional time, facilities, and dollars to conduct process evaluation is consequently decreased.

From the perspective of evidence-based practice, process evaluation is important in the use and patient-centered modification of clinical practice guidelines (CPGs). A well-constructed CPG includes not only the specific intervention—teaching a patient how to take his discharge medication, for example—but also includes the evidence-based process that should be used to provide that teaching.

Formal development of a CPG requires a high level of rigor and is intended for guiding care to all patients who have similar characteristics and learning needs. As will be discussed later in this chapter, CPG development is conducted as evaluation research. Evaluation of the process of using a CPG, however, is focused on the fit of a CPG for a specific learner or learners. To the extent that a patient is the same as those studied in development of the CPG, the patient's nurse will follow the guideline as written. To the extent that the patient has unique behaviors or responses to teaching, the nurse will use informal process evaluation to vary from the guideline so the patient is able to learn.

Evidence-based practice is not a cookbook approach to providing health care. Similarly, CPGs are not intended to be followed without regard for the individual learner. This does not mean that variance from a CPG is determined in a haphazard manner based on what may be convenient at the moment. As attention to practice-based evidence evolves, the importance of the conscientious use of internal evidence gathered from process evaluation will become an increasingly critical component of every teaching–learning experience.

For instance, Watters and Moran (2006) describe a coordinated approach to care of patients recovering from hip fractures that explains how an interdisciplinary team implemented and modified a hip fracture protocol to be evidence-based and appropriate for a geriatric cohort. An example of process evaluation to examine the benefit of fitting an education intervention to the learner is provided by Schreurs, Colland, Kuijer, Ridder, and van Elderen (2003). Using self-regulation theory to support an emphasis on personal goal setting, these clinicians worked with patients to develop an action plan for self-management of their asthma, diabetes, or heart failure, then continuously reevaluated and adjusted the plan based on patients' success in managing symptoms and maintaining adherence to treatment regimens. Findings demonstrated that both patients and nurses caring for these patients were satisfied with the education.

The importance of evidence-based practice to process evaluation encompasses staff education as well as patient education. Covell (2005) describes the use of the Iowa model of evidence-based practice to evaluate and modify guidelines for teaching basic cardiac life support (BCLS) to nursing staff. Guided by the Iowa model, nurse educators and staff examined their practice environment and searched the literature, then drafted new guidelines for teaching BCLS that were evidence based plus reflected key environmental factors. Using process evaluation to revise their guidelines during implementation, nurse educators identified the need for additional equipment and regularly scheduled refresher training for instructors as well as for staff.

Content Evaluation

The purpose of *content evaluation* is to determine whether learners have acquired the knowledge or skills taught during the learning experience. Abruzzese (1992) described content evaluation as taking place immediately after the learning experience to answer the guiding question, "To what degree did the learners learn what was imparted?" or "To what degree did learners achieve specified objectives?" Asking a patient to give a return demonstration and asking participants to complete a cognitive test at the completion of a 1-day seminar are common examples of content evaluation.

Content evaluation is depicted in the RSA model as the level in between process and outcome evaluation levels. In other words, content evaluation can be considered as focusing on how the teaching–learning process affected immediate, short-term outcomes. To answer the question, "Were specified objectives met as a result of teaching?" requires that the evaluation be designed differently from an evaluation to answer the question, "Did learners achieve specified objectives?" Evaluation designs will be discussed in some detail later in this chapter. An important point to be made here, however, is that evaluation questions must be carefully considered and clearly stated because they dictate the basic framework for design and conduct.

The scope of content evaluation is limited to a specific learning experience and to specifically stated objectives for that experience. Content evaluation occurs at a circumscribed point in time, immediately after completion of teaching, but encompasses all teaching–learning activities included in that specific learning experience. Data are obtained from all learners targeted in a specific class or group. For example, if both parents and the juvenile diabetic are taught insulin administration, all three are asked to complete a return demonstration. Similarly, all nurses

attending a workshop are asked to complete the cognitive posttest at the end of the workshop.

Resources used to teach content can also be used to carry out evaluation of how well that content was learned. For example, equipment included in teaching a patient how to change a dressing can be used by the patient to perform a return demonstration. In the same manner, a pretest used at the beginning of a continuing education seminar can be readministered as a posttest at seminar completion to measure change.

From the perspective of evidence-based practice, content evaluation, like process evaluation, is focused on collecting internal evidence to determine whether objectives for a specific group of learners were met. Internal evidence must include both baseline data and immediate outcome data so that any change in learning can be demonstrated.

Lott (2006) describes an example of content evaluation in her description of one hospital's creation of a new nursing services orientation program. Nurses in the staff development department developed an evaluation tool to measure satisfaction of new employees with their nursing orientation experience. Because lack of knowledge about policies in a hospital where nurses had not worked before would have been an unmeaningful baseline, data collected from employees prior to implementation of the new program served as baseline data. These baseline data were compared with data using the same tool given to employees completing the new program. Knowledge of policies and procedures was improved for those employees who participated in the new program. Skill acquisition was evaluated by pre- and postdemonstrations, however, it was evaluated in a manner consistent with traditional content evaluation.

Outcome (Summative) Evaluation

The purpose of *outcome or summative evaluation* is to determine the effects or outcomes of teaching efforts. Its intent is to sum what happened as a result of education. Guiding questions in outcome evaluation include the following:

- Was teaching appropriate?
- Did the individual(s) learn?
- Were behavioral objectives met?
- Did the patient who learned a skill before discharge use that skill correctly once home?

Just as process evaluation occurs concurrently with the teaching–learning experience, outcome evaluation occurs after teaching has been completed or after a program has been carried out. Outcome evaluation measures the changes that result from teaching and learning.

Abruzzese (1992) differentiated outcome evaluation from content evaluation by focusing outcome evaluation on measuring more long-term change that "persists after the learning experience" (p. 243). Changes can include institution of a new process, habitual use of a new technique or behavior, or integration of a new value or attitude. Which changes you will measure usually will be dictated by the objectives established as a result of your initial needs assessment.

The scope of outcome evaluation depends in part on the changes being measured, which, in turn, depend on the objectives established for the educational activity. As mentioned earlier, outcome evaluation focuses on a longer time period than does content evaluation. Whereas evaluating accuracy of a patient's return demonstration of a skill prior to discharge may be appropriate for content evaluation, outcome evaluation should include measuring a patient's competency with a skill in the home setting after discharge. Similarly, nurses' responses on a workshop posttest may be sufficient for content evaluation, but if the workshop objective states that nurses will be able to incorporate their knowledge into practice on the unit, outcome evaluation should include measuring nurses' knowledge or behavior some time after they have returned to the unit. Abruzzese (1992) suggested that outcome data be collected 6 months after baseline data to determine whether a change has really taken place.

Resources required for outcome evaluation are more costly and sophisticated than those for process or content evaluation. Compared to the resources required for the first two types of evaluation in the RSA model, outcome evaluation requires greater expertise to develop measurement and data collection strategies, more time to conduct the evaluation, knowledge of baseline data establishment, and ability to collect reliable and valid comparative data after the learning experience. Postage to mail surveys and time and personnel to carry out observation of nurses on the clinical unit or to complete patient/family telephone interviews are specific examples of resources that may be necessary to conduct an outcome evaluation.

From an evidence-based practice perspective, outcome evaluation might arguably be considered as where the rubber meets the road. Once a need for change has been identified, the search for evidence upon which to base that change commonly begins with a structured clinical question that will guide an efficient search of the literature. This question is also known as a PICO question. The letters *P*, *I*, *C*, and *O* stand for patient or population, intervention, comparison, and outcome, respectively.

For example, nurses caring for an outpatient population of adults with heart failure might discover that many patients are not following their prescribed treatment regimen. Upon questioning these patients, the nurses learn that a majority of the patients do not recognize symptoms resulting from failure to take their medications on a consistent basis. To efficiently search the literature for ways in which they might better educate their patients, the nurses would pose the following PICO question: Does nurse-directed patient education on symptoms and related treatment for heart failure provided to adult outpatients with heart failure result in improved compliance with treatment regimens? In this example, the *P* is adult outpatients with heart failure, the *I* is the nurse-directed patient education on symptoms and related treatment for heart failure, the *C* is inferred as education currently being provided—or lack of education, if that is the case—and the *O* is improved compliance with treatment regimens.

A literature search identified an article by Gonzalez and colleagues (2005) that described an education intervention highly relevant to the PICO question posed by the nurses. As presented in the article, nurse-guided education demonstrated significant improvements in understanding of disease, symptoms, purpose of medications, and self-monitoring among 298 outpatients with heart failure. Data were collected at baseline and at one-year follow-up appointments. Although self-management and knowledge did improve, treatment compliance remained approximately the same. Results from the evaluation published in this article would inform the nurses' practice and would provide useful suggestions for them to consider. By itself, this article would not be sufficient to dictate change in practice.

Ideally, several well-conducted studies providing external evidence directly relevant to a PICO question should be reviewed prior to making a practice change, especially if that change is resource intensive or, if unsuccessful, might increase patient risk. The Gonzalez and colleagues (2005) study is an excellent example of practice-based internal evidence resulting from a 1-year evaluation of specified patient outcomes. Such reports should be considered judiciously, but should not be overlooked by nurses searching for evidence to suggest how they might address clinical issues in their own setting.

Another example of an outcome evaluation was a study conducted by Aldana and colleagues (2006) to examine effectiveness of a worksite diabetes prevention program. Using a sample of at-risk employees who did not have diabetes and who were interested in participating, a team of occupational health nurses and researchers conducted a 1-year program using a protocol and curriculum from the United States National Institutes of Health (NIH). Outcomes, including weight, body mass index, oral glucose tolerance testing, fasting insulin, and aerobic fitness were measured at baseline, after 6 months, after 12 months, and after 2 years. Positive outcomes demonstrated the effectiveness of the NIH protocol and curriculum. Aldana and colleagues (2006) provide not only an example of outcome evaluation, but also an example of evaluation of a CPG—in this case the NIH Diabetes Prevention Program—that was modified for use in a specific setting.

Impact Evaluation

The purpose of *impact evaluation* is to determine the relative effects of education on the institution or the community. Put another way, the purpose of impact evaluation is to obtain information that will help decide whether continuing an educational activity is worth its cost. Examples of questions appropriate for impact evaluation include "What is the effect of an orientation program on subsequent nursing staff turnover?" and "What is the effect of a cardiac discharge teaching program on long-term frequency of rehospitalization among patients who have completed the program?"

The scope of impact evaluation is broader, more complex, and usually more long term than that of process, content, or outcome evaluation. For example, whereas outcome evaluation would focus on whether specific teaching resulted in achievement of specified outcomes, impact evaluation would go beyond that to measure the effect or worth of those outcomes. In other words, outcome evaluation would focus on a course objective, whereas impact evaluation would focus on a course goal. Consider, for instance, a class on the use of body mechanics. The objective is that staff members will demonstrate proper use of body mechanics in providing patient care. The goal is to decrease back injuries among the hospital's direct-care providers. This distinction between outcome and impact evaluation may seem subtle, but it is important to the appropriate design and conduct of an impact evaluation.

Resource requirements for conducting an impact evaluation are extensive and may be beyond the scope of an individual nurse educator. Literature on evaluation (Abruzzese, 1992; Hamilton, 1993; Waddell, 1992) describes impact evaluation as being most like evaluation research. (The distinction between evaluation and evaluation research will be addressed later in this chapter.) One example of impact evaluation conducted as research is described by Eklund, Sonn, and Dahlin-Ivanoff (2004). Consistent with the scope and focus of an impact evaluation, the investigators examined long-term outcomes of a health education program for elderly persons with visual impairment on perceived security in performance of daily activities. The study was conducted, not at the site of the education, but where the elderly lived in the community. Using a randomized controlled study design, both observational and survey data were collected over a 28-month period.

Good science is rarely inexpensive and never quick; good impact evaluation shares the same characteristics. The resources needed to design and conduct an impact evaluation generally include reliable and valid instruments, trained data collectors, personnel with research and statistical expertise, equipment and materials necessary for data collection and analysis, and access to populations who may be culturally or geographically diverse. Because impact evaluation is so expensive and time intensive, this type of evaluation should be targeted toward courses and programs where learning is critical to patient well-being or to safe, high-quality, cost-effective healthcare delivery (Puetz, 1992).

Conducting an impact evaluation may seem a monumental task, but it should not let that stop someone from undertaking the effort. Rather, one should plan ahead, proceed carefully, and obtain the support and assistance of colleagues. Keeping in mind the purpose for conducting an impact evaluation should be helpful in maintaining the level of commitment needed throughout the process. The current managed care environment requires justification for every health dollar spent. The value of patient and staff education may be intuitively evident, but the positive impact of education must be demonstrated if it is to be funded.

A recent literature search conducted to determine the state of the evidence on impact evaluation in patient education found that the term *impact* is used generically to describe both evaluations of patient outcomes resulting from education and evaluations of long-term impact from education. What is important to remember when reviewing this literature is not what term the authors use, but what they have as their purpose for evaluation. As noted earlier, the purpose of an outcome evaluation is to determine whether an educational intervention resulted in intended behavior change, whereas the purpose of an impact evaluation is to determine whether long term education goals are met. As evidence-based practice continues to grow, impact evaluations will become especially useful in examining the long-term effectiveness of different educational interventions used to disseminate CPGs to healthcare providers.

Program Evaluation

The purpose of *program evaluation* can be generically described as "designed and conducted to assist an audience to judge and improve the worth of some object" (Johnson & Olesinski, 1995, p. 53). The object in this case is an educational program. Using the framework of the RSA model (Abruzzese, 1992), the purpose of total program evaluation is to determine the extent to which all activities for an entire department or program over a specified period of time meet or exceed goals originally established.

Guiding questions appropriate for a total program evaluation from this perspective might be "To what extent did programs undertaken by members of the nursing staff development department during the year accomplish annual goals established by the department?" or "How well did patient education activities imple- mented throughout the year meet annual goals established for the institution's patient education program?"

The scope of program evaluation is broad, generally focusing on overall goals rather than on specific objectives. While the term program could be defined as an individual educational offering (Albanese & Gjerde, 1987), the resource requirements for conducting a program evaluation generally are too extensive to justify the effort on less than a broad scale. Abruzzese (1992) described the scope of program evaluation as encompassing all aspects of educational activity (e.g., process, content, outcome, impact) with input from all the participants (e.g., learners, teachers, institutional representatives, community representatives). The time period over which data are collected may extend from several months to 1 or more years, depending on the time frame established for meeting the goals to be evaluated.

Resources required for program evaluation may include the sum of resources necessary to conduct process, content, outcome, and impact evaluations. A program evaluation may require significant expenditures for personnel if the evaluation is conducted by an individual or team external to the organization. Additional resources required may include time, materials, equipment, and personnel necessary for data entry, analysis, and report generation.

Suhayda and Miller (2006) provide an excellent example of the scope of program evaluation to establish organized, data-driven, ongoing quality improvement across multiple programs offered by one college of nursing. Using Stufflebeam's content, inputs, process, and product (CIPP) model, the entire infrastructure of the college was included in evaluation of activities ranging from the admissions process to budget decisions to student certification and licensure pass rates. Data tracking was accomplished using a specifically developed data action form completed by members of the evaluation committee with input from program directors, faculty, and students as well as a broad spectrum of stakeholders both internal and external to the college (e.g., accreditation board reviewers).

As stated earlier, the RSA model remains useful as a general framework for categorizing basic types of evaluation: process, content, outcome, impact, and program. As depicted in the model, differences between these types are, in large part, a matter of degree. For example, process evaluation occurs most frequently; program evaluation occurs least frequently. Content evaluation focuses on immediate effects of teaching; impact evaluation concentrates on more long-term effects of teaching. Conduct of process evaluation requires fewer resources compared with impact and program evaluation, which re-

quire extensive resources for implementation. The RSA model further illustrates one way that process, content, outcome, and impact evaluations can be considered together as components of total program evaluation.

Clinical examples of how different types of evaluation relate to one another can be found in Haggard's (1989) description of three dimensions in evaluating teaching effectiveness for the patient and in Rankin and Stallings's (2005) four levels of evaluation of patient learning. The three dimensions described by Haggard and the four levels identified by Rankin and Stallings are consistent with the basic types of evaluation included in Abruzzese's RSA model, as shown in **Table 14–1**. As can be seen from Table 14–1, models developed from an education theory base, such as the RSA model, have much in common with models developed from a patient care theory base, exemplified by the other two models.

Table 14–1 COMPARISON OF LEVELS/TYPES OF EVALUATION ACROSS STAFF/PATIENT EDUCATION EVALUATION MODELS

Abruzzese (1992)	Haggard (1989)	Rankin and Stallings (2005)
Process	Patient assimilation of information during teaching	Patient-education intervention
Content	Patient information retention after teaching	Patient/family performance following learning
Outcome	Patient use of information in day-to-day life	Patient/family performance at home
Impact	N/A	Overall self-care and health maintenance
Program	N/A	N/A

At least one important point about the difference between the RSA and other models needs to be mentioned, however. That difference is depicted in the learner evaluation model shown in **Figure** 14–2. This learner-focused model emphasizes the continuum of learner status determined from needs assessment to learner performance over time once an adequate level of participation has been regained or achieved. Both models have value in focusing and planning any type of evaluation but are especially important for impact and program evaluations.

Designing the Evaluation

The design of an evaluation is created within the framework, or boundaries, already established by focusing the evaluation. In other words, the design must be consistent with the purpose, questions, and scope and must be realistic given available resources. Evaluation design includes at least three interrelated components: structure, methods, and instruments.

Design Structure

An important question to be answered in designing an evaluation is "How rigorous should the evaluation be?" The obvious answer is that all evaluations should have some level of rigor. In other words, all evaluations should be systematic and carefully and thoroughly planned or structured before they are conducted. How rigor is translated into design structure depends on the questions to be answered by the evaluation, the complexity of the scope of the evaluation, and the expected use of evaluation results. The more the questions address cause and effect, the more complex the scope. Likewise, the more critical and broad-reaching the expected use of results, the more the evaluation design should be structured from a research perspective.

EVALUATION VERSUS RESEARCH

Evaluation and research are neither synonymous nor mutually exclusive activities. The extent to which they are either very different

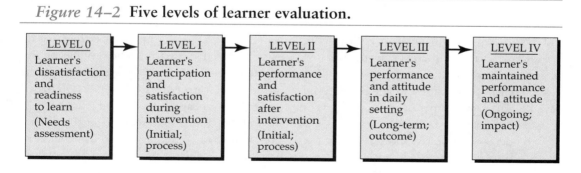

Figure 14–2 **Five levels of learner evaluation.**

LEVEL 0	LEVEL I	LEVEL II	LEVEL III	LEVEL IV
Learner's dissatisfaction and readiness to learn (Needs assessment)	Learner's participation and satisfaction during intervention (Initial; process)	Learner's performance and satisfaction after intervention (Initial; process)	Learner's performance and attitude in daily setting (Long-term; outcome)	Learner's maintained performance and attitude (Ongoing; impact)

Source: Based on Rankin, S. H., & Stallings, K. D. (2005). *Patient education in health and illness* (5th ed.). Philadelphia: Lippincott Williams & Wilkins.

or indistinguishable from each other depends on the type of evaluation and type of research considered. Ruzicki (1987) made the following distinction between the two:

> While both research and evaluation involve objective, systematic collection of data, evaluation is conducted to make decisions in a given setting. Research is designed so that it can be generalized to other settings and replicated in other settings. Furthermore, research seeks new knowledge, examines cause and effect relationships, tests hypotheses, whereas evaluation determines mission achievement, examines means-end processes, and assesses attainment of objectives. (p. 234)

For example, this argument holds true when comparing basic research to process evaluation. Basic research is defined as tightly controlled experimental studies of cause and effect conducted for the purpose of generating new knowledge. This new knowledge may or may not eventually influence practice. Process evaluation occurs concurrently with an educational intervention and is conducted in an uncontrolled or real-world setting for the purpose of making change as soon as the need for change is identified. As described earlier in this chapter, this distinction between research and evaluation is analogous to the distinction between external and internal evidence (Melnyk & Fineout-Overholt, 2005).

Differences between research and evaluation have become less distinct over the past several years with the advent of applied research, with the acceptance of qualitative measures and methods as legitimate research, and with the increasing importance given to results of outcome, impact, and program evaluations. This importance is likely to increase as more credibility, and therefore attention, is given to practice-based

evidence—or internal evidence—as a legitimate support for evidence-based decision making.

The purpose for conducting applied research is to positively affect change in practice. There is little difference between this purpose and the purpose for conducting evaluation. *Evaluation research*, which is one type of applied research, can be defined as "a process of applying scientific procedures to accumulate reliable and valid data on the manner and extent to which specified activities produce outcomes or effects" (Hamilton, 1993, p. 148).

Using this definition, Hamilton identifies program accreditation, program cost analysis, and outcome of treatment as appropriate for use of evaluation research designs and methods. Hamilton further describes impact evaluation as appropriate for use of quasi-experimental and experimental research design structures. A number of other authors support some use of research designs and data collection methods for outcome, impact, and program evaluations (Albanese & Gjerde, 1987; Berk & Rossi, 1990; Eklund et al., 2004; Holzemer, 1992; Puetz, 1992; Templeton & Coates, 2004; Waddell, 1992).

Of course, not all outcome, impact, and program evaluations should be conducted as research studies. Some important differences do exist between evaluation and evaluation research. One of the most significant relates to the influence of a primary audience. As discussed earlier in this chapter, the primary audience, or the individual or group requesting the evaluation, is a major component in focusing an evaluation. The evaluator must design and conduct the evaluation consistent with the purpose and related questions identified by the primary audience. Evaluation research, by contrast, does not have an identified primary audience. The researcher has autonomy to develop a protocol to answer a question posed by the researcher.

A second difference between evaluation and evaluation research is one of timing. The necessary timeline for usability of evaluation results may not be sufficient to prospectively develop a research proposal and obtain institutional review board approval prior to beginning data collection.

Given the discussion of evaluation versus evaluation research, how are decisions about level of rigor of an evaluation actually translated into an evaluation structure? The structure of an evaluation design depicts the number of groups to be included in the evaluation, the number of evaluations or periods of evaluation, and the time sequence between an educational intervention and evaluation of that intervention. A group can comprise one individual, as in the case of one-to-one nurse–patient teaching, or several individuals, as in the case of a nursing in-service program or workshop.

A process evaluation might be conducted during a single-patient education activity where the educator observes patient behavior during instruction/demonstration and engages the patient in questions and answers upon completion of each new instruction. Because the purpose of process evaluation is to facilitate better learning while that learning is going on, education and evaluation occur concurrently in this case.

Evaluation also may be conducted immediately after an educational intervention. This structure is probably the most commonly employed in conducting educational evaluations, although it is not necessarily the most appropriate. If the purpose of conducting the evaluation is to determine whether after a class learners know specific content that they did not know before attending that class, then a structure that

begins with collection of baseline data is more appropriate. Collection of baseline data via a pretest, which can be compared with data collected via a posttest at one or more points in time after learners have completed the educational activity, provides an opportunity to measure whether change has occurred. The ability to measure change in a particular skill or level of knowledge, for example, also requires that the same instruments be used for pre- and posttest data collection at both points in time. Data collection will be discussed in more detail later in this chapter.

If the purpose of conducting an evaluation is to determine whether learners know content or can perform a skill as a result of an educational intervention, the most appropriate structure will include at least two groups: one receiving education and one not receiving education. Both groups are evaluated at the same time, even though only one group receives education. The group receiving the new education program is called the treatment or experimental group, and the group receiving standard care or the traditional education program is called the comparison or control group. The two groups may or may not be equivalent. Equivalent groups are those with no known differences between them prior to some intervention, whereas nonequivalent groups may be different from one another in several ways. For example, patients on nursing unit A may receive an educational pamphlet to read prior to attending a class, while patients on nursing unit B attend the class without first reading the pamphlet. Because patients on the two units probably are different in many ways—age and diagnosis, for example—besides which educational intervention they received, they would be considered nonequivalent groups.

Use of the term *nonequivalent* is common to discussions of traditional research designs. Quasi-experimental designs, such as nonequivalent control group designs, should be among those considered in planning an outcome, impact, or program evaluation. Especially if the purpose of an evaluation is to demonstrate that an education program caused fewer patient returns to the clinic or fewer nurses to leave the institution, for example, the evaluation structure must have the rigor of evaluation research.

Another type of quasi-experimental design, called a time-series design, might include only one group of learners from which evaluative data are collected at several points in time both before and after receiving an educational intervention. If data collected before the education consistently demonstrate lack of learner ability to comply with a treatment regimen, whereas data collected after the education consistently demonstrate a significant improvement in patient compliance with that regimen, the evaluator could argue that the education was the reason for the improvement in this case.

In more recent years, pluralistic designs have appeared in the literature as approaches especially suited for evaluation of projects that have a community base, that include participants from diverse settings or perspectives, or that require both program processes and outcomes to be included in the evaluation (Billings, 2000; Gerrish, 2001; Hart, 1999; Suhayda & Miller, 2006). As the term implies, a pluralistic design uses a variety of sources and methods for obtaining evaluative data, often including both qualitative and quantitative evidence. Because these designs are comprehensive, resource intensive, and long term in nature, they are most appropriate for program evaluation.

This chapter does not provide an exhaustive description of evaluation designs. Rather, it is intended to increase awareness of the value and usefulness of these designs, especially when the results of an evaluation will be used to make major financial or programmatic decisions. The literature on evaluation of nursing staff education and patient education has become an increasingly rich source of examples of how to conduct rigorous evaluation.

A literature search that includes many or all of the following journals is a must for planning evaluation of healthcare education in a cost-conscious and outcome-focused healthcare environment: *Canadian Journal of Nursing Research, Clinical Effectiveness in Nursing, Evaluation and the Health Professions, Evidence-Based Nursing, Journal of Continuing Education in Nursing, Adult Education Quarterly, Health Education Quarterly, Nurse Educator, Journal of Nursing Staff Development, Health Education Research, Nursing Research, Patient Education and Counseling, Research in Nursing and Health, Journal of Advanced Nursing,* and *Worldviews on Evidence-Based Nursing.*

Evaluation Methods

Evaluation focus provides the basis for determining the evaluation design structure. The design structure, in turn, provides the basis for determining evaluation methods. Evaluation methods include those actions that are undertaken to carry out the evaluation according to the design structure. All evaluation methods deal in some way with data and data collection. Answers to the following questions will assist in selection of the most appropriate, feasible methods for conducting a particular evaluation in a particular setting and for a specified purpose:

- What types of data will be collected?
- From whom or what will data be collected?
- How, when, and where will data be collected?
- By whom will data be collected?

TYPES OF DATA TO COLLECT

Evaluation of healthcare education includes collection of data about people, about the educational program or activity, and about the environment in which the educational activity takes place. Process, outcome, impact, and program evaluations require data about all three: the people, the program, and the environment. Content evaluations may be limited to data about the people and the program, although this limitation is not necessary.

Types of data that are collected about people can be classified as physical, cognitive, affective, or psychomotor. Data that are collected about educational activities or programs generally include such program characteristics as cost, length, number of educators required, amount and type of materials required, teaching–learning methods used, and so on. Data that are collected about the environment in which a program or activity is conducted generally include such environmental characteristics as temperature, lighting, location, layout, space, and noise level.

Given the possibility that an unlimited and overwhelming amount of data could be collected, how do you decide what data should be collected? The most straightforward answer to this question is that data that will answer evaluation questions posed in focusing the evaluation should be collected. The likelihood that one will collect the right amount of the right type of data to answer evaluation questions can be

significantly improved by (1) remembering that any data collected must be used, and (2) using operational definitions.

An operational definition of a word or phrase is a definition that is written in measurement terms. Functional health status, for example, can be theoretically defined as an individual's ability to independently carry out activities of daily living without self-perceived undue difficulty or discomfort. Functional health status can be operationally defined as an individual's composite score on the SF-36 survey instrument (Stewart, Hays, & Ware, 1988; Ware, Davies-Avery, & Donald, 1978). The SF-36, which has undergone years of extensive reliability and validity testing with a wide variety of patient populations and in several languages, is generally considered the gold standard for measuring functional health status from the individual's perspective. Continuously updated information about the SF-36 as well as different versions of the actual instrument can be found on the Internet at http://www.sf-36.org.

Similarly, patient compliance can be theoretically defined as the patient's regular and consistent adherence to a prescribed treatment regimen. For use in an outcome evaluation of a particular educational activity, patient compliance might be operationally defined as the patient's demonstration of unassisted and error-free completion of all steps in the sterile dressing change as observed in the patient's home on three separate occasions at 2-week time intervals.

These examples show that an operational definition states exactly what data will be collected. In the first example, measurement of functional health status will require collection of patient survey data using a specific self-administered questionnaire. The second example provides even more information about data collection than does the first, by including where and how many times the patient's performance of the dressing change is to be observed, as well as stating that criteria for compliance include both unassisted and error-free performance on each occasion.

In addition to being categorized as describing people, programs, or the environment, data can be categorized as quantitative or qualitative. Quantitative data are numeric and generally are expressed in statistics such as mean, median, ratio, F statistic, t statistic, or chi-square. Numbers can be used to answer questions of how much, how many, how often, and so on in terms that are commonly understood by the audience for the evaluation. Mathematical analysis can demonstrate with some level of precision and reliability whether a learner's knowledge or skill has changed since completing an educational program, for example, or how much improvement in a learner's knowledge or skill is the result of an educational program.

Qualitative data include feelings, behaviors, words, and phrases and generally are expressed in themes or categories. Qualitative data can be described in quantitative terms, such as percentages or counts, but this transformation eliminates the richness and insight that the use of qualitative data can offer. Qualitative data can be used as background to better interpret quantitative data, especially if the evaluation is intended to measure such value-laden or conceptual terms as satisfaction or quality.

Any evaluation may be strengthened by collecting both quantitative and qualitative data. For example, an evaluation to determine whether a stress reduction class resulted in decreased work stress for participants could include participants' qualitative expressions of how stressed they feel plus quantitative pulse and blood pressure readings. Because collection of both quantitative and qualitative data, while intuitively appealing, is resource-intensive, one must be certain that the focus of the evaluation justifies such an undertaking.

From Whom or What to Collect Data

Data can be collected directly from the individuals whose behavior or knowledge is being evaluated, from surrogates or representatives of these individuals, or from documentation or databases already created. Whenever possible, researchers should plan to collect at least some data directly from individuals being evaluated. In the case of process evaluation, data should be collected from all learners and all educators participating in the educational activity. Content and outcome evaluations should include data from all learners.

Because impact and total program evaluations have a broader scope than do the first three types of evaluation, collecting data from all individuals who participated in an educational program over an extended period of time may be impossible. This is because data collectors may not be able to locate every participant or they may lack sufficient resources to gather data from such a large number of people.

When all participants cannot be counted or located, data may be collected from a subset, or sample, of participants who are considered to represent the entire group. If an evaluation is planned to collect data from a sample of participants, participants who are representative of the entire group should be included. A random selection of participants from whom data will be collected will minimize bias in the sample but cannot guarantee representativeness.

For example, an impact evaluation was conducted to determine whether a five-year program supporting home-based health education actually improved the general health status of individuals in the community served by the program. If all members of the community could be counted, a random sample of community members could be generated by first listing and numbering all members' names, then drawing numbers using a random numbers table until a 10% sample was obtained. Such a method for selecting the sample of community members would eliminate intentional selection of those individuals who were the most active program participants and who might therefore have a better health status than does the community as a whole. At the same time, the 10% random sample could unintentionally include only those individuals who did not participate in the health education program. Data collected from this sample of nonparticipants would be equally as misleading as data collected from the first sample. A more representative sample for this evaluation should include both participants and nonparticipants, ideally in the same proportions in the sample as in the community.

Preexisting databases should never be used as the only source of evaluative data unless they were created for the purpose of that evaluation. Even though these data were collected for a different purpose, they may be helpful for providing additional information to the primary audience for the evaluation. Data already in existence generally are less expensive to obtain than are original data. The decision whether to use preexisting data depends on whether they were collected from people of interest in the current evaluation and whether they are consistent with operational definitions used in the current evaluation.

How, When, and Where to Collect Data

Methods for how data can be collected include the following:

- Observation
- Interview
- Questionnaire or written examination
- Record review
- Secondary analysis of existing databases

Which method is selected depends, first, on the type of data being collected and, second, on available resources. Whenever possible, data should be collected using more than one method. Using multiple methods will provide the evaluator, and consequently the primary audience, with more complete information about the program or performance being evaluated than could be accomplished using a single method.

Observations can be conducted by the evaluator in person or can be videotaped for viewing at some later time. In the combined role of educator–evaluator, the nurse educator who is conducting a process evaluation can directly observe a learner's physical, verbal, psychomotor, and affective behaviors so that they can be responded to in a timely manner. Use of videotape or a nonparticipant observer also can be beneficial for picking up the educator's own behaviors of which the educator is unaware, but which might be influencing the learner.

The timing of data collection, or when data collection takes place, has already been addressed both in discussion of different types of evaluation and in descriptions of evaluation design structures. Process evaluation, for example, generally occurs during and immediately after an educational activity. Content evaluation takes place immediately after completion of education. Outcome evaluation occurs some time after completion of education when learners have returned to the setting where they are expected to use new knowledge or perform a new skill. Impact evaluation generally is conducted from weeks to years after the educational program because the purpose of impact evaluation is to determine what change has occurred within the community or institution as a whole as a result of an educational intervention.

Timing of data collection for program evaluation is less obvious than for other types of evaluation, in part because a number of different descriptions of what constitutes a program evaluation can be found both in the literature and in practice. As discussed earlier, Abruzzese (1992) described data collection for program evaluation as occurring over a prolonged period because program evaluation is itself a culmination of process, content, outcome, and impact evaluations already conducted.

Where an evaluation is conducted can have a major effect on evaluation results. Those conducting an evaluation must be careful not to make the decision about where to collect data on the basis of convenience for the data collector. An appropriate setting for conducting a content evaluation may be in the classroom or skills laboratory where learners have just completed class instruction or training. An outcome evaluation to determine whether training has improved the nurse's ability to perform a skill with patients on the nursing unit, however, requires that data collection—in this case, observation of the nurse's performance—be conducted on the nursing unit.

Similarly, an outcome evaluation to determine whether discharge teaching in the hospital enabled the patient to provide self-care at home requires that data collection, or observation of the patient's performance, be conducted

in the home. What if available resources are insufficient to allow for home visits by the evaluator? To answer this question, keep in mind that the focus of the evaluation is on performance by the patient, not performance by the evaluator. Training a family member, a visiting nurse, or even the patient to observe and record patient performance at home is preferable to bringing the patient to a place of convenience for the evaluator.

WHO COLLECTS DATA

Evaluative data are most commonly collected by the educator who is conducting the class or activity being evaluated because that educator is already present and interacting with learners. Combining the role of evaluator with that of educator is one appropriate method for conducting a process evaluation because evaluative data are integral to the teaching–learning process. Inviting another educator or a patient representative to observe a class can provide additional data from the perspective of someone who does not have to divide his or her attention between teaching and evaluating. This second, and perhaps less biased, input can strengthen legitimacy and usefulness of evaluation results.

Data can also be collected by the learners themselves, by other colleagues within the department or institution, or by someone from outside the institution. Puetz's (1992) description of data collection using a participant evaluation team is an example of data collection that includes learners. The evaluation team is composed of a small number of randomly selected individuals who are scheduled to attend an educational program. Team members are introduced to other program participants at the beginning of the class, join other participants during the program, and collect data through self-report as well as through observation and interaction with others during breaks.

The individuals chosen to carry out data collection become an extension of the evaluation instrument. If the data that are collected are to be reliable, unbiased, and accurate, the data collectors must be unbiased and sufficiently expert at the task. Use of unbiased expert data collectors is especially important for collecting observation and interview data, because these data in part depend on the subjective interpretation by the data collector.

Also, data collectors can influence in other ways the information that is obtained. For example, if staff nurses are asked to complete a job satisfaction survey and their head nurse is asked to collect the surveys for return to the evaluator, what problems might occur? Might some staff nurses be hesitant to provide negative scores on certain items, even though they hold a negative opinion? Likewise, physiological data can be altered, however unintentionally, by the data collector. For example, an outcome evaluation might be conducted to determine whether a series of biofeedback classes given to young executives can reduce stress as measured by pulse and blood pressure. How might some executives' pulse and blood pressure results be affected by a data collector who is extremely physically attractive or overtly acting rushed or frustrated?

Use of trained data collectors from an external agency is, in most cases, not a financially viable option. The potential for a data collector to bias data can be minimized using a number of less expensive alternatives, however. First, the number of data collectors should be limited as much as possible, as this step will automatically decrease person-based variation. Also, individuals assisting with data collection should wear similar conservative clothing and speak in a moderate tone. Because moderate tone, for example, may not be interpreted the same way by everyone, at least one practice session or dry run should be held with all data collectors prior to actually conducting the evaluation. In addition, data collection should be conducted by someone who has no vested interest in results and who will be perceived as unbiased and nonthreatening by those providing the data. Furthermore, providing interview scripts to be read verbatim by the interviewer can ensure that all patients or staff being interviewed will be asked the same questions.

With the advent of continuous quality improvement based on evidence as an expectation of daily activity in healthcare organizations, nurses and other professionals are obligated to become more knowledgeable about principles of measurement and ways to implement measurement techniques in their work setting (Joint Commission on Accreditation of Healthcare Organizations, 2006). One benefit that this change in practice has for the nurse educator is that more people within the organization have some expertise in data collection and are motivated to help with data collection activities. Another potential benefit is that data collection activities already are likely to be a part of practice. Not only might the nurse educator have readily available individuals to assist with data collection, but the educator also might have readily available and usable instruments and data.

Use of a portfolio as a method for evaluation of an individual's learning over time has been documented in the literature for more than 30 years, primarily from an academic perspective (Appling, Naumann, & Berk, 2001; Ball, Daly, & Carnwell, 2000; Cayne, 1995; Roberts, Priest, & Bromage, 2001). Although formal education of nursing students is not the focus of this text, other uses of portfolios are relevant to the role of the practice-based nurse as educator. Individual completion of a professional portfolio is a current requirement for recertification in some nursing specialties in the United States and for periodic registration in the United Kingdom (Ball et al., 2000; Serembus, 2000). In light of the increasing demands on today's professionals to maintain currency in their competence to practice, Serembus suggests that a practice portfolio may soon be a requirement for relicensure in the United States.

Given the importance of a nurse's portfolio to his or her career status, the nurse educator may find several colleagues asking for assistance in creating and maintaining a portfolio that will provide a strong base of evaluative evidence demonstrating that nurse's continuing professional development and consequent impact on practice. Perhaps the best suggestion the nurse educator might offer—and heed—is to clarify the focus of the portfolio as determined by the requiring organization (in this case, the primary audience) as stated in that organization's criteria for portfolio completion. Is the focus more on process evaluation, outcome evaluation, or both? Specifically, is the nurse expected to demonstrate reflective practice? If so, what does the organization accept as evidence of reflective practice?

One reason why focus clarification is so challenging is because there is no consistent description of how portfolios are to be used or what they are to contain. In its simplest form, a practice portfolio comprises a collection of information and materials about one's practice that have been gathered over time. The issue of whether this collection is intended to demonstrate previous learning or whether the process of collecting is

itself a learning experience continues to foster debate (Cayne, 1995; Roberts et al., 2001).

Central to this issue is the notion of reflective practice. First coined by Schön (1987), the term reflective practice still does not have a commonly agreed-upon definition (Cotton, 2001; Hannigan, 2001; Teekman, 2000). Schön describes two key components of reflective practice as reflection-in-action and reflection-on-action. Reflection-in-action occurs when the nurse introspectively considers a practice activity while performing it so change for improvement can be made at that moment. Reflection-on-action occurs when the nurse introspectively analyzes a practice activity after its completion so as to gain insights for the future (Cotton, 2001). From an evaluation perspective, these components are similar to formative and summative evaluation, indicating that reflective practice has more than one focus.

Given the complexity of attempting to address multiple foci with the use of a single evaluation method—the practice portfolio—it is not surprising that use of portfolios has inspired such controversy. To the extent that a portfolio is required to include physical documentation as evidence of reflective practice (an introspective activity), the argument by some that portfolios are not adequately reliable or valid for use in evaluation of learning is not at all surprising (Ball et al., 2000; Cayne, 1995).

Evaluation Instruments

In the selection, modification, or construction of evaluation instruments, some key points must be considered. Whenever possible, an evaluation should be conducted using existing instruments, because instrument development requires considerable expertise, time, and expenditure of resources. Construction of an original evaluation instrument, whether it is in the form of a questionnaire or a type of equipment, also requires rigorous testing for reliability and validity. Timely provision of evaluative information for making decisions rarely allows the luxury of the several months to several years needed to develop a reliable, valid instrument.

The initial step in instrument selection is to conduct a literature search for evaluations similar to the evaluation being planned. A helpful place to begin is with the same journals listed earlier in this chapter. Instruments that have been used in more than one study should be given preference over an instrument developed for a single use, because instruments used multiple times generally have been more thoroughly tested for reliability and validity. Once a number of potential instruments have been identified, each instrument must be carefully critiqued to determine whether it is, in fact, appropriate for the evaluation planned.

First, the instrument must measure the performance being evaluated exactly as that performance has been operationally defined for the evaluation. For example, if satisfaction with a continuing education program is operationally defined to include a score of 80% or higher on five specific program components (such as faculty responsiveness to questions, relevance of content, and so on), then the instrument selected to measure participant satisfaction with the program must include exactly those five components and must be able to be scored in percentages.

Second, an appropriate instrument should have documented evidence of its reliability and validity with individuals who are as closely matched as possible with the people from whom data will be collected. When evaluating the ability of older adult patients to complete activities of daily living, for example, one would not want to use an instrument developed for evaluating the ability of young orthopedic patients to complete routine activities. Similarities in reading level and visual acuity also should exist if the instrument being evaluated is a questionnaire or scale that participants will complete themselves.

Existing instruments being considered for selection also must be affordable, must be feasible for use in the location planned for conducting data collection, and should require minimal training on the part of data collectors.

The evaluation instrument most likely to require modification from an existing tool or development of an entirely new instrument is a cognitive test. The primary reason for constructing such a test is that it must be consistent with content actually covered during the educational program or activity. The intent of a cognitive test is to be comprehensive and relevant and to fairly test the learner's knowledge of content covered. Using a test blueprint is one of the most helpful methods for ensuring comprehensiveness and relevance of test questions. A blueprint enables the evaluator to be certain that each area of course content is included in the test and that content areas emphasized during instruction are similarly emphasized during testing.

Barriers to Evaluation

If evaluation is so crucial to healthcare education, why is evaluation often an afterthought or even overlooked entirely? The reasons given for not conducting evaluations are many and varied but rarely, if ever, insurmountable. To overcome barriers to evaluation, they first must be identified and understood; then the evaluation must be designed and conducted in a way that will minimize or eliminate as many identified barriers as possible.

Barriers to conducting an evaluation can be classified into three broad categories:

1. Lack of clarity
2. Lack of ability
3. Fear of punishment or loss of self-esteem

LACK OF CLARITY

Lack of clarity most often results from an unclear, unstated, or ill-defined evaluation focus. Undertaking any action is difficult if the performer does not know the purpose for taking that action. Undertaking an evaluation certainly is no different. Often evaluations are attempted to determine the quality of an educational program or activity, yet quality is not defined beyond some vague sense of goodness. What is goodness and from whose perspective will it be determined? Who or what has to demonstrate evidence of goodness? What will happen if goodness is or is not evident? Inability to answer these or similar questions creates a significant barrier to conducting an evaluation. Not knowing the purpose of an evaluation or what will be done with evaluation results, for example, can become a barrier for even the most seasoned evaluator.

Barriers in this category have the greatest potential for successful resolution because the best solution for lack of clarity is to provide clarity. Recall that evaluation focus includes five components: (1) audience, (2) purpose, (3) questions, (4) scope, and (5) resources. To overcome a potential lack of clarity, all five components must be identified and made available to those conducting the evaluation.

A clearly stated purpose must explain why the evaluation is being conducted. Part of the answer to this question consists of a statement detailing what decisions will be made on the basis of evaluation results. Clear identification of who constitutes the primary audience is as important as a clear statement of purpose. It is from the perspective of the primary audience that terms such as quality should be defined and operationalized. While the results of the evaluation will provide the information on which decisions will be made, the primary audience will actually make those decisions.

LACK OF ABILITY

Lack of ability to conduct an evaluation most often results from insufficient knowledge of how to conduct the evaluation or insufficient or inaccessible resources needed to conduct the evaluation. Clarification of evaluation purpose, questions, and scope is often the responsibility of the primary audience. Clarification of resources, however, is the responsibility of both the primary audience and the individuals conducting the evaluation.

The primary audience members are accountable for providing the necessary resources—personnel, equipment, time, facilities, and so on—to conduct the evaluation they are requesting. Unless these individuals have some expertise in evaluation, they may not know what resources are necessary. The persons conducting the evaluation, therefore, must accept responsibility for knowing what resources are necessary and for providing that information to the primary audience. The person asked or expected to conduct the evaluation may be as uncertain about necessary resources as is the primary audience, however.

Lack of knowledge of what resources are necessary or lack of actual resources may form a barrier to conducting an evaluation that can be difficult, although not impossible, to overcome. Lack of knowledge can be resolved or minimized by enlisting the assistance of individuals with needed expertise through consultation or contract (if funds are available), through collaboration, or indirectly through literature review.

Lack of other resources—time, money, equipment, facilities, and so on—should be documented, justified, and presented to those requesting the evaluation. Alternative methods for conducting the evaluation, including the option of making decisions in the absence of any evaluation, also should be documented and presented.

FEAR OF PUNISHMENT OR LOSS OF SELF-ESTEEM

Evaluation may be perceived as a judgment of personal worth. Individuals being evaluated may fear that anything less than a perfect performance will result in punishment or that their mistakes will be seen as evidence that they are somehow unworthy or incompetent as human beings. These fears form one of the greatest barriers to conducting an evaluation.

Unfortunately, the fear of punishment or of being seen as unworthy may not easily be overcome, especially if the individual has had past negative experiences. Consider, for example, traditional quality assurance monitoring, where results were used to correct deficiencies through punitive measures. As another example, many times an educator has interpreted learner dissatisfaction with a teaching style as learner dislike for the educator as a person. Or many times pediatric patients' parents said, "If you don't do it right, the doctor won't let you go home . . . and we will be very disappointed in you." And every one of us probably has experienced test anxiety at some point in our own education.

The first step in overcoming this barrier is to realize that the potential for its existence may be close to 100%. Individuals whose performance or knowledge is being evaluated are not likely to say overtly that evaluation represents a threat to them. Rather, they are far more likely to demonstrate self-protective behaviors or attitudes that can range from failure to attend a class that has a posttest, to providing socially desirable answers on a questionnaire, to responding with hostility to evaluation questions. An individual may intentionally choose to fail an evaluation as a method for controlling the uncertainty of success.

The second step in overcoming the barrier of fear or threat is to remember that "the person is more important than the performance or the product" (Narrow, 1979, p. 185). If the purpose of an evaluation is to facilitate better learning, as in process evaluation, the focus is on the process. For example, in teaching a patient how to perform urinary self-catheterization using the same clean technique as she will use at home, the educator has carefully and thoroughly explained each step in the process of urinary self-catheterization, observing the patient's intent expression and frequent head nods during the explanation. When the patient tries to demonstrate the steps, however, she is unable to begin. Why? One answer may be that the use of an auditory teaching style does not match the patient's visual learning style. Another possibility might be that too many distractions are present in the immediate environment, making concentration on learning all but impossible.

A third step in overcoming the fear of punishment or threatened loss of self-esteem is to point out achievements, if they exist, or to continue to encourage effort if learning has not been achieved. The nurse educator should give praise honestly, focusing on the task at hand.

Finally, and perhaps most importantly, communication of information can help prevent or minimize fear. Lack of clarity exists as a barrier for those who are the subjects of an evaluation as much as for those who will conduct the evaluation. If learners or educators know and understand the focus of an evaluation, they may be less fearful than if such information is left to their imaginations.

Also, failure to provide and protect certain information may be unethical or even illegal. For example, any evaluative data about an individual that can be identified with that specific person should be collected only with the individual's informed consent. The ethical and legal importance of informed consent as a protection of human rights must be a central concern and responsibility of anyone involved in collecting data for evaluation purposes.

Conducting the Evaluation

To conduct an evaluation means to implement the evaluation design by using the instruments chosen or developed according to the methods selected. How smoothly an evaluation is implemented depends primarily on how carefully and thoroughly the evaluation was planned. Planning is not a complete guarantee of success, however. Three methods to minimize the effects of unexpected events that occur when carrying out an evaluation are to:

1. Conduct a pilot test first
2. Include extra time
3. Keep a sense of humor

Conducting a pilot test of the evaluation entails trying out the data collection methods, instruments, and plan for data analysis with a few individuals who are the same as or very similar to those who will be included in the full evaluation. A pilot test must be conducted if any newly developed instruments are planned for the evaluation, so as to assess reliability, validity, interpretability, and feasibility of those new instruments. Also, a pilot test should be carried out prior to implementing a full evaluation that will be expensive or time consuming to conduct or on which major decisions will be based. Process evaluation generally is not amenable to pilot testing unless a new instrument will be used for data collection. Pilot testing should be considered prior to conducting outcome, impact, or program evaluations, however.

Ream, Richardson, and Evison (2005) describe a pilot test conducted to evaluate the feasibility of a multidisciplinary education and support group program for patients with cancer treatment-related fatigue. Results provided important information about how to involve team members from different disciplines to best meet patients' needs from a patient-centered perspective. Because only six patients were included in the pilot, findings were not intended to show a significant effect of the education; rather they were intended to indicate whether a more expanded program might be beneficial.

Including extra time during the conduct of an evaluation means leaving room for the unexpected delays. Almost invariably, more time is needed than anticipated for evaluation planning, data collection, and translation of evaluation results into reports that will be meaningful and usable by the primary audience.

Because those delays not only will occur but also are likely to occur at inconvenient times during the evaluation, keeping a sense of humor is vitally important. An evaluator with a sense of humor is more likely to maintain a realistic perspective in reporting results that include negative findings, too. An audience with a vested interest in positive evaluation results may blame the evaluator if results are lower than expected.

Analyzing and Interpreting Data Collected

The purposes for conducting data analysis are twofold: (1) to organize data so that they can provide meaningful information, and (2) to provide answers to evaluation questions. Data and information are not synonymous terms. That is, a mass of numbers or a mass of comments does not become information until it has been organized into coherent tables, graphs, or categories that are relevant to the purpose for conducting the evaluation.

Basic decisions about how data will be analyzed are dictated by the nature of the data and by the questions used to focus the evaluation. As described earlier, data can be quantitative or qualitative. Data also can be described as continuous or discrete. Age and level of anxiety are examples of continuous data; gender and diagnosis are examples of discrete data. Finally, data can be differentiated by level of measurement. All qualitative data are at the nominal level of measurement, meaning they are described in terms of categories such as health focused versus illness focused. Quantitative data can be at the nominal, ordinal, interval, or ratio level of measurement. The level of measurement of the data determines what statistics can be used to analyze those data. A useful suggestion for deciding how data will be analyzed is to enlist the assistance of someone with experience in data analysis.

Analysis of data should be consistent with the type of data collected. In other words, all data analysis must be rigorous, but not all data analysis needs to include use of inferential statistics. For example, qualitative data, such as verbal comments obtained during interviews and written comments obtained from open-ended questionnaires, are summarized, or themed, into categories of similar comments. Each category or theme is qualitatively described by directly quoting one or more comments that are typical of that category. These categories then may be quantitatively described using descriptive statistics such as total counts and percentages.

Different qualitative methods for analyzing data are emerging as they gain legitimacy in a scientific environment once ruled by traditional experimental quantitative methods. One use of qualitative methods in evaluation is called fourth-generation evaluation (Hamilton, 1993). Perhaps most beneficial in conducting a process evaluation, fourth-generation evaluation focuses on teacher–learner interaction and observation of that interaction by the teachers and learners present. Evaluation is an integral component of the education process; that is, evaluation helps construct the education. Data collection, analysis, and use of results occur concurrently. Teacher and learner questions and responses are observed and recorded during an education program. These observations are summarized at the time of occurrence and throughout the program, and then are used to provide immediate feedback to participants in the educational activity.

The first step in analysis of quantitative data consists of organization and summarization using statistics such as frequencies and percentages that describe the sample or population from which the data were collected. A description of a population of learners, for example, might include such information as response rate and frequency of learner demographic characteristics. **Table 14–2** presents an example of how such information might be displayed.

The next step in analysis of quantitative data is to select the statistical procedures appropriate

Table 14–2 Demographic Comparison of Survey Respondents to Total Course Participants Using Group Averages

Learner Demographics	Survey Respondents ($n = 50$)	All Course Participants ($n = 55$)
Age	27.5 years	25.5 years
Length of time employed	3.5 years	7.5 years
Years of post-high school education	2.0 years	2.0 years

for the type of data collected that will answer questions posed in planning the evaluation. Again, a good suggestion is to enlist the assistance of an expert.

Reporting Evaluation Results

Results of an evaluation must be reported if the evaluation is to be of any use. Such a statement seems obvious, but many times an evaluation was reportedly being conducted, but its results were never announced. Many times people participate in an evaluation but never see the final report. How many times have nurses conducted an evaluation but not provided anyone with a report on findings? Almost all of us, if we are honest, would have to answer this question with a number greater than zero.

Reasons for not reporting evaluation results are diverse and numerous. The four major reasons for why evaluative data may often never get from the spreadsheet to the customer are:

1. Ignorance of who should receive the results
2. Belief that the results are not important or will not be used

3. Inability to translate results into language useful for producing the report
4. Fear that results will be misused

Following a few guidelines when planning an evaluation will significantly increase the likelihood that results of the evaluation will be reported to the appropriate individuals or groups, in a timely manner, and in usable form. These guidelines include:

- Be audience focused.
- Stick to the evaluation purpose.
- Use data as intended.

Be Audience Focused

The purpose for conducting an evaluation is to provide information for decision making by the primary audience. The report of evaluation results must, therefore, be consistent with that purpose. One rule of thumb to use: Always begin an evaluation report with an executive summary or an abstract that is no longer than one page. No matter who the audience members are, their time is important to them.

A second rule of thumb is to present evaluation results in a format and language that the audience can use and understand without additional interpretation. This statement does not mean that technical information should be excluded from a report to a lay audience; rather, it means that such information should be written using nontechnical terms. Graphs and charts generally are easier to understand than are tables of numbers, for example. If a secondary audience of technical experts also will receive a report of evaluation results, the report should include an appendix containing the more detailed or technically specific information in which they might be interested.

A third rule of thumb is that the evaluator should make every effort to present results in person as well as in writing. A direct presentation provides an opportunity for the evaluator to answer questions and to assess whether the report meets the needs of the audience.

A final rule to follow is that the evaluation should include specific recommendations or suggestions for how evaluation results might be used. Often the primary audience will expect these as part of the evaluation. Even if the evaluator is not directly asked to provide specific recommendations, however, doing so may increase the likelihood that the results actually will be used.

Stick to the Evaluation Purpose

Evaluators should keep the main body of an evaluation report focused on information that fulfills the purpose for conducting the evaluation. They should provide answers to the questions asked. They should also include the main aspects of how the evaluation was conducted, but avoid a diary-like chronology of the activities of the evaluators.

Use Data as Intended

Evaluators should maintain consistency with actual data when reporting and interpreting findings. A question not asked cannot be an-swered, and data not collected cannot be interpreted. If evaluators did not measure or observe a teacher's performance, for example, they should not draw conclusions about the adequacy of that performance. Similarly, if the only measures of patient performance were those conducted in the hospital, they must not interpret successful inpatient performance as successful performance by the patient at home or at work.

These examples may seem obvious, but conceptual leaps from the data collected to the conclusions drawn from those data are an all-too-common occurrence. One suggestion that decreases the opportunity to overinterpret data is to include evaluation results and interpretation of those results in separate sections of the report.

A discussion of any limitations of the evaluation is an important part of the evaluation report. For example, if several patients were unable to complete a questionnaire because they could not understand it or because they were too fatigued, the report should say so. Knowing that evaluation results do not include data from patients below a certain educational level or physical status will help the audience realize that they cannot make decisions about those patients based on the evaluation. Discussion of limitations also will provide useful information for what not to do the next time a similar evaluation is conducted.

State of the Evidence

A recent search of the Cumulative Index to Nursing & Allied Health Literature (CINAHL) database using the keywords *evaluation*, *patient education*, and *nursing* identified 254 articles. Applying *research*, *English language*, and *2002–2007* as inclusion criteria limited the number of articles to a total of 100. A review of titles and abstracts of these 100 articles to exclude those that did not specifically focus on the evaluation process itself still identified 45 articles directly relevant to the state of evidence in evaluation of patient education.

A search conducted in the same manner, but replacing the keyword *patient education* with two keywords, *inservice education* and *continuing education*, resulted in identification of 56 articles. Using the same search criteria, but changing the time frame to articles published prior to 1992, the year that evidence-based practice first appeared in the literature, no relevant articles were found.

Considering the fact that this search was limited to only those articles published in one database, in English, and during only a 6-year period, the findings were impressive. Clearly a body of evidence exists and is growing.

One reason why a body of literature on evaluation has come into being is because journal review boards have accepted evaluation projects and internal evidence generated by such projects as important for publication. Many of the articles providing evidence on evaluation of patient and staff development education are not research articles—articles providing external evidence resulting from studies conducted to provide generalizable results. For example, Smith and colleagues (2005) describe their project for evaluating patient satisfaction with discharge education, cautioning that their outcomes data cannot be generalized beyond their specific setting. Practice-based evidence from such projects should be considered carefully because patients in one setting may not respond in the same manner as would patients in another setting. However, this information is still valuable for informing practice.

DeSilets (2007) comments that research on evidence-based education activities is still lim-ited. She does summarize one study, however, in which health teams who received an evidence-based educational session demonstrated more appropriate outcome behaviors than did health teams who received traditional education. Other studies and examples of educational evaluation found in the literature have been presented throughout this chapter.

Published evidence can now be found on such topics as content and instructiveness of patient education materials (Johansson, Salentera, Katajisto, & Leino-Kilpi, 2004), computer-based instruction versus instructor-led instruction for nursing staff education (Walker, Harrington, & Cole, 2006), and use of educational videos versus written handouts for patients recovering from surgery (Klein-Fedyshin, Burda, Epstein, & Lawrence, 2005). These studies and others are evaluative in nature and, although rigorous, do not meet traditional criteria for experimental research. Nevertheless, the results of these studies are important for informing nursing practice.

Summary

Conducting evaluation in healthcare education involves gathering, summarizing, interpreting, and using data to determine the extent to which an educational activity is efficient, effective, and useful for those who participate in that activity as learners, teachers, or sponsors. The following five types of evaluation were discussed in this chapter: (1) process, (2) content, (3) outcome, (4) impact, and (5) program evaluations. Each of these types focuses on a specific purpose, scope, and questions to be asked of an educational activity or program to meet the needs of those who ask for the evaluation or who can benefit from its results. Each type of evaluation also requires some level of available resources for the evaluation to be conducted.

The number and variety of evaluation models, designs, methods, and instruments are experiencing an exponential growth as the importance of evaluation becomes more evident in today's healthcare environment. A number of guidelines, rules of thumb, and suggestions have been included in this chapter's discussion of how a nurse educator might go about selecting the most appropriate model, design, methods, and instruments for a particular type of evaluation.

The importance of evaluation as internal evidence has gained even greater momentum with the movement toward evidence-based practice. Perhaps the most important point to remember was made at the beginning of this chapter: Each aspect of the evaluation process is important, but all of them are meaningless if the results of evaluation are not used to guide future action in planning and carrying out educational interventions.

REVIEW QUESTIONS

1. How is the term *evaluation* defined?
2. How does the process of evaluation differ from the process of assessment?
3. How is evidence-based practice related to evaluation?
4. How does internal evidence differ from external evidence?
5. What is the first and most crucial step in planning any evaluation?
6. What are the five basic components included in determining the focus of an evaluation?
7. What are the five basic types (levels) of evaluation in order from simple to complex identified in Abruzzese's RSA evaluation model?
8. How does *formative evaluation* differ from *summative evaluation,* and what is another name for each of these two types of evaluation?
9. What is the purpose of each type (level) of evaluation as described by Abruzzese in her RSA evaluation model?
10. What data collection methods can be used in conducting an evaluation of educational interventions?
11. What are the three major barriers to conducting an evaluation?
12. When and why should a pilot test be conducted prior to implementing a full evaluation?
13. What are three guidelines to follow in reporting the results of an evaluation?

References

Abruzzese, R. S. (1992). Evaluation in nursing staff development. In R. S. Abruzzese, *Nursing staff development: Strategies for success* (pp. 235–248). St. Louis, MO: Mosby–Year Book.

Albanese, M. A., & Gjerde, C. L. (1987). Evaluation. In H. VanHoozer et al. (Eds.), *The teaching process: Theory and practice in nursing* (pp. 269–308). Norwalk, CT: Appleton-Century-Crofts.

Aldana, S., Barlow, M., Smith, R., Yanowitz, F., Adams, T., Loveday, L., et al. (2006). A worksite diabetes prevention program: Two-year impact on employee health. *American Association of Occupational Health Nursing Journal, 54*(9), 389–395.

Appling, S. E., Naumann, P. L., & Berk, R. A. (2001). Using a faculty evaluation triad to achieve evidence-based teaching. *Nursing and Health Care Perspectives, 22*(5), 247–251.

Ball, E., Daly, W. M., & Carnwell, R. (2000). The use of portfolios in the assessment of learning and competence. *Nursing Standard, 14*(43), 35–37.

Berk, R. A., & Rossi, P. H. (1990). *Thinking about program evaluation.* Newbury Park, CA: Sage.

Billings, J. R. (2000). Community development: A critical review of approaches to evaluation. *Journal of Advanced Nursing, 31*(2), 472–480.

Cayne, J. (1995). Portfolios: A developmental influence? *Journal of Advanced Nursing, 21*(2), 395–405.

Cotton, A. H. (2001). Private thoughts in public spheres: Issues in reflection and reflective practices in nursing. *Journal of Advanced Nursing, 36*(4), 512–559.

Covell, C. L. (2005). BCLS certification of the nursing staff: An evidence-based approach. *Journal of Nursing Care Quality, 21*(1), 63–69.

DeSilets, L. D. (2007). The value of evidence-based continuing education. *The Journal of Continuing Education in Nursing, 38*(2), 52–53.

Dilorio, C., Price, M. E., & Becker, J. K. (2001). Evaluation of the neuroscience nurse internship program: The first decade. *Journal of Neuroscience Nursing, 33*(1), 42–49.

Eklund, K., Sonn, U., & Dahlin-Ivanoff, S. (2004). Long-term evaluation of a health education programme for elderly persons with visual impairment. A randomized study. *Disability & Rehabilitation, 26*(7), 401–409.

Gerrish, K. (2001). A pluralistic evaluation to explore people's experiences of stroke services in the community. *Health & Social Care in the Community, 7*(4), 248–256.

Gonzalez, B., Lupon, J., Herreros, J., Urrutia, A., Altimir, S., Coll, R., et al. (2005). Patient's education by nurse: What we really do achieve? *European Journal of Cardiovascular Nursing, 4*(2), 107–111.

Haggard, A. (1989). Evaluating patient education. In A. Haggard (Ed.), *Handbook of patient education* (pp. 159–186). Rockville, MD: Aspen.

Hamilton, G. A. (1993). An overview of evaluation research methods with implications for nursing staff development. *Journal of Nursing Staff Development, 9*(3), 148–154.

Hannigan, B. (2001). A discussion of the strengths and weaknesses of "reflection" in nursing practice and education. *Journal of Clinical Nursing, 10*(2), 278–283.

Hart, E. (1999). The use of pluralistic evaluation to explore people's experiences of stroke services in the community. *Health & Social Care in the Community, 7*(4), 248–256.

Holzemer, W. (1992). Evaluation methods in continuing education. *Journal of Continuing Education in Nursing, 23*(4), 174–181.

Johansson, K., Salentera, S., Katajisto, J., & Leino-Kilpi, H. (2004). Written orthopedic patient education materials from the point of view of empowerment by education. *Patient Education and Counseling, 52,* 175–181.

Johnson, J. H., & Olesinski, N. (1995). Program evaluation: Key to success. *Journal of Nursing Administration, 25*(1), 53–60.

Joint Commission on Accreditation of Healthcare Organizations. (2006). *Accreditation manual for hospitals.* Oakbrook Terrace, IL: Joint Commission on Accreditation of Healthcare Organizations.

Klein-Fedyshin, M., Burda, M. L., Epstein, B. A., & Lawrence, B. (2005). Collaborating to enhance patient education and recovery. *Journal of the Medical Librarians Association, 93*(4), 440–445.

Koch, T. (2000). "Having a say": Negotiation in fourth-generation evaluation. *Journal of Advanced Nursing, 31*(1), 117–125.

Lott, T. F. (2006). Moving forward: Creating a new nursing services orientation program. *Journal for Nurses in Staff Development, 22*(5), 214–221.

Melnyk, B. M., & Fineout-Overholt, E. (2005). *Evidence-based practice in nursing & healthcare: A guide to best practice.* Philadelphia: Lippincott, Williams & Wilkins.

Narrow, B. (1979). *Patient teaching in nursing practice: A patient and family-centered approach.* New York: Wiley.

Puetz, B. E. (1992). Evaluation: Essential skill for the staff development specialist. In K. J. Kelly (Ed.), *Nursing staff development: Current competence, future focus.* Philadelphia: Lippincott.

Rankin, S. H., & Stallings, K. D. (2005). *Patient education in health and illness* (5th ed.). Philadelphia: Lippincott Williams & Wilkins.

Ream, E., Richardson, A., & Evison, M. (2005). A feasibility study to evaluate a group intervention for people with cancer experiencing fatigue following treatment. *Clinical Effectiveness in Nursing, 9*, 178–187.

Roberts, P., Priest, H., & Bromage, C. (2001). Selecting and utilizing data sources to evaluate health care education. *Nurse Researcher, 8*(3), 15–29.

Ruzicki, D. A. (1987). Evaluating patient education— A vital part of the process. In C. E. Smith (Ed.), *Patient education: Nurses in partnership with other health professionals*. Orlando, FL: Grune & Stratton.

Schön, D. A. (1987). *Educating the reflective practitioner. Towards a new design for teaching and learning in the professions*. London: Jossey-Bass.

Schreurs, K. M. G., Colland, V. T., Kuijer, R. G., Ridder, D. T. D., & van Elderen, T. (2003). Development, content, and process evaluation of a short self-management intervention in patients with chronic diseases requiring self-care behaviours. *Patient Education and Counseling, 51*, 133–141.

Serembus, J. F. (2000). Teaching the process of developing a professional portfolio. *Nurse Educator, 25*(6), 282–287.

Smith, C. E., Rebeck, S., Schaag, H., Kleinbeck, S., Moor, J. M., & Bleich, M. R. (2005). A model for evaluating systemic change: Measuring outcomes of hospital discharge education redesign. *Journal of Nursing Administration, 35*(2), 67–73.

Stewart, A. L., Hays, R. D., & Ware, J. E. (1988). The MOS short-form general health survey: Reliability and validity in a patient population. *Medical Care, 26*(7), 724.

Suhayda, R., & Miller, J. M. (2006). Optimizing evaluation of nursing education programs. *Nurse Educator, 31*(5), 200–206.

Teekman, B. (2000). Exploring reflective thinking in nursing practice. *Journal of Advanced Nursing, 31*(5), 1125–1135.

Templeton, H., & Coates, V. (2004). Evaluation of an evidence-based education package for men with prostate cancer on hormonal manipulation therapy. *Patient Education and Counseling, 55*, 55–61.

Waddell, D. (1992). The effects of continuing education on nursing practice: A meta-analysis. *Journal of Continuing Education in Nursing, 23*(4), 164–168.

Walker, B. L., Harrington, S. S., & Cole, C. S. (2006). The usefulness of computer-based instruction in providing educational opportunities for nursing staff. *Journal for Nurses in Staff Development, 22*(3), 144–149.

Walker, E., & Dewar, B. J. (2000). Moving on from interpretivism: An argument for constructivist evaluation. *Journal of Advanced Nursing, 32*(3), 713–720.

Ware, J. E., Jr., Davies-Avery, A., & Donald, C. A. (1978). *Conceptualization and measurement of health for adults in the health insurance study: Vol. V. General health perceptions*. Santa Monica, CA: RAND.

Watters, C. L., & Moran, W. P. (2006). Hip fractures— A joint effort. *Orthopaedic Nursing, 25*(3), 157–167.

Tests to Measure Readability and Comprehension and Tools to Assess Instructional Materials

How to Use the Spache Grade-Level Score Formula

1. For short passages, test the entire piece. For longer passages, test a minimum of three randomly selected samples of 100 words each. (If the 100-word mark in the sample falls after the midpoint of the sentence, count the sentence as a part of the sample.)

2. Average sentence length (a) can be determined by counting the number of words in the sample and dividing by the number of sentences. If a sentence is punctuated by a period, question mark, exclamation point, semicolon, or colon, count it as an independent sentence.

3. Count the number of words not on the Dale list (b) according to the following guidelines:
   - Count a word only once, even if it appears again or with variable endings later in the sample.
   - Do not count first names.
   - Do not count plurals or possessive endings of nouns.
   - Do not count regular verb forms (*-ing, -ed, -es*), but do count irregular verb forms.
   - Count adjective or adverb endings (*-ly, -er, -est*).
   - Count a group of words that consists of repetition of a single word (e.g., "oh, oh, oh"; "look, look, look") as a single sentence regardless of punctuation.
   - Do not count familiar letters like A, B, C.

4. Apply the formula:

$$GL = 0.141(a) + 0.086(b) + 0.839$$

where GL is grade level, (a) is average sentence length, and (b) is the number of words not listed on the Dale list.

In other words, multiply the average sentence length in a sample of 100 words (a) by 0.141. Then multiply the percent of words outside the Dale easy word list (b) by 0.086. To these figures, add a constant, 0.839. The sum represents the estimated reading difficulty of the book. This will be a figure such as 2.267, which, when rounded off as 2.3, designates a book equal in difficulty to readers of school textbooks commonly used in the third month of second grade. When using this formula, it is suggested that at least three samples from the reading material be scored and the results averaged for a more reliable estimate of reading difficulty (Spache, 1953; Spadero, 1983).

How to Use the Flesch–Kincaid Scale

1. To test a whole piece of writing, take three to five 100-word samples of an article or twenty-five to thirty 100-word samples of a book. For short pieces, test the entire selection. Do not pick good or typical samples, but choose every third paragraph or every other page. In a 100-word sample, find the sentence that ends nearest to the 100-word mark; that may be, for example, at the 94th or the 109th word. Start each sample at the beginning of a paragraph, but do not use an introductory paragraph as part of the sample. Count contractions and hyphenated words as one word; count numbers and letters separated by space as words.
2. Figure the average sentence length (SL) by counting the number of words and dividing by the number of sentences. In counting sentences, follow units of thought marked off by periods, colons, semicolons, question marks, or exclamation points.
3. Determine word length (WL) by counting the number of syllables in each word in the sample as they are normally read aloud (i.e., two syllables for $ ["dollars"] and four syllables for *1918* ["nineteen-eighteen"]. It helps to read silently aloud while counting. Divide the syllables by the number of words in the sample and multiply by 100.
4. Determine the average WL by multiplying it by 0.846 and the average SL by multiplying it by 1.015. Then apply the formula:

$$RE = 206.835 - 0.846 \, (WL) - 1.015 \, (SL)$$

where RE is the reading ease score, after WL and SL have been subtracted from 206.835 (Flesch, 1948; Spadero, 1983; Spadero et al., 1980).

The reading ease score ranges from zero (practically unreadable) to 100 (very easy for any literate person) with interpretations in between (**Table A–1**).

Table A–1 Reading Ease Scores

Reading Ease Score	Syllables per 100 Words	Average Sentence Length	Difficulty Level	Grade Level
0–30	192 or more	29 or more	Very difficult	College grad
30–50	167	25	Difficult	College
50–60	155	21	Fairly difficult	10–12
60–70	147	17	Standard	8–9
70–80	139	14	Fairly easy	7
80–90	131	11	Easy	6
90–100	123 or less	8 or less	Very easy	5

Source: Adapted from Flesch, R. (1948). A new readability yardstick. *Journal of Applied Psychology,* 32(3), 230; and Spadero, D. C. (1983). Assessing readability of patient information materials. *Pediatric Nursing,* 9(4), 275.

How to Use the Fog Formula

1. Count 100 words in succession (W). If the selection is long, choose several samples of 100 words from the text, and average the results.
2. Count the number of complete sentences (S). If the 100th word falls past the midpoint of a sentence, include this sentence in the count.
3. Divide the words (W) by the number of sentences (S).
4. Count the number of words having three or more syllables (A), but do not count verbs ending in -ed or -es that make a word have a third syllable; do not count capitalized words, and do not count combinations of simple words, such as *butterfly*.
5. Apply the formula:

$$GL = (W/S + A) \times 0.4$$

In other words, to find the GL (grade level), divide the number of words (W) by the number of complete sentences (S) in the sample 100-word passage, add the number of words having three or more syllables (A), and multiply the result by a constant of 0.4 (Gunning, 1968; Spadero, 1983; Spadero et al., 1980).

How to Use the Fry Readability Graph

1. Select three 100-word sample passages from near the beginning, middle, and end of a book, article, pamphlet, or brochure. Skip all proper nouns as part of the 100-word count.

Fewer than three samples and passages of less than 30 sentences can be used, but the user should be aware that there is necessarily a sacrifice in both reliability and validity.

2. Count the total number of sentences in each 100-word sample (estimating to the nearest 10th of a sentence for partial sentences).

3. Average the sentence counts of the three sample passages.

4. Count the total number of syllables in each 100-word sample. Count one syllable per vowel sound; for example, *cat* has one syllable, *blackbird* has two, and *continental* has four. Caution: Do not be fooled by word size (e.g., *polio* [three syllables], *through* [one syllable]). Endings such as *-y, -ed, -el,* or *-le* usually make a syllable (e.g., *ready* [two syllables], *bottle* [two syllables]). Graph users sometimes have trouble determining syllables. The clue is to believe what you hear (speech sounds), not what you see (e.g., *wanted* is a two-syllable word, but *stopped* is a one-syllable word). Count proper nouns, numerals, and initials or acronyms as words. A word is a symbol or group of symbols bounded by a blank space on either side. Thus, *1945, &,* and *IRS* are all words. Each symbol should receive a syllable count of one (i.e., the date 1945 is one word with five syllables, and the initials *IRS* is one word with three syllables).

5. Average the total number of syllables for the three samples.

6. Plot on the graph the average sentence count and the average word count to determine the appropriate grade level of the material. For example,

	Number of Syllables	Number of Sentences
First 100 words	153	6.3
Second 100 words	161	5.9
Third 100 words	<u>139</u>	<u>5.2</u>
Average count =	453 ÷ 3 = 151	17.4 ÷ 3 = 5.8

In the example, the average number of syllables is 151, and the average number of sentences is 5.8. When plotted on the graph (**Figure A–1**), the point falls within the approximate grade level of 9, which shows the materials to be at the ninth-grade readability level. If the point when plotted falls in the gray area, grade-level scores are invalid (Fry, 1968; Fry, 1977; Spadero et al., 1980).

How to Use the SMOG Formula

Passages Longer Than 30 Sentences

1. Count 10 consecutive sentences near the beginning, 10 consecutive sentences from the middle, and 10 consecutive sentences from the end of the selection to be assessed. A sentence is any independent unit of thought punctuated by a period, question mark, or exclamation point. If a sentence has a colon or semicolon, consider each part as a separate sentence.

Figure A–1 Fry readability graph—extended.

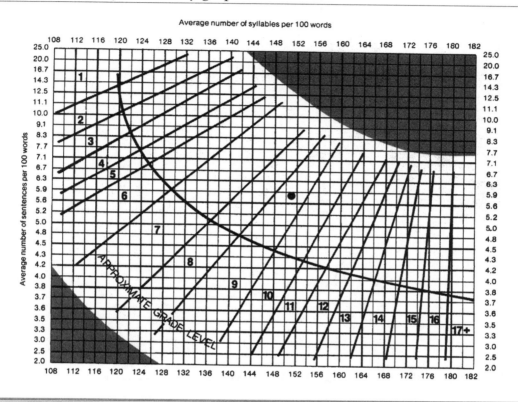

Average number of syllables per 100 words

Source: Edward Fry, Rutgers University Reading Center, New Brunswick, NJ.

2. From the 30 randomly selected sentences, count the words containing three or more syllables (polysyllabic), including repetitions. Abbreviated words should be read aloud to determine their syllable count (e.g., *Sept.* = *September* = three syllables). Letters or numerals in a string beginning or ending with a space or punctuation mark should be counted if, when read aloud in context, at least three syllables can be distinguished. Do not count words ending in *-ed* or *-es* if the ending makes the word have a third syllable. Hyphenated words are counted as one word. Proper nouns should be counted.

3. Approximate the reading grade level from the SMOG conversion table (**Table A–2**), or calculate the reading grade level by estimating the nearest perfect square root of the number of words with three or more syllables and then adding a constant of 3 to the square root. For example, if the total number of polysyllabic words was 53, the nearest perfect

Table A–2 SMOG Conversion Table

Word Count	Grade Level
0–2	4
3–6	5
7–12	6
13–20	7
21–30	8
31–42	9
43–56	10
57–72	11
73–90	12
91–110	13
111–132	14
133–156	15
157–182	16
183–210	17
211–240	18

Source: Developed by Harold C. McGraw, Office of Educational Research, Baltimore County Public Schools, Towson, MD.

square would be 49. The square root of 49 would be 7. By adding a constant of 3, the reading level would be tenth grade.

Figure A–2 is an example of how to count all the words containing three or more syllables in a set of 10 sentences taken from one of the many pamphlets designed and distributed by the National Cancer Institute.

In Figure A–2, there are 20 words with three or more syllables. Note, the word *United* is not counted as a three-syllable word because only the *-ed* ending makes it polysyllabic (see rule 2). For this passage of 10 sentences, the grade level is 11th grade using the conversion table (**Table A–3**) for samples with fewer than 30 sentences. That is, 10 sentences × 3 (conversion number) = 60, which falls at the 11th grade level on Table A–2 as per the rules in the next section for passages shorter than 30 sentences.

Figure A–2 Example of counting words with three or more syllables.

¹Mastectomy: A Treatment for Breast Cancer

²You've been diagnosed as having breast cancer and your doctor has recommended a mastectomy. ³If you're like most women, you probably have many concerns about this treatment for breast cancer. ⁴Surgery of any kind is a frightening experience, but surgery for breast cancer raises special concerns. ⁵You may be wondering if the surgery will cure your cancer, how you'll feel after surgery—and how you're going to look.

⁶It's not unusual to think about these things. ⁷More than 100,000 women in the United States will have mastectomies this year. ⁸Each of them will have personal concerns about the impact of the surgery on her life.

⁹This booklet is designed to ease some of your fears by letting you know what to expect—from the time you enter the hospital to your recovery at home. ¹⁰It may also help the special people in your life who are concerned about your well-being.

Source: National Cancer Institute of the National Institutes of Health, Public Health Service, U.S. Department of Health and Human Services, pamphlet entitled *Mastectomy: A Treatment for Breast Cancer* (1987, p. 1).

Passages Shorter Than 30 Sentences

1. Count the number of sentences in the material and the number of words containing three or more syllables.
2. In the left-hand column of Table A–3, locate the number of sentences. Then in the column opposite, locate the conversion number.
3. Multiply the word count found in step 1 by the conversion number. Locate this number in Table A–2 to obtain the corresponding grade level.

   Example: If the material is 25 sentences long and 15 words of three or more syllables were counted in this material, the conversion number in Table A–3 for 25 sentences is 1.2. Multiply the word count of 15 by 1.2 to get 18. For the word count of 18, the grade level in Table A–2 is 7. Therefore, the material is at a seventh-grade reading level.

Table A–3 SMOG Conversion for Samples with Fewer Than 30 Sentences

Number of Sentences in Sample Material	Conversion Number
29	1.03
28	1.07
27	1.1
26	1.15
25	1.2
24	1.25
23	1.3
22	1.36
21	1.43
20	1.5
19	1.58
18	1.67
17	1.76
16	1.87
15	2.0
14	2.14
13	2.3
12	2.5
11	2.7
10	3

How to Use the Cloze Test

How to Construct a Cloze Test

1. Select a prose passage (one without reference to figures, tables, charts, or pictures) from printed educational materials currently in use such as pamphlets, brochures, manuals, or

instruction sheets. Be sure the material is typical of what is normally given to patients but has not been previously read by them. The chosen passage should include whole paragraphs so that readers benefit from complete units of thought.

2. Leave the first and last sentences intact, and delete every fifth word from the other sentences for a total of about 50 word deletions. Do not delete proper nouns, but delete the word following the proper noun. Replace all deleted words with a line or blank space, all of equal length.

3. Ask the reader to fill in the blanks with the *exact* word replacements.

How to Score a Cloze Test

1. Count as correct only those words that *exactly* replace the deleted words (synonyms are not to be counted as a correct answer).

2. Inappropriate word endings such as *-s, -ed, -er,* and *-ing* should be counted as incorrect.

3. The raw score is the number of exact word replacements.

4. Divide the raw score by the total number of blank spaces to determine the percentage of correct responses. For example, if the passage has 50 blanks and the patient correctly filled in 25 blanks (10 were incorrect responses and 15 spaces were left blank), divide 25 by 50, and the percentage score would be 50%.

5. A score of 60% or above indicates the patient is fully capable of understanding the material. A score of 40–60% indicates the patient needs supplemental instruction. A score below 40% indicates that the material as written is too difficult for the patient to understand.

The following are the words that were deleted from the sample cloze test in **Figure A–3**.

1. it	13. heart	25. all	37. vessels
2. heart	14. cause	26. supplying	38. pumping
3. kidney	15. a	27. oxygen	39. creates
4. cases	16. blood	28. its	40. pressure
5. causes	17. to	29. to	41. moment
6. chemistry	18. the	30. your	42. or
7. a	19. work	31. through	43. are
8. have	20. muscle	32. the	44. you
9. high	21. pump	33. oxygen	45. arteries
10. remain	22. your	34. begins	46. constrict
11. been	23. from	35. by	47. even
12. risk	24. it	36. the	48. blood

Note: Words are listed in missing order. Hyphenated words are counted as one word; words in parentheses are counted as a word.

Figure A–3 Sample cloze test.

High Blood Pressure

High blood pressure, also called hypertension, affects 37 million Americans—many of them older than 55. A dangerous, silent killer, __1__ can lead to stroke, __2__ attack and heart or __3__ failure. Yet, in most __4__, no one knows what __5__ high blood pressure. Body __6__, emotions, heredity, overweight, and __7__ high-sodium (salt) diet may __8__ something to do with __9__ blood pressure, but scientists __10__ uncertain. It has long __11__ recognized as a major __12__ factor in stroke and __13__ attack—cardiovascular diseases which __14__ nearly 1 million deaths __15__ year.

To understand high __16__ pressure, it is necessary __17__ know something about how __18__ heart and blood vessels __19__. Your heart is a __20__ that acts like a __21__. The left side of __22__ heart receives oxygen-rich blood __23__ the lungs and pumps __24__ through the arteries to __25__ parts of your body, __26__ it with nutrients and __27__. Blood that has distributed __28__ nutrients and oxygen returns __29__ the right side of __30__ heart which pumps it __31__ the pulmonary artery to __32__ lungs where it absorbs __33__, and then the process __34__ again.

The force exerted __35__ your blood flowing against __36__ walls of the blood __37__ is blood pressure. The __38__ action of your heart __39__ the force. Your blood __40__ varies from moment to __41__ depending upon the situations __42__ activities in which you __43__ involved. For example, when __44__ become excited, the small __45__ that nourish your tissues __46__. The heart must pump __47__ harder to force the __48__ through the arteries, causing __49__ blood pressure to rise. __50__ the blood pressure will __51__ to normal when you __52__. Because of these changes in blood pressure, the doctor will usually take several blood pressure readings over a period of time before making a diagnosis of high blood pressure.

Source: Adapted from American Heart Association. (1983). An older person's guide to cardiovascular health, Dallas, TX: National Center. The information from this booklet is not current and is used for illustrative purposes only.

Figure A–4 Suitability assessment of materials (SAM) scoring sheet.

2 points for superior rating
1 point for adequate rating
0 points for not suitable rating
N/A if the factor does not apply to this material

FACTOR TO BE RATED	SCORE	COMMENTS
1. CONTENT		
(a) Purpose is evident	_____	_____
(b) Content about behaviors	_____	_____
(c) Scope is limited	_____	_____
(d) Summary or review included	_____	_____
2. LITERACY DEMAND		
(a) Reading grade level	_____	_____
(b) Writing style, active voice	_____	_____
(c) Vocabulary uses common words	_____	_____
(d) Context is given first	_____	_____
(e) Learning aids via "road signs"	_____	_____
3. GRAPHICS		
(a) Cover graphic shows purpose	_____	_____
(b) Type of graphics	_____	_____
(c) Relevance of illustrations	_____	_____
(d) Lists, tables, etc. explained	_____	_____
(e) Captions used for graphics	_____	_____
4. LAYOUT AND TYPOGRAPHY		
(a) Layout factors	_____	_____
(b) Typography	_____	_____
(c) Subheads (chunking) used	_____	_____
5. LEARNING STIMULATION, MOTIVATION		
(a) Interaction used	_____	_____
(b) Behaviors are modeled and specific	_____	_____
(c) Motivation—self-efficacy	_____	_____
6. CULTURAL APPROPRIATENESS		
(a) Match in logic, language, experience	_____	_____
(b) Cultural image and examples	_____	_____

Total SAM score: _____

Total possible score: _____, Percent score: _____%

Source: Doak, Doak, & Root (1996), *Teaching patients with low literacy skills*, p. 51. Reprinted with permission from Lippincott.

Guidelines for Writing and Evaluating Printed Education Materials (PEMs)

To Reduce Reading Level and Increase Reading Ease, Do the Following:

1. Write in conversational style with an active voice in the present tense using the second person pronoun *you* or *your*.
2. Use short, simple vocabulary of one- or two-syllable words; avoid multisyllabic words.
3. Spell out words rather than using abbreviations or acronyms, unless they are familiar to the reader or defined.
4. Organize information into chunks or series of numbered and bulleted lists; use statistics sparingly; a question and answer format is an interactive approach to presenting single units of information.
5. Keep sentences short (20 words maximum); avoid complex grammatical sentence structures that contain colons, semicolons, commas, and dashes.
6. Focus on familiar terms; avoid technical jargon and medical terminology; define or spell out difficult words phonetically; include a glossary if medicalese is necessary.
7. Use words consistently (repetition) throughout text; avoid synonyms.
8. Use exact terms; avoid value judgment words with many interpretations.
9. Put the most important information first by prioritizing the need to know.
10. Use advance organizers to cue the reader about the topic being presented.
11. Limit the use of connective words that lengthen and make sentences more complex.
12. Make the first sentence of a paragraph the topic sentence.
13. Reduce concept density by including only one idea per sentence and limiting each paragraph to a single message or action.
14. Keep the density of words low (do not exceed 30–40 characters per line).
15. Provide adequate white space for margins and between lines and paragraphs (use double spacing).
16. Justify left margins and keep right margins unjustified.
17. Use arrows or numbers that give direction and organization to layouts.
18. Select large print (minimum of 12–14-point font) and simple style type (serif); avoid italics, all capital letters, and fancy lettering.
19. Rely on bold print or underlining to emphasize key points or words.
20. Attract attention with consistent use of appealing colors to highlight and organize topics.
21. Use a simple, short title that clearly indicates the subject being presented.
22. Keep the length of the document short; avoid including details and extraneous information.
23. Avoid glossy paper to reduce glare; rely on bold primary colors (not pastels) and black print on white paper for the older audience.

24. Use simple, realistic illustrations that convey the intended message; never superimpose typed words on a background design.
25. Include a summary at the end to review key points of information.
26. Put reading grade level (RGL) on the back of the tool for future reference.
27. Determine readability, comprehension, and reading skills by applying at least two formulas or tests.

A. Readability Formulas	B. Comprehension Tests	C. Reading Skills Tests
1. SMOG	1. Cloze procedure	1. WRAT
2. Fog	2. Listening test	2. REALM
3. Fry		3. TOFHLA

References

Doak, C. C., Doak, L. G., & Root, J. H. (1996). *Teaching patients with low literacy skills* (2nd ed.). Philadelphia: Lippincott.

Flesch, R. (1948). A new readability yardstick. *Journal of Applied Psychology, 32*(3), 221–233.

Fry, E. (1968). A readability formula that saves time. *Journal of Reading, 11*, 513–516, 555–579.

Fry, E. (1977). Fry's readability graph: Clarifications, validity, and extension to level 17. *Journal of Reading, 21*, 242–252.

Gunning, R. (1968). The fog index after 20 years. *Journal of Business Communications*, 6, 3–13.

Spache, G. (1953). A new readability formula for primary-grade reading materials. *Elementary School Journal, 53*(7), 410–413.

Spadero, D. C. (1983). Assessing readability of patient information materials. *Pediatric Nursing, 9*(4), 274–278.

Spadero, D. C., Robinson, L. A., & Smith, L. T. (1980). Assessing readability of patient information materials. *American Journal of Hospital Pharmacy, 37*, 215–221.

Resources and Organizations for Special Populations

BLINDNESS

American Diabetes Association
1701 N. Beauregard Street
Alexandria, VA 22311
800-342-2383
www.diabetes.org

American Foundation for the Blind
11 Pen Plaza, Suite 300
New York, NY 10001
800-232-5463
www.afb.org

National Braille Press
88 St. Stephen Street
Boston, MA 02115
617-266-6160; 888-965-8965
E-mail: orders@nbp.org
www.nbp.org

National Library Service for the Blind and
Physically Handicapped
1291 Taylor Street N.W.
Washington, DC 20542
202-707-5100
www.loc.gov/nls/index.html

Resource Persons for Diabetes and Vision
Impairment
VIP Special Interest Group
AADE
444 N. Michigan Avenue
Suite 1240
Chicago, IL 60611-3901
www.diabeteseducation.org
*List of members of American Association of
Disabled Educators (AADE) who possess
specialized skills with visually impaired
persons.*

DEAFNESS

The National Academy of Gallaudet
  College
800 Florida Avenue
Washington, DC 20002-3695
www.gallaudet.edu

Helen Keller National Center
11 Middleneck Road
Sands Point, NJ 11020-1299
516-944-8900
www.hknc.org

National Institutes of Health
National Institute on Deafness and Other
  Communication Disorders
31 Center Drive, MSC 2320
Bethesda, MD 20892-2320
800-241-1044
E-mail: nidcdinfo@nidcd.nih.gov
*Training programs; assistance in developing
training programs' publications on working
with deaf patients.*

Registry of Interpreters for the Deaf, Inc.
333 Commerce Street
Alexandria, VA 22314
703-838-0030
www.rid.org
*Information on interpreting and interpreters;
referral to local agencies and state chapters of
the Registry of Interpreters for the Deaf for
assistance in locating interpreters.*

The Library of Congress
101 Independence Avenue, S.E.
Washington, DC 20540
General Information: 202-707-5000
www.loc.gov

DISABILITY SERVICES

Americans with Disabilities Act, ADA
P.O. Box 66738
Washington, DC 20035
800-514-0383
en.wikipedia.org/wiki/Americans_with_
Disabilities_Act

National Council on Disability
1331 F. Street N.W.
Suite 850
Washington, DC 20004
202-272-2004

HEAD INJURY

Brain Injury Association of America
800-444-6443
www.biausa.org

National Brain Injury Research Treatment
  and Training Foundation
434-220-4824
www.nbirtt.org

HEALTHCARE-RELATED FEDERAL AGENCIES

National Institute on Disability and
  Rehabilitation Research (NIDRR)
U.S. Department of Education
400 Maryland Avenue S.W.
Room 3060
Washington, DC 20202
202-245-7640
www.ed.gov/about/offices/list/osers/nidrr

National Center for Medical
  Rehabilitation Research, NIHD, NIH
800-370-2943
www.nichd.nih.gov/about/ncmrr

LEARNING DISABILITIES

A.D.D. Warehouse
300 N.W. 70th Avenue
Suite 102
Plantation, FL 33317
305-792-8944
www.addwarehouse.com/shopsite_sc/
store/html/index.html

Association for Children and Adults With
Learning Disabilities
4156 Library Road
Pittsburgh, PA 15234
412-341-8077
www.ldanatl.org

Attention Disorders Association of
Parents and Professionals Together
(ADAPPT)
P.O. Box 293
Oak Forest, IL 60452
312-361-4330
www.adappt.org

MENTAL HEALTH

Mental Health America
2000 N. Beauregard Street, 6th Floor
Alexandria, VA 22311
703-684-7722
800-969-6642
TTY Line 800-433-5959

National Mental Health Association
(NMHA)
1012 Prince Street
Alexandria, VA 22314-2971
www.nmha.org

National Institute of Mental Health
(NIMH)
Public Information and Communications
Branch
6001 Executive Boulevard
Room 8184, MSC 9663
Bethesda, MD 20892-9663
301-443-4513
866-615-6464
301-443-8431 (TTY)
866-415-8051 (TTY toll free)
E-mail: nimhinfo@nih.gov
www.nimh.nih.gov

DEVELOPMENTAL DISABILITIES

National Institute of Child Health and
Human Development
P.O. Box 3006
Rockville, MD 20847
800-370-2943
TTY: 1-888-320-6942
E-mail:
NICHDInformationResourceCenter@
mail.nih.gov
www.nichd.nih.gov

NEUROMUSCULAR DISORDERS

ALS Association National Office
27001 Agoura Road
Suite 150
Calabassa Hills, CA 91301-5104
800-782-4747
www.alsa.org

Epilepsy Foundation of America
4351 Garden City Drive
Suite 500
Landover, MD 20785
301-459-3700
800-332-1000
www.epilepsyfoundation.org

Myasthenia Gravis Foundation of America
1821 University Avenue W.
Suite S256
St. Paul, MN 55104
651-917-6256
800-541-5454
E-mail: mgfa@myasthenia.org
www.myasthenia.org

Multiple Sclerosis Foundation
6350 North Andrews Avenue
Fort Lauderdale, FL 33309-2130
Administrative Offices, Fund Raising,
   Donations, Advertising
800-225-6495
954-776-6805
E-mail: admin@msfocus.org

Program Services Assistance, MS Helpline
888-MSFOCUS
954-776-6805
E-mail: support@msfocus.org
www.msfocus.org

Muscular Dystrophy Association—USA
National Headquarters
3300 E. Sunrise Drive
Tucson, AZ 85718
1-800-FIGHT-MD (344-4863)
E-mail: mda@mdausa.org
www.mdausa.org

Parkinson's Disease Foundation, Inc.
1359 Broadway
Suite 1509
New York, NY 10018
800-457-6676
212-457-6676
E-mail: info@pdf.org
www.pdf.org

SPINAL CORD

Paralyzed Veterans of America
801 Eighteenth Street N.W.
Washington, DC 20006-3517
800-555-9140
E-mail: info@pva.org
www.pva.org

National Spinal Cord Injury Association
6701 Democracy Boulevard
Suite 300-9
Bethesda, MD 20817
800-962-9629
301-214-4006
Email: info@spinalcord.org
www.spinalcord.org

STROKE

National Stroke Association
9707 E. Easter Lane Building B
Centennial, CO 80112
800-STROKES or 800-787-6537
E-mail: Info@stroke.org
www.stroke.org

National Institute of Neurological
   Disorders and Stroke (NINDS)
P.O. Box 5801
Bethesda, MD 20824
www.ninds.nih.gov

ASSISTIVE TECHNOLOGY

ABLEDATA
8630 Fenton Street
Suite 930
Silver Springs, MD 20910
800-227-0216
E-mail: abledata@verizon.net
www.abledata.com

Alliance for Technology Access
1304 Southpoint Boulevard
Suite 240
Petaluma, CA 94954
707-778-3011
E-mail: ATAinfo@ATAccess.org
www.ataccess.org

AUGMENTATIONS AND ALTERNATIVE COMMUNICATION

American Speech-Language-Hearing
Association (ASHA)
10801 Rockville Pike
Rockville, MD 20852
888-321-ASHA
www.asha.org

International Society for Augmentative and
Alternative Communication (ISAAC)
49 The Donway West, Suite 308
Toronto, ON M3C 3M9
Canada
416-385-0351
www.isaac-online.org

GENERAL

Centers for Disease Control and
Prevention
1600 Clifton Road
Atlanta, GA 30333
404-639-3311
Public Inquiries: 404-639-3534
800-311-3455
www.cdc.gov

Health Resources and Services
Administration
301-443-3376
www.hrsa.gov

Disability Resources, Inc.
Four Glatter Lane
Centereach, NY 11720-1032
631-585-0290
www.disabilityresources.org

Teaching Plans

Postcircumcision Care

Purpose: To provide mothers of male newborns with the information necessary to perform post-circumcision care.

Goal: The mother will independently manage postcircumcision care for her baby boy.

Objectives	Content Outline	Method of Instruction	Time Allotted	Resources	Method of Evaluation
Following a 20-minute teaching session, the mother will be able to:					

1. Demonstrate procedure for postcircumcision care with each diaper change (psychomotor)	A. Definition of circumcision
	B. Circumcision care
	  1. Washing penis
	  2. Applying petroleum jelly and gauze
	  3. Diapering baby
		Demonstration
		
		Return demonstration
			10 minutes	Written/ pictorial flip chart
				Infant doll
				Washcloth
				Warm water
				Petroleum jelly
				Gauze
				Diaper
					Observation of return demonstration

Objectives	Content Outline	Method of Instruction	Time Allotted	Resources	Method of Evaluation
2. Identify three reasons to call the doctor or nurse (cognitive)	Postcircumcision complications 1. bleeding 2. weak or absent stream of urine 3. drainage 4. swollen penis 5. baby acts sick or more fussy than expected	1:1 instruction	5 minutes	Written/pictorial flip chart	Posttest
3. Express any concerns about circumcision care (affective)	A. Summarize common concerns B. Explore feelings	Discussion	5 minutes	White board	Question and answer

Source: Developed as part of teaching project assignment by Eleanor P. McLees, BSN, RN, CNM and Julie-Lynn Corsoniti, BS, RN in NSG 561 course during Spring 2007 semester at Le Moyne College, Syracuse, NY.

Safe Sleep Positioning of Infants

Purpose: Provide parents with information on safe sleep conditions of infant after discharge from the NICU.

Goal: Parents will maintain safe sleep conditions at home for infant to reduce the risk of SIDS.

Objectives and Subobjectives	Content Outline	Method of Instruction	Time Allotted	Resources	Method of Evaluation
Following a 15-minute teaching session, the parents will be able to:					
1. Explain what SIDS is, its causes, and ways to prevent it with 100% accuracy (cognitive)	Introduce the Back to Sleep Campaign concept Review SIDS definition, including incidence				
– Define sudden infant death syndrome (SIDS)	Discuss risk factors (preterm, low birth weight, smoking, prone/side sleeping, soft bedding, cosleeping, cold months, males)	1:1 instruction	5 minutes	PEM on back to sleep	Pre- and Posttest

Objectives and Subobjectives	Content Outline	Method of Instruction	Time Allotted	Resources	Method of Evaluation
– Identify the most common risk factors – State six ways to reduce SIDS	Review risk reduction—back to sleep, no smoking, no soft bedding, no cosleeping, pacifiers, do not overheat				
2. Demonstrate proper safe sleep techniques with 100% accuracy (psychomotor) – Choose crib items that are safe and unsafe – Position baby in crib with proper clothing	Typical shower gifts to avoid—loose blankets, toys, crib bumpers, rolls, pillows Crib set-up, swaddle blanket for warmth	Demonstration, return demonstration	5 minutes	Portable crib with crib bumpers, quilts, toys, rolls, pacifier, loose blankets, dolls, baby clothes	Skills checklist for return demonstration
3. Express any concerns about placing infant on his or her back to sleep (affective)	Summarize common concerns such as choking, flat heads, inability to sleep as well	Discussion	5 minutes	Worksheets listing concerns filled out by participants prior to discussion session	Completed worksheets on observation of level of learner participation in discussion

Source: Developed as part of a teaching project assignment by Christine A. Aris, CNNP, RN and Carol A. Weeks, BS, RN in NSG 461 course during Spring 2007 semester at Le Moyne College, Syracuse, NY.

Use of Incentive Spirometer

Purpose: To provide patients in a preoperative open-heart surgery class with the information and skills necessary to properly use an incentive spirometer.

Goal: Patients will use the incentive spirometer as directed to prevent postoperative pulmonary complications.

Objectives	Content Outline	Method of Instruction	Time Allotted	Resources	Method of Evaluation
Following three 15-minute consecutive group sessions, the patients will:					
1. Name two postoperative complications that can potentially be prevented by their proper use of the incentive spirometer (cognitive: knowledge level)	a. *Pneumonia*: Inflammation of lungs caused by bacterial growth secondary to an excessive build-up of secretions. b. *Atelectasis*: A collapsed or airless condition of the lung caused by excessive secretions.	Lecture	15 minutes	Simple anatomical poster of lungs within the chest cavity	Posttest

2. Return demonstrate the eight steps in proper use of incentive spirometer (psychomotor: guided response level)	a. Use analogy of drinking a thick liquid through a straw
	
	b. The eight steps in using incentive spirometer:
	  1. Slide arrow to the number ordered by your doctor
	  2. Blow out all of the air from your lungs
	  3. Hold mouthpiece and close your lips around it
	  4. Suck air in through the mouthpiece (like a straw)
	  5. Watch the blue flow rate guide and see the blue riser move up
		Demonstration and return demonstration	15 minutes	Milkshake
				Small cups
				Straws
				
				Incentive spirometers for each patient to practice with
				
				PEM on incentive spirometer
					Observation of return demonstration

Objectives	Content Outline	Method of Instruction	Time Allotted	Resources	Method of Evaluation
	6. when the blue flow rate guide rises between the two arrows, hold it there for 6 seconds				
	7. look at the number where the blue riser stops				
	8. blow out and repeat				
3. Explain their feelings regarding mastery of incentive spirometer use preoperatively (affective: responding level)	Discussion of the patients' overall feelings towards use of the incentive spirometer prior to surgery	Group discussions: Patients break into small groups, each group discusses feelings and selects a presenter and then each group presenter summarizes feelings and shares them with the larger group	15 minutes	Paper and pencils to document responses	Question and answer

Source: Developed as part of a teaching project assignment by Diane G. Mather, BS, RN and Diane S. McDermott, BS, RN, CNOR in NSG 561 course during Spring 2007 semester at Le Moyne College, Syracuse, NY.

Glossary

4MAT system A learning style model based on Kolb's model combined with right–left brain research.

abstract conceptualization A term used by Kolb as one of two ways of processing information; known as the thinking mode.

accommodator One of the four learning style types according to Kolb's theory, combining the learning modes of concrete experience and active experimentation.

acculturation Describes an individual's adaptation to the customs, values, beliefs, and behaviors of a new country or culture.

active experimentation A term used by Kolb as one of two ways of processing information; known as the doing mode.

adherence Commitment or attachment to health-promoting regimens.

affective domain One of three domains in the taxonomy of behavioral objectives; deals with attitudes, values, and beliefs.

ageism Prejudice against the older adult that perpetuates the negative stereotyping of aging as a period of decline.

aids *See* instructional materials/tools.

analogue A type of model that uses analogy to explain something by comparing it to something else. The model performs like the real object, although its actual appearance may differ. A dialysis machine and the use of a description of a pump to explain how the kidneys and heart work respectively are examples of analogues.

andragogy The art and science of helping adults learn; a term coined by Knowles to describe his theory of adult learning.

animistic thinking The tendency of preschoolers to endow inanimate objects with life and consciousness; the belief that objects possess human characteristics.

appearance As an important feature of instructional tools, it is the way printed and display materials look to the reader. Appearance is a vital element in determining the effectiveness of media in capturing and holding the learner's attention through adequate use of white space, minimal use of words to convey the message, use of illustrations to break up blocks of print, and use of contrasts in color or shading.

assess To gather, summarize, and interpret pertinent data about the learner to make a decision or plan.

assessment The process of systematically collecting data to determine the relative magnitude, importance, or value of needs, problems, and strengths of the learner to decide a direction for action.

assessment phase The first phase of the educational cycle, which provides the foundation for the rest of the educational process.

assimilation The willingness of a person emigrating to a new culture to gradually adopt and incorporate the characteristics of the prevailing culture.

assimilator One of the four learning style types, according to Kolb's theory, combining the learning modes of abstract conceptualization and reflective observation.

assistive technologies   Technological tools (computers and communication devices) available for people with disabilities that provide access to education, employment, recreation, and communication opportunities that allow them to live as independently as possible.

asynchronous   A message that can be sent via the computer at the convenience of the sender and the message will be read when the receiver is online and ready to read it; messages that can be sent and responded to any time, day or night.

attention deficit hyperactivity disorder (ADHD)   A disorder of children with prominent attentional difficulties as demonstrated by inattention and impulsivity that are signs of developmentally inappropriate behavior.

audio learning resources   Instructional tools whose chief characteristic is exploitation of the learners' sense of hearing as a mechanism for teaching. Audiotapes and recorders are examples.

audiovisual materials (tools)   Nonprint instructional media that can influence all three domains of learning and stimulate the senses of hearing and/or sight to help convey the message to the learner. This category includes five major types: projected, audio, video, telecommunications, and computer formats.

augmentative and alternative communication   Devices, such as the computer, that allow people who are unable to speak or whose speech is difficult to understand to be able to communicate with others, which has added a whole new dimension and quality to their lives.

augmented feedback   An opinion or conveyance of a message through oral or body language by the teacher to the learner about how well he or she performed a psychomotor skill.

autonomy   The right to self-determination.

avoidance conditioning   A type of negative reinforcement whereby an unpleasant stimulus is anticipated rather than directly applied and the person receiving the reinforcement avoids doing something he or she does not want to do when faced with a fearful event.

barriers to teaching   Those factors that impede the nurse's ability to deliver educational services.

behavioral (learning) objectives   Intended outcomes of the education process that are action oriented rather than content oriented and learner centered rather than teacher centered.

behaviorist learning   One of the five major learning theories. According to behaviorists, the focus for learning is mainly on what is directly observable, and learning is viewed as the product of the stimulus conditions (S) and the responses (R) that follow. It is sometimes termed the S-R model of learning.

beneficence   The principle of doing good.

blogs   One of the newest forms of online communication, also known as Web logs or Web diaries, is an increasingly popular mechanism for individuals to share information and/or experiences about a given topic that include images, media objects, and links allowing for public responses.

bodily-kinesthetic intelligence   A term used by Gardner to describe children who learn by processing knowledge through bodily sensations.

brain preference indicator (BPI)   A learning style instrument used to determine hemispheric dominance.

breach of contract   Failure, without legal excuse, to perform a promise. Violation of a binding agreement or obligation in the performance of professional duties.

causal thinking   The ability of school-aged children to understand cause and effect through logic, concrete thinking, and inductive and deductive reasoning.

causality   The ability to grasp a cause-and-effect relationship between two paired, successive events, which is an elementary concept that begins to develop during toddlerhood.

chronic illness   A disease or disability that is permanent and can never be completely cured. It constitutes the number one medical malady of people in this country and affects the physical, psychosocial, economic, and spiritual aspects of an individual's life.

cloze procedure   A standardized test to measure comprehension of written materials (particularly recommended for health education literature) based on systematically deleting every fifth word from a portion of a text and having the reader fill in the blanks.

cognitive ability   The extent to which information can be processed, indicative of the level at which the learner is capable of learning; of major importance when designing instruction.

cognitive development   A cognitive perspective on learning focuses on the qualitative changes in perceiving, thinking, and reasoning as individuals grow and mature based on how external events are conceptualized, organized, and represented within each person's mental framework or schema. The process of acquiring more complex and adaptive ways of thinking as an individual grows from infancy to adulthood according to Piaget's four stages of cognitive maturation: sensorimotor, preoperational, concrete operations, and formal operations.

cognitive domain   One of three domains in the taxonomy of behavioral objectives; deals with aspects of behavior focusing on the way in which someone thinks in acquiring facts, concepts, principles, etc.

cognitive-emotional perspective   A cognitive theory recognizing that emotions must be considered within a cognitive framework to adequately consider affect as an aspect of conceptual change.

cognitive learning   One of the five major learning theories. According to a cognitive theorist's perspective, in order to learn, individuals change as a result of the way they perceive, process, interpret, and organize information based on what is already known; the reorganization of information leads to new insights and understanding.

commercially prepared materials   Predesigned, cost-effective printed educational materials that are widely available on a wide range of topics for purchase by educators as supplements to teaching and learning, such as brochures, pamphlets, books, posters, etc.

compliance   Submission or yielding to predetermined goals through regimens prescribed or established by others.

comprehension   The degree to which individuals understand what they have read or heard; the ability to grasp the meaning of a verbal or nonverbal message.

computer-assisted instruction (CAI)   An individualized instructional method of self-study using the high technology of the computer to deliver an educational activity. The interactive capability of CAI holds enormous potential for reinforcing learning, primarily in the cognitive domain, and its efficacy is dependent on programmatic software, hardware, and the learner's familiarity with and motivation to use this technology.

computer literacy   The ability to use the necessary computer hardware and software to meet the needs for information.

concept mapping   A contemporary nursing educational strategy that can be used to promote motivation by enabling the learner to integrate previous learning with newly acquired knowledge through diagrammatic mapping, which facilitates the gaining of complex knowledge with visual links.

concordance   A consultative process that is characterized by mutual respect for the client's and the professional's beliefs and that allows for negotiation to take place about the best course of action for the client.

concrete experience   A term used by Kolb to describe a dimension of perceiving; known as the feeling mode.

concrete operations period   As defined by Piaget, this is the third stage in the cognitive development of children in middle to late childhood (ages 6 to 11 years) who are capable of logical thought processes and the ability to reason but are still incapable of abstract thinking.

confidentiality   A binding social contract or covenant; a professional obligation to respect privileged information between the health professional and the client.

conservation   The ability to recognize that the properties of an object stay the same even though its appearance and position may change, which is a concept mastered during middle to late childhood.

constructivism   *See* social constructivism.

consumer informatics   A discipline that analyzes consumers' needs for information, studies and implements methods of making information accessible to consumers, and models and integrates consumer preferences into medical information systems. Also referred to as consumer health informatics.

content   The actual information that is communicated to the learner through various teaching methods and tools.

content evaluation   A systematic assessment taking place immediately after the learning experience to determine the degree to which learners have acquired the knowledge or skills taught during a teaching–learning session.

contracting   A popular, relatively recent means of facilitating learning through informal or formal agreements that delineate and promote learning objectives.

converger   One of the four learning style types according to Kolb's theory, combining the learning modes of abstract conceptualization and active experimentation.

corpus callosum   The connector between the two hemispheres of the brain.

cosmopolitan orientation   Persons with a worldly perspective on life who are receptive to new ideas and opportunities to learn new ways of doing things; a component of experiential readiness.

cost benefit   Money well spent. Cost of services (e.g., education) ensures return of satisfied clients and stability of the economic base of a healthcare facility.

cost-benefit analysis   The relationship between cost and outcomes that can be expressed in monetary terms; also called a cost-benefit ratio.

cost-benefit ratio   Relationship (expressed as a ratio) of program costs to economic benefits gained by the healthcare institution.

cost-effectiveness analysis   The efficiency of an educational offering when an actual monetary value cannot be assigned to a program.

cost recovery   Occurs when revenues generated are equal to or greater than expenditures.

cost savings   Monies realized through decreased use of expensive services, shortened lengths of stay, or fewer complications resulting from preventive services or patient education.

crystallized intelligence   The intellectual ability developed over a lifetime, which includes such elements as vocabulary, general information, understanding of social interactions, arithmetic reasoning, and capacity to evaluate experiences, which tends to increase over time as a person ages.

cuing   Using prompts and reminders to get a learner to perform routine tasks by focusing on an appropriate combination of time and situation.

cultural assessment   An organized, systematic appraisal of beliefs, values, and practices of an individual or group to determine client needs as a basis for planning nursing care interventions.

cultural awareness   The process of becoming sensitive to the interactions with other cultural groups by examining one's biases and prejudices toward others of another culture or ethnic background.

cultural competence   The ability to demonstrate knowledge and understanding of another person's culture and accept and respect cultural differences by adapting interventions to be congruent with that specific culture when delivering care.

cultural diversity   Interacting with others who represent different cultures from one's own culture.

cultural encounter   The process of exposing oneself in nursing practice to cross-cultural interactions with clients of diverse cultural backgrounds.

cultural knowledge   The process of acquiring an educational foundation about various cultural worldviews.

cultural literacy   The ability of knowing how to communicate with someone from another culture without having to explain undertones, voice intonations, and message contexts during a conversation.

cultural relativism   The values and behaviors every human group assigns to its conventions, which arise out of its own historical background and can only be accurately interpreted and understood in the light of that group's cultural worldview.

cultural skill   The process of learning how to conduct an accurate cultural assessment.

culturally competent model of care   A model for conducting a thorough and sensitive cultural assessment that includes the four components of cultural awareness, cultural knowledge, cultural skill, and cultural encounter.

culture   A complex concept that is an integral part of each person's life and includes knowledge, beliefs, values, morals, customs, traditions, and habits acquired by the members of a society.

defense mechanisms   Employed to protect the self when an individual's ego is threatened; short-term use is a way of coming to grips with reality, but long-term reliance allows individuals to avoid reality and may act as a barrier to learning and transfer.

delivery system   The physical form of instructional materials, including durable equipment used to present these materials, such as film and projectors, audiotapes and tape players, and computer programs and computers.

demonstration   An instructional method by which the learner is shown by the teacher how to perform a particular psychomotor skill.

demonstration materials   Tools that stimulate the senses by combining sight with touch, smell, and sometimes even taste with the advantage of helping to teach cognitive and psychomotor skill development. Major forms of media in this category include many types of nonprint media, such as models, real equipment, diagrams, charts, posters, displays, photographs, and drawings.

deontological   The ethical notion of the Golden Rule promulgated by the 16th-century philosopher Kant.

desirable needs   Learning needs of the client that are not life dependent but related to well-being

and can be met by the overall ability of nursing staff to provide quality care.

determinants of learning   Consist of learning needs, readiness to learn, and learning styles.

developmental disability   A disorder that manifests itself during the developmental period when a child demonstrates subaverage general intellectual functioning with concurrent deficits in adaptive behaviors. Sometimes referred to as mental retardation or developmental delay.

developmental stages   Milestones marking changes in the physical, cognitive, and psychosocial growth of an individual over time from infancy to old age.

dialectical thinking   The ability to search for complex and changing understandings to find a variety of solutions to any given situation (to see the bigger picture) which is characteristic of middle-aged adults.

digital divide   The gap between those individuals who have access to information technology resources and those who do not.

direct costs   Tangible, predictable costs associated with expenditures for personnel, equipment, etc.

disability   Inability to perform some key life functions; often used interchangeably with the term functional limitation.

discrimination learning   The ability to differentiate, with more and varied practice, among similar stimuli.

displays   Type of demonstration materials, frequently regarded as static, which may be permanently installed or portable. Included in this category are whiteboards, flip charts, and posters.

distance learning   A flexible telecommunications method of instruction using video or computer technology to transmit live, online, or taped messages directly between the instructor and the learner, who are separated from one another by time and/or location.

distributed practice   Learning information over successive periods of time, which is much more effective for remembering facts and forging memories than massed practice or cramming, which does not allow for long-term recall of information.

diverger   One of the four learning style types according to Kolb's theory, combining the learning modes of concrete experience and reflective observation.

domains of learning   Cognitive, psychomotor, and affective are the three domains in which learning occurs.

Dunn and Dunn learning style inventory   A self-reporting instrument that is used in the identification of how individuals prefer to function, learn, concentrate, and perform in learning activities.

duty   Responsibility; professional expectation.

dysarthria   Difficulty with voluntary muscle control of speech due to damage to the central or peripheral nervous system that controls muscles essential to speaking and swallowing. Types of dysarthria include flaccid, spastic, ataxic, hypokinetic, or mixed. Persons with degenerative neurologic diseases often suffer with this disorder.

education   An overall umbrella term used to describe the process, including the components of teaching and instruction, of producing observable or measurable behavioral changes (in knowledge, attitudes, and/or skills) in the learner through planned educational activities.

education process   A systematic, sequential, planned course of action that parallels the nursing process and consists of two interdependent operations, teaching and learning, which form a continuous cycle to include assessment of the learner, establishment of a teaching plan, implementation of teaching methods and tools, and evaluation of the learner, teacher, and education program.

educational contracting   *See* learning contract.

educational objectives   *See* instructional objectives.

educator role   The teaching role a nurse assumes in supporting, encouraging, and assisting the learner to put learning of behaviors (knowledge, skills, and attitudes) into meaningful parts and wholes to reach an optimum potential of functioning.

edutainment   Computer games as educational software that are disguised in a game format.

e-learning   An abbreviation for electronic learning, which professional development and training organizations have capitalized on by using the power of computer technology to provide learning solutions for workforce training; it involves the use of technology-based tools and processes to provide for customized learning anytime or anywhere.

e-mail   An Internet-based activity that is a quick, inexpensive, and increasingly popular way to communicate asynchronously via the computer.

embedded figures test (EFT)   A test designed to measure how a person's perception of the environment (field independence/dependence) is influenced by the context in which it appears.

emoticons   Symbols commonly used to represent emotions, such as a :) (smiley face) or ;) (winking), by people who are sending e-mail messages.

emotional readiness   A state of psychological willingness to learn, which is dependent on such factors as anxiety level, support system, motivation, risk-taking behavior, frame of mind, and psychosocial developmental stage.

escape conditioning   An individual's response that causes an unpleasant or uncomfortable stimulation to cease.

ethical   A term that refers to the norms or standards of behavior of healthcare professionals.

ethics   Guiding principles of human behavior.

ethnic group   A population of people, also referred to as a subculture, that has different experiences from those of the dominant culture.

ethnicity   A dynamic and complex concept referring to how members of a group perceive themselves and how, in turn, they are perceived by others in relation to the population subgroup's common heritage of customs, characteristics, language, and history.

ethnocentrism   A concept in which the belief is held that one's own culture is superior and all other cultures are less sophisticated.

ethnomedical   A cultural orientation delineating the nature and consequences of illness problems and disease interventions rather than adhering to the biomedical orientation of defining diseases and illness interventions. In this context, the concept of illness incorporates the relationship of humans with their universe, bridging culture with a sensitivity toward the daily practices inherent within specific ethnic groups.

evaluation research   Scientific inquiry applied to a specific program or activity to determine processes, outcomes, and/or their relationship.

evaluation   A systematic and continuous process by which the significance of something is judged; the process of collecting and using information to determine what has been accomplished and how well it has been accomplished to guide decision making.

evidence-based practice (EBP)   The conscientious use of current best evidence in making decisions about client care; most EBP models gather evidence from systematic reviews of clinically relevant, randomized controlled trials upon which to base practice decisions, especially about treatment.

experiential readiness   A state of willingness to learn based on such factors as an individual's past experiences with learning, cultural background, previous coping mechanisms, locus of control, orientation, and level of aspiration.

expressive aphasia   An absence or impairment of the ability to communicate through speech or writing due to a dysfunction in the Broca's area of the brain, which is the center of the cortex that controls motor abilities.

external evidence   Evidence derived from research that is generalizable beyond a particular study setting or sample.

external locus of control   An individual's motivation to learn comes from outside oneself, attributing success or failure of an action to luck, the nature of the task, or to the efforts of someone else.

extraversion-introversion (E-I)   Terms used to describe behavior that reflects an orientation to either the outside world of people or to the inner world of concepts and ideas; one of four dichotomous preference dimensions in the Myers-Briggs type indicator.

extrinsic feedback   A response provided by the teacher through the sharing of opinion or the conveying of a message through body language about how well a learner has performed; often used in relation to psychomotor skill performance.

field dependence   One of two styles of learning in the cognitive domain identified by Witkin in which a person's perception of the environment is immersed in and influenced by the surrounding field.

field independence   One of two styles of learning in the cognitive domain identified by Witkin in which a person's perception of the environment is separate from the surrounding field.

fixed costs   Predictable and controllable expenses that remain stable over time.

Flesch-Kincaid scale   An objective, statistical measurement tool for readability of written materials between fifth grade and college level, based on a count of the two basic language elements of average sentence length in words of selected samples and of average word length measured as syllables per 100 words of sample.

fluid intelligence   The intellectual capacity to perceive relationships, to reason, and to perform abstract thinking, which declines over time as degenerative changes occur with aging.

focus groups   Optimally 4 to 12 potential learners grouped together for the purpose of identifying points of view or knowledge about a certain topic. A facilitator leads the discussion by asking questions.

Fog Index   A formula appropriate for use in determining readability of materials from fourth grade to college level based on average sentence length and the percentage of multisyllabic words in a 100-word passage.

formal operations period   As defined by Piaget, this is the fourth and final stage of cognitive development in which the adolescent (ages 12 to

19 years) is capable of abstract thought, internalization of ideas, complex logical reasoning, and understanding causality.

formal settings Scheduled sessions in which teaching and learning take place.

format The general physical appearance of a book, pamphlet, or other printed materials, which includes such characteristics as the type face, the margins, the organization of information, the quality of the paper, etc.

formative evaluation Also referred to as process evaluation. It is a systematic and continuous assessment of success of the teaching process made during the implementation of materials, methods, and activities to control, ensure, or improve the quality of performance in delivery of an educational program.

four-step appraisal of needs A systematic approach for assessing learning needs of caregivers and the healthcare organizations in which they practice.

Fry readability graph A measurement tool for testing the readability of materials (especially books, pamphlets, and brochures) at the level of first grade through college by using a graph to plot the number of syllables of words and the number of sentences in three 100-word samples.

functional illiteracy The lack of fundamental education skills needed by adults to read, write, or comprehend information to function effectively in today's society; the inability to read well enough to understand and interpret written information for use as intended.

functional magnetic resonance imaging (fMRI) A type of advanced technology that has revolutionized the field of neuroscience by making colorful images of the brain on computer monitors to determine the possible areas of nerve activity involved in the processes of thinking, emotions, and recall.

gaming An instructional method requiring the learner to participate in a competitive activity (which may or may not reflect reality) with preset rules.

Gardner's eight types of intelligence A theory that describes the styles of learning in children.

gender bias A preconceived notion about the abilities of women and men that prevent individuals from pursuing their own interests and achieving their potentials.

gender gap The behavioral and biological differences between males and females.

gender-related cognitive abilities A comparison between the sexes as to how males and females act, react, and perform in situations affecting every sphere of life as a result of genetic and environmental influences on behavior.

gender-related personality behaviors The observed differences between the sexes in personality and affective behaviors thought to be largely determined by culture, but to some extent is a result of interaction between environment and heredity.

gerogogy The art and science of teaching the older adult.

Gestalt perspective The oldest of psychological theories that emphasizes the importance of perception in learning from a cognitive perspective, with a focus on the configuration or organization of a pattern of stimuli rather than of discrete stimuli. It reflects the maxim that "the whole is greater than the sum of the parts."

goal A desirable outcome to be achieved by the learner at the end of the teaching–learning process; goals are global and more future oriented and long term in nature than the specific, short-term objectives that lead step by step to the final achievement of a goal.

group discussion A commonly employed method of instruction whereby a group of learners (ideally 3 to 20 people) gather together to exchange information, feelings, and opinions with each other and the teacher; the activity is learner centered and subject centered.

habilitation Includes all the activities and interactions that enable individuals with a disability to develop new abilities to achieve their maximum potential.

hardware   Part of the delivery system for many types of media (e.g., computers, projectors, tape players).

health belief model   A framework or paradigm used to explain or predict health behavior composed of the interaction between individual perceptions, modifying factors, and likelihood of action.

health education   A participatory educational approach, often used interchangeably with the term *patient education* or *client education*, aimed at preventing disease, promoting positive health, and incorporating the physical, mental, and social aspects of learning needs.

health literacy   Refers to how well an individual can read, interpret, and comprehend health information for maintaining an optimal level of wellness.

health promotion model   A framework that describes the interaction of health-promoting factors including cognitive perceptual factors, modifying factors, and likelihood of participation in health-promoting behaviors.

healthcare-related setting   One of three classifications of instructional settings, in which healthcare-related services are offered as a complementary function of a quasi-health agency. Examples: American Heart Association, American Cancer Society, Muscular Dystrophy Association, and Leukemia Society of America.

healthcare setting   One of three classifications of instructional settings, in which the delivery of health care is the primary or sole function of an institution, organization, or agency. Examples: hospitals, visiting nurse associations, public health departments, outpatient clinics, physician offices, health maintenance organizations, extended-care facilities, and nurse-managed centers.

healthcare team   An interdisciplinary group of healthcare professionals and nonprofessionals who provide services to the patient and family members in an attempt to maximize optimal health and well-being of the client to whom their activities are directed.

hearing impairment   A complete loss or a reduction in sensitivity to sounds by persons who are deaf or hard of hearing.

hidden costs   Costs that cannot be predicted or accounted for until after the fact.

hierarchy of needs   Theory of human motivation based on integrated wholeness of the individual and levels of satisfaction of basic human needs organized by potency.

humanistic learning   One of the five major learning theories, which views learning as being facilitated by curiosity, needs, a positive self-concept, and open situations where freedom of choice and individuality are promoted and respected.

ideology   Thoughts, attitudes, and beliefs that reflect the social needs and desires of an individual or ethnocultural group.

illiteracy   The total inability of adults to read, write, or comprehend information or whose reading and writing skills are at or below the fourth-grade level.

illusionary representations   A category of instructional materials that depict realism, such as dimensionality. Examples are photographs, drawings, and audiotapes, which depend on imagination to fill in the gaps and offer the learner experiences that simulate reality.

iloralacy   The inability to understand simple oral language.

imaginary audience   A type of social thinking that explains the pervasive self-consciousness of adolescents who may feel embarrassed because they believe everyone is looking at them, which has considerable influence over their behavior.

impact evaluation   The process of assessing outcomes or effects of an educational activity that extend beyond the activity itself to address organizational and/or societal effects.

indirect costs   Costs that may be fixed but are not necessarily directly related to an educational activity (e.g., heating, electricity, housekeeping).

informal settings   Unplanned or spontaneous sessions in which teaching and learning take place.

informatics *See* consumer informatics.

Information Age   The present period of time, in which sweeping advances in computer and information technology have transformed the economic, social, and cultural life of society.

information literacy   The ability to access, evaluate, organize, and use information from a variety of sources.

information processing   A cognitive perspective that emphasizes thinking processes: thought, reasoning, the way information is encountered and stored, memory functioning, and information retrieved.

input disabilities   A general category of learning disability that refers to the process of receiving and recording information in the brain, which includes visual, auditory, perceptual, and integrative processing, such as dyslexia and short- and long-term memory disorders.

instruction   Often used interchangeably with teaching. Involves the communicating of information about a specific skill in the cognitive, affective, or psychomotor domain with the objective of producing learning.

instructional materials/tools   The resources or vehicles used to help communicate information, which include both print and nonprint media, to aid teaching and learning by stimulating the various senses, such as vision and hearing. These are intended to supplement, not replace, actual teaching. Synonymous terms are *educational aids* and *audiovisual materials*.

instructional method   The way information is taught that brings the learner into contact with what is to be learned; a technique or approach used by the teacher to communicate and share information with the learner. Examples of methods include lecture, group discussion, one-to-one instruction, etc.

instructional objectives   Intended outcomes of the education process that are in reference to an aspect of a program or a total program of study that are content oriented and teacher centered; also referred to as educational objectives.

instructional setting   A situation or area in which health teaching takes place as classified on the basis of what relationship health education has to the primary function of an organization, agency, or institution in which the teaching occurs.

instructional strategy   *See* teaching strategy.

internal evidence   Evidence that is not generated from research but is appropriate for use when, for example, it is derived from a systematically conducted evaluation.

internal locus of control   Individuals are motivated from within to learn, attributing success or failure to their own ability or effort.

Internet   A huge global computer network, of which the World Wide Web is a component, established to allow transfer (exchange) of information from one computer to another; it provides a diverse range of services used to deliver information to large numbers of people and to enable people to communicate with one another, such as via e-mail, real-time chat, or electronic discussion groups.

interpersonal intelligence   A term used by Gardner to describe children who learn best in groups.

intrapersonal intelligence   A term used by Gardner to describe children who learn well with independent, self-paced instruction.

intrinsic feedback   A response that is generated within the self, giving learners a sense of or a feel for how they have performed; often used in relation to a psychomotor skill performance.

judging-perceiving (J-P)   Terms used to describe behavior that reflects the way a person comes to a conclusion about something or becomes aware of something; one of four dichotomous preference dimensions in the Myers-Briggs type indicator.

justice   The equal distribution of benefits and burdens.

knowledge deficit   A gap in what a learner needs or wants to know; this category of nursing diagnosis can include learning needs in the cognitive, affective, and psychomotor domains.

knowledge readiness   A state of willingness to learn dependent on such factors as the learner's present knowledge base, the level of learning capability, and the preferred style of learning.

Kolb's learning style inventory An experiential learning model that includes four modes of learning reflecting the dimensions of perception and processing.

LAD (Literary Assessment for Diabetes) A reading skills test to measure word recognition in adult patients with diabetes. This standardized test, modeled after the REALM test, consists of lists of common words used when teaching self-care management of diabetes.

law A clearly stated pronouncement of a binding custom, enforceable by a controlling body.

layout The arrangement of printed and/or graphic information on a flat surface. Effective use of white space, graphics, and wording will depend heavily on this arrangement.

learner characteristics One of the three major variables that refers to the learner's perceptual abilities, reading ability, self-direction, and learning style, which must be considered when making appropriate choices of instructional materials.

learning A conscious or unconscious permanent change in behavior as a result of a lifelong, dynamic process by which individuals acquire new knowledge, skills, and/or attitudes that can be measured and can occur at any time or in any place due to exposure to environmental stimuli.

learning contract A mutually agreed-on specific plan of action between the learner and educator clearly defining the specific behavioral objectives and predetermined goal to be achieved as a result of instruction. Also referred to as an educational contract.

learning curve Also sometimes referred to as the experience curve, it is a record of an individual's improvement in psychomotor skill development made by measuring his or her ability at different stages during a specified time period, which includes six stages: negligible progress, increasing gains, decreasing gains, plateau, renewed gains, and approach to limit.

learning disability (LD) A generic term that refers to a heterogeneous group of disorders manifested by significant difficulties with learning. Inattention and impulsivity are signs indicating developmentally inappropriate behavior.

learning needs Gaps in knowledge that exist between a desired level of performance and the actual level of performance; what the learner needs or wants to know.

learning styles The manner by which (how) individuals perceive and then process information. Certain characteristics of style are biological in origin, whereas others are sociologically developed as a result of environmental influences.

learning theory A coherent framework and set of integrated constructs and principles that describe, explain, or predict how people learn.

lecture The oldest, most commonly used, and most traditional instructional method by which the teacher verbally transmits information in a highly structured format directly to a group of learners.

left-brain thinking The left hemisphere of the brain is vocal and analytic, which is used for verbalization and reality-based, logical thinking according to Sperry.

legal A term that refers to rules governing behavior or conduct of healthcare professionals that are enforceable under threat of punishment or penalty, such as a fine, imprisonment, or both.

legally blind A person's vision is 20/200 or less in the better eye with correction, or if visual field limits in both eyes are within 20 degrees diameter.

linguistic intelligence A term used by Gardner to describe children who have highly developed auditory skills and think in words.

listening test A standardized test to measure comprehension using a selected passage from an instructional material written at approximately the fifth-grade level that is read aloud at a normal rate to determine what a person understands and remembers when listening.

ListServ An automated mailing list software program that copies messages and distributes them to all subscribers.

literacy   The ability of adults to read, understand, and interpret information written at the eighth-grade level or above. An umbrella term used to describe socially required and expected reading and writing abilities; the relative ability of persons to use printed and written material commonly encountered in daily life.

literate   The ability to write and to read, understand, and interpret information written at the eighth-grade level or above.

locus of control (LOC)   The location of control of behaviors as either self-directed or directed by others. Persons with internal or external locus of control differ particularly in the degree of responsibility taken for their own actions (*see also* internal locus of control and external locus of control).

logical-mathematical intelligence   A term used by Gardner to describe children who are strong in exploring patterns, categories, and relationships of objects.

low literacy   The ability of adults to read, write, and comprehend information between the fifth- and the eighth-grade level of difficulty (also referred to as marginally literate or marginally illiterate).

m-learning   Stands for mobile learning, which is a new strategy that takes advantage of the many wireless, portable, and handheld devices, such as MP3 players, that can access course materials, search the Web, listen to lectures, and record experiences and assignments.

malpractice   Failure to exercise an accepted degree of professional skill or knowledge by one rendering professional services that results in injury, loss, or damage to the recipient of those services.

mandatory needs   Requisites to be learned for survival or situations where the learner's life or safety is threatened.

marginally literate   A term to describe a person with low literacy skills; also known as marginally illiterate.

massed practice   Learning information all at once, which is much less effective for remembering facts than learning information over successive periods of time; similar to cramming.

media characteristics   One of the three major variables that refers to the form through which information will be communicated that must be considered when making appropriate choices of instructional materials.

media/medium   The form in which information or ideas are conveyed to learners.

message   *See* content.

metacognition   A person's understanding of his/her way of learning. A concept related to cognitive learning theory.

models   Three-dimensional instructional tools that allow the learner to immediately apply knowledge and psychomotor skills by observing, examining, manipulating, handling, assembling, and disassembling objects while the teacher provides feedback. Replicas, analogues, and symbols are all types of models that enhance instruction by means that range from concrete to abstract.

moral   A term that refers to an internal value system, a certain moral fabric, that is expressed externally in ethical behaviors of healthcare professionals; often used interchangeably with the terms *morality* and *morals*.

motivation   A psychological force that moves a person to take action in the direction of meeting a need or goal, evidenced by willingness or readiness to act.

motivational axioms   Premises on which an understanding of motivation is based, such as a state of optimum anxiety, learner readiness, realistic goal setting, learner satisfaction/success, and uncertainty-reducing or uncertainty-maintaining dialogue.

motivational incentives   Factors that influence motivation in the direction of the desired goal.

motivational interviewing   A method of staging readiness to change for the purpose of promoting desired health behaviors, which is an individualized, flexible, client-centered approach that is supportive, empathetic, and goal directed.

musical intelligence   A term used by Gardner to describe children who are talented in playing musical instruments, singing, dancing, and keeping rhythm and who often learn best with music playing in the background.

Myers-Briggs type indicator (MBTI)   A self-report inventory that uses forced-choice questions and word pairs to measure four dichotomous dimensions of behavior.

needs assessment   The process of determining through data collection what a person, group, organization, or community must learn or wants to learn to provide appropriate education programs to meet the required or desired needs of the learners.

negligence   Doing or nondoing of an act, pursuant to a duty, that a reasonable person in the same circumstances would or would not do; the acting or the nonacting is the proximate cause of injury to another person or property.

noncompliance   Nonsubmission or resistance of the individual to follow a prescribed, predetermined regimen.

nonhealthcare setting   One of three classifications of instructional settings in which health care is an incidental or supportive function of an organization, such as a business, industry, and school system.

nonmalfeasance   The notion of doing no harm.

nonprint instructional materials   Include the full range of audio and visual instructional materials, including demonstrations and displays.

numeracy   The ability to read and interpret numbers.

nurse–client negotiations model   A model developed for the purpose of cultural assessment and planning for care of culturally diverse people that recognizes discrepancies existing between notions of the nurse and client about health, illness, and treatments. This model is used to bridge the gap between the scientific perspectives of the nurse and the cultural perspectives of the client.

nurse practice acts   Legal provisions of each state defining nursing and the standards of nursing practice, including patient teaching as a professional responsibility to protect the public from incompetent practitioners.

nursing process   A model for nursing practice using the problem-solving approach, which includes the phases of assessment, nursing diagnosis, planning, implementation, and evaluation of patient care that parallels the educational process.

object permanence   Toward the end of the second year of life, a child realizes that objects and events exist even when they cannot be seen, heard, or touched.

objective   A specific, single, unidimensional behavior that is short term in nature, which should be achievable at the conclusion of one teaching session or within a matter of a few days following a series of teaching sessions.

obstacles to learning   Those factors that negatively affect the ability of the learner to attend to and process information.

one-to-one instruction   A common instructional method for exchange of information whereby the teacher delivers individual verbal instruction of learning activities in a format designed specifically to meet the needs of a particular learner.

operant conditioning   Focuses on the behavior of an organism as a result of a positive or negative reinforcer (stimulus or event) applied after a response that strengthens the probability that the response will be performed again; nonreinforcement and punishment decrease the likelihood that a response will continue to be performed.

oral literacy   The ability to comprehend the spoken word.

outcome   The result of actions that may be intended or unintended; synonymous with *stated goals*.

outcome evaluation   *See* summative evaluation.

output disabilities   A general category of learning disability that refers to orally responding and performing physical tasks, which include language and motor disorders.

pacing   The speed at which information is presented to a learner.

parochial orientation   Persons who demonstrate close-mindedness in thinking, conservativeness, and less willingness to learn new material and who place trust in traditional authority figures; a component of experiential readiness.

patient education   A process of assisting consumers of health care to learn how to incorporate health-related behaviors (knowledge, skills, and/or attitudes) into everyday life with the purpose of achieving the goal of optimal health.

pedagogy   The art and science of helping children to learn.

PEMs   *See* printed education materials.

personal fable   A type of social thinking that leads adolescents to believe that they are invulnerable or invincible, which can result in them engaging in risk-taking behavior.

physical maturation   Change in an individual's physical characteristics as a result of normal body growth and development during the aging process.

physical readiness   A state of willingness to learn that is dependent on such factors as measures of physical ability, complexity of task, health status, gender, and environmental effects.

pooled ignorance   Lack of knowledge or information about issues or problems during a group discussion session, whereby clients cannot adequately learn from one another if they do not possess a basic, accurate understanding of a subject to draw on for purposes of discourse.

portfolio   A method for evaluation of an individual's learning over time.

positron emission tomography (PET)   A type of technology that has revolutionized the field of neuroscience by making images of the brain to detect which possible areas of the brain are used for cognating, feeling, and remembering.

possible needs   Nice to know information that is not essential at a given point in time or in situations in which learning is not directly related to daily activities.

posters   A type of display that combines print and nonprint media to help convey a message.

post-formal operations period   The ability to learn during middle adulthood that goes beyond Piaget's last stage of cognitive development (formal operations) to include searching for complex and changing understandings to find a variety of solutions to any given situation or problem; to be able to see the bigger picture.

poverty circle (cycle of poverty)   A process whereby parents who are of low income and educational level produce children of low income and educational attainment, who grow up and repeat the process with their own children; a situation in which generation after generation are born into poverty by many factors, such as poor health care, limited resources, family stress, and low-paying jobs.

practice-based evidence   Evidence derived from practice rather than from research, such as the results of a systematically conducted evaluation, clients' responses to care delivered on the basis of clinical expertise, or a systematically conducted quality improvement project.

precausal thinking   Unawareness by children in early childhood (3 to 5 years of age) of causation by invisible and mechanical forces.

preoperational period   As defined by Piaget, this is the second key milestone in the cognitive development of children when in the early childhood stage (3–5 years) are acquiring language skills and gaining experience but thinking is precausal, animistic, egocentric, and intuitive, with only a vague understanding of relationships and multiple classifications of objects.

presentation   The form in which the message (content) is put forth, occurring along a continuum from real objects to symbols.

primary characteristics of culture   Factors that influence an individual's identification with an ethnic group and that cause the individual to share a group's worldview, such as nationality, race, color, gender, age, and religious affiliation.

printed education materials (PEMs)   As the most common type of teaching tools, these include handouts, leaflets, books, pamphlets, brochures, and instruction sheets, which may be purchased or instructor developed.

process evaluation *See* formative evaluation.

Prochaska's change model *See* stages of change model.

productivity environmental preference survey (PEPS) The assessment tool used in the adult version of the Dunn and Dunn learning style inventory.

program evaluation A systematic assessment to determine the extent to which all activities for an entire department or program over a specified time period have accomplished the goals originally established.

programmed instruction A type of self-study tool, usually printed or computerized, that takes the learner through the learning task step by step.

projected learning resources Audiovisual instructional formats that depend primarily on the learners' sense of sight as the means through which messages are received. These resources require equipment to project images, usually in a darkened room, and include movies, PowerPoint slides, overhead transparencies, and others.

propositional reasoning The ability to think abstractly and use complex logical reasoning, which begins in the adolescent stage of development.

protection motivation theory A linear motivational theory that explains behavioral change in terms of threat and coping appraisal, which leads to intent and ultimately to action.

psychodynamic learning One of the five major learning theories. Largely a theory of motivation stressing emotions rather than cognition and responses; this perspective emphasizes the importance of conscious and unconscious forces derived from earlier childhood experiences and conflicts that guide and change behavior.

psychomotor domain One of three domains in the taxonomy of behavioral objectives, which is concerned with the physical activities of the body,

such as coordination, reaction time, and muscular control, related to the acquisition of a skill or task.

psychosocial development The process of psychological and social adjustment as an individual grows from infancy to adulthood according to Erickson's eight stages of the psychological and social maturation of humans: trust versus mistrust; autonomy versus shame and doubt; initiative versus guilt; industry versus inferiority; identity versus role confusion; intimacy versus isolation; generativity versus self-absorption and stagnation; and ego integrity versus despair.

Purnell model for cultural competence A popular organizing framework for understanding the complex phenomenon of culture and ethnicity that provides a comprehensive, systematic, and concise approach to assist healthcare providers in delivering holistic, culturally competent, and therapeutic interventions.

reachable moment A unique opportunity described by Beddoe when nurses provide emotional support to clients; the time when a nurse truly connects with clients by directly meeting them on mutual terms without the nurse being inhibited by prejudice or bias, setting the stage for the teachable moment.

readability The level of reading difficulty at which printed teaching tools are written. A measure of those elements in a given text of printed material that influence with what degree of success a group of readers will be able to read and understand the information; the ease, or, conversely, the difficulty, with which a person can understand or comprehend the style of writing of a selected printed passage.

readiness to learn The time when the learner is receptive to learning and is willing and able to participate in the learning process; preparedness or willingness to learn.

reading Also known as word recognition, it is the process of transforming letters into words and being able to pronounce them correctly.

realia   The most concrete form of stimuli that can be used to deliver information. Example: a real person or a model being used to demonstrate a procedure such as breast self-examination.

REALM (rapid estimate of adult literacy in medicine)   A reading skills test to measure a client's ability to read medical and health-related vocabulary.

receptive aphasia   An absence or impairment of the ability to comprehend what is read or heard due to a dysfunction in the Wernicke's area of the brain, which controls sensory abilities. Although hearing is unimpaired, the person is unable to understand the significance of the spoken word and is unable to communicate verbally.

reflective observation   A term used by Kolb to describe a dimension of perceiving; known as the watching mode.

reflective practice   A notion of evaluation that includes the two components of reflection-in-action, when the nurse introspectively considers a practice activity while performing it so change for improvement can be made at that moment (formative evaluation), and reflection-on-action, when the nurse introspectively analyzes a practice activity after completion so as to gain insights for the future (summative evaluation).

rehabilitation   The relearning of previous skills, which often requires an adjustment to altered functional abilities and altered lifestyle.

religiosity   An individual's adherence to beliefs and ritualistic practices associated with religious institutions.

repetition   A technique that strengthens learning by aiding in retention of information of new or difficult material through reinforcement of important points.

replica   A facsimile constructed to scale that resembles the features or substance of the original object. It may be examined or manipulated by the learner to get an idea of how something works. Example: resuscitation dolls.

resistance   What people oppose talking about or learning, which is an indicator of underlying emotional difficulties that must be dealt with for them to move ahead emotionally and behaviorally.

respondeat superior   Master–servant rule: "let the master respond and answer."

respondent conditioning   Emphasizes the importance of stimulus conditions and the associations formed in the learning process, whereby, without thought or awareness, learning takes place when a newly conditioned stimulus (CS) becomes associated with a conditioned response (CR); also termed *classical* or *Pavlovian conditioning*.

return demonstration   An instructional method by which the learner attempts to perform a psychomotor skill, with cues or prompting as needed from the teacher.

revenue generation   Income realized over and above costs; also called profit.

right-brain thinking   The right hemisphere of the brain is emotional, visual-spatial, and nonverbal, in which thinking is intuitive, subjective, relational, holistic, and time free, according to Sperry.

role modeling   The use of self as a role model, often overlooked as an instructional method, whereby the learner acquires new behaviors and social roles by identification with the role model.

role playing   A method of instruction by which learners participate in an unrehearsed dramatization, acting out an assigned part of a character as they think the character would act in reality.

SAM (suitability assessment of materials)   An evaluation instrument designed to measure the appropriateness of print materials, illustrations, and video- and audiotaped instructions for a given client population.

secondary characteristics of culture   Factors that influence an individual's identification with an ethnic group and that cause the individual to share a group's worldview, such as SES (socioeconomic status), physical characteristics, educational status, occupational status, and place of residence.

selective attention   The process of recognizing and selecting appropriate or inappropriate stimuli.

self-composed instructional materials   Printed instructional materials composed by individual instructors for the purpose of supplementing teaching.

self-efficacy theory   A framework that describes the belief that one is capable of accomplishing a specific behavior.

self-instruction   A method of instruction used by a teacher to provide or design teaching materials and activities that guide the learner in independently achieving the objectives of learning.

self-study materials   Written materials that are designed to allow the learner to independently master understanding of concepts or tasks.

sensing-intuition (S-N)   Describes how individuals perceive the world, either directly through the five senses or indirectly by way of the unconscious; one of four dichotomous preference dimensions in the Myers-Briggs type indicator.

sensorimotor period   As defined by Piaget, this is the first key milestone in the cognitive development of children in the age group of infancy to toddlerhood when learning is enhanced through movement and manipulation of objects in the environment via visual, auditory, tactile, olfactory, taste, and motor stimulation.

sensory deficits   A category of common physical disabilities that includes, in particular, hearing and visual impairments.

silent epidemic   A term used to describe the literacy problem in the United States; also known as the silent barrier or silent disability.

simulation   A method of instruction whereby an artificial or hypothetical experience that engages the learner in an activity reflecting real-life conditions but without the risk-taking consequences of an actual situation is created.

simulation laboratories   A type of learning laboratory that contains real equipment in a lifelike setting, but that allows the learner to practice manipulating and using this equipment as a prelude to performing a task in a real-life situation. Frequently used to supplement the learning of psychomotor skills.

skill inoculation   The opportunity for repeated practice of a behavioral task.

SMOG formula   A relatively easy-to-use, popular, valid test of readability based on a set number of sentences and polysyllabic words in printed material from grade four to college level.

social cognition   An increasingly popular perspective within cognitive theory that highlights the influence of social factors on perception, thought, motivation, and behaviors.

social constructivism   An increasingly popular perspective within cognitive theory proposing that individuals formulate or construct their own versions of reality and that learning and human development are richly colored by the social and cultural context in which people find themselves.

social learning   One of five major learning theories, this theory is seen as a mixture of behaviorist, cognitive, and psychodynamic influences; much of learning is a social process that occurs by observation and watching other people's behavior to see what happens to them. Role modeling is a central concept of this theory, with cognitive or psychodynamic aspects of internal processing and motivation sometimes considered in the learning process.

socioeconomic status (SES)   Variation in health status, health behavior, or learning abilities among individuals of different social and economic levels.

software   Computer programs and other instructional materials such as videotapes, CDs, and overhead transparencies.

Spache grade-level score   A readability formula specifically designed to judge materials written for children at grade levels below the fourth grade (elementary grades first through third).

spatial intelligence   A term used by Gardner to describe children who learn by images and pictures.

spirituality   A belief in a higher power, a sacred force that exists in all things.

spontaneous recovery   A response, which appears to be extinguished, reappears at any time (even years later), especially when stimulus conditions are similar to those in the initial learning experience.

staff education   A process of assisting nursing staff personnel to acquire knowledge, skills, or attitudes in nursing practice for the purpose of maintaining or improving their ability to deliver quality care to the consumer.

stages of change model   A model developed by Prochaska that forms the phenomenon of health behaviors of the learner, particularly applied to addictive and problem behaviors, and includes the six distinct stages of change: precontemplation, contemplation, preparation, action, maintenance, and termination.

stereotyping   An oversimplified conception, opinion, or belief about some aspect of an individual or group.

stimulus generalization   The tendency of initial learning experiences to be easily applied to other similar stimuli.

subculture   An ethnocultural group of people who have experiences different from those of the dominant culture.

subobjective   A specific statement of a short-term behavior that is written to reflect an aspect of the main objective leading to the achievement of the primary objective.

suitability assessment of materials   See SAM.

summative evaluation   Systematic assessment of the degree to which individuals have learned or objectives have been met as a result of education intervention; also referred to as outcome evaluation.

support system   Resources and significant others, such as family and friends, on whom the patient relies or is dependent for information or assistance in managing activities of daily living and who

may serve as a positive or negative influence on teaching efforts.

syllogistic reasoning   The ability to consider two premises and draw a logical conclusion from them, which is a cognitive skill developed in middle to late childhood.

symbol   A type of model that conveys a message to the learner through the use of abstract constructs, like words, that stand for the real thing. Cartoons and printed materials are examples of symbolic forms of a message.

symbolic representations   Numbers and words, symbols written and spoken to convey ideas or represent objects, which are the most common form of communication and yet are the most abstract types of messages.

systematic desensitization   A technique based on respondent conditioning that is used by psychologists to reduce fear or anxiety by unlearning or extinguishing it through teaching relaxation techniques or introducing a fear-producing stimulus at a nonthreatening level.

tailoring   Coordinating a patient's treatment regimens into his or her daily schedule by allowing new tasks to be associated with old behaviors.

task characteristics   One of the three major variables defined by the behavioral objectives in the cognitive, affective, and psychomotor domains of learning, which must be considered when making appropriate choices of instructional materials.

taxonomic hierarchy   See taxonomy.

taxonomy   A form of hierarchical classification of cognitive, affective, and psychomotor domains of behaviors according to their degree or level of complexity.

teachable moment   As defined by Havighurst, that point in time when the learner is most receptive to a teaching situation; it can occur at any time that a patient, family member, staff member, or nursing student has a question or needs information.

teaching   As one component of the educational process, it is a deliberate, intentional act of communicating information to the learner in response to identified learning needs with the objective of producing learning to achieve desired behavioral outcomes.

teaching plan Overall blueprint or outline for instruction clearly defining the relationship between the essential components of behavioral objectives, instructional content, teaching methods and tools, time frame for teaching, and methods of evaluation that fit together in a logical pattern of flow to achieve a predetermined goal.

teaching strategy An overall plan of action for instruction that anticipates barriers and resources of the learning experience to achieve specific behavioral objectives.

telecommunications Technological devices for the deaf (TDD).

telecommunications learning resources Instructional tools used to help convey information via electrical energy from one place to another such as telephones, televisions, and computers.

teleological The ethical notion purported by Mill that, given the alternatives, choices should be made that result in the greatest good for the greatest number of people.

telepractice The provision of nursing, medical, and other types of technology-facilitated healthcare services to clients at a distance.

theory of reasoned action A framework that is concerned with prediction and understanding of human behavior within a social context.

therapeutic alliance model An interpersonal provider-client model that addresses the continuum of compliance, adherence, and collaboration in therapeutic relationships.

therapeutic relationship A principle of humanistic theory that emphasizes the healing nature of a relationship between health professionals and their clients.

thinking-feeling (T-F) An approach used by individuals to arrive at judgments through impersonal, logical, subjective, or empathetic processes; one of four dichotomous preference dimensions in the Myers-Briggs type inventory.

TOFHLA (test of functional health literacy in adults) A relatively new instrument for measuring patients' literacy level by using actual hospital materials, such as prescription labels, appointment slips, and informed consent documents, to determine their reading and numeracy skills.

tools *See* instructional materials/tools.

transcultural nursing A formal area of study and practice comparing and analyzing different cultures and subcultures with respect to cultural care, health practices, and illness beliefs with the goal of using these insights to provide culture-specific and culture-universal care to diverse groups of people.

transfer of learning The effects of learning one skill on the subsequent performance of another related skill; includes self-transfer, near transfer, and far transfer.

transference Occurs when individuals project their feelings, conflicts, and reactions, especially those developed during childhood, onto authority figures and others in their lives.

triad communication A technique of involving a third person, such as a family member, significant other, or caregiver, in the communication pattern of the nurse and the client to serve as a listener and learner in the teaching situation for the purpose of assisting the client in understanding content, encouraging family or caregiver involvement and support, and enhancing client compliance with treatment regimens.

variable costs Not predictable, volume-related expenses.

VARK learning style A model that describes four categories or preferences—visual, aural, read/write, and kinesthetic—that reflect learning style experiences.

veracity Truth telling; honesty.

vicarious reinforcement A concept from social learning theory that involves determining whether role models are perceived as rewarded or punished for their behavior.

visual impairment   A reduction or complete loss of vision due to infection, accident, poisoning, or congenital degeneration of the eye(s). *See* legally blind.

whole brain thinking   When learners are able to use both brain hemispheres in developing their thought processes; a duality of thinking.

worldview   The way individuals or groups of people look at the universe to form values and beliefs about their lives and the world around them.

World Wide Web   A computer network of information servers around the world that are connected to the Internet; it is a technology-based educational resource that was created as a virtual space for the display of information.

WRAT (wide range achievement test)   A word recognition screening test used to assess a person's ability to recognize and pronounce a list of words out of context as a criterion for measuring comprehension of written materials. The level I test is designed for children ages 5–12 years; level II is intended to test persons over 12 years of age.

Index